1997
YEAR BOOK OF
SURGERY®

Statement of Purpose

The Year Book Service

The Year Book series was devised in 1901 by practicing health professionals who observed that the literature of medicine and related disciplines had become so voluminous that no one individual could read and place in perspective every potential advance in a major specialty. In the final decade of the 20th century, this recognition is more acutely true than it was in 1901.

More than merely a series of books, Year Book volumes are the tangible results of a unique service designed to accomplish the following:

- to *survey* a wide range of journals of proven value
- to *select* from those journals papers representing significant advances and statements of important clinical principles
- to provide *abstracts* of those articles that are readable, convenient summaries of their key points
- to provide *commentary* about those articles to place them in perspective

These publications grow out of a unique process that calls on the talents of outstanding authorities in clinical and fundamental disciplines, trained literature specialists, and professional writers, all supported by the resources of Mosby, the world's preeminent publisher for the health professions.

The Literature Base

Mosby and its editors survey more than 1,000 journals published worldwide, covering the full range of the health professions. On an annual basis, the publisher examines usage patterns and polls its expert authorities to add new journals to the literature base and to delete journals that are no longer useful as potential Year Book sources.

The Literature Survey

The publisher's team of literature specialists, all of whom are trained and experienced health professionals, examines every original, peer-reviewed article in each journal issue. More than 250,000 articles per year are scanned systematically, including title, text, illustrations, tables, and references. Each scan is compared, article by article, to the search strategies that the publisher has developed in consultation with the 270 outside experts who form the pool of Year Book editors. A given article may be reviewed by any number of editors, from one to a dozen or more, regardless of the discipline for which the paper was originally published. In turn, each editor who receives the article reviews it to determine whether or not the article should be included in the Year Book. This decision is based on the article's inherent quality, its probable usefulness to readers of that Year Book, and the editor's goal to represent a balanced picture of a given field in each volume of the Year Book. In addition, the editor indicates when to include figures and tables from the article to help the YEAR BOOK reader better understand the information.

Of the quarter million articles scanned each year, only 5% are selected for detailed analysis within the YEAR BOOK series, thereby assuring readers of the high value of every selection.

The Abstract

The publisher's abstracting staff is headed by a seasoned medical professional and includes individuals with training in the life sciences, medicine, and other areas, plus extensive experience in writing for the health professions and related industries. Each selected article is assigned to a specific writer on this abstracting staff. The abstracter, guided in many cases by notations supplied by the expert editor, writes a structured, condensed summary designed so that the reader can rapidly acquire the essential information contained in the article.

The Commentary

The YEAR BOOK editorial boards, sometimes assisted by guest commentators, write comments that place each article in perspective for the reader. This provides the reader with the equivalent of a personal consultation with a leading international authority—an opportunity to better understand the value of the article and to benefit from the authority's thought processes in assessing the article.

Additional Editorial Features

The editorial boards of each YEAR BOOK organize the abstracts and comments to provide a logical and satisfying sequence of information. To enhance the organization, editors also provide introductions to sections or individual chapters, comments linking a number of abstracts, citations to additional literature, and other features.

The published YEAR BOOK contains enhanced bibliographic citations for each selected article, including extended listings of multiple authors and identification of author affiliations. Each YEAR BOOK contains a Table of Contents specific to that year's volume. From year to year, the Table of Contents for a given YEAR BOOK will vary depending on developments within the field.

Every YEAR BOOK contains a list of the journals from which papers have been selected. This list represents a subset of the more than 1,000 journals surveyed by the publisher and occasionally reflects a particularly pertinent article from a journal that is not surveyed on a routine basis.

Finally, each volume contains a comprehensive subject index and an index to authors of each selected paper.

The 1997 Year Book Series

Year Book of Allergy, Asthma, and Clinical Immunology: Drs. Rosenwasser, Borish, Gelfand, Leung, Nelson, and Szefler

Year Book of Anesthesiology and Pain Management®: Drs. Tinker, Abram, Chestnut, Roizen, Rothenberg, and Wood

Year Book of Cardiology®: Drs. Schlant, Collins, Engle, Gersh, Kaplan, and Waldo

Year Book of Chiropractic®: Dr. Lawrence

Year Book of Critical Care Medicine®: Drs. Parrillo, Balk, Calvin, Franklin, and Shapiro

Year Book of Dentistry®: Drs. Meskin, Berry, Jeffcoat, Leinfelder, Roser, Summitt, and Zakariasen

Year Book of Dermatologic Surgery®: Drs. Greenway, Papadopoulos, and Whitaker

Year Book of Dermatology®: Drs. Sober and Fitzpatrick

Year Book of Diagnostic Radiology®: Drs. Federle, Clark, Gross, Latchau, Madewell, Maynard, and Young

Year Book of Digestive Diseases®: Drs. Greenberger and Moody

Year Book of Drug Therapy®: Drs. Lasagna and Weintraub

Year Book of Emergency Medicine®: Drs. Wagner, Dronen, Davidson, King, Niemann, and Roberts

Year Book of Endocrinology®: Drs. Bagdade, Braverman, Horton, Kannan, Landsberg, Molitch, Morley, Nathan, Odell, Poehlman, Rogol, and Ryan

Year Book of Family Practice®: Drs. Berg, Bowman, Davidson, Dexter, and Scherger

Year Book of Geriatrics and Gerontology®: Drs. Beck, Burton, Rabins, Reuben, Roth, Shapiro, and Whitehouse

Year Book of Hand Surgery®: Drs. Amadio and Hentz

Year Book of Hematology®: Drs. Spivak, Bell, Ness, Quesenberry, Wiernik, and Blume

Year Book of Infectious Diseases: Drs. Keusch, Barza, Bennish, Poutsiaka, Skolnik, and Snydman

Year Book of Medicine®: Drs. Klahr, Cline, Petty, Frishman, Greenberger, Malawista, Mandell, and O'Rourke

Year Book of Neonatal and Perinatal Medicine®: Drs. Fanaroff, Maisels, and Stevenson

Year Book of Nephrology, Hypertension, and Mineral Metabolism: Drs. Schwab, Bennett, Emmett, Hostetter, Kumar, and Toto

Year Book of Neurology and Neurosurgery®: Drs. Bradley and Wilkins

Year Book of Nuclear Medicine®: Drs. Gottschalk, Blaufox, Neumann, Strauss, and Zubal

Year Book of Obstetrics, Gynecology, and Women's Health: Drs. Mishell, Herbst, and Kirschbaum

Year Book of Occupational and Environmental Medicine®: Drs. Emmett, Frank, Gochfeld, and Hessl

Year Book of Oncology®: Drs. Ozols, Cohen, Glatstein, Loehrer, Tallman, and Wiersma

Year Book of Ophthalmology®: Drs. Augsburger, Cohen, Eagle, Flanagan, Grossman, Laibson, Maguire, Nelson, Penne, Rapuano, Sergott, Spaeth, Tipperman, and Ms. Salmon

Year Book of Orthopedics®: Drs. Sledge, Poss, Cofield, Dobyns, Griffin, Springfield, Swiontkowski, Wiesel, and Wilson

Year Book of Otolaryngology–Head and Neck Surgery®: Drs. Paparella and Holt

Year Book of Pathology and Laboratory Medicine: Drs. Mills, Bruns, Gaffey, and Stoler

Year Book of Pediatrics®: Dr. Stockman

Year Book of Plastic, Reconstructive, and Aesthetic Surgery®: Drs. Miller, Cohen, McKinney, Robson, Ruberg, Smith, and Whitaker

Year Book of Podiatric Medicine and Surgery®: Dr. Kominsky

Year Book of Psychiatry and Applied Mental Health®: Drs. Talbott, Ballenger, Breier, Frances, Meltzer, Schowalter, and Tasman

Year Book of Pulmonary Disease®: Dr. Petty

Year Book of Rheumatology®: Drs. Sergent, LeRoy, Meenan, Panush, and Reichlin

Year Book of Sports Medicine®: Drs. Shephard, Alexander, Drinkwater, Eichner, George and Torg

Year Book of Surgery®: Drs. Copeland, Bland, Deitch, Eberlein, Howard, Luce, Seeger, Souba, and Sugarbaker

Year Book of Thoracic and Cardiovascular Surgery®: Drs. Ginsberg, Wechsler, and Williams

Year Book of Urology®: Drs. Andriole and Coplen

Year Book of Vascular Surgery®: Dr. Porter

1997

The Year Book of SURGERY®

Editor-in-Chief

Edward M. Copeland, III, M.D.

The Edward R. Woodward Professor and Chairman, Department of Surgery, University of Florida College of Medicine; Director, University of Florida Shands Cancer Center, Gainesville, Florida

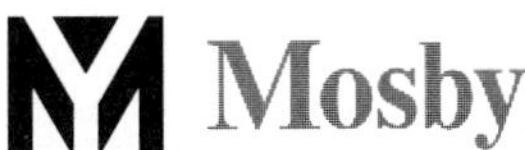

St. Louis Baltimore Boston Carlsbad Naples New York Philadelphia Portland London Madrid Mexico City Singapore Sydney Tokyo Toronto Wiesbaden

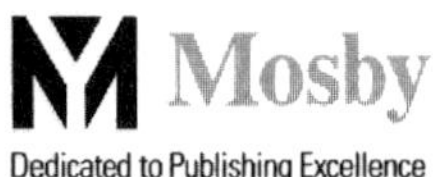

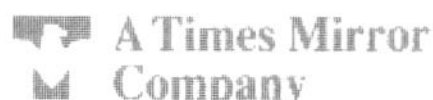

Vice President and Publisher: Carol Trumbold
Director, Editorial Development: Gretchen C. Murphy
Assistant Developmental Editor, Continuity: Vivienne Heard
Acquisitions Editor: Gina G. Wright
Illustrations and Permissions Coordinator: Steven J. Ramay
Project Manager, Editing: Kirk Swearingen
Senior Project Manager, Production: Joy Moore
Manager Literature, Services: Idelle Winer
Information Specialist: Kathleen Moss, R.N.
Circulation Manager: Lynn D. Stevenson

1997 EDITION

Printed in the United States of America
Composition by Reed Technology and Information Services, Inc.
Printing/binding by Maple-Vail

Mosby–Year Book, Inc.
11830 Westline Industrial Drive
St. Louis, MO 63146

International Standard Serial Number: 0090-3671
International Standard Book Number: 0–8151-9742-X

Editors

Editorial Board

Kirby I. Bland, M.D.

J. Murray Beardsley Professor and Chairman, Department of Surgery, Professor of Medical Sciences, Brown University School of Medicine; Surgeon-in-Chief, Rhode Island Hospital, Providence, Rhode Island

Edwin A. Deitch, M.D.

Professor and Chairman, Department of Surgery, UMD-New Jersey Medical School, Newark, New Jersey

Timothy J. Eberlein, M.D.

Richard E. Wilson Professor of Surgery, Harvard Medical School; Vice-Chairman for Research, Department of Surgery, Chief, Division of Surgical Oncology, Director, Biologic Cancer Therapy Program, Brigham and Women's Hospital, Surgical Director, Breast Evaluation Center, Dana Farber Cancer Institute, Boston, Massachusetts

Richard J. Howard, M.D., Ph.D.

Professor of Surgery, University of Florida College of Medicine, Shands Hospital at the University of Florida, Gainesville, Florida

Edward A. Luce, M.D.

Kiehn-Desprez Professor and Chief of Plastic Surgery, Case-Western Reserve and University Hospital, Cleveland, Ohio

James M. Seeger, M.D.

Professor and Chief, Section of Vascular Surgery, Department of Surgery, University of Florida College of Medicine, Gainesville, Florida

Wiley W. Souba, M.D., Sc.D.

Chief, Division of Surgical Oncology, Deputy Director, Massachusetts General Hospital Cancer Center, Director, Surgical Oncology Research Laboratories; Director, Nutrition Support Service, Massachusetts General Hospital; Professor of Surgery, Harvard Medical School; Professor of Nutrition, Harvard School of Public Health, Boston, Massachusetts

David J. Sugarbaker, M.D.

Associate Professor of Surgery, Harvard Medical School; Chief, Division of Thoracic Surgery, Brigham and Women's Hospital, Chief of Surgical Services, Dana Farber Cancer Institute, Boston, Massachusetts

Contributing Editors

Joseph F. Amaral, M.D.

Associate Professor of Surgery, Brown University School of Medicine; Director of Laparoscopic Surgery, Rhode Island Hospital, Providence, Rhode Island

William G. Cioffi, M.D.

Associate Professor of Surgery, Brown University School of Medicine; Chief of Trauma and Burns, Rhode Island Hospital, Providence, Rhode Island

Francois I. Luks, M.D.

Associate Professor of Surgery and Pediatrics, Brown University School of Medicine; Pediatric Surgeon, Hasbro Children's Hospital and Rhode Island Hospital, Providence, Rhode Island

Victor E. Pricolo, M.D.

Associate Professor of Surgery, Brown University School of Medicine; Chief of Gastrointestinal Surgery, Rhode Island Hospital, Providence, Rhode Island

H. Hank Simms, M.D.

Associate Professor of Surgery, Brown University School of Medicine; Chief, Division of Surgical Critical Care, Department of Surgery, Rhode Island Hospital, Providence, Rhode Island

Table of Contents

Journals Represented

Mosby and its editors survey nearly 1,000 U.S. and foreign medical and allied health journals. From these journals, the Editors select the articles to be abstracted. Journals represented in this YEAR BOOK are listed below.

Acta Cytologica
American Journal of Clinical Pathology
American Journal of Gastroenterology
American Journal of Medicine
American Journal of Neuroradiology
American Journal of Pathology
American Journal of Physiology
American Journal of Respiratory and Critical Care Medicine
American Journal of Roentgenology
American Journal of Surgery
American Surgeon
Anesthesia and Analgesia
Anesthesiology
Annals of Otology, Rhinology, and Laryngology
Annals of Plastic Surgery
Annals of Surgery
Annals of Surgical Oncology
Annals of Thoracic Surgery
Annals of the Royal College of Surgeons of England
Archives of Otolaryngology—Head and Neck Surgery
Archives of Pathology and Laboratory Medicine
Archives of Surgery
British Journal of Cancer
British Journal of Surgery
British Medical Journal
Burns
Canadian Journal of Surgery
Cancer
Cancer Research
Chest
Clinical Cancer Research
Clinical Infectious Diseases
Clinical Orthopaedics and Related Research
Critical Care Medicine
Dermatologic Surgery
Diseases of the Colon and Rectum
European Journal of Surgery
European Journal of Vascular and Endovascular Surgery
European Respiratory Journal
Gastroenterology
Gastrointestinal Endoscopy
Head and Neck
Health Affairs
Hepatology
Infection Control and Hospital Epidemiology
International Journal of Cancer
International Journal of Radiation, Oncology, Biology, and Physics

Investigative Radiology
Journal of Burn Care and Rehabilitation
Journal of Cardiovascular Surgery
Journal of Clinical Immunology
Journal of Clinical Investigation
Journal of Clinical Oncology
Journal of Computer Assisted Tomography
Journal of Cranio-Maxillo-Facial Surgery
Journal of Immunology
Journal of Infectious Diseases
Journal of Internal Medicine
Journal of Laryngology and Otology
Journal of Neurology
Journal of Neurosurgery
Journal of Pediatric Surgery
Journal of Pediatrics
Journal of Surgical Oncology
Journal of Surgical Research
Journal of Thoracic and Cardiovascular Surgery
Journal of Trauma: Injury, Infection, and Critical Care
Journal of Vascular Surgery
Journal of the American College of Surgeons
Journal of the American Medical Association
Journal of the National Cancer Institute
Laboratory Investigation
Lancet
Laryngoscope
Mechanisms of Ageing and Development
Nephrology, Dialysis, Transplantation
New England Journal of Medicine
Nutrition
Otolaryngology–Head and Neck Surgery
Pediatric Radiology
Plastic and Reconstructive Surgery
Proceedings of the National Academy of Sciences
Quintessence International
Scandinavian Journal of Plastic and Reconstructive Hand Surgery
Spine
Stroke
Surgery
Transplantation
World Journal of Surgery
Wound Repair and Regeneration

Standard Abbreviations

The following terms are abbreviated in this edition: acquired immunodeficiency syndrome (AIDS), cardiopulmonary resuscitation (CPR), central nervous system (CNS), cerebrospinal fluid (CSF), computed tomography (CT), deoxyribonucleic acid (DNA), electrocardiography (ECG), health maintenance organization (HMO), human immunodeficiency virus (HIV), intensive care unit (ICU), intramuscular (IM), intravenous (IV), magnetic resonance (MR) imaging (MRI), and ribonucleic acid (RNA).

Note

The YEAR BOOK OF SURGERY is a literature survey service providing abstracts of articles published in the professional literature. Every effort is made to assure the accuracy of the information presented in these pages. Neither the editor nor the publisher of the YEAR BOOK OF SURGERY can be responsible for errors in the original materials. The editors' comments are their own opinions. Mention of specific products within this publication does not constitute endorsement.

To facilitate the use of the YEAR BOOK OF SURGERY as a reference tool, all illustrations and tables included in this publication are now identified as they appear in the original article. This change is meant to help the reader recognize that any illustration or table appearing in the YEAR BOOK OF SURGERY may be only one of many in the original article. For this reason, figure and table numbers appear to be out of sequence within the YEAR BOOK OF SURGERY.

1 General Considerations

Introduction

The financing of medical education is threatened because of the dependence on ever-decreasing clinical income and the planned reduction in federal funding for resident education. Our profession continues to attract the best students, who are still able to find jobs on completion of training. In the near future, however, income will be lower but debt accumulated during medical training will be the same or higher. This financial burden may be a deterrent to some qualified students to enter medicine.

The resurgence of for-profit medicine has been associated with multiple cost reduction strategies such as the recommendation for elimination of the clear liquid diet and intraoperative blood transfusion for spinal surgical procedures. Guidelines for blood transfusion, the treatment of deep vein thrombosis as an outpatient, and clinical pathways for specific surgical disciplines are also aimed at reducing costs. The simple act of obtaining a proper history has been shown to result in a reduction in the incidence of postoperative bleeding in patients ingesting cyclooxygenase inhibitors.

There are situations where the expenditure of minimal funds in the present might prevent medical costs in the future. Examples are prospective peer review of pathologic diagnoses and new diagnostic tests that will provide early diagnosis or prevention of diseases that are costly to treat when clinically manifested.

Quality of care and outcome are important to measure, especially when traditional medical management principles are being restricted. Obligations and responsibilities of the managed care company and the contracting physician should be understood fully. Also, in malpractice cases, physicians are often their own worst enemies because of the unqualified "expert" witness.

Transmission of hepatitis B virus from surgeon to patient has now been documented, and the technique of double gloving should be re-evaluated. The safety of the infusion of stored blood and the reinfusion of unwashed wound drainage blood is under further evaluation.

An interesting report on Operation Desert Storm indicates that this battlefield may not have been such a dangerous place after all.

Edward M. Copeland III, M.D.

Review of US Medical School Finances, 1993–1994

Ganem JL, Beran RL, Krakower JK (Assoc of American Med Colleges, Washington, DC)

JAMA 274:723–730, 1995 1–1

Background.—Each year, the finances of United States medical schools accredited by the Liaison Committee on Medical Education are reviewed. Medical school revenues and expenditures for fiscal year 1993–1994, including a review of patterns in the financing of medical education in the previous 3 years, were reviewed.

Current Finances.—For all medical schools in the year considered, total revenues were $27,509 million, a 6% inflation-adjusted increase over 1992–1993. After adjustment for inflation, revenue obtained from government appropriations, parent universities, endowments, and grants and contracts decreased. There was a $581 million increase in revenues from practice plans—which contributed one third of all revenues—for a 7% inflation-adjusted increase. Hospital revenues totaled $3,659 million, a 20% increase after adjustment for inflation. However, after exclusion of 15 schools that had not previously reported hospital revenues, this increase fell to 5%. Revenues from grants and contracts totaled $8,411 million, or 31% of total revenues. Federal grants and contracts totaled $5,819 million, for an inflation-adjusted increase of 4%. Indirect costs recovered for grants and contracts totaled $1,768 million. Tuition and fee revenue was $1,130 million, for an inflation-adjusted increase of 5%. The total revenues of public and private medical schools were similar, within 5% of each other. Public medical schools obtained more revenue from governmental appropriations, whereas private medical schools got more revenue from other sources. The mean revenue from practice plans for private schools was 43% higher than that for public schools.

Expenditures, excluding transfers, totaled $26,854 million, representing a 6% increase. Total revenues exceeded total expenditures by $665 million. The medical schools retained $252 million for future operations, after transferring $403 million for debt retirement, capital acquisitions, and other funds.

Trends in Finances.—The previous 3 years have seen a 19% increase in medical school revenues, with an inflation-adjusted annual growth rate of 4%. From 1991–1992 to 1993–1994, the number of graduate students increased by 11%, full-time clinical faculty by 10.5%, and basic science faculty by 5.5%. Practice plan revenues increased for each of the 3 years, but the rate of increase has been declining. The 3-year period saw a 9% increase in federal research grants and contracts, exclusive of indirect cost recoveries. Total expenditures increased by 13% from 1991–1992 to

1993–1994. In 1994 and 1995, average faculty salaries declined in many instances when assessed by region, department, and rank. Compared with the previous year, the average number of salaries that declined after adjustment for inflation more than doubled.

Discussion.—Medical school revenues continue to increase. However, with the rise of managed care and governmental pressures to reduce health care spending, the continued growth of academic medical centers is in doubt.

▶ The data for 1993–1994 show all sources of revenue for medical schools increasing, except for governmental appropriations, university support, training grants, and contracts. The number of faculty members also increased proportionately, to use up this increase in revenue. The period 1996–1997 will find most sources of revenue decreasing but faculty size remaining the same. Most medical schools have become accustomed to an ever increasing source of revenue, primarily from patient care, and are having a hard time adjusting to the necessity of having to downsize. Also, the complexity of a medical school makes it hard to downsize without an across-the-board budget cut, which, of course, penalizes the frugal, productive departments out of proportion to the nonproductive ones. Financially productive faculty then leave the medical school and a vicious cycle is created.

E.M. Copeland III, M.D.

The Initial Employment Status of Physicians Completing Training in 1994

Miller RS, Jonas HS, Whitcomb ME (American Med Assoc, Chicago; Assoc of American Med Colleges, Washington, DC)

JAMA 275:708–712, 1996 1–2

Background.—In the near future, the United States will have a serious oversupply of physicians. It has been reported that physicians who complete residency in some specialties have problems finding suitable work, and that some established physicians have seen a serious decline in the number of patients they treat. The career status of physicians who completed residency training in the 1993–1994 academic year was examined.

Methods.—A survey was completed by 3,090 directors of residency programs. The survey included questions about total number of graduates, number of physicians working full time in their specialty, and number of physicians who had trouble finding employment.

Results.—Of nearly 16,000 physicians who completed residency in 1 of 26 specialties, 63% were potentially seeking employment. Of those not seeking employment, 93% were pursuing additional training. The percentage of physicians who did not find a full-time job in their specialty ranged from 0% in urology to almost 11% in pathology; the percentage was 5.5% in rheumatology. The total percentage of physicians who did not find a full-time job in their specialty was 3%. About 70% of graduates seeking employment obtained a position in their specialty. Physicians in more general specialties, such as family practice and internal medicine, have less trouble finding a position in their field. Program directors in nongeneral specialties believed that it will become more difficult to find a full-time position.

Conclusions.—The full-time employment opportunities for physicians in some specialties are becoming more limited in some parts of the United States. These findings may be helpful to medical students and members of the academic medical community who make decisions about the supply of physicians and the relationship to graduate medical education.

▶ Although generalist physicians had the fewest problems finding employment in their chosen specialty, I wonder how long this advantage will last. Physician's assistants (PAs) are now allowed to write orders in many states and their training programs are becoming more sophisticated. The same can be said for nurse practitioners. As a child, my life was saved by the family practitioner in a small town in Georgia and, obviously, I am forever grateful. Most of my visits to the doctor, however, could have been managed by a current day PA.

A figure in the original article shows no area of the country underserved by surgeons but does identify the problem areas for employment to be the Pacific and New England. Graduates of the University of Florida Program have no difficulty finding jobs in the South-Atlantic and these jobs are in some very nice places to live. From the standpoint of finding jobs for our residents, I hope the rest of the country continues to ignore the opportunities here.

E.M. Copeland III, M.D.

Physician Earnings in a Changing Managed Care Environment

Simon CJ, Born PH (Univ of Illinois at Chicago; American Med Assoc, Chicago)

Health Aff (Millwood) 15:124–133, 1996 1–3

Introduction.—Although physician income had risen annually by 5.9% since 1982, it dropped by 4% between 1993 and 1994 in the managed care environment. The number of physicians holding at least 1 managed care contract has risen from 43% in 1986 to 83% in 1995.

Changes in Physician Income.—After adjusting for inflation, physician income rose at an annual rate of 2.2% between 1985 and 1994. Physicians earning the most money had the largest increases in income between 1985 and 1991 (4%) and the largest decreases in income between 1993 and 1994 (6%). Although incomes of all physician groups fell during this period, the decline in income for subspecialists was the smallest.

Specialty Earnings Trends.—Annual, inflation-adjusted income growth rates divided into 3 time periods—rapid growth but low market penetration of managed care (1985 to 1989); the spread of physician network plans (1989 to 1993); and expanded market penetration and extensive contracting with physicians (1993 and 1994)—show a consistent decline in income growth.

Geographic Variation.—There is a weak association between managed care market penetration and decline in physicians' earnings, with income growth being highest and managed care penetration being lowest in the South Central states, whereas the opposite situation prevails in the Pacific, Mountain, and New England states. Both rate of growth and level of market penetration are expected to have an effect on income growth.

Other Factors Affecting Physician's Incomes.—More than one quarter of physicians' incomes came from Medicare in 1995. Although Medicare payments to family or general practitioners increased by 19% from 1991 to 1993, reimbursements to surgeons and internists fell by 6%. These reimbursement changes are consistent with the income patterns but do not explain the most recent income drops.

Conclusion.—Although many income changes can be explained by the rise of managed care, the reasons for the loss of income to specialists with the least amount of managed care are not clear. Obviously, other factors are having an impact on physicians' incomes.

▶ There is little question that managed care has reduced physician income, and this article provides excellent documentation. Interestingly, the income for all specialties, including general internal medicine, has fallen recently, and family practice income is only elevated marginally. When will these savings be passed on to the consumers (patients)? Probably not until patients become disenchanted with the new system that restricts medical services and limits freedom of choice. "Organized" medicine is not well enough organized to effect the distribution of savings from health care dollars nor to protect patients' rights. For now, only patients—through their power to vote—can change unpleasant circumstances. Signs of a patient revolt are beginning to appear. Who would like to lead them?

E.M. Copeland III, M.D.

Columbia/HCA and the Resurgence of the For-Profit Hospital Business

Kuttner R (Cambridge, Mass)

N Engl J Med 335:362–367,446–451, 1996 1–4

Introductions.—For-profit hospitals have emerged as a growth industry for the 1990s. One corporation alone, Columbia/HCA Healthcare Corporation, now accounts for nearly half of for-profit hospital beds in the United States and 7% of all beds. The profitability of such chains can be ascribed to their cost-consciousness, their avoidance of unprofitable services and patients, their internal "re-engineering," and their financial incentives for physicians. The medical, ethical, and public policy issues raised by the renewed growth of for-profit hospitals were reviewed.

Growth of For-Profit Hospitals.—For-profit hospitals have little room for the tacit "cross-subsidies" of nonprofits, such as uncompensated care, unprofitable admission, research, education, or public health. Although the marketplace theoretically avoids declines in quality, the health care system is full of imbalances of information and captive "customers." The main strategy at Columbia/HCA is to attract patients through its referral networks, even when it is not the lowest-cost provider. If its market share in a given area is high enough, insurers have no choice but to deal with Columbia/HCA. The available data on the new wave of for-profit hospitals suggest that they provide less charity care than nonprofits and that they skim off the most profitable admissions. There are also key questions about possible declines in quality of care related to cost-cutting measures, such as the purchase of cheaper supplies and the replacement of nurses with lower-skilled personnel. Columbia/HCA and other chains are answerable only to their stockholders. As long as their cash flow remains sufficient, they should be able to perpetuate expansion. There is, however, growing resistance to such expansion.

Objections.—Many questions have been raised about the acquisition of not-for-profit hospitals by for-profit chains, including the legitimacy of the initial sale. Columbia/HCA relies on secrecy to acquire community hospitals as cheaply as possible, and thus discourages competitive bids. The increased resistance to the growth of for-profit hospitals is part of a growing backlash against market intrusions into health care. Such opposition has had a substantial impact on Columbia/HCA—over 30 deals that were pending have been killed or altered in the past year. Columbia/HCA claims that its emphasis on market discipline has created a rational and efficient health care system. However, unlike previous prepaid group plans, the money saved by cost-cutting at Columbia/HCA goes toward dividends to stockholders and future acquisitions, not to improved patient care. Also, the system integration relied on by Columbia/HCA actually works counter to market forces by preventing customers from shopping around. All of these trends lead to a growing convergence between nonprofit and for-profit hospitals, as the nonprofits act more like the for-profits in order to compete.

Discussion.—The resurgence of for-profit hospitals is discussed, with a focus on the preeminent example of Columbia/HCA. The future will see for-profit and nonprofit hospitals become either more alike or more different. If they become more alike, further pressures on patient care and physician autonomy can be expected, with increased conflict between the physician's professional and entrepreneurial roles.

▶ Corporate competition has resulted in much needed cost savings in health care delivery in both for-profit and non-profit hospitals. To date, I am unaware of a body of data that convincingly indicates that quality of care has been negatively affected. There are 2 potential major problems. First, the cost savings may not be passed on to the patient and may be used to pay exorbitant salaries and bonuses to the administrators of these new corporations (or to pay shareholders). Second, if cost cutting continues, quality may soon be sacrificed (convenience for both the patient and physician already has). There is a level below which the elimination of medical services will result in an increase in morbidity and mortality for many illnesses. This threshold should be identified.

E.M. Copeland III, M.D.

The Clear Liquid Diet Is No Longer a Necessity in the Routine Postoperative Management of Surgical Patients

Jeffery KM, Harkins B, Cresci GA, et al (Med College of Georgia, Augusta; Eisenhower Army Med Ctr, Augusta, Ga)

Am Surg 62:167–170, 1996 1–5

Introduction.—The return of normal bowel function has been the accepted signal to advance from a liquid diet after abdominal surgery. There is little scientific evidence, however, to support the need for restricting patients with abdominal surgery to a liquid diet in the presence of a postoperative ileus. The recent interest in challenging traditional views regarding the immediate postoperative diet has prompted this large, prospective randomized investigation.

Methods.—All patients from 3 large medical centers scheduled to undergo elective or emergent abdominal surgery were randomized to receive either a clear liquid or regular diet in the immediate postoperative period. Patients in the clear liquid diet group were advanced to a regular diet as tolerated. Patients were followed postoperatively for nausea, vomiting, abdominal distention, and other signs of dietary intolerance.

Results.—Of 241 patients, 106 were assigned to a regular diet and 135 to a clear liquid diet for the first postoperative meal. The regular diet group received significantly more calories and protein than the patients in the clear liquid diet group. The most common symptoms of dietary intolerance were nausea and vomiting. Eight (7.5%) patients in the regular diet group and 11 (8.1%) patients in the clear liquid diet group developed intolerance. All patients in the clear liquid diet group and 6 patients in the regular diet group were placed on "nothing by mouth" status. The remaining 2 patients in the regular diet group were placed on a liquid diet until symptoms resolved. There were no significant differences in dietary intolerance according to type of surgery performed. There were no significant between-group differences in diet-associated morbidity.

Conclusion.—Findings suggest there was no increased morbidity associated with the use of a regular meal as the first postoperative meal. Patients should proceed cautiously, and eat only food that is appealing in the immediate postoperative period. It will be interesting to see if hospital stays are significantly shorter because of the additional nutritional support received when a regular diet is served.

▶ For my entire career, I have been hesitant to give a regular diet as a first meal after an abdominal procedure, even though our laboratory demonstrated a return of basic myoelectrical rhythm of the small bowel within 18 hours of several intra-abdominal procedures including small bowel anastomosis.[1] Enough studies now exist for me to eliminate "clear" and "full" liquids from my initial feeding regimen, and I am sure hospital stay has been shortened.

E.M. Copeland III, M.D.

Reference

1. Carmichael MJ, Weisbrodt NW, Copeland EM: Effect of abdominal surgery on intestinal myoelectric activity in the dog. *Am J Surg* 133:34–38, 1997.

Efficacy and Cost Considerations of Intraoperative Autologous Transfusion in Spinal Fusion for Idiopathic Scoliosis With Predeposited Blood

Siller TA, Dickson JH, Erwin WD (Baylor College of Medicine, Houston)

Spine 21:848–852, 1996 1–6

Background.—The use of intraoperative autologous transfusion (IAT) —a procedure that necessitates considerable planning, trained technicians, and monetary resources—has increased in recent years. The cost effectiveness and actual reduction of homologous blood exposure attributable to IAT have not, however, been demonstrated in previous studies. Guidelines regarding which procedures and patient populations would be best served by IAT also are not available. The efficacy of IAT in reducing the need for homologous blood, as well as its effects on postoperative hematocrit, were therefore investigated in healthy adolescents undergoing spinal fusion for scoliosis.

Patients and Methods.—One hundred five patients (average age, 14.1 years) with adolescent idiopathic scoliosis were included in the study. Of these, 55 patients underwent posterior instrumentation and fusion with the use of an IAT device. The remaining 50 patients underwent the same procedure but without the IAT device. Hypotensive anesthesia was used in all patients to reduce blood loss, and all operations were performed by the same 2 surgeons. All patients predonated at least 1 unit of autologous blood before surgery, with blood collection done on preoperative day 14 and preoperative day 7. The Haemonetics Cell Saver or the Baylor Autologous Transfusions devices were used during intraoperative autologous transfusions, and were operated by trained technicians according to manufacturers' guidelines.

Results.—Age, weight, number of predeposited units, surgical duration, number of levels fused, estimated blood loss, and preoperative hematocrits were similar between patient groups. Patients in the IAT group predeposited an average of 1.9 units of autologous blood, compared with 2.0 units among controls. The total number of transfusions (autologous, directed donor, and homologous) were significantly less in the IAT group, at 1.45 units/patient or 80 units/55 patients vs. 1.96 units/patient or 98 units/50 patients in the control group. The average number of predeposited autologous blood transfused was 1.78 units/patient among controls, which was significantly greater than the 1.34 units/patients among the IAT patients. Directed donor blood transfusions were not significantly different between groups, with the IAT group averaging 0.03 units/patient (2 patients), compared with 0.1 units/patient (5 patients) in the control group. The number of nondirected homologous blood transfused also was not significantly different between groups, with the IAT patients averaging 0.07 units/patient (4 units overall in 2 patients) compared with 0.08 units/patient (4 units overall in 3 patients) among the controls. Postoperative hematocrits were slightly, but not significantly, higher in the controls compared with the IAT group, most likely reflecting the increased use of predeposited blood among controls. The percentage of unused/wasted predeposited autologous blood also was found to be substantially less in the control group, at 6% vs. 25% in the IAT patients.

Conclusion.—The use of IAT did not result in a decreased use of homologous blood in this patient population. The increased use of available predonated autologous blood, which averaged 0.5 units/patient more in the control group, was enough to counter any possible advantage of IAT. It is concluded that in patients with adolescent scoliosis, blood requirements for spinal instrumentation and fusion can be met with better cost efficiency and as reliably with predonated adequate autologous blood.

► The results of this study argue for predeposited autologous blood transfusion and against IAT in a healthy patient population. This lack of benefit brings into question the value of IAT in general. Certainly, for patients in whom the blood might be contaminated with bile, ascitic fluid, or other substances, the use of IAT should be seriously questioned unless blood loss is to be so massive that transfusion requirements cannot be met with predeposited autologous blood.

E.M. Copeland III, M.D.

Surgical Red Blood Cell Transfusion Practice Policies

Spence RK, for the Blood Management Practice Guidelines Conference (Staten Island Univ, New York)

Am J Surg 170:3S–14S, 1995 1–7

Background.—Surgical transfusion has become a complex decision-making process in recent years. To address the problems related to the appropriate use of red blood cell (RBC) transfusion in the surgical patient, a consensus conference was held in Dallas, Texas in January, 1995. The proceedings of the 2-day conference are summarized here.

Outcomes of Surgical Transfusion.—Four important outcomes were identified by the consensus participants. The primary reason for surgical blood transfusion is to provide additional oxygen delivery to either correct or prevent the development of tissue hypoxia. The patient must have a

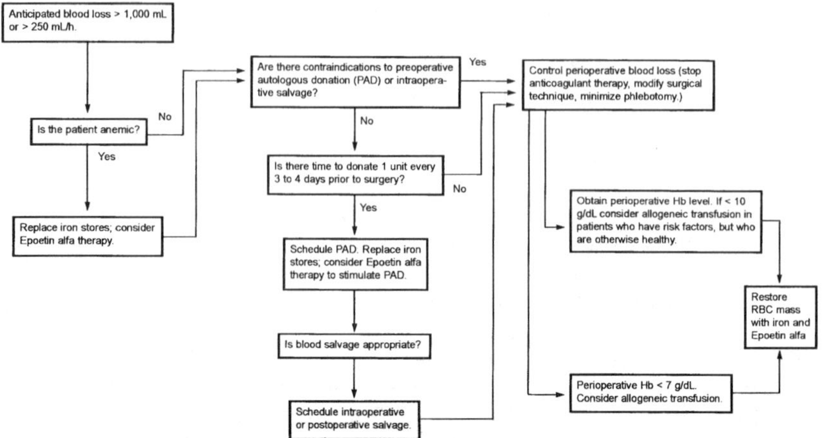

FIGURE 1.—Blood management algorithm for elective surgery. (Reprinted by permission of the publisher from Spence RK, for the Blood Management Practice Guidelines Conference: Surgical red blood cell transfusion practice policies. AMERICAN JOURNAL OF SURGERY, 170:3S–14S, copyright 1995 by Excerpta Medica Inc.)

clinically defined need for improved oxygen delivery. The risks of RBC transfusion must be minimized, physicians and patients need to be educated about transfusion practices and their risks and benefits, and nonblood management techniques (such as those used for Jehovah's Witness patients) should be optimized.

Surgical Transfusion Practice Policies.—Eleven policies were proposed as standards to be followed whenever possible: (1) the need for transfusion is to be assessed on a case-by-case basis; (2) blood should be transferred 1 unit at a time and followed by an assessment of further need; (3) exposure to allogeneic blood should be limited to appropriate need; (4) perioperative blood loss is to be prevented or controlled; (5) consideration of autologous blood as an alternative to allogeneic transfusion; (6) maximization of oxygen delivery; (7) increase or restoration of RBC mass by means other than RBC transfusion; (8) involvement of the patient in the transfusion decision; (9) documentation of reasons for and results of the transfusion decision in the patient's record; (10) development of hospital transfusion policies and procedures as a cooperative effort among various specialists; and (11) regular reassessment of transfusion policies, scheduled yearly or more often.

Discussion.—These policies are offered as a supplement and guide to sound clinical judgment and experience in surgical transfusion decisions. Blood management for elective surgery is described in an algorithm (Fig 1), and appendices to the report present definitions and background for the development of practice policies and outline blood management policies for Jehovah's Witness patients.

▶ This article is recommended to all surgeons for its summary of the data on the level of acceptable hemoglobin prior to transfusion for multiple sets of circumstances. The flow chart that accompanies the article should be studied as a common sense approach to blood transfusion.

E.M. Copeland III, M.D.

A Multicentre Comparison of Once-daily Subcutaneous Dalteparin (Low Molecular Weight Heparin) and Continuous Intravenous Heparin in the Treatment of Deep Vein Thrombosis

Luomanmäki K, Grankvist S, Hallert C, et al (Univ of Helsinki; Huddinge Hosp, Stockholm; Norköping Hosp, Stockholm; et al)

J Intern Med 240:85–92, 1996 1–8

Purpose.—The low-molecular weight heparins have the potential to simplify the initial treatment of deep vein thrombosis (DVT). The low-molecular weight heparin dalteparin was compared with unfractionated heparin (UFH) for acute treatment of patients with DVT.

Methods.—The open, randomized trial included 330 patients with suspected DVT. Each patient underwent ascending contrast venography within 12 hours after the start of treatment and again after 6–10 days of treatment. Patients with pulmonary embolism, recent DVT, or sequelae of previous DVT in the same leg were excluded, as were those who had previously been treated with UFH. Patients assigned to dalteparin received a single subcutaneous injection of 5,000 IU, followed by a fixed dose of 200 IU/kg^{-1} once daily. Those assigned to UFH received an IV bolus injection of 5,000 IU, followed by continuous infusion of 20,000–40,000 $IU/24\ hr^{-1}$, adjusted to the activated partial thromboplastin time. All patients received oral anticoagulant therapy as well. Heparin therapy continued for 5–10 days, until the results of the oral anticoagulant test were within the normal range. The main outcome measure was a change in the quantitative venographic score (Marder score) from before to after heparin therapy. The occurrence of pulmonary embolism or bleeding complications was assessed, and a follow-up examination was performed about 6 months after admission.

Results.—The 2 groups were fairly well matched, except for a higher incidence of malignancy in the UFH group. Patients in both groups were treated for a mean of 6.5 days after randomization. Improvement in the Marder score occurred in 51% of patients in the dalteparin group vs. 62% of those in the UFH group. The Marder score either improved or remained unchanged in 88% of patients treated with dalteparin and 93% of those treated with UFH. Eight patients in each group achieved complete clot lysis. Both groups achieved pain relief at a median of 3.5 days. Six patients in each group had bleeding complications. Recurrent DVT was confirmed in 2 patients in each group.

Conclusions.—Once-daily subcutaneous injection with the low-molecular weight heparin dalteparin is as effective as conventional UFH for the initial treatment of patients with DVT. The ease of dalteparin treatment suggests that it could be given on an outpatient basis. This could lead to substantial cost savings in the treatment of DVT.

▶ The clinical value of low-molecular weight heparin (LMWH) in the treatment of established DVT compares favorably with the use of IV heparin therapy. The efficacy of a single subcutaneous injection of LMWH in the treatment of DVT eliminates the cumbersome equipment required for continuous IV therapy, eliminates multiple laboratory studies, improves patient comfort, and makes possible the treatment of DVT on an outpatient basis. The future cost of treating a patient with DVT should be substantially reduced.

E.M. Copeland III, M.D.

Resource Utilization and Pathways: Meeting the Challenge of Cost Containment

Edwards WH Sr, Edwards WH Jr, Martin RS III, et al (Vanderbilt Univ, Nashville, Tenn; St Thomas Hosp, Nashville, Tenn)

Am Surg 62:830–834, 1996 1–9

Introduction.—The challenge for health care in the 1990s is to find new ways of delivering cost-effective care while maintaining the quality of care. One way of meeting this challenge is clinical pathways, which are designed to coordinate, plan, deliver, monitor, and review care by a multidisciplinary team for a defined, homogeneous patient population. In response to concerns about the availability of monitored beds and the monitoring needs of patients undergoing vascular surgery, one hospital recently created a specialized vascular unit to care for those patients throughout their hospitalization. This unit's 4.5-year experience using clinical pathways for cerebral revascularization (CVR) or femoral revascularization (FR) was reviewed.

Methods.—The experience included a total of 2,023 procedures—848 CVRs and 1,175 FRs—in 1,524 patients. Data for the analysis were gathered from the medical records, clinical evaluation, and telephone interviews. All patients were treated according to previously developed clinical protocols. The patients were monitored for at least 1–3 hours in the postanesthesia recovery room. If they were in stable condition, they were then transferred to the nonmonitored vascular surgery unit. Neurovascular and vital signs were checked every 2 hours through the first night and then every 4 hours until discharge. The patients began ambulation on the day after surgery. Preparations for discharge began before surgery; by the end of the experience, many CVR patients were discharged on the first day.

Results.—Seventy-three patients (3.6%) were observed in the ICU for management of cardiac or blood pressure problems. Twenty-six patients (1.2%) were transferred from the vascular unit to the ICU because of complications. Most patients with postoperative hypertension were successfully managed with sublingual nifedipine. Forty-six patients were readmitted to the hospital in the month after surgery, but only 3 within the first 10 days. The mean length of stay decreased from 5.69 to 3.26 days for patients with CVRs and from 10.67 to 4.49 days for patients with FRs. Expressed in 1995 dollars, the adjusted mean cost for a patient with CVR decreased from $7,223 to $4,490, a saving of $2,733, a 37.8% reduction. Costs for patients with FRs decreased from $14,332 to $5,541, a 59% reduction.

Conclusions.—In the study vascular unit, clinical pathways have reduced costs while maintaining quality of care for patients undergoing CVR and FR. The multidisciplinary, collaborative practice model used in this study offers a plan of hour-to-hour, day-to-day, and phase-to-phase patient care. Continuity of nursing care throughout hospitalization is an important aspect of this care plan; the response of nurses has been highly enthusiastic. Intensive care unit utilization for patients undergoing vascular surgery can be significantly reduced without increasing morbidity or mortality.

▶ No question, clinical pathways have led to cost savings with no decrease in quality of care. The key to success of this program is the dedicated vascular surgical service established by the hospital in conjunction with the vascular surgeons. Thereby, all physicians, nurses, physicians' assistants, nurse practitioners, clerks, and discharge planners are focused daily on the same treatment protocols. Common sense dictates that such a program will be successful. This institution's organization around a clinical discipline should serve as a model, not just for vascular surgery, but for multiple specialty services. Then, in a teaching institution, the only major patient care variable becomes the resident rotating through the service, a situation diametrically opposed to the traditional resident rotations, whereby the residents were expected to maintain quality and continuity of care, though they might not have ever before been on the specialty service.

E.M. Copeland III, M.D.

Unplanned Reoperation for Bleeding

Scher KS (Family Health Plan Cooperative, Milwaukee, Wis)

Am Surg 62:52–55, 1996 1–10

Background.—Any operation can be complicated by bleeding. The incidence of postoperative bleeding complications after elective surgical procedures was investigated.

Methods and Findings.—After 6,499 elective surgical procedures, 30 patients (0.46%) needed at least 1 additional operation to control bleeding. A specific bleeding site was identified in 10 patients (0.15%). Twenty patients (0.31%) had diffuse bleeding. In all 30 patients hemorrhage occurred despite normal prothrombin and partial thromboplastin times and adequate platelet counts. In 95% of the patients, diffuse bleeding was associated with the preoperative use of aspirin and/or nonsteroidal anti-inflammatory drugs (NSAIDs). None of the patients with a discrete bleeding point detected during reoperation were taking aspirin and/or NSAIDs.

TABLE 2.—Comparison of Outcome

Parameters	Diffuse bleeding	Specific bleeding point	*P*
ICU use	14 (70%)	2 (20%)	<0.05
ICU stay (days)	9.3 ± 16.1	1.5 ± 3.8	<0.02
Hospital stay (days)	22.7 ± 17.8	8.0 ± 7.6	<0.01
Hospital charges ($)	24,441 ± 29.869	6661 ± 8469	<0.01

(Courtesy of Scher KS: Unplanned reoperation for bleeding. *Am Surg* 62:52–55, 1996.)

Patients with diffuse bleeding needed more than 1 reoperation more often than patients with a specific site. Many subsequent reoperations were performed to manage infections that developed after the first reoperation to control bleeding. Diffuse bleeding was associated with significantly increased use of the ICU, length of ICU stay, total hospital stay, and hospital charges (Table 2).

Conclusions.—Postoperative bleeding, especially when it is diffuse, significantly increases hospital stay and costs. Obtaining routine screening coagulation profiles does not prevent bleeding. A medication history should be taken before elective surgery, with special attention given to the recent use of aspirin and NSAIDs. Surgery may be delayed until the antiplatelet effects of these agents have ceased.

▶ This study is missing the denominator. How many of the patients who had no postoperative bleeding were taking aspirin or NSAIDs? The health risks of these compounds for patients who undergo elective operations is unknown. Consequently, the cost–benefit ratio of doing platelet function tests on ingestors of these preparations is unknown. Nevertheless, in the small percentage of patients who bled postoperatively in this study, two thirds were associated with ingestion of cyclo-oxygenase inhibitors. Such bleeding could be eliminated by obtaining a proper history and by complete abstinence preoperatively from these compounds for 4 to 10 days because small quantities of aspirin will inhibit platelet function in susceptible patients.

E.M. Copeland, III, M.D.

Prospective Peer Review in Surgical Pathology

Lind AC, Bewtra C, Healy JC, et al (Creighton Univ, Omaha, Neb)

Am J Clin Pathol 104:560–566, 1995 1–11

Objective.—Quality assurance (QA) in surgical pathology is usually performed by retrospective audit of randomly selected cases. The benefit and feasibility of incorporating prospective peer review of diagnostic biopsy specimens were examined as part of QA in surgical pathology.

Methods.—During a 6-month study period in 1993–94, a total of 4,869 diagnostic biopsies were performed, of which 2,694 (55%) were reviewed by a second pathologist before the release of the surgical pathology report.

The cases included diagnostic biopsies of the skin, gastrointestinal tract, female genital tract, head and neck, breast, lung, and other sites. Errors detected were classified as major errors, diagnostic discrepancies, minor errors, or clerical errors. The results of this study were compared with those obtained in a retrospective audit.

Results.—Prospective review of 2,694 diagnostic biopsies yielded 380 errors. Thirty-two were classified as major with a potential for inappropriate patient care, 104 as diagnostic discrepancies, 192 as minor errors, and 52 as clerical errors. The 32 major errors represented 1.2% of all cases reviewed and included 17 gynecologic cases, 7 dermatologic, 5 gastrointestinal, 2 head and neck, and 1 pulmonary case. Peer review of the cases increased the mean overall turnaround time from 1.44 days to 1.50 days. The average time spent in performing prospective peer review was 4 hours/day, and the average time spent on peer review per case was 11.7 minutes. Retrospective review of 480 of 5,556 cases in an earlier 6-month period revealed 8 (1.7%) major errors. The cost of finding each major error would be $2,000 to $3,000, based on a total reimbursement cost of $150,000 per pathologist.

Conclusions.—Prospective peer review increases the accuracy of diagnostic biopsies while it only slightly increases the workload and not significantly increases the turnaround time.

► The estimated cost of $2,500 to discover an error in pathologic diagnosis must be weighed against the magnitude and type of errors made in an individual hospital. Interhospital variability makes such a study valuable to any individual hospital. At Creighton University, most errors were gynecologic and dermatologic and not life threatening. A compromise at this institution might be to review specimens from only these 2 clinical areas. In other hospitals, the identified problems might be in a different class of histological diagnoses or with a specific physician. The results of such an audit would provide a sense of security for patients and physicians, making it well worth the incremental increase in costs.

E.M. Copeland III, M.D.

The Impact of Diagnostic Testing on Therapeutic Interventions

Verrilli D, Welch HG (Urban Inst, Washington, DC; Veterans Affairs Med Ctr, White River Junction, Vt; Dartmouth Med School, Hanover, NH)

JAMA 275:1189–1191, 1996 1–12

Introduction.—Much of the effort to contain health care costs has targeted therapeutic interventions, big-ticket items that are easily identified and open to consensus decisions. Because diagnosis precedes therapy, the decision to diagnose may also provide a way to control the increase of therapeutic interventions. Longitudinal data from Medicare were used to examine the relationship between diagnostic tests and the therapeutic interventions they may trigger.

Methods.—Summary information was obtained for all physician claims submitted from 1987 through 1993 and available through Medicare's National Claims History and Part B files. Seven diagnostic test-therapeutic intervention pairs were selected for investigation. The portion of the variance in therapeutic intervention that could be explained by diagnostic testing was determined by simple linear regression.

Results.—The data examined represent physician services received by approximately 30 million elderly Americans in each of the 7 years under review. Use of all diagnostic tests expanded rapidly, with the greatest growth seen in prostate biopsy. Abdominal US, with the slowest growth, increased approximately 40% over 7 years. Much of the variance in the rates of therapeutic intervention was accounted for by the increase in diagnostic testing. Only abdominal US was not related to increases in its therapeutic pair. In the case of cardiac catheterization, 1 revascularization procedure was performed for every 1.5 diagnostic tests.

Discussion.—The rate of testing appears to be closely related to the rate of therapeutic interventions. Increases in diagnostic tests were not accompanied by rapid increases in disease rates. Because more diagnoses are made when more tests are ordered, the management of the growth of diagnostic testing may be as important in the reduction of health care costs as the management of the increase in therapeutic interventions.

▶ The increase in therapeutic intervention, based on an increase in diagnostic testing, makes outcome studies in the treatment of diseases such as ductal carcinoma in situ (DCIS) and prostate cancer discovered when subclinical even more important, especially when the treatments are expensive (radiation therapy for DCIS) and/or morbid (radical prostatectomy). Soon, genetic tests will be able to diagnose diseases before they occur. The treatment of diagnosed patients will add another layer of expense to the health care system. Of course, if early treatment is able to cure or eliminate the diseases that the tests are designed to accurately diagnose, then a cost savings will accrue in the long run, because it is less expensive to eliminate a disease than to treat it when clinically manifest.

E.M. Copeland III, M.D.

Physician Liability Under Managed Care

Manuel BM (Boston Univ)

J Am Coll Surg 183:537–546, 1996 1–13

Introduction.—A substantial portion of the U.S. population is enrolled in a managed care plan. For the physician, the most pernicious effect of managed care has been the expansion of physician liability. In any managed care company relationship, contract provisions are key. The insurance and indemnification section of a contract should be reviewed by a professional liability insurance carrier for the physician.

Contract Liabilities.—The obligations and responsibilities of the managed care company and physician should be clearly stated. The physician can be at risk when there is a failure to conform to the contract requirements, even when there is no negligence. In some instances, however, when there is a negligence, the contract can protect a physician. Under the Employee Retirement Income Security Act, employee-sponsored health plans are exempt from liability. Even in instances when the parties have never met, a contractual relationship between the company and its physicians and subscribers may create a doctor-patient relationship. Many plans use risk sharing and may include "withhold pools," which can affect all physicians equally in the plan, or physician capitation, in which the primary physician is at risk for the entire health care costs of the patient. Physicians should avoid contracts with "gag rules," which may be unethical, as they prohibit physicians from communicating with patients about the financial incentives, quality of care, and procedural and administrative issues.

Other Liabilities.—Physicians should watch for a plan that can assign or transfer the physician's contract to another plan without notice and approval. Language should include "neither party may assign the contract without the written consent of the other party." The termination policy of the plan should be clear. To avoid claims of abandonment, notification and transfer of patients must be addressed when a physician resigns. With the insolvency indenture policy, a physician is still under obligation to continue treating patients who are receiving treatment when a managed care company becomes insolvent. The contract should specify, however, how long the physician is obligated to accept new patients. Hold harmless clauses stipulate that surgeons are required to indemnify managed care companies for claims resulting from surgical negligence. In gatekeeper liability, the physician should be sure that the company's plan has enough specialists or out-of-plan specialists.

More Liabilities.—In practice liability, a physician's ultimate responsibility to the patient must override the limitations on treatment imposed by a third-party payer, as managed care companies can be held legally accountable when defects in the design of cost-containment mechanisms cause medically inappropriate decisions. Even if a plan may delay care by requiring additional consultations or tests, the liability for the delay of care may be placed on the physician. Practice guidelines in a plan should be created by physicians.

▶ For those of us who still live in areas not heavily penetrated by capitated care, this article is especially instructive (and frightening). Unfortunately, most of the recommendations in this article were learned from a bad experience. Hopefully, there will soon be a patient revolt against the restriction of quality and quantity of health care dictated by some managed care contracts. I sense a rising dissatisfaction from the patient perspective. Physicians have known this dissatisfaction for some time now.

E.M. Copeland III, M.D.

Shattuck Lecture—Evaluating the Health Risks of Breast Implants: The Interplay of Medical Science, the Law, and Public Opinion
Angell M
N Engl J Med 334:1513–1518, 1996 1–14

Introduction.—The safety of silicon-gel–filled breast implants has become a controversial and important public health question. Examination of this controversy reveals the interference of litigation, fear, bias, and greed in the scientific process of investigation, which has resulted in a reaction against science on the part of the public.

History.—Breast implants became available in the early 1960s. In 1976, the devices came under the authority of the Food and Drug Administration (FDA). The FDA required evidence of safety from breast implant manufacturers in 1988 after anecdotal reports of an association between breast augmentation and systemic disease, and multi–million dollar lawsuits were filed. In 1991, an FDA advisory panel was convened. Based on the findings of the panel, the FDA banned silicon-gel–filled breast implants, except in clinical trials of breast reconstruction after cancer surgery. However, the FDA commissioner reported that there was no scientific evidence either supporting or denying a link between breast implants and systemic disease. Nonetheless, lawsuits against manufacturers of breast implants proliferated, culminating in a $4.25 billion class-action settlement from the manufacturers to be set aside for the lawyers, the women claiming current implant-related illness, and women with future claims.

Scientific Evidence.—Breast implants have been placed in about 1% of American women, and connective tissue disease has been diagnosed in about 1% of American women, yielding a coincidental expected prevalence of both in 10,000 women. Therefore, a link between breast implants and connective tissue disease would be supported by a greater-than-expected prevalence of disease in women with implants. Several epidemiologic studies undertaken since the ban have failed to establish this link.

The Law.—Science presented in the courtroom was not related to the emerging scientific evidence. It is likely that the use of expert witnesses was the most instrumental factor in the dissociation between scientific evidence and courtroom evidence. The credentials defining expert witnesses are too broadly defined, and the opinions they offer need not be supported by evidence from the literature. These witnesses are chosen by and coached by the lawyers. Other features of the legal system subvert the use of scientific evidence, including the threat of large damages, leading to settlement out of court, and the use of juries to consider highly technical matters, leading to sympathy verdicts.

Consequences.—As a result of the experience with breast implants, suppliers of raw materials are reluctant to sell to medical device manufacturers. Tort law has had an impact on the conduct of research studies by threatening patient confidentiality by clinicians under subpoena. The history of breast implants reflects the public distrust and misunderstanding of science.

Conclusion.—The courts have ignored scientific processes and evidence, underscoring this same weakness in the general public. Therefore, the educational system at all levels must promote a better understanding of science and scientific thinking, including understanding evidence, chance, error, and the value of skepticism.

▶ This article should be read by all physicians who participate as expert witnesses for either the defense or the plaintiff. Almost anybody can be called an "expert" without much other than a medical degree as documentation. The public cannot be expected to believe the scientific evidence if "medical experts" decry it to win the case for their employers (the lawyers). The first step is for physicians to uphold scientific evidence in court as credible before criticizing lay jurors for ignoring it.

E.M. Copeland III, M.D.

Transmission of Hepatitis B Virus to Multiple Patients From a Surgeon Without Evidence of Inadequate Infection Control

Harpaz R, von Seidlein L, Averhoff FM, et al (Natl Ctr for Infectious Diseases, Atlanta, Ga; Univ of California at Los Angeles; Los Angeles County Health Dept)

N Engl J Med 334:549–554, 1996 1–15

Purpose.—A hepatitis B virus (HBV) outbreak, associated with an infected thoracic-surgery resident was described and possible mechanisms of transmissions were investigated.

Methods.—Chart reviews, interviews, and serologic testing of thoracic surgery patients were performed at the 2 hospitals where the infected resident had worked from July 1991 to July 1992. Hepatitis B surface antigen (HBsAg) subtypes and DNA sequences were obtained from the resident and from infected patients.

Findings.—Among the infected surgeon's 144 available patients, 13% had acute HBV infection. One of the 2 hospitals at which he had worked during this period was chosen for further study. At this hospital, none of the 124 patients of other thoracic surgeons had evidence of recent infection with HBV. No other common source of HBV infection was detected. The HBsAg subtype and partial HBV DNA sequences from the surgeon matched those from infected patients. Infection transmission was associated with cardiac transplantation, but not other surgical procedures. The infected surgeon was positive for hepatitis B e antigen and had high serum HBV DNA levels. The surgeon and hospital were in compliance with recommended infection-control procedures.

Conclusion.—Although the surgeon's technical skills were not a problem, his high levels of serum HBV DNA, combined with paper-cut–like lesions on his fingers during suturing could have contributed to disease transmission if glove failure occurred. This tragic outbreak could have been avoided had the surgeon been inoculated with HBV vaccine.

► This report is a bit frightening because transmitting HBV from surgeon to patient has been thought unlikely. Tying sternal wires can produce small cuts in the skin, even though the gloves do not appear to be violated. I suspect that these small cuts combined with the high titer of HBV in the surgeon at the time of the cluster infections were the causal factors in this situation, just as the authors suggest. Because transmission of HBV to patients from infected surgeons is apparently rare, I would hate to see all surgeons with prior HBV infections barred from the operating room (especially in the absence of disability insurance coverage). Nevertheless, the public must be protected. Possibly, there is an HBV titer above which the infected surgeon should not operate. If so, this titer should be determined immediately.

E.M. Copeland III, M.D.

Subjective Effects of Double Gloves on Surgical Performance
Wilson SJ, Uy A, Sellu D, et al (Royal Hosp, Muscat, Oman)
Ann R Coll Surg Engl 78:20–22, 1996 1–16

Introduction.—Although double gloving has been shown to be an effective prevention of infection transmission by needlestick injuries and blood contact, it is frequently not used. There has been little study of the effects of double gloving on surgical technique. This factor was investigated by comparing the subjective ratings of comfort, sensitivity, and dexterity during surgery of 3 combinations of double gloving and single gloving.

Methods.—General, vascular, pediatric, orthopedic, and urologic surgeons performed the same type of operation 4 times with the following glove protocols in random order: single gloving or double gloving with the normal-sized gloves worn inside and gloves a half size larger worn outside, larger gloves worn inside and normal gloves worn outside, and normal-sized gloves worn inside and outside. After each operation, the surgeon rated comfort, sensitivity, instrument handling, needle loading, knot tying, and tissue handling. Glove perforations were assessed by filling the gloves with water and squeezing.

Results.—Compared with single gloving, all of the double gloving methods were found to impair all of the subjective measures of comfort, sensitivity, and dexterity. The method of wearing normal-sized gloves over larger gloves was preferred for all of the measured variables, but the differences were not statistically significant. All 3 double gloving methods were associated with significantly fewer glove perforations, compared with single gloving.

Conclusions.—Double gloving was associated with significantly impaired perceived sensation and dexterity. However, it was an effective technique for preventing glove perforations. Therefore, it must become acceptable to sacrifice some sensation and dexterity to protect against blood contamination and infection.

▶ The technique of double gloving has been around for a long time but has not enjoyed widespread appeal. Multiple studies have shown that double gloving reduces the glove puncture rate and skin exposure to the patient's body fluids. Therefore, at the very least, any surgeon with an open wound of the hand would be wise to double glove, as would all nurses and technicians who scrub on routine surgical procedures.

E.M. Copeland III, M.D.

Time-dependent Histamine Release From Stored Human Blood Products

Nielsen HJ, Edvardsen L, Vangsgaard K, et al (Hvidovre Univ, Copenhagen)
Br J Surg 83:259–262, 1996 1–17

Purpose.—Perioperative allogeneic blood transfusion has potentially detrimental effects that have been attributed to immunosuppressive mechanisms. Previous studies have shown that perioperative histamine$_2$ receptor antagonist administration reduces postoperative immunosuppression. The hypothesis of a time-dependent spontaneous histamine release from stored human blood products and its role in the detrimental effects of blood transfusion was studied.

Methods.—One unit of blood was obtained from each of 18 unpaid randomly selected healthy donors. The 18 units were prepared as whole blood (6 units), plasma-reduced whole blood (6 units), and plasma- and buffy coat-reduced saline-adenine-glucose-mannitol (SAGM) blood (6 units). All units were stored in the blood bank under standard conditions for 35 days at 4°C. Plasma histamine and total cell-bound histamine concentrations were analyzed with an enzyme-linked immunosorbent assay in blood samples drawn from the stored units at baseline, and on days 2, 5, 9, 14, 21, 28, and 35 after initial storage. In addition, 4.5 mL SAGM blood samples were drawn from 56 randomly selected units immediately before they were used for clinical transfusion.

Results.—The median plasma histamine concentration in the 18 donors was 4.8 nmol/L. The median total cell-bound histamine concentration was 417.0 nmol/L in whole blood, 475.0 nmol/L in plasma-reduced whole blood, and undetectable in SAGM blood. Spontaneous histamine release increased in a time-dependent manner between the time of storage and day 35 from a median of 6.7 nmol/L to 175.0 nmol/L in whole blood, from 18.8 nmol/L to 328.5 nmol/L in plasma-reduced whole blood, and from 0.5 nmol/L to 2.2 nmol/L in SAGM blood. A significant concentration of free histamine was found in 7 of the 56 randomly selected blood samples obtained from units of SAGM blood that had been stored from 10 to 23 days.

Conclusions.—Histamine is released from whole blood and plasma-reduced whole blood in a time-dependent manner during storage at 4°C under standard conditions. Histamine release is rarely detected in SAGM blood. However, it remains to be determined whether histamine released from stored blood plays a significant role in the detrimental effects of perioperative blood transfusion.

► The immunosuppression secondary to blood transfusions has been recognized for some time and has been held partially responsible for postoperative infectious complications and distant metastasis in patients with cancer. No doubt, the reasons for this immunosuppression are more complex than just histamine release during blood storage, but the hypothesis is certainly intriguing since H_2 receptor blockade is a pharmacologic reality.

E.M. Copeland III, M.D.

Unwashed Wound Drainage Blood: What Are We Giving Our Patients?
Southern EP, Huo MH, Mehta JR, et al (Johns Hopkins Univ, Baltimore, Md; Waterbury Hosp Health Ctr, Conn; Yale Univ, New Haven, Conn)
Clin Orthop 320:235–246, 1995 1–18

Purpose.—Reinfusion of postoperative sanguineous wound drainage has been proposed as a means of replacing perioperative blood loss in patients undergoing total joint arthroplasty. However, the retransfusion of unwashed filtered wound drainage blood is not free of complications. The composition of unwashed postoperative wound drainage blood was studied in patients undergoing total joint arthroplasty.

Patients.—Nine women and 4 men (43–72 years of age) undergoing arthroplasty or total knee arthroplasty were enrolled in the study. The Solcotrans Orthopaedic Drainage Reinfusion System (Smith Nephew Richards, Inc., Memphis, Tenn) was used for the postoperative collection and reinfusion of wound drainage blood. A standard enzyme-linked immunosorbency assay was used to measure tumor necrosis factor-α, interleukin-1α, interleukin-6, and interleukin-8 levels in peripheral blood samples collected in the recovery room and at 6 hours postoperatively, and in postoperative wound drainage blood samples collected immediately and 6 hours postoperatively.

Results.—The estimated mean intraoperative blood loss was 620 mL, the mean volume of reinfused drainage blood collected in the Solcotrans device was 417 mL, and the mean initial hematocrit of the drainage blood was 24.3%. None of the patients experienced any adverse reactions attributable to the reinfusion of wound drainage blood. At 6 hours postoperatively both peripheral and drainage blood samples showed a significant increase in cytokine concentrations.

Recommendations.—A review of the literature confirmed that unwashed salvaged wound drainage blood was a dilute erythrocyte product lacking in normal clotting factors and containing numerous undesirable biologically active components. The routine use of predeposited autologous blood instead of wound drainage blood was highly recommended.

▶ As the authors state, "salvaged drainage blood has been shown to be a dilute erythrocyte product lacking in normal clotting factors with many known undesirable biologically active molecules. . . ." The reinfusion of unwashed wound drainage fluid never made much sense to me, especially when autologous blood is potentially available for an elective procedure. Our group showed multiple growth factors present in drainage from mastectomy wounds.[1] The risk of reinfusion of such a heterogeneous mixture of known and unknown potentially biologically active compounds should be questioned. The authors found no untoward effects in the 13 patients studied, but the literature is replete with multiple reports of complications that range from mild fever to shock from the reinfusion of unwashed filtered postoperative wound drainage blood.

E.M. Copeland III, M.D.

Reference

1. Rotatori DS, Coffee HH, Copeland EM, Schultz ES: Growth factors are present in human wound fluid. *Surg Forum* 4:627, 1990.

Comparative Mortality Among US Military Personnel in the Persian Gulf Region and Worldwide During Operations Desert Shield and Desert Storm

Writer JV, DeFraites RF, Brundage JF (Walter Reed Army Inst of Research, Washington, DC; US Army Ctr for Health Promotion and Preventative Medicine, Aberdeen Proving Ground, Md)

JAMA 275:118–121, 1996 1–19

Introduction.—There have been concerns about possible adverse health effects related to service in the 1991 Persian Gulf War. In a retrospective review of United States military personnel on active duty during the 1-year period of preparation, combat, and post-war recovery, investigators sought to characterize nonbattle deaths and determine whether the death rate in the Persian Gulf region was higher than expected.

Methods.—Service records were examined for the period from August 1, 1990 through July 31, 1991. Included were all members of the 4 service branches who were on active duty at the start of the study period, or who entered active service through the year. Person-years of exposure to the Persian Gulf region were calculated for all personnel, and rates for non–battle-related deaths were compared with rates for active duty troops deployed in other areas of the world.

Results.—During the study period, 688,702 individuals on active duty were deployed to the Persian Gulf region. Compared with troops who served in other regions, those in the Persian Gulf were younger and were more likely to be nonwhite, male, enlisted, in the reserve or national guard, and in the army. There were 1,662 nonbattle deaths among active-duty military personnel from August 1990 through July 1991; 225 (13.9%) occurred in the Persian Gulf region. Deaths that were a direct result of battle in the 6-week combat period numbered 147. Most nonbattle deaths (81.3%) were the result of unintentional trauma. Illness accounted for 30 deaths, most of which were classified as cardiovascular or unexpected/undefined. The number of observed deaths from illness was similar to the number that would have been expected for military personnel serving elsewhere.

Conclusion.—This first comprehensive study of deaths among United States troops who served in the Persian Gulf War showed no excess risk for unexpected/undefined deaths; most of the deaths in this category were subsequently determined at autopsy to have some underlying processes predisposing to sudden death. No evidence was found that deaths were the result of exposure to hazards unique to the Persian Gulf.

▶ Morbidity and mortality during a war-time conflict receive much more publicity and appear to be more of a sociological problem than the same injury rate to the same sex and age group in civilian life. In fact, the military may be a safer place to be for a certain segment of the population than in their local neighborhoods.

E.M. Copeland III, M.D.

2 Critical Care

Introduction

Several potentially important articles describing advances in the biology, prevention, or treatment of pulmonary failure and the adult respiratory distress syndrome (ARDS) were chosen. The first 3 of these articles deal with modes of ventilation. As described in last year's selections, one new experimental ventilatory strategy was the use of partial liquid ventilation. Based on the success of liquid ventilation in numerous animal models of respiratory failure, this technique began to be tested clinically, and the results of the first published clinical trial appear promising. Specifically, the results of a phase I clinical trial of partial liquid ventilation in adult patients with ARDS demonstrated that this new ventilatory technique improved both pulmonary gas exchange and pulmonary compliance without any measurable deleterious hemodynamic effects. Thus the early optimistic results of animal studies are supported by this limited clinical trial. The next study evaluated pressure-limited vs. volume-limited ventilation in patients with acute lung injury. You might wonder why this article was chosen, since pressure-controlled ventilation has generally become recognized as a superior option to volume-controlled ventilation in patients at increased risk of barotrauma. The answer is that the current study had an important twist. In this study, for the first time the flow pattern (waveform) was considered and proved to be a more important variable in preventing barotrauma than was the mode of ventilation. What the authors showed was that volume-ventilation using a decelerating waveform in place of the standard square waveform was as effective as pressure-controlled ventilation in preventing barotrauma. Since volume-controlled ventilation is a more reliable way of providing a consistent tidal volume than pressure-controlled ventilation is, this observation is of potential importance in patients with elevated airway pressure who are difficult to oxygenate. Another area of ventilatory support receiving increased attention is that of permissive hypercapnia. Since the pH can drop rather profoundly with this ventilatory strategy and no consensus has emerged on the level to which the pH should be allowed to decrease before bicarbonate therapy should be administered, an experimental study documenting that there are adverse physiologic consequences of acute changes in PCO_2 and pH and that these can be prevented by correcting the pH was chosen.

In patients with acute respiratory failure, the diagnosis of pneumonia is notoriously difficult and frequently requires the use of either bronchoscopic-directed bronchoalveolar lavage (BAL) or protected-brush bronchoscopy. These techniques, while relatively accurate, are expensive and time-consuming. Consequently, a well-controlled clinical study documenting that both these procedures can be performed without bronchoscopy with a high accuracy rate was chosen. A number of other clinical trials evaluating a wide range of topics and controversies were also chosen for inclusion. For example, a meta-analysis comparing the efficacy of stress ulcer prophylaxis regimens (antacids, H_2-receptor antagonists, or sucralfate) indicated that both sucralfate and H_2 blockers are essentially equally effective. A second area of controversy was clarified by a meta-analysis of 23 prospective randomized clinical trials. This study indicated that selective gut decontamination is likely to improve the survival of ICU patients, but only in the subset of high-risk patients whose predicted mortality rates exceed 30% to 40%. As reflected in the next article, the controversy of driving patients to achieve supranormal levels of oxygen delivery and consumption continues, but not as loud nor for much longer as the facts continue to emerge indicating that in a fully volume-resuscitated patient, oxygen-based parameters are more useful as predictors of outcome than as end points for resuscitation.

As uncontrolled sepsis, septic shock, ARDS, and multiple organ failure remain the most common causes of death in the ICU, studies evaluating new therapies and investigating the mechanisms of these disorders are of unique importance. Based on the concept that proinflammatory substances such as cytokines and oxidants contribute to organ injury, at least in part, through neutrophil-mediated endothelial cell damage, a number of agents directed against these putative mediators continue to be tested in clinical trials. Several phase I and II clinical trials as well as some preclinical studies were selected to illustrate the current level of activity in this important area. As reflected in the selected abstracts, the administration of liposomal prostaglandin E_1 in patients with ARDS was clearly beneficial, as was treating patients with septic shock with an antibody that inhibits neutrophil adherence to the endothelium (E-selectin). However, the administration of a monoclonal antibody directed against tumor necrosis factor did not improve the outcome in patients with severe sepsis or septic shock. Several preclinical experimental studies investigating other putative ways of treating endotoxic and hemorrhagic shock were included both to illustrate research directions being pursued as well as to raise a note of caution about the potential serious clinical limitations of these studies.

One particularly intriguing clinical study indicates that there may be a genetic factor involved in the predisposition of certain septic patients to organ failure. The concept that certain patients may have a predisposition to the development of an excessive inflammatory response while other patients do not may help explain the clinical paradox of why some patients live and others die after seemingly similar insults. This concept of genetic predisposition to cellular and hence organ death or dysfunction was further extended by an experimental study documenting that the genetically controlled response of a cell to a series of insults will determine whether the cell lives or dies. Perhaps I am being overly optimistic, but I am beginning to believe that insights from cellular biology may lead to clinically effective molecular medicine.

The last 2 articles chosen this year include one describing a new way to assess organ dysfunction in ICU patients, termed the logistic organ dysfunction system, and a study dealing with the costs of futile care in the ICU. Both these articles contain important information for physicians caring for ICU patients.

Edwin A. Deitch, M.D.

Initial Experience With Partial Liquid Ventilation in Adult Patients With the Acute Respiratory Distress Syndrome

Hirschl RB, Pranikoff T, Wise C, et al (Univ of Michigan, Ann Arbor)
JAMA 275:383–389, 1996 2–1

Background.—The initial reports of spontaneous liquid breathing of perfluorocarbon in animals appeared in 1966. More recently, laboratory studies of partial liquid ventilation (PLV)—in which the lungs are filled with perfluorocarbon and mechanically ventilated—to improve gas exchange in acute respiratory distress syndrome (ARDS) have been reported. An initial clinical experience with PLV in adult patients with ARDS was evaluated.

Methods.—The uncontrolled, phase I study included 10 consecutive patients who required extracorporeal life support (ECLS) for severe respiratory failure. The predicted survival rate for this category of patients was 10% to 20% without ECLS and 50% to 60% with ECLS. The patients were started on PLV 1–11 days after the start of ECLS. The dependent zone of the lung was filled with perflubron by tracheal instillation, followed by gas ventilation of the lung. As the alveolar gas/perfluorocarbon oxygen tensions increased, oxygen gas was distributed through the airways into alveoli. As alveolar gas/perfluorocarbon CO_2 levels decreased, CO_2 elimination occurred. The patients underwent volatilized perflubron replacement each day for 1–7 days, with a median cumulative dose of 38 mL/kg. The results of PLV were assessed in terms of physiologic shunt and static pulmonary compliance.

Results.—Chest radiographs showed diffuse opacification and aeration of the lungs immediately after perflubron administration. Median physiologic shunt decreased from 0.72 to 0.46 in the 72 hours after PLV started. At the same time, median static pulmonary compliance corrected for patient weight increased from 0.16 to 0.27 mL/cm of water per kilogram. Half of the patients survived. There was 1 case of pneumothorax and 1 case of mucus plug formation that may have been related to PLV.

Conclusions.—Initial clinical experience with the use of PLV for adults with severe ARDS demonstrated no gain in survival, as expected in a group of patients with such severe lung injury. However, the safety of administering perflubron into the lungs of patients receiving ECLS while maintaining gas exchange is demonstrated. Phase III studies of PLV for patients with respiratory insufficiency who are not receiving ECLS are being conducted.

▶ This phase I clinical trial describes the first adult human clinical trial of PLV in patients with severe ARDS. Previously, liquid ventilation with perfluorocarbons has been shown to be effective in numerous animal models of acute lung injury and ARDS indicating that this ventilatory strategy might have clinical benefit. Thus, at last, a clinical trial. Because this was a phase I safety-oriented trial, only 10 patients were enrolled and there were no controls. Nonetheless, the use of the perfluorocarbon did appear to improve both pulmonary gas exchange and compliance without any measurable deleterious hemodynamic effects.

The most likely explanations for the beneficial effects of the perfluorocarbon solution appear to be related to its mechanical properties as well as its ability to carry large amounts of oxygen and carbon dioxide. Perfluorocarbons have a high density and low viscosity, which allows then to reach atelectatic regions of the lung. These same properties help to clear exudate from the peripheral airways and alveoli, thereby improving ventilation/perfusion matching. In essence, these compounds appear to recruit previously closed lung units and thus improve gas exchange. Hopefully, as more clinical trials are carried out and reported, the results will continue to be positive and 1 more tool in the fight against ARDS will be available. Personally, I am very optimistic.

E.A. Deitch, M.D.

Comparison of Volume Control and Pressure Control Ventilation: Is Flow Waveform the Difference?

Davis K Jr, Branson RD, Campbell RS, et al (Univ of Cincinnati, Ohio)
J Trauma: Injury Infect Crit Care 41:808–814, 1996 2–2

Background.—Currently, pressure-limited, time-cycled ventilation is widely advocated for treating adult respiratory distress syndrome (ARDS). However, previous studies comparing pressure-limited and volume-limited ventilation have been methodologically flawed. Thus, in the current study, volume-limited ventilation with a square flow waveform or a decelerating flow waveform was compared with pressure-limited ventilation to determine whether a decelerating inspiratory flow waveform is responsible for improvements in gas exchange during pressure control ventilation for acute lung injury.

Methods.—Twenty-five patients with acute lung injury that required mechanical ventilation, sedation, and paralysis were studied. Positive-end expiratory pressure was 10 cm water or greater; ventilator frequency, 8 beats/min or greater; inspired oxygen concentration, 0.5 or greater; and peak inspiratory pressure, 40 cm water or greater. Ventilation was done at a tidal volume of 10 mL/kg. Respiratory frequency was set to maintain a pH of greater than 7.3 and $PaCO_2$ of less than 50 mm Hg. Positive end-expiratory pressure was set to maintain PaO_2 greater than 70 mm Hg or SaO greater than 93% with an FiO_2 of 0.5 or less. In a random order, ventilator mode was switched from volume control with a square flow waveform, pressure control ventilation with a decelerating flow waveform, or volume control ventilation with a decelerating flow waveform.

Findings.—During volume control ventilation with a square flow waveform, PaO_2 was reduced and peak inspiratory pressure increased compared with volume control with a decelerating flow waveform and pressure control ventilation. In addition, mean airway pressure was lower with volume control with a square flow waveform compared with volume control with a decelerating flow waveform and pressure control ventilation. Hemodynamic parameters did not differ.

Conclusions.—Both pressure control ventilation and volume control ventilation with decelerating flow waveform improved oxygenation at a lower peak inspiratory pressure and greater mean airway pressure than did volume control ventilation with a square flow waveform. The reported advantages of pressure control ventilation over volume control ventilation with a square flow waveform can be achieved with volume control ventilation with a decelerating flow waveform.

▶ Is it the waveform or the ventilatory mode that makes pressure-controlled ventilation a better option than volume-controlled ventilation in patients at increased risk of barotrauma (i.e., elevated airway pressures)? This is the key question asked in this prospective, controlled, crossover clinical trial that compared pressure-controlled ventilation with volume-controlled ventilation with both a decelerating and a square waveform. This article was selected because the results of the study support the authors' conclusion that the waveform is more important than the mode of ventilation in improving oxygenation and in potentially limiting barotrauma. The take-home message is that one can gain many of the benefits of pressure-controlled ventilation using a volume-controlled mode if the waveform utilized is decelerating rather than square. Because volume-controlled ventilation is a more reliable way of providing a consistent tidal volume than pressure-controlled ventilation, this observation is of potential importance in patients who have elevated airway pressures and in patients who are difficult to oxygenate.

E.A. Deitch, M.D.

Correction of Blood pH Attenuates Changes in Hemodynamics and Organ Blood Flow During Permissive Hypercapnia

Cardenas VJ Jr, Zwischenberger JB, Tao W, et al (Univ of Texas, Galveston; Shriners Burns Inst, Galveston, Tex)

Crit Care Med 24:827–834, 1996 2–3

Introduction.—Permissive hypercapnia in patients who have adult respiratory distress syndrome (ARDS) attempts to limit ventilatory-induced lung injury by restricting airway pressures. This approach is meant to prevent alveolar overdistention and "permits" PCO_2 to vary without definite intervention. This reduction in delivered volume can lead to clinically important systemic hypercapnia and associated respiratory acidosis in patients who have severe ARDS. Significant changes in hemodynamics, such as increased cerebral blood flow, increased intracranial pressure, and changes in regional organ perfusion, can then occur. It is not certain whether these changes can be diminished by systemic control of blood pH. The effect of correcting arterial blood pH with sodium bicarbonate on cardiac output, intracranial pressure, and carotid, mesenteric, and renal blood flow was evaluated during acute permissive hypercapnia.

Methods.—Six Marino ewes were randomly assigned to a pH-corrected group, and 5 were assigned to a pH-uncorrected group. One week before experimentation, a pulmonary artery catheter, femoral arterial and venous catheters, and a catheter in the third cerebral ventricle were placed in the ewes. Ultrasonic flow probes were placed on the left carotid, superior mesenteric, and left renal arteries. During experimentation, ewes were anesthetized and then underwent endotracheal intubation with mechanical ventilation. The arterial blood pH was allowed to decrease without treatment in the pH-uncorrected group by reducing minute ventilation to precipitate hypercapnia. The target $PaCO_2$ was 80 mm Hg. Sodium bicarbonate, 14.4 mEq/kg, was administered intravenously as a bolus to correct arterial blood pH to 7.40 in the pH-corrected group. Measurements were taken at baseline and every hour during hypercapnia.

Results.—As blood $PaCO_2$ increased to 81.2 mm Hg, the arterial blood pH decreased from 7.41 to 7.14 in the pH-uncorrected group. The blood pH was maintained at 7.37 in the pH-corrected group as $PaCO_2$ was increased to 80.3 mm Hg. There were significant increases in intracranial pressure, cardiac output, and organ blood flow that remained throughout in the pH-uncorrected group. These increases were not observed in the pH-corrected group.

Conclusion.—Increases in regional blood flow and intracranial pressure occur in the presence of acute hypercapnia. These physiologic responses are attenuated when sodium bicarbonate is used to correct pH. When uncorrected respiratory acidosis is allowed to develop slowly, it is generally well tolerated. This strategy should be used with caution in patients with ARDS who also have cardiovascular or neurologic disease.

► Based on uncontrolled prospective and retrospective clinical reports, many intensivists have perceived that the use of permissive hypercapnia improves the survival of patients with severe ARDS, compared with other ventilatory options. In some of these clinical series, the acute increase in PCO_2 has been profound; some patients have an arterial pH of less than 7.10. Although some authors propose the use of bicarbonate to keep the arterial pH at 7.24 or greater, others have allowed it to remain between 7.10 and 7.20.

Because acute changes in PCO_2 and pH can have adverse physiologic consequences, it is important to understand the physiologic consequences of this ventilatory strategy. Thus, this excellent and sophisticated experimental study on the hemodynamic effects of compensated and uncompensated hypercapnia is valuable. Although this study contains a large amount of information, the most important finding to my way of thinking was the observation that acute hypercapnia was associated with a significant increase in cerebral blood flow and, more importantly, a major increase in intracranial pressure (i.e., it increased from 9 to 26.8 mm Hg). Equally important, the authors documented that the use of sodium bicarbonate to correct the pH prevented this hypercapnia-induced increase in intracranial pressure. Because many patients with ARDS may have associated changes in CNS function, or even CNS injury, the take home message is that pH should be corrected when permissive hypercapnia is used, especially in patients with evidence of CNS dysfunction.

E.A. Deitch, M.D.

Comparison of Nonbronchoscopic Techniques With Bronchoscopic Brushing in the Diagnosis of Ventilator-associated Pneumonia

Wearden PD, Chendrasekhar A, Timberlake GA (West Virginia Univ, Morgantown)

J Trauma: Injury Infect Crit Care 41:703–707, 1996 2–4

Background.—Ventilator-associated pneumonia (VAP) carries a very high mortality rate, often exceeding 50%. Inappropriate use of empirical antibiotics further increases mortality rate and the incidence of more virulent organisms. Protected specimen brushing (PSB) with bronchoscopy is currently the diagnostic method of choice for VAP. However, this is a time-consuming, labor-intensive, costly procedure. The diagnostic accuracy of quantitative cultures acquired through nonbronchoscopic PSB and nonbronchoscopic bronchoalveolar lavage (BAL) were compared with those obtained by bronchoscopic PSB in surgical patients thought to have VAP.

Methods.—Fifteen ventilated patients in the surgical ICU were included in the prospective, crossover, controlled trial. Ventilator-associated pneumonia was suspected on the basis of leukocytosis, purulent sputum, and chest radiographic findings. In all patients, nonbronchoscopic PSB and BAL were followed by bronchoscopic PSB. Positive culture results were defined as the presence of more than 10^4 colony-forming units per milliliter.

Findings.—Bronchoscopic PSB and nonbronchoscopic BAL were in perfect agreement. Bronchoscopic and nonbronchoscopic PSB had a 93% concordance. The nonbronchoscopic procedures required significantly less time than the bronchoscopic (Table 3).

Conclusions.—Nonbronchoscopic PSB and BAL are as accurate as bronchoscopic PSB for diagnosing VAP in surgical intensive care patients. The nonbronchoscopic techniques are also faster and less costly.

TABLE 3.—Procedure Time, Concordance, and Charges

Procedure	Time	Concordance (%)	Charges
Bronchoscopic PSB	10.3 ± 0.38		$632
Blind PSB	0.5 ± 0.38	93	$ 82
Blind BAL	2.1 ± 0.38	100	$207
Tracheal aspirate		47	$ 72

Note: Procedure time is represented in minutes with SEM, concordance of culture data with bronchoscopic PSB, and patient charges for each procedure. Blind indicates nonbronchoscopic.

Abbreviations: PSB, protected specimen brush; *BAL,* bronchoalveolar lavage.

(Courtesy of Wearden PD, Chendrasekhar A, Timberlake GA: Comparison of nonbronchoscopic techniques with bronchoscopic brushing in the diagnosis of ventilator-associated pneumonia. *J Trauma* 41(4):703–707, 1996.)

▶ The diagnosis of ventilator-associated pneumonia using standard radiographic and tracheal culturing techniques is notoriously inaccurate. This difficulty in correctly identifying patients with pneumonia has led many clinicians to use protected-brush bronchoscopy or bronchoscopic-directed bronchoalveolar lavage as a way of more accurately diagnosing pneumonia. The results of the study presented above indicate that nonbronchoscopic PSB and BAL are as accurate as bronchoscopic techniques, plus they are faster and cheaper.

A famous pundit once said, show me a simple solution to a complex problem and I will show you an answer that is wrong. In this case, the pundit and not the answer appears to be wrong. The data presented in this article support the authors' basic conclusion that correctly performed nonbronchoscopically obtained specimens provide as accurate microbiological data as do bronchoscopically collected specimens. Because this practical approach appears to be so much quicker and cheaper, it may be the way to go. Thus, I recommend that you read the material and methods section of the article and give it a try.

E.A. Deitch, M.D.

Phenotypic and Functional Analysis of Pulmonary Microvascular Endothelial Cells From Patients With Acute Respiratory Distress Syndrome

Grau GE, Mili N, Lou JN, et al (Univ Med Ctr, Geneva)

Lab Invest 74:761–770, 1996 2–5

Background.—The mechanisms involved in the pathogenesis of acute respiratory distress syndrome (ARDS) have not been elucidated. Previous studies have shown that endothelial dysfunction, particularly in pulmonary microvessels, plays a critical role in ARDS. Therefore the phenotypic and functional alterations in pulmonary microvascular endothelial cells (MVECs) of patients with ARDS were investigated.

Methods.—Pulmonary MVECs were isolated and purified from lung tissue obtained from 5 patients with severe ARDS and 4 patients who underwent lobectomy for bronchial carcinoma. Surface molecules on the MVECs were measured with monoclonal antibodies and flow cytometry.

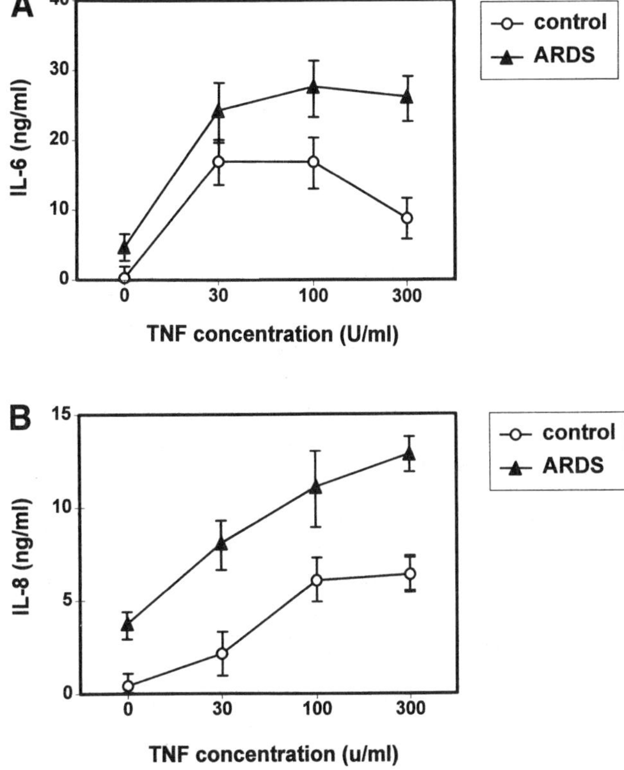

FIGURE 4.—Inducible interleukin-6 (*IL-6*) (**A**) and IL-8 (**B**) production by pulmonary microvascular endothelial cells from patients with acute respiratory distress syndrome (*ARDS*) and from controls after tumor necrosis factor (*TNF*) stimulation. Cytokines were measured in the supernatants by enzyme-linked immunosorbent assay. Results are presented as means ± SD. For both cytokines, Mann-Whitney $P < 0.05$ in resting conditions and at each TNF concentration tested. (Courtesy of Grau GE, Mili N, Lou JN, et al: Phenotypic and functional analysis of pulmonary microvascular endothelial cells from patients with acute respiratory distress syndrome. *Lab Invest* 74(4):761–770, 1996.)

Cytokine expression was measured by using an enzyme-linked immunosorbent assay. These measurements were repeated after overnight exposure to varying concentrations of tumor necrosis factor (TNF) or lipopolysaccharide.

Results.—Endothelial cell leukocyte adhesion molecule type 1 was expressed by none of the control MVECs and by the MVECs of only 2 ARDS patients. When compared with the control cells, the ARDS MVECs expressed significantly more intercellular adhesion molecule type 1 (ICAM-1), vascular adhesion molecule type 1, CD14, and tumor necrosis factor receptor p75 (TNF-R2). Expression of TNF receptor p55 (TNF-R1) was not significantly upregulated in the ARDS MVECs. Stimulation by TNF induced a dose-dependent upregulation in ICAM-1 expression in both control and ARDS MVECs, which somewhat reduced the differences between them. Lipopolysaccharide stimulation did not induce significant upregulation in ICAM-1 expression in control MVECs and only weakly increased ICAM-1 expression in ARDS MVECs. The ARDS MVECs demonstrated significantly greater constitutive expression of both interleukin-6 (IL-6) (9.5–26 times greater) and IL-8 (4.5–16 times greater) than did control MVECs. The differences were reduced but remained significant with TNF stimulation (Fig 4).

Conclusions.—Pulmonary MVECs in patients with ARDS have significant phenotypic and functional differences from pulmonary MVECs in subjects without ARDS in that they demonstrate spontaneous overexpression of some adhesion molecules and increased production of pro-inflammatory and anti-inflammatory cytokines. ICAM-1 and TNF-R2 may be particularly involved in the pathogenesis of ARDS, and the endothelium may be the main source of the cytokines typically seen in the bronchoalveolar lavage fluid obtained from these patients. Monitoring these phenotypic and functional parameters in pulmonary MVECs may increase understanding of the mechanisms of acute lung injury and allow an accurate evaluation of medication efficacy.

▶ This elegant basic science study on pulmonary MVECs provides important insight into the pathogenesis of ARDS. Their basic finding was that MVECs from ARDS patients were significantly different from control endothelial cells in terms of both increased cell surface adhesion molecule expression and the capacity to produce the cytokines IL-6 and IL-8. This study is important for several reasons. First of all, it is the first study of its kind performed on patients. Second, the authors tested MVECs rather than large-vessel endothelial cells. This second point is critical since animal and cell culture studies suggest that MVECs respond to inflammatory stimuli differently than macrovascular endothelial cells. Finally, these studies support the concept that activation of MVECs plays a *primary* role in the pathogenesis of ARDS by recruiting and activating neutrophils.

E.A. Deitch, M.D.

Increased Interleukin-8 Concentrations in the Pulmonary Edema Fluid of Patients With Acute Respiratory Distress Syndrome From Sepsis

Miller EJ, Cohen AB, Matthay MA (Univ of Texas, Tyler; Univ of California, San Francisco)

Crit Care Med 24:1448–1454, 1996 2–6

Background.—Interleukin-8 (IL-8), a chemokine secreted by various types of cells in response to inflammatory stimuli, has been implicated in mediating the early phase of acute lung injury. High concentrations of IL-8 have been found in the bronchoalveolar lavage fluid and pulmonary edema fluid of patients with acute respiratory distress syndrome (ARDS). Because the mechanisms mediating acute lung injury may differ among the different clinical disorders involved in the etiology of ARDS, the possibility that septic and nonseptic causes of ARDS could be differentiated by the concentrations of IL-8 in the pulmonary edema fluid was investigated.

Methods.—Pulmonary edema fluid and plasma samples were obtained from 35 adult patients with pulmonary edema, including 16 patients with septic ARDS, 9 patients with nonseptic ARDS, and 8 patients with hydrostatic pulmonary edema. Interleukin-8 and total protein concentrations were measured in both the plasma and edema fluid samples. Neutrophils were also quantified in the edema fluid samples.

Results.—The pulmonary edema fluid from the septic ARDS group had significant greater IL-8 concentrations than in either of the other 2 patient groups. The septic ARDS group also had a significantly greater IL-8/total protein ratio in the edema fluid than did the other 2 groups. In all patients with ARDS, the neutrophil count was significantly correlated with the IL-8 concentration.

Conclusions.—Interleukin-8 may be an important mediator of acute lung inflammation, particularly in patients with ARDS with a septic etiology. The markedly excessive concentration of IL-8 in the pulmonary edema fluid of these patients early in the course of ARDS suggests the potential efficacy of anti–IL-8 antibody therapy.

▶ The key findings of this study were that pulmonary IL-8 levels were higher in lung fluid from septic ARDS patients than nonseptic ARDS patients or patients with other causes of respiratory failure at a time when blood IL-8 levels were similar between the 3 groups. Now, what might this mean? First, these results strongly suggest that the lung itself is the source of the neutrophil-attracting agent IL-8. Second, measuring blood levels of IL-8 may not be accurate or clinically helpful. When the results of this study are combined with those of the abstract by Grau et al. (Abstract 2–5), it appears that IL-8 might be a pivotal mediator in the pathogenesis of ARDS, and if so, blocking IL-8 production or neutralizing IL-8 activity might be a successful clinical strategy. Since monoclonal antibodies against IL-8 are potentially available and have been shown to be protective in animal models of acute lung injury, this strategy can be tested. However, since the lung appears to be the primary source of IL-8 in patients with ARDS, it would appear that for this type of therapy to be effective, it will need to be administered directly to the lung and not intravenously.

E.A. Deitch, M.D.

Stress Ulcer Prophylaxis in Critically Ill Patients: Resolving Discordant Meta-analyses

Cook DJ, Reeve BK, Guyatt GH, et al (McMaster Univ, Hamilton, Ontario, Canada; Univ Hosp Bergmannsheil, Bochum, Germany)

JAMA 275:308–314, 1996 2–7

Purpose.—Stress ulcer prophylaxis has been the subject of several systematic reviews. However, these studies have produced some inconsistent results. An updated review of stress ulcer prophylaxis in the critical care unit is presented, including a meta-analysis performed to resolve previous inconsistencies.

Methods.—The review included randomized clinical trials comparing the use of various prophylactic drugs, including antacids, histamine$_2$-receptor antagonists, or sucralfate, with each other or with no treatment. Only studies of critically ill adults using gastrointestinal (GI) bleeding or pneumonia as outcome measures were included. The analysis included 57 unique trials representing 7,218 critically ill patients with a wide range of medical and surgical diagnoses.

Results.—Histamine$_2$-receptor antagonist treatment reduced the risk of overt GI bleeding and clinically important bleeding. In addition, antacids tended to decrease the risk of overt bleeding compared with no treatment. The rate of clinically important bleeding tended to be lower with histamine$_2$-receptor antagonists and antacids than with sucralfate. However, histamine$_2$-receptor antagonists tended to increase the risk of pneumonia compared with no prophylaxis. In addition to reducing the nosocomial pneumonia rate, sucralfate was also associated with a lower mortality than antacids or histamine$_2$-receptor antagonists.

Conclusions.—An up-to-date review of the evidence suggests that histamine$_2$-receptor antagonist treatment decreases the rate of clinically important GI bleeding in critically ill adults. Sucralfate may be just as effective in reducing the bleeding rate while also reducing the risk of nosocomial pneumonia and death. The net effect of sucralfate vs. no prophylaxis remains to be determined.

▶ Perhaps the answer is in. Based on this meta-analysis, it appears that, as far as stress ulcer prophylaxis is concerned, one can treat according to one's bias and still be correct. For example, if you fear the development of pneumonia more than stress bleeding, use sucralfate. On the other hand, if you fear bleeding more than pneumonia, use a histamine-$_2$ receptor antagonist. Nonetheless, for my money, I will continue to use sucralfate inasmuch as there is a survival trend in its favor.

E.A. Deitch, M.D.

Does Selective Decontamination of the Digestive Tract Reduce Mortality for Severely Ill Patients?

Sun X, Wagner DP, Knaus WA (George Washington Univ, Washington, DC)

Crit Care Med 24:753–755, 1996 2–8

Introduction.—Selective decontamination of the digestive tract has been investigated as a means to prevent nosocomial infections and to reduce mortality and morbidity in critically ill patients. Studies have demonstrated a reduction in bacterial colonization and infection; however, data on mortality are less certain. The relationship between mortality risk and

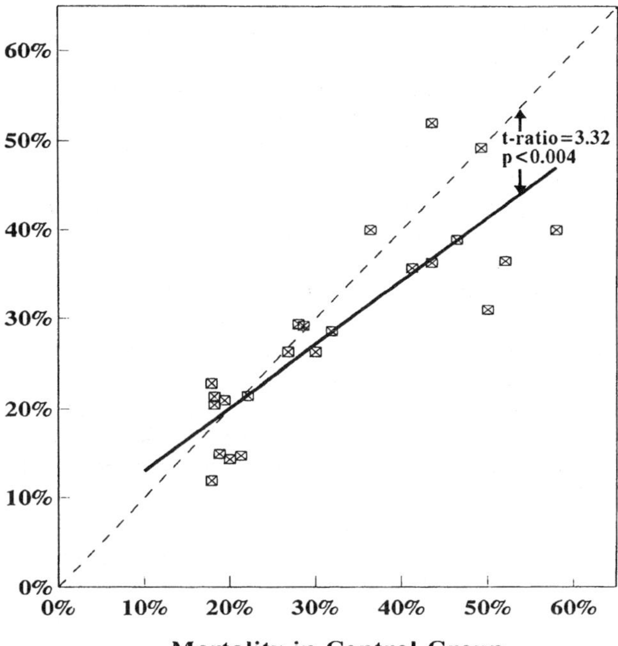

FIGURE 1.—Relationship of mortality rates between selective decontamination of the digestive tract (*SDD*) treatment and control groups in 23 randomized, controlled trials from Trialists' Collaborative Group. *Squares* indicate individual trial. The *dashed line* is the 45-degree line, which indicated no difference between mortality rates in treatment and control groups. All trials below this line had a lower mortality rate in the selective decontamination of the digestive tract–treated group than in the control group. The *solid line* is the regression line, which is is drawn through all trials. The difference between this regression line and the 45-degree line is tested by *t*-test for statistical significance (regression coefficient, 0.70; *t*-ratio for difference from 1.0, 3.32; degrees of freedom; 21; $P < 0.004$). (Courtesy of Sun X, Wagner DP, Knaus WA: Does selective decontamination of the digestive tract reduce mortality for severely ill patients? *Crit Care Med* 24(5):753–755, 1996.)

the effect of selective decontamination of the digestive tract was assessed with the use of data collected for a meta-analysis.

Methods.—Data from 23 studies, collected for a meta-analysis, were analyzed. Baseline mortality risk was determined from the mortality rates among control groups in the studies. The effect of selective decontamination of the digestive tract on mortality was evaluated as a function of baseline risk. A weighted least-squares regression analysis across all 23 trials was used to determine reduction in mortality rates. Mortality rates in the selective decontamination–treated group was graphed against the mortality rates in control groups. A 45-degree line represented no difference in mortality rates between the 2 groups. Trials that did show a reduction in mortality rate with selective decontamination would produce a regression line below the 45-degree line. A 2-tailed test of significance was used to test the difference between the slope of the regression line and that of the 45-degree line.

Results.—A total of 4,142 patients were included in the 23 trials. As mortality rates in the control groups increased, mortality rates in the groups that received selective decontamination were significantly more likely to decrease (Fig 1). An observed t value of 3.32 was found which indicated that selective decontamination was more effective in reducing mortality in patients at higher risk for mortality.

Conclusion.—Selective decontamination of the digestive tract produced a reduction in mortality rate in patients at high risk for mortality. As the risk of mortality in the control groups increased, mortality risk in the treatment group decreased significantly.

▶ This article was chosen because it illustrates the importance of using sophisticated data interpretation to help clarify a controversial and confusing clinical subject, i.e., the use of selective decontamination of the digestive tract (SDD) to reduce mortality. It also shows how the entry criteria used to enroll patients in clinical trials can have profound effects on the conclusions of those trials. Specifically, this meta-analysis indicates that SDD is likely to improve survival only in those patient populations where the risk of death exceeds 30% to 40%. Because the risk of death is an important factor in identifying patients likely to benefit from SDD, this study also highlights the need for accurate scoring systems that allow prediction of mortality at a time early enough to institute this therapy.

E.A. Deitch, M.D.

The Use of Oxygen Consumption and Delivery as Endpoints for Resuscitation in Critically Ill Patients

Durham RM, Neunaber K, Mazuski JE, et al (St Louis Univ, Mo)

J Trauma 41:32–40, 1996 2–9

Background.—Studies have recently suggested that in hypoperfusion states, resuscitation based on oxygen consumption and delivery indicators is associated with a better outcome than resuscitation based on conventional indicators such as pulmonary capillary wedge pressure (PCWP), right ventricular end-diastolic volume index (RVEDVI), mean arterial pressure, and cardiac index. Although improved outcome has been reported for patients who reached VO_2I (oxygen consumption index)/DO_2I (oxygen delivery index) goals, it is also possible that those patients with sufficient volume resuscitation who still fail to increase VO_2I/DO_2I have poor physiologic reserve and, therefore, a poor outcome. The use of above-normal values for VO_2I/DO_2I was prospectively compared with the use of conventional indicators as resuscitation end points for critically ill patients.

Methods.—Fifty-eight critically ill patients underwent randomization into 2 groups. In the first group (27 patients), an attempt was made to maintain a VO_2I of at least 150 or a DO_2I of at least 600 mL/min/m_2. The second group (31 patients) received resuscitation based on conventional indicators. The volume resuscitation procedures and the PCWP goals were the same in both groups. Physicians were "blinded" to the oxygen consumption and delivery indices in the second group. Age, Injury Severity Score, and Acute Physiology and Chronic Health Evaluation (APACHE II) scores were not significantly different between these 2 groups.

Results.—There were 3 deaths in the first group and 2 deaths in the second group caused by organ failure (OF). Another patient in the second group died of refractory shock within the first 24 hours. Two of the 3 patients in the first group who died had failed to achieve VO_2I/DO_2I goals within the first 24 hours. There was no significant difference in mortality between these 2 groups, even when the patients who failed to meet their resuscitation goals in the first group were excluded. Excluding the patient who died of shock, OF occurred in 67% of patients in the first group and 73% of patients in the second group. There was no significant difference in length of ventilator support, ICU stay, or hospital stay between these 2 groups. There was no significant difference in OF incidence between those patients who achieved the VO_2I goal and those who could not achieve this goal. Organ failure occurred in 59% of those patients with an average DO_2I of at least 600 mL/min/m^2, and in 88% of those who could not maintain this indicator at that level within the first 24 hours.

Conclusion.—There was no significant outcome difference between critically ill patients resuscitated based on conventional indicators as compared with those resuscitated using VO_2I/DO_2I, when the volume resuscitation protocols were similar. When the data from both groups of patients were examined together, achievement of the oxygen delivery goal was associated with a decreased incidence of OF. Therefore when volume resuscitation is sufficient, DO_2I may be useful as a prognostic indicator rather than as a resuscitation goal.

► Since Shoemaker, in the 1980s, first proposed the importance of ICU patients achieving supranormal levels of oxygen delivery and consumption to improve survival, this concept has been widely debated. Today, the debate continues, but not as loud nor for much longer as the facts continue to emerge. That is because well-controlled studies such as this one are showing similar results and reaching similar conclusions. In other words, I strongly concur with the authors' major conclusion which is that "given adequate volume resuscitation, oxygen-based parameters are more useful as predictors of outcome than as endpoints for resuscitation."

This conclusion has practical consequences. Specifically, it means that it is important to volume resuscitate and to assess hemodynamic (PCWP and RVEDVI) as well as oxygen delivery and consumption variables. It also means that reasonable attempts to increase these parameters are worthwhile (i.e., it provides important prognostic information), but fanatical attempts to drive these hemodynamic variables where they will not go or to higher and higher levels just because the patients are sick are ill conceived.

E.A. Deitch, M.D.

Liposomal Prostaglandin E_1 in Acute Respiratory Distress Syndrome: A Placebo-controlled, Randomized, Double-blind, Multicenter Clinical Trial

Abraham E, Park YC, Covington P, et al (Univ of Colorado, Denver; Liposome Company, Princeton, NJ; Pharmaceutical Product Development, Morristown, NC; et al)

Crit Care Med 24:10–15, 1996 2–10

Background.—The mortality rate of patients with acute respiratory distress syndrome (ARDS) remains high. Prostaglandin E_1 (PGE_1 produces vasodilation, downregulates inflammatory responses, and blocks platelet aggregation. The safety and efficacy of liposomal PGE_1 (TLC C-53) was evaluated in a randomized, prospective, multicenter, double-blind, placebo-controlled phase II clinical trial.

Methods.—Twenty-five patients with ARDS were prospectively randomly assigned to be infused for 60 minutes every 6 hours for 7 days with either drug or placebo. The starting dose was 0.15 μg/kg/hr, which was increased every 12 hours until intolerance developed, invasive monitoring was halted, or the maximum dose of 3.6 μg/kg/hr was reached. Patients received aggressive care throughout the study period. The outcome measurements were PaO_2/FIO_2, dynamic pulmonary compliance, ventilator dependence on day 8, and 28-day mortality.

Results.—On day 8, all 8 patients in the placebo group required mechanical ventilation, whereas 8 of 17 in the treatment group were no longer on the ventilator. The PaO_2/FIO_2 improved more in the treatment group, and this reached significance on day 3 (Fig 1). Lung compliance increased significantly more in the treatment group than in the placebo group by day 8. The 28-day mortality rate was 6% in the treatment group and 25% in the placebo group, but this difference did not reach significance because of the small sample size. Drug-related adverse events were reported in 82% of the treatment group, but half of these were localized infusion site irritations. TLC C-53 was well tolerated hemodynamically.

Conclusions.—In a small group of patients with ARDS, the liposomal PGE_1, TLC-53, was associated with improved oxygenation, increased lung compliance, and decreased ventilator dependency compared with placebo. The trend in mortality rates with this drug was favorable but did not reach significance because of small sample size. Larger clinical studies will be required to confirm the beneficial effects of TLC C-53 in the treatment of patients with ARDS.

► For those who have followed the literature on this subject, you might say, not PGE_1 again. Didn't a prospective randomized clinical trial show that it did not work? The answer is yes. But, in that trial PGE_1 was given as a free drug in solution rather than contained in liposomes as in the current study. Why might PGE_1 be more clinically effective in liposomes than as a free suspension? The answer appears to be twofold. First, more PGE_1 can be administered safely when it is in liposomes and, second, PGE_1 in liposomes seems

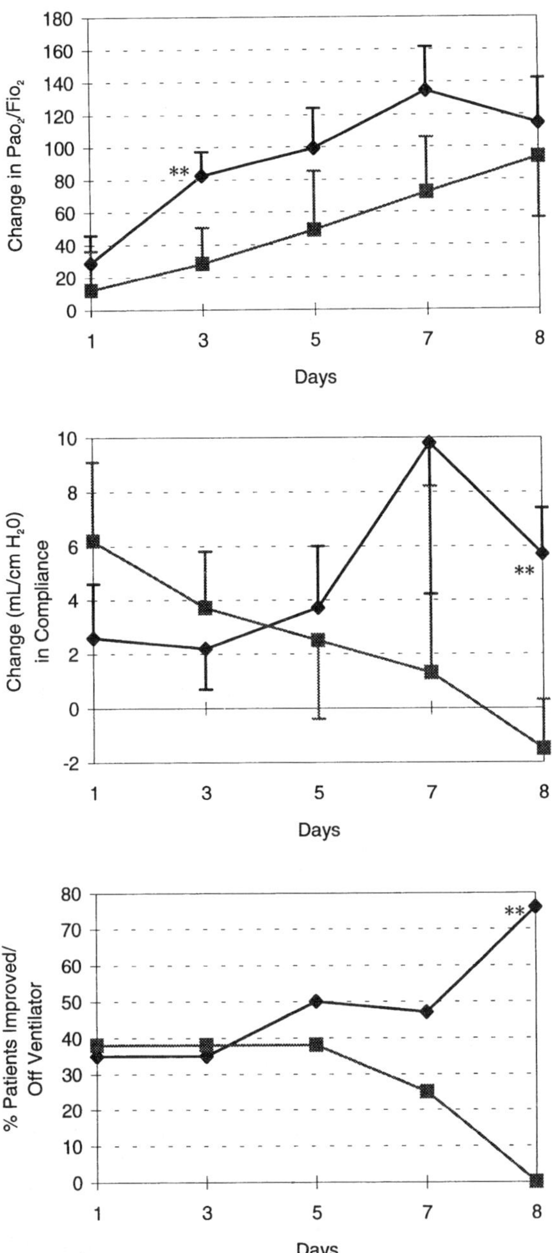

FIGURE 1.—Top, change from baseline in Pao_2/Fio_2 for the liposomal prostaglandin E_1 (TLC C-53) group (*diamonds*) and the placebo group (*squares*) (***P* =0.05). **Middle,** change from baseline in lung compliance for the TLC-53 group (*diamonds*) and the placebo group (*squares*) (***P* = 0.01). **Bottom,** percentage of patients with improvement in pulmonary status, defined by being off the ventilator or a 25% or more increase from baseline in lung compliance for the TLC-53 group (*diamonds*) and the placebo group (*squares*) (***P* = 0.001). Data are mean ± SD for baseline and mean ± SEM for changes. (Courtesy of Abraham E, Park YC, Covington P, et al: Liposomal prostaglandin E_1 in acute respiratory distress syndrome: A placebo-controlled, randomized, double-blind, multicenter clinical trial. *Crit Care Med* 24(1):10–15, 1996.)

to be more effective at decreasing neutrophil-mediated lung injury than is free PGE_1.

Although the benefit of liposomal PGE_1 on survival was not shown in this small study ($P = 0.23$), the overall mortality rate in the PGE_1 group was 6% vs. 25% in the control group, suggesting that survival might have been statistically improved if a larger patient group was studied. Thus, future trials are required to verify these preliminary beneficial results and to determine the potential role of this drug in the treatment of ARDS.

E.A. Deitch, M.D.

Administration of an Antibody to E-Selectin in Patients With Septic Shock

Friedman G, Jankowski S, Shahla M, et al (Erasme Univ, Brussels, Belgium; Free Univ of Brussels, Belgium; Cytel Corp, San Diego, Calif)

Crit Care Med 24:229–233, 1996 2–11

Background.—Measures to inhibit leukocyte adherence to the endothelium could be useful in the treatment of septic shock. Although animal studies of antibodies to the CD11b/CD18 glycoprotein complex showed some protective effects, these antibodies tended more to aggravate than reduce the septic response. Endothelial leukocyte adhesion molecule (E-selectin) is an inducible molecule that is expressed on the endothelial surface after induction by cytokines and bacterial toxins and binds leukocytes. Treatment with an anti–E-selectin antibody has the potential to preserve leukocytes' ability to phagocytize bacteria and bacterial products while preventing adherence of leukocytes to the endothelium. The safety and pharmacokinetics of a murine monoclonal antibody to E-selectin were studied in patients with septic shock.

Methods.—The open-label, phase II pilot study included 9 patients with newly developed septic shock who survived the first 24 hours. All received standard therapy for septic shock. In addition, they received an IV bolus of CY1787, a recently developed murine monoclonal antibody to E-selectin. The patients received 1 of 3 doses of CY1787: 0.1 mg/kg, 0.33 mg/kg, or 1.0 mg/kg.

Results.—The E-selectin antibody treatment was well tolerated. It was followed by resolution of the signs of shock in all patients and by complete reversal of organ failure in 8 of the 9. All 9 patients survived through 28 days of follow-up. The PaO_2/FIO_2 ratio increased from 146 ± 38 mm Hg to 205 ± 45 mm Hg within 2 hours after CY1787 administration, and to 250 ± 58 mm Hg within 12 hours (Fig 1). Patients receiving the highest dose of CY1787 were quicker to wean from catecholamine therapy and to progress to resolution of organ failure. Eight patients were found to have antimouse antibodies, which were usually transient.

Conclusions.—The anti-E-selectin antibody CY1787 appears to be a safe and promising new treatment for septic shock. The side effects of this treatment include the possibility of increased susceptibility to bacterial

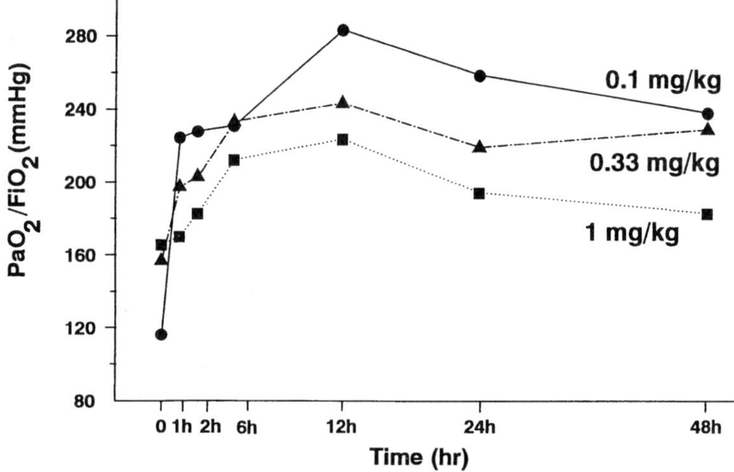

FIGURE 1.—Time course of the PaO_2/FIO_2 ratio in each dose group. *Dotted line* (*squares*), 1 mg/kg-dose; *dashed line* (*triangles*). 0.33 mg/kg-dose; *solid line* (*circles*), 0.1 mg/kg-dose. For the 9 patients, all values are $P < .05$ from baseline. (Courtesy of Friedman G, Jankowski S, Shahla M, et al: Administration of an antibody to E-selectin in patients with septic shock. *Crit Care Med* 24(2):229–233, 1996.)

infection. The resulting reduction in morbidity and mortality will have to be assessed in larger studies.

▶ The concept that neutrophil-mediated endothelial cell damage can lead to organ dysfunction and failure has led to a search for agents to limit neutrophil-endothelial cell interactions. The initial strategy was to test agents that decreased neutrophil attachment to endothelial cells by binding directly to the neutrophils. Although this approach was successful in reducing organ damage in multiple animal models, it had the untoward effect of impairing the animal's ability to control an infectious challenge. Consequently, attention has turned toward blocking receptors expressed on activated endothelial cells (such as E-selectin) that potentiate neutrophil adherence. The conceptual advantage of this strategy is that it does not impair neutrophil antibacterial function.

Although uncontrolled, this phase II clinical trial using a mouse monoclonal antibody against E-selectin appears quite promising, in so far as all 9 patients manifested a rapid improvement in pulmonary function, resolution of their shock state, and all survived. Hopefully, subsequent, well-controlled phase III studies will show equal effectiveness. Until then, stay tuned.

E.A. Deitch, M.D.

Assessment of the Safety and Efficacy of the Monoclonal Anti-Tumor Necrosis Factor Antibody-Fragment, MAK 195F, in Patients With Sepsis and Septic Shock: A Multicenter, Randomized, Placebo-Controlled, Dose-Ranging Study

Reinhart K, Wiegand-Löhnert C, Grimminger F, et al (Friedrich-Schiller-Univ, Jena, Germany; Steglitz Univ, Berlin; Univ of Gieβen, Germany; et al)
Crit Care Med 24:733–742, 1996 2–12

Background.—Sepsis and septic shock are still responsible for much morbidity and mortality among the critically ill. Evidence has accumulated linking the proinflammatory cytokines, such as tumor necrosis factor-α (TNF-α) and interleukin 6 (IL-6), to the pathogenesis of sepsis and septic shock. Administration of TNF can produce many of the adverse changes observed in sepsis and septic shock. Therefore MAK 195F, an Fab-fragment of a murine monoclonal antibody directed against human TNF, was developed as a treatment for sepsis and septic shock in critically ill patients. The safety and efficacy of MAK 195F were determined in a phase II trial of patients with severe sepsis.

Methods.—A prospective, randomized, open, placebo-controlled, dose-ranging clinical trial was conducted at 16 academic medical center ICUs in 6 European countries. The study group consisted of 122 patients with severe sepsis or septic shock who received standard supportive and antimicrobial therapy and were randomly assigned to receive 0.1, 0.3, or 1.0 mg/kg of MAK 195F or placebo. This treatment was administered in 9 doses at 8-hour intervals during a 3-day period.

Results.—There were no significant differences in mortality between the placebo group and any of the groups receiving MAK 195F. Retrospective stratification of patients by baseline serum IL-6 concentrations demonstrated that in patients with baseline IL-6 concentrations greater than 1,000 pg/mL, MAK 195F appeared to have a beneficial effect on mortality in a dose-dependent manner. An elevated level of circulating IL-6 was a prognostic mortality indicator in placebo group patients and in patients at the 2 lower dosages of MAK 195F, but not in the high-dose group. The levels of circulating IL-6 decreased within the first 24 hours in all treatment groups but not in the placebo group. In all treatment groups, MAK 195F was well tolerated by patients. Antimurine antibodies developed in 40% of all patients receiving MAK 195F.

Conclusion.—The murine monoclonal anti–TNF fragment, MAK 195F, was well tolerated but did not increase survival in a study population with severe sepsis or septic shock. When the data were retrospectively stratified by baseline IL-6 serum concentrations, patients with baseline serum IL-6 levels of greater than 1,000 pg/mL appeared to have reduced mortality when treated with MAK 195F. These results must be confirmed in a prospective clinical study involving patients with severe sepsis or septic shock and elevated levels of serum IL-6.

▶ Another failed clinical trial—or is it? While acknowledging that anti-TNF antibodies did not increase overall survival, a subgroup of patients—those with IL-6 levels of greater than 1,000 pg/mL—were identified in whom anti-TNF antibodies improved survival. To quote the famous philosopher Yogi Berra; "this is *déjà vu* all over again." Previous clinical trials with various immunomodulators have had similar results, that is, no improvement was observed between the experimental and control groups for the entire patient group. However, in the post hoc dredging of the data to find something positive to say, a subgroup was found in whom the therapy was effective. Armed with this encouraging information, further trials were instituted focusing on the retrospectively identified subgroup, only to fail. Will the effects of therapy in this subgroup of patients with high IL-6 levels identified in this study be any different? Perhaps.

As discussed in an editorial accompanying this article,[1] this may be because some patients dying of sepsis have impaired immune responses while others have overactive immune responses. Because the goal of anticytokine therapy is to help control an overexuberant immunoinflammatory response, only those patients whose immune response is overactive would be expected to benefit. In this light, are the authors correct? Did the subgroup of patients with an excessive IL-6 response do better because they were the subgroup with an excessive immunoinflammatory response and consequently the subgroup in which anticytokine therapy should work? Unfortunately, the answer to this critically important question must await better and more rapid techniques of identifying and separating patients with sepsis who have an excessive immunoinflammatory response from those who do not. I hope so because in the absence of this type of explanation for why immunomodulatory therapy has failed, we appear to have reached a dead end.

E.A. Deitch, M.D.

Reference

1. Dellinger RP: Post hoc analyses in sepsis trials: A formula for disappointment? *Crit Care Med* 24:727–729, 1996.

A Clinical Study on the Significance of Platelet-activating Factor in the Pathophysiology of Septic Disseminated Intravascular Coagulation in Surgery

Ono S, Mochizuki H, Tamakuma S (Natl Defense Med College, Saitama, Japan)

Am J Surg 171:409–415, 1996 2–13

Objective.—The differences between septic disseminated intravascular coagulation (septic DIC) in patients with surgical sepsis and disseminated intravascular coagulation (DIC) in patients with advanced cancer without infection were studied, focusing on the roles of endotoxin and platelet-activation factor.

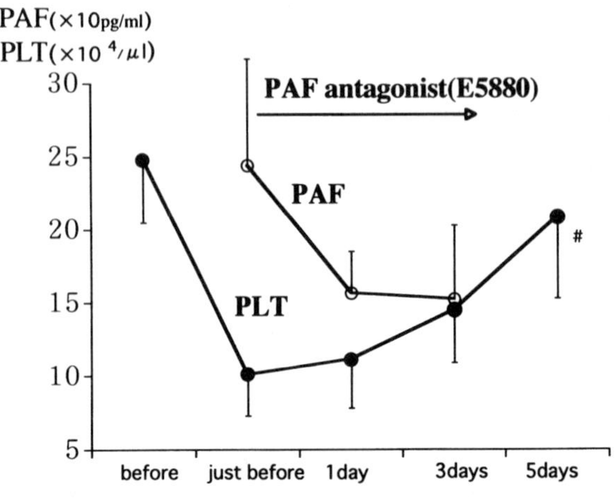

FIGURE 6.—Changes in platelet counts (*PLT*) and platelet-activating factor (*PAF*) blood concentrations in cases of disseminated intravascular coagulation at diagnosis, before PAF antagonist (E5880) administration (before), and 1, 3, and 5 days after administration of the antagonist. (Reprinted by permission of the publisher from Ono S, Mochizuki H, Tamakuma S: A clinical study on the significance of platelet-activating factor in the pathophysiology of septic disseminated intravascular coagulation in surgery. *AMERICAN JOURNAL OF SURGERY* 171:409–415, 1996, copyright 1996 by Excerpta Medica Inc.)

Methods.—Coagulation test values were measured in 36 patients with DIC. In 13 of these patients, platelet-activating factor and endotoxin concentrations were also measured. Platelet-activating factor antagonist was given IV to 7 patients with sepsis.

Results.—In patients with septic DIC, blood platelet-activating factor and endotoxin levels were higher than in non-septic patients with DIC. Furthermore, in patients with cancer and DIC, these levels were near normal. Only in patients with septic DIC was there a strong positive correlation between blood concentrations of platelet-activating factor and endotoxin. There also was a negative correlation between the concentration of platelet-activating factor and platelet counts in patients with sepsis. After platelet-activating factor antagonist was administered, platelet counts increased gradually (Fig 6).

Conclusions.—In patients with septic DIC, levels of platelet-activating factor are inversely correlated with platelet counts. Platelet-activating factor antagonist has inhibitory effects on characteristic changes of septic DIC. Because conventional treatment seems unable to control thrombocytopenia, platelet-activating factor antagonists may soon have a role in treating septic DIC.

▶ The potential roles of cytokines such as interleukin-1, interleukin-6, and tumor necrosis factor have received a lot of attention as key mediators in patients with sepsis. However, as immunotherapy directed against these agents has failed, other "suspects" have continued to emerge.

This article deals with such a suspect, platelet-activating factor. Platelet-activating factor's multiple pro-inflammatory properties plus its ability to promote platelet aggregation and clot formation in the microcirculation indicate that this cytokine is of potential importance in the development of organ failure. Consequently, this study was chosen because it provides direct evidence for elevated platelet-activating factor levels as a major cause of DIC in patients with sepsis, plus it documents the ability of a platelet-activating factor antagonist to improve coagulation function and increase circulating platelet levels. Because DIC is related more to platelet-activating factor than other cytokines studied, it is possible that failure of anticytokine clinical trials (e.g., anti–tumor necrosis factor, anti–interleukin-1, etc.) may be partly related to a failure of these agents to prevent thrombosis of the microcirculation and subsequent microvascular thrombosis-related organ injury. As the ability to measure platelet-activating factor levels increases (currently they are very difficult to measure), the role of this putative factor in the adverse effects of sepsis will be better clarified.

As an aside, I do not believe that monotherapy directed against platelet-activating factor, or any other pro-inflammatory agent, will be fully successful clinically. However, I do believe that ultimately a clinically beneficial "anti-mediator" cocktail containing agents effective against a number of mediators will emerge. Studies such as this one will help us determine what this cocktail should contain.

E.A. Deitch, M.D.

Antibodies Against CD14 Protect Primates From Endotoxin-induced Shock

Leturcq DJ, Moriarty AM, Talbott G, et al (RW Johnson Pharmaceutical Research Inst, San Diego, Calif; Harborview Med Ctr, Seattle; Univ of Washington, Seattle; et al)

J Clin Invest 98:1533–1538, 1996 2–14

Background.—Lipopolysaccharide (LPS), located in the outer membrane of gram-negative bacteria, is thought to be an important initiating factor in gram-negative septic shock syndrome. A complex with the LPS-binding protein is formed in plasma and engages a specific receptor, CD14, on the surface of myeloid cells, resulting in the production of potent proinflammatory cytokines. The importance of the CD14 pathway in vivo was tested in a primate model similar to human septic shock.

Methods and Results.—Cynomolgus monkeys were pretreated with 1 of 2 inhibitory anti-CD14 mAbs and challenged with IV endotoxin, 375 μg/kg/hr, for 8 hours. Anti-CD14 treatment successfully prevented profound hypotension, decreased plasma cytokine levels, and inhibited the lung epithelial permeability changes that occurred in monkeys given LPS and an isotype-matched control antibody.

Conclusions.—The importance of the CD14 pathway was demonstrated for the first time in this primate model. Inhibiting this pathway would be a novel therapeutic approach in the treatment of gram-negative septic shock syndrome.

▶ The mechanisms by which LPS (endotoxin) activates immune as well as nonimmune cell populations involves the binding of LPS plus a specific LPS-binding protein either directly to cells that express the CD14 receptor on their surface (immune cells), or to soluble CD14 in the cell populations that do not express membrane-bound CD14 (endothelial and epithelial cells). Thus, CD14, whether cell-bound or soluble, is a critical factor in LPS-induced cell activation and/or injury. For this reason, development of antibodies that neutralize CD14 might be effective in abrogating the adverse systemic consequences of LPS as well as of bacteria. On the basis of this well-done study of experimental endotoxic shock in primates, this may be the case.

Although this preclinical study is important and the results are encouraging, a word of caution is in order before one goes out and buys the stock of this company. The model used in this study (slow IV injection of LPS) does not fully mimic clinical infection, because in clinical infection, circulating LPS levels increase gradually over a longer period of time and the patients have sustained other insults. Although I am pessimistic, based on the failure of clinical trials testing other agents directed at blocking the inflammatory response, hope springs eternal. Perhaps this approach will work in patients. It certainly makes biological sense, because the interaction of LPS with CD14 is the most proximal step in LPS's cascade of effects on the host. Time will tell.

E.A. Deitch, M.D.

Effect of Human Hemoglobin on Systemic and Regional Hemodynamics in a Porcine Model of Endotoxemic Shock

Aranow JS, Wang H, Zhuang J, et al (Harvard Med School, Boston)

Crit Care Med 24:807–814, 1996 2–15

Introduction.—Evidence is growing to support the theory that arterial hypotension and decreased systemic vascular resistance in human sepsis are precipitated by increased production of nitric oxide. A nitric acid scavenging agent might minimize these deleterious effects. Hemoglobin is an effective hemoglobin scavenger. The effects of hemoglobin on systemic hypotension and organ perfusion were evaluated in a porcine model of normodynamic endotoxemic shock.

Methods.—Fourteen male Yorkshire pigs were randomly assigned to 1 or 2 groups. After anesthesia, the pigs underwent a tracheostomy and were mechanically ventilated with 100% oxygen. Continuous measurements were taken of pulmonary artery, aortic, and central venous pressures; mucosal blood flow; and mucosal pH. Several hemodynamic measures were recorded throughout the study. After baseline values were taken, endotoxemia was induced by infusion of *Escherichia coli* lipopolysaccaride from 0 to 90 minutes. Group 1 pigs were infused with cross-linked human hemoglobin (150 mg/kg), and group 2 control pigs received an infusion of dextran (150 mg/kg) starting at 30 minutes.

Results.—The mean arterial pressure decreased significantly in both groups after infusion of endotoxin. The baseline cardiac index was maintained in both groups. From 60 to 120 minutes, the mean arterial pressure was significantly higher in control animals, compared with test animals. There were no significant between-group differences in systemic vascular resistance index, renal blood flow, mesenteric blood flow, systemic oxygen delivery, or systemic oxygen extraction. The ileal blood flow was significantly lower in hemoglobin-treated vs. control animals. Endotoxin-induced arterial hypoxemia and pulmonary hypertension were significantly exacerbated in the hemoglobin-treated group, compared with the control group.

Conclusion.—A significant exacerbation of endotoxin-induced pulmonary hypertension and arterial hypoxemia was observed in hemoglobin-treated pigs, compared with control animals, even though it improved mean arterial pressure.

► As we search for new therapies to maintain blood pressure in patients who have septic shock, we must be careful not to judge a book by its cover. This appears to be the case with agents to scavenge (i.e., hemoglobin) nitric oxide as well as nitric oxide blockers. As shown in this experimental study, therapy with low-dose hemoglobin solutions, although effective at increasing the mean arterial blood pressure, impairs intestinal mucosal perfusion and significantly increases endotoxin-induced pulmonary hypertension and arterial hypoxemia. This is not good. Thus, the current study, as well as other recent studies, clearly supports the concept that nitric oxide has beneficial effects in septic or endotoxic shock and highlights the potential clinical downside of nitric oxide elimination in hypotensive septic patients, even though the blood pressure may be improved.

E.A. Deitch, M.D.

Effects of Nonanticoagulant Heparin on Cardiovascular and Hepatocellular Function After Hemorrhagic Shock

Wang P, Ba ZF, Reich SS, et al (Michigan State Univ, East Lansing; Glycomed, Alameda, Calif)

Am J Physiol 270:H1294–H1302, 1996 2–16

Background.—Animal studies have demonstrated that heparin treatment has beneficial effects on cell and organ function after hemorrhage, sepsis, and ischemia-reperfusion. Unfortunately, heparin's anticoagulant properties would interfere with any potential clinical applications. Whether a novel nonanticoagulant heparin, GM1892, would have beneficial effects on cell and organ function in a rat model of hemorrhage, sepsis, and ischemia-reperfusion was determined.

Methods.—Male Sprague-Dawley rats underwent laparotomy to induce trauma. Hemorrhage was then induced, and the rats were bled to and maintained at an average arterial pressure of 40 mm Hg until 40% of the maximal bleedout volume was returned as Ringer lactate (RL) solution. These rats were resuscitated with RL at 3 times the lost volume over a 45-minute period, then infused with a double volume of RL plus 7 mg/kg of GM1892 or saline over a 1-hour period. At 2 and 4 hours after resuscitation, cardiac output, hepatocellular function, and microvascular blood flow were monitored.

Results.—Cardiac output, hepatocellular function, and microvascular blood flow in the liver, spleen, and small intestine significantly declined in these rats after hemorrhage and resuscitation. In those rats who were treated with GM1892, these parameters were restored. Mucosal ulceration, sloughing, congestion, and hemorrhage were detected 4 hours after resuscitation in the liver, kidney, and small intestine of saline-treated animals, but these changes were significantly less noticeable in GM1892-treated animals. Treatment with GM1892 also normalized plasma prostaglandin E_2 levels, which were elevated in the saline-treated rats. Of 16 rats that also underwent cecal excision to induce sepsis, 83% died. Of 16 rats who were treated with GM1892 after cecal excision, only 44% died.

Conclusion.—Administration of the nonanticoagulant heparin, GM1892, in a rat model of trauma-hemorrhage and resuscitation resulted in significantly improved hepatocellular function, cardiac output, and microvascular blood flow and decreased morphologic abnormalities in various organ systems. Mortality from sepsis was also reduced. Therefore GM1892 may be a useful adjunctive treatment in the management of trauma and hemorrhagic shock.

▶ During the last several years, heparin and heparin-like compounds have been found to possess a remarkable number of beneficial properties. The administration of heparin improves cellular and organ function in hemorrhage, sepsis, and ischemia-reperfusion models. This protective effect seems to be related in part to heparin's ability to prevent endothelial cell dysfunction, and furthermore this beneficial effect of heparin appears to be independent of its anticoagulant effect.

This study provides further data in support of the beneficial effects of nonanticoagulant heparin-type molecules in clinically relevant models of hemorrhagic shock and infection. As surprising as it may seem, heparin-like molecules may soon become part of the therapeutic regimen of high-risk trauma and ICU patients because of their organ-protective effects.

E.A. Deitch, M.D.

A Genomic Polymorphism Within the Tumor Necrosis Factor Locus Influences Plasma Tumor Necrosis Factor-α Concentrations and Outcome of Patients With Severe Sepsis

Stüber F, Petersen M, Bokelmann F, et al (Christian-Albrechts-Univ Kiel, Germany; Univ Hosp, Essen, Germany)

Crit Care Med 24:381–384, 1996 2–17

Purpose.—Previous studies have suggested that the circulating concentration of tumor necrosis factor α (TNF-α) is correlated with outcome in patients with sepsis, mortality being higher in patients with higher TNF-α concentrations. A biallelic *Nco* I restriction fragment length polymorphism in the first intron of TNF-β has been described in patients with autoimmune diseases, and TNF-α secretion may be increased in subjects who are homozygous for the TNFB2 allele. The genotype distribution and allele frequency of the *Nco* I polymorphism was assessed in patients with severe sepsis.

Methods.—The prospective study included 40 consecutive patients with severe sepsis in a postoperative ICU. Polymerase chain reaction was used to amplify a 782 bp fragment of genomic DNA that included the polymorphic site of the restriction enzyme *Nco* I within the TNF locus. Then, *Nco* I digestion of the amplified product and agarose gel electrophoresis were performed to determine each patient's genotype, as defined by the alleles TNFB1 and TNFB2. The information on genotype was evaluated in terms of the survival rate, occurrence of multiple organ dysfunction, and plasma TNF-α concentration.

Results.—Sixty-six percent of patients had the TNFB2 allele and 34% had the TNFB1 allele. Forty-eight percent of patients were TNFB1/TNFB2 heterozygotes, 42% were TNFB2 homozygotes, and 10% were TNFB1 homozygotes. The allelic and genotypic findings were comparable in the patients with sepsis and in a group of normal subjects. Eighty-three percent of the patients had multiple organ failure and 58% died. The TNFB2 allele was significantly more frequent in the patients who died ($P < .005$), and

TABLE 3.—Survival of Patients with Severe Sepsis Related to Tumor Necrosis Genotypes

Genotype	Survivors	Non-survivors
Homozygous TNFB2/TNFB2	2	15
Heterozygous TNFB1/TNFB2	12	7
Homozygous TNFB1/TNFB1	3	1

Note: Patients homozygous for the allele tumor necrosis factor (TNF)B2 showed a significantly reduced survival rate compared with heterozygous patients ($P = .0022$; Fisher's Exact test, two-sided).

(Courtesy of Stüber F, Petersen M, Bokelmann F, et al: A genomic polymorphism within the tumor necrosis factor locus influences plasma tumor necrosis factor-α concentrations and outcome of patients with severe sepsis. *Crit Care Med* 24(3):381–384, 1996.)

mortality was significantly higher in TNFB2 homozygotes than in TNFB1/TNFB2 heterozygotes (Table 3). Circulating TNF-α concentrations and Multiple Organ Failure scores were higher in TNFB2 homozygotes than in TNFB1/TNFB2 heterozygotes.

Conclusions.—Patients with the biallelic *Nco* I polymorphism in the TNF locus appear to have an elevated TNF-α response and a high risk of poor outcome in sepsis. Information on the TNF-β *Nco* I polymorphism could be useful in selected patients with sepsis for intensive monitoring or prophylactic treatment, or in studying the effectiveness of anti-TNF treatment strategies.

▶ Molecular genetics to the rescue. Technology aside, the take-home message from this study is that individuals with a genetic predisposition for high TNF production appear to be at increased risk for having organ dysfunction develop and dying during episodes of severe sepsis.

In my opinion, this simple but elegant genetic study will be the first of many such studies that will help unravel the clinical paradox of why some patients live and others die after seemingly similar insults. I also believe these future studies will document that certain individuals have a genetic predisposition to having organ dysfunction develop during periods of severe stress, just as certain individuals have a genetic predisposition to cancer. Remember, it's all in the genes.

E.A. Deitch, M.D.

Effect of Heat Shock and Endotoxin Stress on Enterocyte Viability Apoptosis and Function Varies Based on Whether the Cells Are Exposed to Heat Shock or Endotoxin First

Xu D-Z, Lu Q, Swank GM, et al (Univ of Medicine and Dentistry of New Jersey, Newark)

Arch Surg 131:1222–1228, 1996 2–18

Background.—Stress-gene responses such as heat shock (HS) and acute phase responses protect cells after exposure to stress. These 2 responses cannot occur at the same time. In endothelial cells, the sequence of stress-gene expression appears to be critical in determining whether cells are protected or injured. Whether the sequence of stress-gene expression affects cellular protection or injury in epithelial cells also was investigated.

Methods.—Rat epithelial cell-6 (IEC-6) cells were exposed either to 25 μg/mL lipopolysaccharide (LPS) for 18 hours, to HS for 90 minutes, to LPS followed by HS, or to HS followed by LPS. After exposure, the cells were assessed for viability, apoptosis, and bacterial translocation (BT).

Findings.—Rat IEC-6 cells exposed to LPS followed by HS had an 83% viability, significantly lower than that of the other groups. These cells also had a higher percentage of apoptotic cells. Three hours after *Escherichia coli* challenge, the LPS-exposed IEC-6 cell monolayers had significantly increased BT compared to control monolayers. By contrast, the cell monolayers exposed to HS followed by LPS had reduced BT. Cells exposed to LPS followed by HS had the highest magnitude of BT.

Conclusions.—Preinduction of HS response can decrease LPS-induced cell injury. By contrast, induction of HS response after LPS challenge may result in reduced enterocyte viability, increased apoptosis, and cellular dysfunction as manifested by BT.

▶ That it is all in the genes has been suspected for a long time. Likewise, it is well accepted that various insults, stimuli, or stresses modulate cell function. However, it has only recently been recognized that whether a particular cellular signal, stimulus, or insult will ultimately protect or injure the cell depends not only on the various stimuli but also on the sequence in which they occur. That the sequence in which the insults occur may be as (and in some cases more) important as the insults themselves is the basic message of this paper. This concept is supported by the authors' experimental observation that a specific cellular response (in these experiments the HS response) can either protect the cell or kill it, depending on what other signals the cell has received.

Although the clinical correlates of these experiments remain to be established, the potential clinical relevance behind this work is that certain insults or stresses experienced by high-risk patients can predispose them to cell death, organ dysfunction, or even multiple-organ failure syndrome when they occur at a time when the cells are "vulnerable." However, the same insults or stresses may have minimal adverse effects or even protective effects depending on what other signals the cells have recently or previously received. Thus, in my opinion, the concept of "tolerizing" or modulating cells so that they become more resistant to the adverse effects of subsequent stressors or clinical insults will be a potential clinical strategy of the future.

E.A. Deitch, M.D.

The Logistic Organ Dysfunction System: A New Way to Assess Organ Dysfunction in the Intensive Care Unit

Le Gall J-R, for the ICU Scoring Group (Hôpital Saint Louis, Paris; Univ of Massachusetts, Amherst; Hôpital Calmette, Lille, France; et al)

JAMA 276:802–810, 1996 2–19

Introduction.—Numerous systems have been developed to assess organ dysfunction. An objectively derived organ dysfunction system was created by using a large database of ICU patients and multiple logistic regression. The system was designed to use sophisticated statistical methods but be simple to apply clinically.

Methods.—Data were obtained on 14,745 ICU patients who had participated in the European/North American Study of Severity Systems. The development sample was 80% of the patient data, and the validation sample was 20% of the patient data. Variables to define organ dysfunction were extracted with regard to 6 organ systems: neurologic, cardiovascular, renal, pulmonary, hematologic, and hepatic. Cut points were first identified to define severity ranges for each variable by using the LOWESS smoothing function with locally weighted least squares. The variables were then analyzed simultaneously in a multiple logistic regression model to determine the relative weight of each level of the variables, which was multiplied by a factor of 10 to determine the points for each severity level. The performance of the final model was evaluated with goodness-of-fit tests and receiver operating characteristic (ROC) curves.

Results.—The logistic organ dysfunction (LOD) system had a score range of 1–22 points. Impairment of the neurologic, cardiovascular, and renal systems was associated with the worst clinical outcomes. Therefore, each of these organ systems received a maximum of up to 5 points for the most severe level of dysfunction, whereas the pulmonary and hematologic systems received a maximum of 3 points and the hepatic system received a maximum of 1 point. Goodness of fit and area under the ROC curve were excellent in both the developmental and validation samples, with the LOD score strongly predicting the probability of hospital mortality.

Conclusions.—The LOD system is an accurate tool for assessment of the severity of organ dysfunction in ICU patients. It considers both the degree of severity within an organ system and the relative severity between organ systems.

▶ This is a very important study because the lack of an accurate organ dysfunction tool in the ICU has potentially limited the accuracy of clinical sepsis trials. Without an accurate scoring system it becomes difficult to fully control for the magnitude of organ dysfunction and the prognosis of patients randomized into the clinical arms of the trial. For this reason, a number of authors have attempted to develop clinical accurate organ dysfunction scales for use in the ICU. Most of these scoring systems are somewhat accurate, but they all have certain weaknesses, the most important being their relative weakness in predicting outcome in individual patients and in certain patient populations.

The logistic organ dysfunction system proposed in this study appears to be an improvement over these previous studies. One reason is that not all the organs are treated equally. That is, the authors have found that dysfunction of certain organ systems (i.e., CNS, cardiovascular, and renal) is a more important predictor of outcome than others (i.e., liver). Second, the variables used are easily obtained and the system is easy to use. Hopefully, the early optimistic findings with this system will be borne out in future studies. Because of the potential utility and importance of this study, I recommend that all clinicians who care for patients in the ICU read this study and try it on their ICU patients. I know I will.

E.A. Deitch, M.D.

Resource Consumption and the Extent of Futile Care Among Patients in a Pediatric Intensive Care Unit Setting

Sachdeva RC, Jefferson LS, Coss-Bu J, et al (Baylor College of Medicine, Houston)

J Pediatr 128:742–747, 1996 2–20

Introduction.—The relationship between medical futility and resource consumption has been explored in ICU populations. Findings are controversial, particularly for pediatric populations. It is not known whether the extent of futile care differs with ICUs or whether pediatric intensivists fail to recognize the extent of futile care delivered in pediatric ICUs (PICUs). The extent of resource consumption and futile care was evaluated prospectively in 353 PICU admissions followed for 1,334 patient-days.

Methods.—Three broad operational definitions were created to determine the maximum extent of resource consumption related to medical futility. The first definition, imminent demise futility, applied to patients with a very high risk of death during current hospitalization. The Pediatric Risk of Mortality Score, which is an objective and validated measure of severity of illness, was used. The second definition, lethal condition futility, applied to patients with diagnoses considered to be incompatible with long-term survival. The third definition, quantitative futility, applied to patients with a high degree of morbidity that could result in poor quality of life. The number of patient days in the PICU and the Therapeutic Intervention System were used to determine resource consumption.

Results.—Thirty-six of the 1,334 patient-days (2.7%) met at least 1 definition of futility. Twenty-three patients (6.5%) had at least 1 day that met at least 1 definition of medical futility. Eighteen of 353 children (5.1%) died in the PICU. Of those who died, 11 met at least 1 definition of medical futility. All remaining children who met at least 1 definition of medical futility for at least 1 day were transferred to a step-down or pediatric unit. Eight of 18 patients who met at least 1 definition of medical futility, but were considered "full code," died. A comparison of medical futile and nonfutile patient-days indicated that there was no significant between-group difference in high resource consumption.

Conclusion.—Few PICU patient-days were associated with futile care, and futile care was not a source of considerable resource consumption, compared with nonfutile care. Clinical decision-making in the PICU should not be directed at reducing resource consumption in patients who meet criteria for medical futility. This approach will not achieve cost savings.

► Emphasis on cost containment and limited ICU bed availability has forced many physicians and hospital administrators to focus on futile care in the ICU, as well as on the use of ICU resources in general. This article is valuable because it dispels the myth (at least in this 1 hospital) that futile care is rampant in the ICU. Although this is a study from a pediatric ICU, similar results were reported recently from an adult medical ICU.[1]

The only way to know what the incidence of "futile" care is in your ICU, however, is to collect the data. To assess this issue meaningfully, one needs to have some acceptable definitions of what constitutes futile care. This article was therefore chosen because the definitions used in this study, plus information from some of the references cited, can be used to establish such a yardstick for those inclined to test their own environment.

E.A. Deitch, M.D.

Reference

1. Halevy A, Neal RC, Brody BA: Low frequency of futility in an adult ICU setting. *Arch Intern Med* 156:100–104, 1996.

3 Burns

Introduction

As we move into the 21st century and articles such as the cloning of a sheep from an adult cell make the headlines of the lay press, it becomes ever more apparent that the era of molecular medicine is upon us. In fact, as illustrated by several of this year's selection of burn articles, studies of molecular mechanisms are providing insights into the effects of thermal injury on the immune and metabolic responses. One particularly intriguing observation is the potential role that burn-induced programmed cell death of immune cells such as lymphocytes plays in the development of an immunocompromised state. The recent recognition that all types of cells can be induced to commit suicide (a process termed *apoptosis,* or programmed cell death) by environmental signals is a major conceptual breakthrough that helps explain a number of previously paradoxical observations. Based on the rapidly growing information on this subject, it appears that stress-induced apoptosis may be a key factor in organ as well as immune failure. Likewise, basic studies of the immune system continue to provide clues on how to improve immune function, such as by the use of certain cytokines like interleukin-12 to specifically bolster host antibacterial defenses after a thermal injury.

Further encouraging experimental information published this year indicates that resuscitation fluids containing antioxidants such as deferoxamine or large doses of vitamin C can ameliorate the systemic and pulmonary consequences of smoke inhalation injury, and complement studies have implicated oxidant production in the pathogenesis of smoke-induced pulmonary injury. Because smoke-induced pulmonary injury is a major factor in mortality after thermal injury, these basic studies have great potential clinical significance. In fact, as reflected in an article investigating the pathogenesis of burn anemia, peroxidation of red blood cells may explain why red blood cell survival is shortened and burn patients become anemic.

Several clinical articles were chosen because of their direct relevance to patient care. One of these articles documented that burn patients do better in a warm environment and that by keeping the ambient temperature hotter than normal (32°C to 35°C), the patient's metabolic response can be reduced by 40% to 50%. Since it can be difficult to meet the nutritional needs of hypermetabolic burn patients, knowing that it is possible to blunt the hypermetabolic response by controlling the room (ambient) temperature assumes significant clinical importance. Although there is some hesitancy in aggressively grafting second-degree facial burns, information indicating that early skin grafting improves the cosmetic response of facial burns continues to emerge. Because of the increased pressure to limit hospital admissions and perform as much outpatient surgery as possible, an interesting article illustrating the technique of using an Unna's boot dressing to facilitate safe outpatient skin grafting of burned hands was chosen. Finally, an article selected highlights the frequently unrecognized but real and persistent cognitive and psychological consequences of electrical injuries.

Edwin A. Deitch, M.D.

Immune Deficiency Following Thermal Trauma Is Associated With Apoptotic Cell Death

Teodorczyk-Injeyan JA, Cembrzynska-Nowak M, Lalani S, et al (Univ of Toronto; Wellesley Hosp, Toronto; Toronto Hosp)
J Clin Immunol 15:318–328, 1995 3–1

Objective.—Recent studies suggest that activation-induced cell death (AICD)—which is morphologically the same as the programmed cell death (PCD) or apoptosis observed during normal development—may govern T cell ontogeny and the results of mature T lymphocyte activation. In patients with burns, specific immune deficiency can occur in the absence of systemic activation of the lymphoid compartment. The possibility that AICD causes immune deficiency and T-cell activation after thermal injury was investigated.

Methods.—The study included 14 patients with extensive burns involving 35% to 90% of total body surface area and inducing immunosuppression. Peripheral blood mononuclear cell (PBMC) cultures were used to assess the relationship between the cellular immune response and cell death. The study included monitoring of the patients' in vivo and in vitro immune parameters, assessment of DNA fragmentation, and in situ identification of apoptotic cell death.

Findings.—As cellular immunity declined, so did cell viability, as demonstrated by propidium iodide staining and dye reduction assays. Apoptotic cell death was demonstrated in culture by the finding of DNA fragmentation after stimulation with the mitogenic lectin phytohemagglutinin (PHA). Apoptosis was demonstrated even in nonstimulated patient cells by the presence of oligonucleosomal bands on agarose gel electrophoresis. Both stimulated and nonstimulated DNA fragmentation were significantly decreased by the addition of exogenous interleukin-2 or phorbol ester (Fig 2). A TdT-based labeling technique showed DNA strand breaks in freshly isolated PBMCs from the patients, demonstrating that up to 60% of circulating lymphocytes were undergoing apoptosis on the periphery.

Conclusions.—Apoptotic cell death is demonstrated in T cells isolated directly from the peripheral blood of burn patients, as well as in in

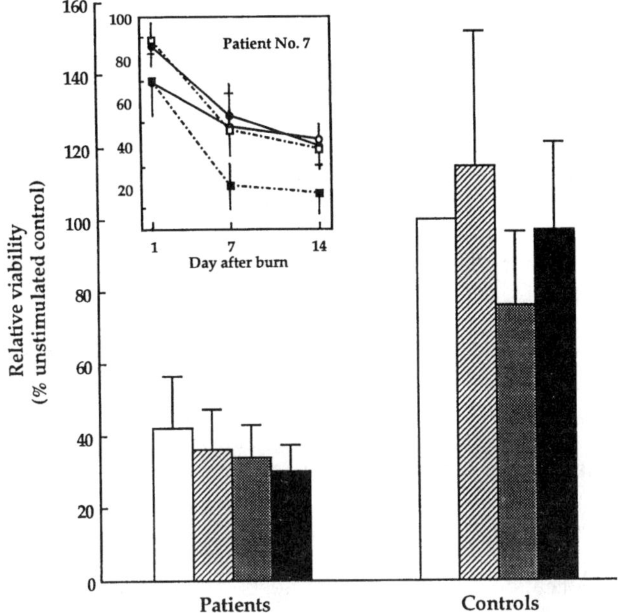

FIGURE 2.—Cell viability in peripheral blood mononuclear cell cultures from 11 patients studied between 1 and 4 weeks after the burn. Cell viability was determined by the dye reduction assay in unstimulated (*open bar*) and phytohemag-glutinin (PHA) (*hatched bar*), PHA and interleukin (IL2) (*dotted bar*), or IL2 only (*solid bar*)-stimulated cultures and is expressed as the percentage of unstimulated control preparations. After activation, a significant ($P < 0.01$–0.05) decrease in cell viability was observed in patient cultures. The inset depicts a gradual decline in cell viability in unstimulated (*open circle*) and PHA (*solid square*)-, PHA and IL2 (*open square*), or IL2 (*solid circle*)-activated cultures from a nonsurviving patient (65% total body surface area) studied for 2 weeks after the burn. (Courtesy of Teodorczyk-Injeyan JA, Cembrzynska-Nowak M, Lalani S, et al: Immune deficiency following thermal trauma is associated with apoptotic cell death. *J Clin Immunol* 15:318–328, 1995.)

vitro-activated T cells. The results suggest that apoptosis, or AICD, may play a key role in inducing or regulating the immune deficiency that occurs after thermal injury. Studies of the mechanisms by which T cell activation in patients with major burns results in apoptosis may lead to new treatment approaches for immune manipulation in burn-induced and other clinical types of specific immune deficiency.

► One never stops being amazed by the inherent elegance of the ways the body has developed to regulate and control its responses to injury and stress. This article correlating postburn T cell immune deficiency with activation-induced apoptotic cell death appears to be such an example of cell regulation. Because of the high incidence of infection-related death, investigators have studied multiple components of the immune system in patients with significant burn injuries for more than 2 decades. These studies have clearly documented that burn patients are immunocompromised; however, the mechanisms underlying this immunocompromised state have remained elusive. This is especially true as far as the pathogenesis of impaired T cell (cellular) immunity is concerned. Thus, the importance of this study is that the authors have found an association between postburn impaired cellular immunity and an increased rate of spontaneous (apoptotic) T cell death. The term apoptosis has been used to describe the process of non-necrotic cell death.

The increasing recognition of the importance of programmed apoptotic cell death in regulating normal tissue development and preventing uncontrolled cellular proliferation has profound biological and clinical implications for injured or stressed patients as illustrated in this paper. Basically, the authors found that the T cells from their patients expressed increased levels of T cell activation markers, yet their immune responses were depressed. In an attempt to explain the paradox of peripheral activation of the lymphoid system and concomitant immunosuppression, they tested the concept that these activated cells were primed for an apoptotic cell death. Based on their results that these T cells were undergoing apoptosis, they concluded that environmentally induced apoptotic cell death is directly involved in the pathogenesis of postburn immunosuppression, and that apoptotic cell death may be 1 mechanism that the body uses to protect itself from an exaggerated T cell immune response.

The take-home message is that cell death by apoptosis is a fundamental process of the normal host, and induction of the apoptotic state may have profound implications in the pathogenesis of immune dysfunction after trauma.

E.A. Deitch, M.D.

Regulation of the Acute Phase Response Genes Alpha$_1$-acid Glycoprotein and Alpha$_1$-antitrypsin Correlates With Sensitivity to Thermal Injury

Gilpin DA, Hsieh C-C, Kuninger DT, et al (Univ of Texas, Galveston)

Surgery 119:664–673, 1996 3–2

Background.—Acute phase reactants carry out protective functions in a systemic response to stress. The plasma concentrations of α_1-acid glycoprotein, α_1-antitrypsin, albumin, and other acute phase reactants change significantly in response to traumatic stimuli. Differences in recovery in rat strains may be associated with their response to stress, as measured by the acute phase response. Whether there is an association between severity of thermal injury and intensity of the acute phase response of positively and negatively regulated acute phase reactant genes in 3 rat strains with varying ability to survive thermal injury was determined.

Methods.—Anesthetized male Buffalo, Sprague-Dawley, and Fischer 344 rats, aged 12–16 weeks, received a 40% total body surface area third-degree scald burn. At 0, 2, 6, 12, 24, and 48 hours after injury, RNA was isolated from liver tissue. Northern blot hybridization with ^{32}P-labeled rat α_1-glycoprotein, rat albumin, and mouse α_1-antitrypsin complementary DNAs was performed. Densitometric analyses were used to measure α_1-glycoprotein, α_1-antitrypsin, and albumin messenger RNAs.

Results.—A positive and negative acute phase response was seen in all 3 rat strains. There were significant differences, however, in the degree and kinetics of these responses among the 3 strains. A more intense positive acute phase response and possible delayed recovery were noted in rats that were more sensitive to thermal injury. There was a correlation between the acute phase response and the ability to survive severe thermal injury.

Conclusions.—All 3 strains of rats exhibited a positive and negative acute phase response, but there were significant differences in the degree and kinetics of the response. This finding indicates that rat strains that are more sensitive to thermal injury have a more intense positive response and a possible delayed response recovery. A more intense and extended acute phase response is associated with sensitivity to severe thermal injury. The protective effect of the acute phase response may result from a rapid appearance and rapid removal.

▶ It's in the genes. That is the basic conclusion of this study, which investigated whether a correlation exists between burn mortality and magnitude of the acute phase response in 3 different strains of rats. For example, the mortality rate of the Buffalo rats was 0%, and they had the least sustained acute phase response; the Sprague-Dawley rats had a 38% mortality rate and the most sustained acute phase response. These results therefore support the concept that heritable genetic factors are an important determinant of whether an animal, or a patient, will survive a serious injury.

E.A. Deitch, M.D.

Injury Induces Rapid Changes in Hepatocyte Nuclear Factor-1:DNA Binding

Burke PA, Luo M, Zhu J, et al (Harvard Med School, Boston)

Surgery 120:374–381, 1996 3–3

Background.—Although transcriptional regulation in the liver is known to be involved in the acute-phase response to injury, little is known about the molecular basis of these transcriptional changes. Many acute-phase genes show binding of the liver-specific transcription factor hepatocyte nuclear factor (HNF)-1 in their 5' upstream region. Changes in HNF-1 binding could play a role in transcriptional regulation of these genes after injury. A mouse model of burn injury was used to determine the effects of injury on HNF-1 binding activity in vivo.

Methods.—A true or sham burn injury was produced in anesthetized mice. After fluid resuscitation, the mice were killed, and liver nuclear extracts were obtained. Electrophoretic mobility shift analysis was performed in the liver extract to determine HNF-1 binding activity, affinity, and off rate.

Results.—Compared to extracts from uninjured animals, the extracts from burned mice showed a 28% decrease in HNF-1 binding activity 1.5 hours after injury. Binding remained depressed after 3 hours. The HNF-

1:DNA dissociation constant at 1.5 hours was 0.60 nmol in the uninjured mice vs. 11.8 nmol in the injured mice. Part of this difference was related to an increased off rate for the HNF-1:DNA complex.

Conclusions.—Burn injury reduces the affinity of HNF-1 for DNA, resulting in significantly decreased HNF-1 binding activity. This could provide the mechanism regulating transcription of acute-phase genes in vivo. The molecular mechanism of the reduced affinity of HNF-1 for DNA is unknown. Further study of transcriptional regulation after injury will help in understanding the molecular basis controlling the response to injury, with possible therapeutic applications.

▶ This article was chosen because it provides important insight into a fundamental physiologic response observed after thermal and mechanical injury and during sepsis; that is, after injury and during periods of significant stress, the classes of proteins produced by the liver change profoundly. Specifically, the production of transport proteins, such as albumin decreases, whereas the production of acute phase proteins increases. How this reprioritization of protein synthesis is regulated by the liver has largely remained a mystery. Thus, this molecular-based study suggesting that the decrease in albumin synthesis is attributable to a decrease in affinity of the transcription factor HNF-1 for DNA is important. Although the direct clinical ramification of this observation remains to be determined, it is very likely that the next generation of therapeutic options will result from the knowledge gained through studies such as this. For this reason, it will be important for clinicians to be aware of the progress being made in unraveling the mechanisms underlying the patient's basic response to injury.

E.A. Deitch, M.D.

Interleukin-12 Treatment Restores Normal Resistance to Bacterial Challenge After Burn Injury

O'Suilleabhain C, O'Sullivan ST, Kelly JL, et al (Harvard Med School, Boston)
Surgery 120:290–296, 1996 3–4

Introduction.—Serious injuries are associated with abnormalities of adaptive immunity, including failure of T lymphocytes to proliferate and produce interleukin-2. This growth factor cytokine, like interferon-γ, is produced by T-helper-1 cells. Studies in burned mice have shown that interleukin-12 (IL-12) treatment improves survival after a septic challenge. The efficacy and mechanism of action of IL-12 treatment in this animal model was studied further.

Methods.—Experiments were done in adult male A/J mice that underwent a 25% full-thickness scald injury or sham burn. On the third day thereafter, the animals received 5 daily injections of IL-12, interferon-γ (IFN-γ) or saline solution. In addition, some received anti-IFN-γ monoclonal antibody. Cecal ligation and puncture (CLP) was done as a septic challenge after 10 days in some animals. Others were killed at day 10 and

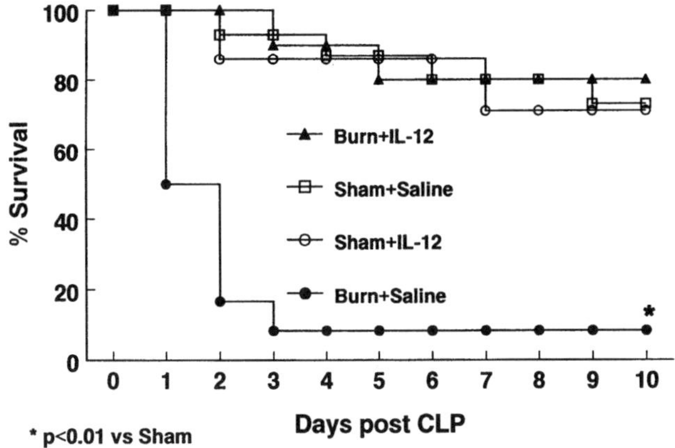

FIGURE 4.—It is apparent that a 25-ng dose of interleukin-12 (*IL-12*) administered to the sham burn group did not affect mortality from cecal ligation and puncture (*CLP*). This dose of IL-12 improved the survival of the burn group to that of the sham burn group. (Courtesy of O'Sulleabhain C, O'Sullivan ST, Kelly JL, et al: Interleukin-12 treatment restores normal resistance to bacterial challenge after burn injury. *Surgery* 120:290–296, 1996.)

studied for cytokine production and messenger RNA expression in CD4-enriched splenocytes stimulated with anti-CD3 antibody or concanavalin A.

Results.—Five days of IL-12 treatment, 25 ng/day, resulted in better survival after CLP in the burn group than in the sham burn control group. Interleukin-12 treatment was less effective when anti-IFN-γ antibody, 500 µg, was given the day before. Survival was somewhat improved by treatment with IFN-γ, 7,000 U. In the sham burn control group, survival was unaffected by IL-12 treatment (Fig 4). The animals sacrificed at the time of CLP showed a marked decreased CD4+ lymphocyte IL-4 production and some increase in IFN-γ production and messenger RNA expression. Interleukin-2 was unaffected, however.

Conclusions.—Treatment with IL-12 improves survival in mice who are subjected to burn injury and septic challenge. This treatment, started shortly after injury, can restore normal resistance to infection at a time when the animal is most susceptible to sepsis. The mechanism of action of IL-12 treatment seems to involve IFN-γ at least in part, but treatment with IFN-γ is less effective.

▶ It was pointed out about 20 years ago that thymus-derived lymphocytes or T cells could be divided into helper T cells, or Th, and suppressor T cells. However, it has only recently been appreciated that not all Th cells are similar. Instead, there appear to be 2 classes of Th cells; Th1 cells are involved in cell-mediated immunity and Th2 cells are involved in humoral or antibody-mediated immunity. As progress in understanding how these 2 classes of Th cells interact during periods of injury or infection has occurred, several important observations have come to light. One such observation is that after burn injury, there is a shift toward the production of cytokines characteristic of Th2 cells, such as interleukin-4 and interleukin-10, at a time when cytokines, such as interleukin-2 or IFN-γ, that are produced by Th1 cells are reduced. On the basis of this observation, the authors in this current study tested the hypothesis that restoration of Th1 cell activity would protect burned animals from an infectious challenge. To increase Th1 cells, they administered IL-12, because this cytokine preferentially increases the production of Th1 cells. Their prediction that increasing Th1 cells would improve survival was verified.

The importance of this study is severalfold. First, it indicates that loss of Th1 cells is important in the increased susceptibility of burned animals to an infectious challenge. Second, the authors documented that Th1 cell activity can be pharmacologically improved. Last, these studies provide further insight into the mechanisms by which the immune system regulates itself after injury. In this case, increased activation of Th2 cells results in the production of cytokines, which decreases Th1 cell activity.

E.A. Deitch, M.D.

Fluid Resuscitation With Deferoxamine Hetastarch Complex Attenuates the Lung and Systemic Response to Smoke Inhalation

Demling R, LaLonde C, Ikegami K (Harvard Med School, Boston)

Surgery 119:340–348, 1996 3–5

Background.—Smoke inhalation is the major cause of death in fires. Respiratory failure is the major cause of morbidity and mortality in burn patients with smoke inhalation who have been resuscitated. The mechanisms of early smoke-induced lung injury and of the early systemic response to smoke inhalation are not completely understood. Evidence indicates that there is increased oxygen free radical activity in lungs exposed to smoke. In addition, large amounts of oxygen radicals are present in common materials in household fires. The role of oxidants in lung injury and systemic hemodynamic changes from smoke inhalation has not been fully defined. The effect of a deferoxamine-hetastarch complex infusion on lung injury and systemic abnormalities resulting from exposure to smoke was investigated.

Methods.—Under anesthesia, 28 adult sheep were given a controlled smoke exposure that produced a peak level of carboxyhemoglobin of 40% to 45%. Eight sheep were resuscitated with lactated Ringer's solution; 7 were resuscitated with 10% deferoxamine-hetastarch solution, 8 mL/kg plus 1 mL/kg/hr; and 5 were resuscitated with a 10% hetastarch solution alone. Responses of the study sheep and 8 control sheep were recorded for 24 hours.

Results.—A shunt fraction of more than 25% and a reduction of 50% in compliance, severe airway inflammation, mucosal slough, atelectasis, and alveolar edema were seen in animals given smoke alone and smoke with hetastarch. There were more lipid peroxides in airway fluid, measured as malondialdehyde. Oxygen consumption increased by 100% early after smoke injury, the net 24-hour positive fluid balance was 3 L, and there was a significant increase in liver lipid peroxidation. Animals given deferoxamine had a significantly diminished lung response and moderate airway damage, lung dysfunction, and minimal systemic changes (including a net positive fluid balance of approximately 1 L), and no liver lipid peroxidation.

Conclusions.—When the iron chelator deferoxamine was administered after smoke inhalation in these animals, there was significantly less injury to the airway from smoke inhalation, as well as significantly less systemic oxygen consumption, fewer fluid requirements, and less systemic oxidant activity measured as liver lipid peroxidation. The release of free iron and the hydroxyl radical production that results are major factors in the etiology of lung injury from smoke inhalation.

► Studies aimed at ameliorating the pulmonary and systemic hemodynamic consequences of smoke inhalation injury are very important, because respiratory failure and pneumonia are the most common causes of death in burn patients who sustain an inhalation injury. Thus, this study, which documents that deferoxamine complexed to hetastarch decreased both the magnitude of the pulmonary injury and the systemic consequences of a severe smoke inhalation injury, was included in this year's edition. Of major potential clinical importance was the fact that deferoxamine was administered after the smoke insult, which suggests that this potential therapy is clinically feasible. The reason deferoxamine worked appeared to be related to its ability to limit production of oxidants. This antioxidant property is important, because smoke contains oxidants and because smoke-induced pulmonary injury or inflammation results in the generation of additional oxidants.

E.A. Deitch, M.D.

Early Effects of Smoke Inhalation on Alveolar Macrophage Functions

Bidani A, Wang CZ, Heming TA (Univ of Texas, Galveston; Shriners Burns Inst, Galveston, Tex)

Burns 22:101–106, 1996 3–6

Introduction.—Efficient functioning of alveolar macrophages (AMs) is crucial in controlling respiratory tract infections, yet AMs can potentially exacerbate the inflammatory response to lung injury by their release of cytotoxic agents that can directly damage lung tissues, as well as chemotactic agents that attract and activate neutrophils, thus leading to bystander cell injury and the production of inflammatory mediators. The responses of AMs to smoke inhalation injury induced by cotton smoke were observed in adult male New Zealand White rabbits.

Methods.—Fourteen rabbits were anesthetized and intubated and then insufflated with cotton smoke. The rabbits underwent 5 cycles of O_2 for 1 minute, followed by smoke insufflation for 1 minute. They were then ventilated with O_2 for 10 minutes, followed by room air for 50 minutes.

Thirteen control animals were insufflated with room air instead of smoke. After the animals were killed, BAL fluid was collected and AMs were analyzed.

Results.—There was a significant 11-fold increase in arterial blood levels of carboxyhemoglobin and a significant decrease in PaO_2 in test animals, compared with controls. At 60 minutes after exposure, smoke-exposed, but not control, animals were found to have tracheobronchial foamy fluid and exudate in the upper airways. The viability of BAL fluid cells recovered within 70 minutes of start of injury was not affected. The absolute number of AMs recovered in each animal was approximately threefold in smoke vs. control animals. The AM morphology was changed by smoke exposure. Compared with cells from controls, scanning electron micrographs showed apparent denudation of plasmalemmal pseudopods in macrophages from test animals. The AM adherence to plastic was approximately 30% less, and Fc receptor–mediated phagocytosis was suppressed by approximately 40% in test animals, compared with controls. Basal superoxide was increased by approximately 60% and basal TNF-α was decreased by approximately 50% in smoke-exposed animals, compared with controls. The cells in smoke-exposed animals had a greater (but not significant) TNF-α release to stimulation with LPS, compared with control cells. The LPS-stimulated TNF-α releases from both smoke-exposed and control AMs were suppressed by phosphodiesterase inhibitors pentoxifylline and theophylline. They were significantly enhanced by the lipoxygenase inhibitor MK886.

Conclusion.—The early responses of AMs to smoke inhalation lung injury are in keeping with activation of superoxide production and the priming of AM for TNF-α release. Findings suggest a functional down-regulation of phagocytosis. Patients who have smoke inhalation lung injury may benefit from early intervention targeted at regulating AM responses, particularly upregulating phagocytosis while preventing hyper-reactivity of oxidant to cytokine release.

▶ This study on AMs adds further evidence to the concept that smoke directly induces an oxidant response within the lung. The findings are consistent with those of Demling et al. (Abstract 3–5), which document that limiting production of oxidants protects against smoke-induced pulmonary injury. In addition, because 1 function of AMs is to ingest bacteria, the observation that phagocytosis is impaired after smoke exposure provides 1 more reason why patients exposed to smoke have such a high incidence of pneumonia. Thus, this experimental study provides potentially important insights into the mechanisms by which smoke leads to pulmonary injury and predisposes to pneumonia.

E.A. Deitch, M.D.

Effects of Early and Delayed Wound Excision on Pulmonary Leukosequestration and Neutrophil Respiratory Burst Activity in Burned Mice
Rennekampff OH, Hansbrough JF, Tenenhaus M, et al (Univ of California, San Diego)
Surgery 118:884–892, 1995 3–7

Introduction.—Many burn patients die of pulmonary failure and pneumonia. The pulmonary complications of burns often take the form of acute respiratory distress syndrome, which has been linked to neutrophil accumulation in the lungs, followed by local release of toxic mediators. Previous studies have suggested that neutrophils may be primed or activated by features in the local environment of the burn wound. The effects of immediate vs. delayed burn wound excision and closure on neutrophil activation and leukosequestration in lung, gut, and liver were studied in mice.

Methods.—In the experimental model, mice were subjected to a 32% total body surface area burn. The burn wound was excised and closed with allograft skin either immediately or 48 hours after the injury. A colorimetric assay was used to measure tissue myeloperoxidase (MPO) as a marker of neutrophil accumulation in tissues. Flow cytometry was performed to measure intracellular H_2O_2 content as an indicator of polymorphonuclear lymphocyte (PMN) respiratory activity.

Results.—Lung tissue showed increased MPO content in the first 8 to 24 hours after burn injury, although liver and gut tissue did not. Animals

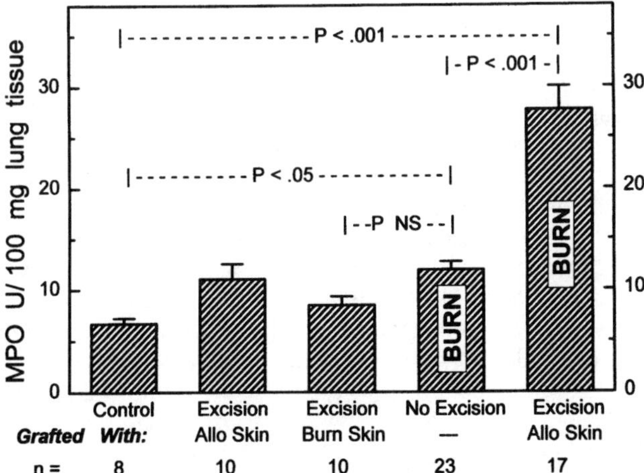

FIGURE 5.—Myeloperoxidase (MPO) levels in lung tissue after immediate postburn excision of burn wound and closure with allograft skin. Control animals included unburned animals that underwent excision of an equivalent-sized (32% total body surface area) piece of dorsal full-thickness skin, followed by closure with allograft skin (**column 2**). The MPO levels were determined 8 hours after burn or excision in all groups. The number of mice in each group is shown in bottom line. *Abbreviation: NS*, not significant. (Courtesy of Rennekampff OH, Hansbrough JF, Tenenhaus M, et al: Effects of early and delayed wound excision on pulmonary leukosequestration and neutrophil respiratory burst activity in burned mice. *Surgery* 118:884–892, 1995.)

undergoing immediate excision of their burn wounds had the greatest levels of MPO in lung tissue ($P < 0.001$). There was no difference in lung MPO levels between unburned animals undergoing skin excision and grafting with unburned vs. burned skin. Delayed burn excision was associated with a moderate increase in lung MPO levels ($P < 0.005$), but not as high as in mice undergoing immediate excision (Fig 5). Influx of PMNs into lung tissue was demonstrated by histologic examination. The mice showed increased PMN H_2O_2 production after burn injury, with an additional increase in the animals undergoing immediate excision.

Conclusions.—Immediate excision of burn wounds is associated with a higher level of pulmonary leukosequestration than the burn itself. Intracellular H_2O_2 content is increased as well. If pulmonary leukosequestration is a contributing factor to lung injury after burns, this may lessen the benefits of very early burn wound excision.

► Most burn surgeons who practice early burn wound excision perform the first operation between 3 and 5 days postburn in patients with moderate or large burns, although earlier excision may be performed in patients with smaller burns (i.e., burns less than 10% to 15% of the body surface area). However, there is an increasing trend toward immediate burn wound excision in patients with larger burns, in whom the burn wound is excised and grafted as soon as possible and, in some cases, even on the day of injury.

The results of this experimental study documenting that burn wound excision performed immediately postburn, or even at 48 hours postburn, is associated with increased sequestration of neutrophils in the lung and increased neutrophil activation is disconcerting. That is, these results indicate that burn surgery performed during the early postburn shock period appears to further activate neutrophils and could therefore result in potentiation of neutrophil-mediated lung injury. Thus, the take-home warning of this controlled study is that very early burn wound excision may have potential adverse consequences for the patient, especially for those with smoke inhalation injuries or preexistent lung disease. These results remind me of recent clinical studies documenting the adverse clinical effects (i.e., increased pulmonary dysfunction) of immediate postinjury fracture fixation in multitrauma patients with chest injuries. Whether immediate burn surgery will potentiate pulmonary dysfunction in certain groups of burn patients as immediate fracture fixation has in trauma patients with chest injuries is not known. However, this experimental study does raise this concern.

E.A. Deitch, M.D.

Reduced Erythrocyte Deformability Related to Activated Lipid Peroxidation During the Early Postburn Period

Bekyarova G, Yankova T, Kozarev I, et al (Varna and Regional Hosp of Silstra, Bulgaria)

Burns 22:291–294, 1996 3–8

Objective.—Burn injury is followed by microcirculatory disturbances and progressive hypoxia, which are linked to morphological alterations in red blood cells and activation of lipid peroxidation. Erythrocyte survival is reduced in patients with burns, and this change is related to high plasma lipid peroxide levels, low glutathione peroxidase activity, and reduced vitamin E content. The role of lipid peroxidation in reduced red blood cell deformability after burns was assessed in rats.

Methods.—Full-thickness burns were produced over 15% to 20% of total body surface area in male Wistar rats. The link between erythrocyte deformability and membrane oxidation during the first 3 days after the injury was studied, including the effects of α-tocopherol (α-T) as a membrane antioxidant.

Results.—The erythrocyte concentration of malonyldialdehyde (MDA) and the level of thiobarbituric acid reactive product in blood were significantly reduced after the burn (Fig 1). Red blood cell superoxide dismutase activity was greatly reduced, and glucose-6-phosphate dehydrogenase was increased. In the 3 days postinjury, erythrocyte deformability was significantly reduced and was negatively correlated with the amount of MDA

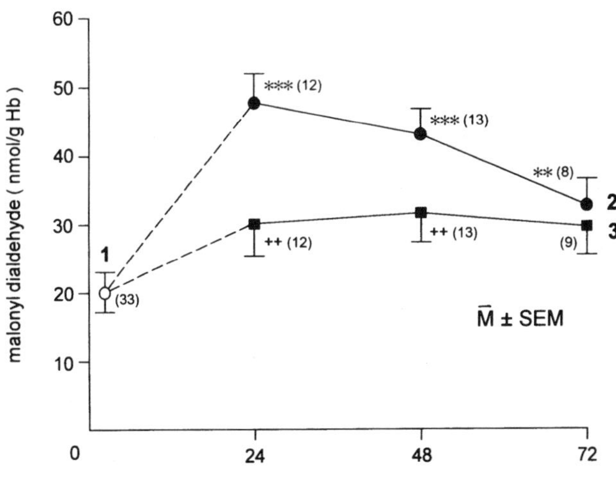

FIGURE 1.—Changes of the content of erythrocyte malonyldialdehyde during the early stage after thermal injury: *1*, controls; *2*, burned untreated; *3*, burned treated with α-tocopherol; ***P2-I < 0.001; **P2-I < 0.01; ++P3-2 < 0.01. (Reprinted from *Burns*, vol 22, Bekyarova G, Yankova T, Kozarev I, et al, Reduced erythrocyte deformability related to activated lipid peroxidation during the early postburn period, pp 291–294, copyright 1996, with permission from Elsevier Science Ltd, The Boulevard, Langford Lane, Kidlington OX5 1GB, UK.)

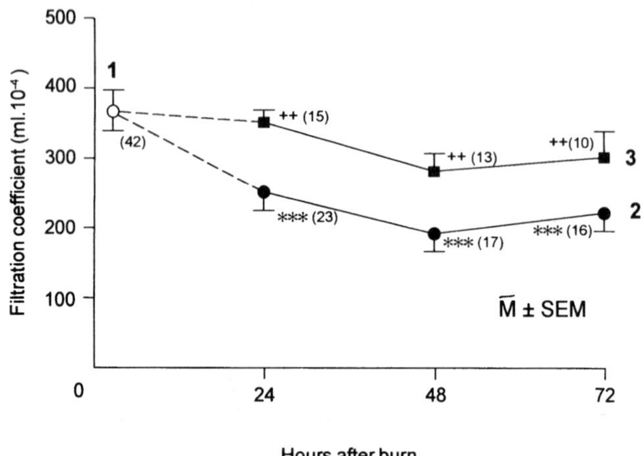

FIGURE 5.—Changes of the filtration coefficient during the early stage after thermal injury: *1*, controls; *2*, burned untreated; *3*, burned treated with α-tocopherol; ***P2-1 < 0.001; ++P3-2 < 0.001. (Reprinted from *Burns*, vol 22, Bekyarova G, Yankova T, Kozarev I, et al, Reduced erythrocyte deformability related to activated lipid peroxidation during the early postburn period, pp 291–294, copyright 1996, with permission from Elsevier Science Ltd, The Boulevard, Langford Lane, Kidlington OX5 1GB, UK.)

accumulated. The filtration coefficient also was reduced after burn injury (Fig 5). Treatment with α-T significantly reduced the MDA accumulation and reduction of superoxide dismutase activity in erythrocytes. This treatment also prevented the postinjury decrease in erythrocyte deformability.

Conclusions.—The decreased erythrocyte deformability observed after burns may involve activation of the peroxidative process. The resulting abnormalities could play a role in the microcirculatory complications that occur after thermal injury. It may be possible to reverse the changes in red blood cell deformability using antioxidant-T treatment.

► It is well known that patients become severely anemic after major thermal injuries and that this anemia is associated with a shortened red blood cell survival time. The question of why red blood cell survival is decreased after burn injury has intrigued physicians caring for patients with burns for years. The importance of this study is that it suggests that the decrease in red blood cell survival time is because these cells become oxidized and, once oxidized, they are less deformable and thus more easily destroyed. For conceptual simplicity, an analogy can be drawn between sickle cells (although the mechanism is different) and red blood cells after thermal injury in that in both instances the cells have become more rigid and therefore less deformable.

Whether the use of agents that decrease red blood cell oxidation and thus prevent the loss of deformability will be effective in reducing the magnitude of burn-induced anemia in patients, in a manner similar to that shown in this animal study, must await clinical trials. It is hoped that this study and other published studies documenting that red blood cell oxidation may be an important factor in the pathogenesis of burn-related anemia will provide the impetus for clinical trials testing this concept.

E.A. Deitch, M.D.

Effect of Ambient Temperature on Metabolic Rate After Thermal Injury

Kelemen JJ III, Cioffi WG Jr, Mason AD Jr, et al (Brooke Army Med Ctr, Fort Sam Houston, Tex; Brown Univ, Providence, RI; US Army Inst, Fort Sam Houston, Tex)

Ann Surg 223:406–412, 1996 3–9

Introduction.—It has been well established that a hypermetabolic response occurs after burn injuries, with the degree of the response proportional to the burn size. One recent study however, reported a decrease in the degree of hypermetabolic response to burn injury. The effects of ambient temperature and the degree of burns on metabolic rate were evaluated.

Methods.—Fifty-two patients who had burns that involved 20% to 97% (mean, 44%) of total body surface area were included. A control group of 8 volunteers was also included. All patients were placed in a metabolic chamber, with the ambient temperature adjusted from 22°C, to 28°C, 32°C, and 35°C. Indirect calorimetry was used to measure the resting energy expenditure (REE). An index of metabolic rate was then calculated from the REE and the estimated basal metabolic rate (BMR).

Results.—The metabolic response (as calculated by REE/BMR) of the control group did not change significantly as the ambient temperature was

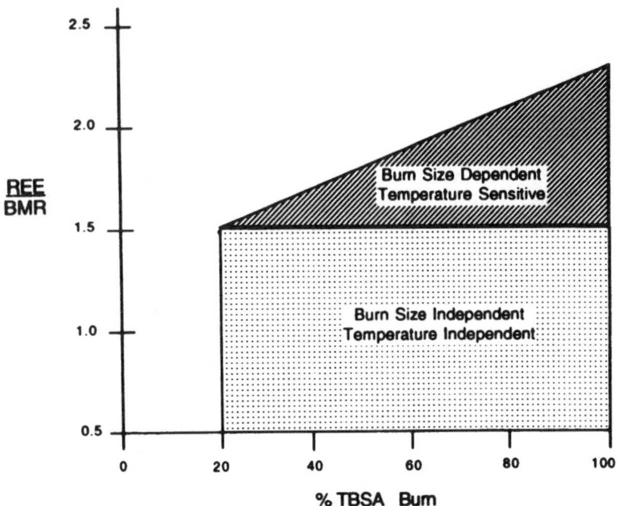

FIGURE 4.—Variation in metabolic rate at room temperature (22°C). (Courtesy of Kelemen JJ III, Cioffi WG Jr, Mason AD Jr, et al: Effect of ambient temperature on metabolic rate after thermal injury. *Ann Surg* 223:406–412, 1996.)

increased. In patients, burn size and ambient temperature were significant determinants of metabolic rate, as calculated by stepwise multivariate regression analysis. Fifty-five percent of the observed variation in metabolic rate was accounted for by these 2 factors. At 32°C and 35°C, the metabolic rate was independent of burn size; at these temperatures, the REE increased by 1.5 times the BMR. In addition to a metabolic response to thermal injury, which is maximal at burns of 20% of total body surface area, a temperature sensitive component that increases as the area of burn increases was suggested (Fig 4).

Conclusion.—At temperatures of 32°C and 35°C, the metabolic rate was independent of the burn size. At lower temperatures (22°C and 28°C), however, the increase in metabolic rate was proportional to the burn size.

▶ This article shows that burn patients like it hot and that by keeping the ambient environment hotter than normal (32–35°C), the patient's metabolic response can be reduced by 40% to 50%. Because burn-induced hypermetabolism leads to a severe catabolic response with muscle wasting, anything that can be done to blunt this hypermetabolic response is good. The reason that burn patients have an increased metabolic response to temperatures that do not cause hypermetabolism in normal volunteers is that a thermal injury disrupts the ability of the skin to control surface temperature by vasoregulatory mechanisms. Not surprisingly, as shown in this study, at temperatures lower than 32°C, the patients experience increased heat loss through the burn wound. What was surprising, and bears emphasis, was that patients with burns as small as 20% of their body surface area also did better metabolically at higher ambient temperatures. Thus, when treating burn patients, remember that even though they have been burned, they like it hot.

E.A. Deitch, M.D.

Progressive Burn Injury Documented With Vimentin Immunostaining

Nanney LB, Wenczak BA, Lynch JB (Vanderbilt School of Medicine, Nashville, Tenn)

J Burn Care Rehabil 17:191–198, 1996 3–10

Introduction.—Determination of burn depth has typically necessitated a 3–4 day waiting period. Earlier diagnosis of burn depth could help focus appropriate treatment in the initial stages of injury and possibly improve patient survival. Indocyanine green fluorescence and laser Doppler flow have been tested as methods for rapid diagnosis of burn depth but are not widely used in clinical practice. Immunohistochemical staining techniques were evaluated for their ability to stain eschar from viable skin differentially and thus assess burn depth objectively in patients who had burn injuries. Partial-thickness burns were analyzed in a porcine model to test the hypothesis that burn injury continues to progress beyond the first 24 hours after burn injury.

Methods.—Forty-three male and 16 female patients, aged 2–73 years, were included. The total body surface area burns ranged from 1% to 76%. Tissue specimens were harvested by serial punch biopsy or excisional tissues on postburn days 1–5 from various body locations. Thirty-two partial-thickness burns were created with the use of a metal template in 4 anesthetized domestic pigs. Burns were examined postburn days 1–4. Human and porcine specimens underwent immunohistochemical staining with the use of vimentin.

Results.—Precise demarcation between burn eschar and viable underlying dermis was observed days 1–5 after burn injury in the patients. The dermal cell populations showed positive immunoreactivity distinct from the overlying nonstained eschar as early as the first day after burn trauma. The ubiquitous distribution of the vimentin 58-kd molecule in mesenchymal cells throughout the dermis made it a useful tool, even in small 3-mm punch biopsy specimens. Regardless of age, sex, and initial burn depth, a progressive pattern of increase in depth of the burn injury was observed during postburn days 2–5 in sequential immunostained biopsy specimens obtained from the patients. The magnitude of wound change varied individually, but all human wounds continued to deepen beyond the first 24 hours after injury. Significant progression in wound depth beyond the first 24 hours after injury was also observed in the porcine model.

Conclusion.—Partial-thickness wounds in human beings and pigs continued to demarcate for several days after burn injury. Findings indicate that vimentin immunomarking is a reliable method for assessing burn depth. This relatively inexpensive technique can be considered an adjunct tool for quantitative determination of burn depth in both clinical and research settings.

▶ The 2 goals of this study were to develop a rapid and simple diagnostic procedure to indicate the depth of a burn in the acute postburn period and to determine whether a burn gets deeper in the first few days after injury. Based on the results presented in this study, it appears that the authors met both goals. Thus, the importance of this article is twofold. First, the authors have documented that burn depth in patients does progress during the first 5 postburn days. Second, they developed a potential clinical test to determine burn depth. If the accuracy of this test holds up with further study, it may provide useful clinical information in the patient who has a burn of indeterminate depth in whom there is a question about whether early excision and grafting should be performed. Let's hope that future clinical studies will validate the accuracy of this histologic test.

E.A. Deitch, M.D.

Assessment of Cosmetic and Functional Results of Conservative Versus Surgical Management of Facial Burns

Fraulin FOG, Illmayer SJ, Tredget EE (Univ of Alberta, Edmonton)
J Burn Care Rehabil 17:19–29, 1996 3–11

Background.—Deep, full- and partial-thickness burns of the face have traditionally been managed conservatively—the wounds are simply allowed to heal during a prolonged period. However, this approach can be associated with severe hypertrophic scarring, which limits the functional and cosmetic results. The results of tangential excision and thick split-thickness grafting (STSG) in patients with deep facial burns were assessed.

Methods.—The study included 40 patients treated for facial burns during a 2-year period. There were 28 adults and 12 children, with a mean follow-up of 18 months. The patients were divided into 4 groups, according to the depth and management of their burns. Group A included 13 patients whose burns healed without surgery in less than 21 days, whereas group B consisted of 11 patients whose burns healed without surgery after 21 days. The 6 patients in group C underwent early debridement and thick STSG within 18 days after the burn, whereas the 10 patients in group D had debridement and thick STSG delayed for more than 18 days. A modified scar assessment scale of 0 to 16 was used to evaluate the facial cosmetic results. Functional problems were assessed by physical examination.

Results.—The cosmetic results were significantly better ($P < 0.01$ on analysis of variance) for patients in group A than for those in the other 3 groups, in whom healing took longer than 21 days. The results were also significantly better in the 2 surgically treated groups than in the patients whose burns took longer than 21 days to heal without surgery ($P < 0.05$). The functional results were similar for patients in groups B, C, and D.

Conclusions.—Surgical management gives better results than conservative management for some patients with facial burns. If the burn is deep and takes a long time to heal spontaneously, the cosmetic results appear to be better with tangential wound excision and resurfacing with thick STSG. The surgical approach does not increase the incidence of functional problems.

▶ The message here is simple. Skin grafting is esthetically and functionally superior to spontaneous healing of deep second-degree burns of the face. Thus, patients whose facial burns are not likely to have healed by 21 days postburn should be operated on as soon as clinically feasible. Unfortunately, although the data are clear and the message is simple, some physicians have been hesitant to recommend early excision and grafting of deep facial burns. Hopefully, as more information documenting the advantages of early skin grafting for facial burns is published, this hesitancy will disappear.

E.A. Deitch, M.D.

Unna's Boot Dressings Facilitate Outpatient Skin Grafting of Hands
Sanford S, Gore D (Med College of Virginia, Richmond)
J Burn Care Rehabil 17:323–326, 1996 3–12

Introduction.—Burns to the hands may be especially difficult to treat and may have significant adverse cosmetic and functional effects. Functional loss from burn injuries may be minimized with rapid wound coverage and early mobilization. In addition, early debridement and skin grafting can speed healing of deep second- and third-degree burns. The use of Unna's boot dressings and splints on upper extremity skin grafts, along with calcium alginate dressings on donor sites, was evaluated in an outpatient setting.

Methods.—Twelve patients, who had a total of 16 hand burns, were included. Eleven patients had burns on the dorsal (10 patients) or dorsolateral (1 patient) aspect of the hand; 1 patient had an isolated palmar burn. Surgery was performed a mean 8 days after burn injury (range 1–26 days). After grafting, antibiotic-impregnated gauze was placed over the grafts. The grafted hands were then wrapped with an Unna's boot paste bandage and an elastic bandage applied over the Unna's boot. A splint was then applied over the bandaged hand (Fig 1). Calcium alginate dressings and ABD pads were applied to the donor sites. Patients were discharged with instructions on postoperative care 4–6 hours after surgery. They returned on postoperative days 2 and 5 for observation, dressing care, and splint removal. Later follow-up was done to assess range of motion, skin condition, and healing.

Results.—Grafts were successful in more than 95% of patients. No infectious complications occurred, and the donor site healed as expected. Only 2 patients had impaired range of motion 2 weeks after surgery. One patient had a previous similar injury, which also required an intensive program to regain normal range of motion. A web-space release was eventually required in the remaining patient.

Conclusion.—The combination of Unna's boot dressings and splints following skin grafting, along with calcium alginate dressings on donor sites, was successful in the outpatient treatment of hand burns. These findings suggest that surgical debridement and skin grafting of a more extensive nature may be successful on an outpatient basis.

▶ Same-day burn surgery. Not only is it possible, it works for both the patient and the physician. In this context, the current article illustrates how to use an Unna's boot dressing in same-day surgery for hand burns. Not only do I fully concur with this approach, but I have been practicing it for years and can say that most patients are grateful not to have to spend days in the hospital.

E.A. Deitch, M.D.

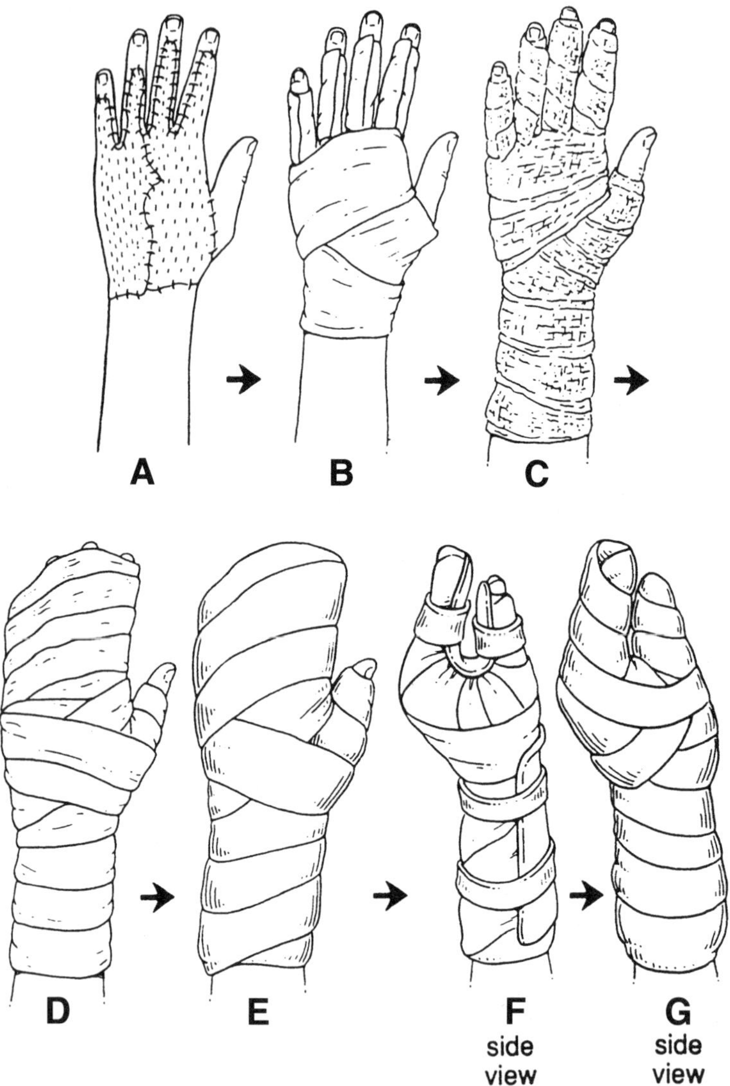

FIGURE 1.—Layers of postoperative dressings after skin grafting. **A,** grafted hand; **B,** bacitracin-impregnated fine-mesh gauze; **C,** Kling wrap; **D,** Unna's boot dressing; **E,** Ace wrap; **F,** splint; **G,** Ace wrap. (Courtesy of Sanford S, Gore D: Unna's boot dressings facilitate outpatient skin grafting of hands. *J Burn Care Rehabil* 17:323–326, 1996.)

Neurologic and Neurobehavioral Effects of Electric and Lightning Injuries

Janus TJ, Barrash J (Univ of Iowa, Iowa City)
J Burn Care Rehabil 17:409–415, 1996 3–13

Background.—Little is known about the neurologic and neuropsychological effects of electric and lightning injuries. One experience was reviewed to determine the presence of acute neurologic dysfunction and cognitive and affective problems in patients sustaining such injuries.

Methods and Findings.—The medical records of 41 patients with injuries from lightning or high-voltage electricity seen at 1 center between 1987 and 1993 were reviewed. Fourteen of these patients were referred for neurologic assessment. Twelve had been injured by high-voltage electricity, and 2 by lightning. Cardiac arrest had occurred after injury in 8 patients. In 10, neurologic problems were noted at the initial assessment. Neuroimaging findings were normal in 8 patients. Four of 6 undergoing electroencephalography had abnormal results. Of the 13 undergoing neuropsychological assessment, 92% had cognitive dysfunction, including impairments in memory, attention, and affective disturbances such as anxiety, depression, irritability, and poor frustration tolerance. Five of 12 patients had multiple episodes of physically aggressive outbursts not present before the injury. Patients with and without cardiac arrest did not differ in neurologic psychological test results.

Conclusions.—These data indicate that a coherent syndrome of cognitive, affective, and behavioral disturbances may be associated with electric and lightning injuries. Patients sustaining such injuries need to be followed up carefully in the long term with neurologic and neuropsychological assessments.

▶ Although a select group of patients is reported in this study, it does highlight the important but insufficiently recognized fact that neurologic and psychological consequences can occur after an electric injury. Essentially all clinicians treating patients who have sustained high-voltage electric injuries notice that a significant number of these patients have difficulty returning to work and/or reintegrating themselves into society. Recognition that persistent psychosocial difficulties, such as depression, increased irritability, aggressive behavior, and memory loss, can occur after an electric injury is critical, because early recognition of the potential emotional and cognitive sequelae of electric injury is the first step in treatment.

E.A. Deitch, M.D.

4 Trauma

Introduction

This year's trauma selections begin with a hot topic in the lay press—air bags: good or bad? As more attention is focused by the lay press on anecdotal stories of injuries caused by air bag deployment, the need for good data evaluating the potential benefits of air bags vs. seat belts has become even more important. The first article in this section contains this critical information and clearly documents the benefits of air bags in reducing both the severity of injury and the cost of trauma care. In fact, air bags were found to be superior to seat belts in preventing injuries in that unrestrained patients (no seat belts) who had air bags had a lower incidence and magnitude of injury than did seat belt–restrained patients whose cars did not have air bags. Speaking of news, as described in the next article, there is a trauma list serve on the Internet that one can join (http://www.trauma.lsumc.edu) called Trauma NET. This forum provides an opportunity for information exchange on all aspects of burn and trauma care.

Quality assessment programs and cost issues continue to occupy the attention of both trauma surgeons, hospitals, and the federal government. One such important quality issue is addressed in the article on delayed diagnoses in trauma patients, and a second study documented that resident-level, cost-directed educational programs can significantly reduce charges (average of $818/day) in a trauma ICU without affecting the quality of patient care. Similarly, it is becoming increasingly clear that percutaneous dilational tracheostomy is both a safe and cost-effective alternative to the performance of a traditional tracheostomy in the operating room.

Studies stressing the accuracy and clinical value of emergency room US in the diagnosis of abdominal and thoracic trauma continue to appear. Consequently, an article documenting how surgeons can learn focused US was included in this year's selection. Other areas of interest that continue to receive attention include criteria for the safe nonoperative management of blunt splenic injury in adults (not safe in patients over 55 years of age), new ventilatory strategies to decrease days on the ventilator and improve the success of weaning, and further information that the early use of specialized enteral diets reduces morbidity and costs in trauma patients. Further work on the deleterious systemic effects of increased intra-abdominal pressure (IAP) related to visceral edema or a tightly closed abdomen continues to appear. In fact, in my opinion, the recent recognition of abdominal compartment syndrome secondary to increased IAP has been one of the important observations made over the last few years.

A spectrum of articles dealing with clinically relevant or biologically important topics in trauma care were also chosen. These include the diagnosis and treatment of blunt carotid artery injuries, the ability of the addition of antibiotics to the peritoneal lavage fluid to reduce the incidence of infection, and the relationship between low antithrombin III levels and the development of thromboembolic phenomena. An interesting prospective study indicated that secondary elective operations should be delayed in trauma patients with persistent signs of an ongoing systemic inflammatory response. In this study, secondary operations in severely injured patients acted like secondary insults and predisposed the patients to the development of organ failure. Finally, 2 basic science articles were chosen, one dealing with the significance of nitric oxide in the pathogenesis of organ injury and mortality after hemorrhagic shock and a study looking at the effect of sex hormones on trauma-induced immunosuppression.

Edwin A. Deitch, M.D.

Airbag Protection Versus Compartment Intrusion Effect Determines the Pattern of Injuries in Multiple Trauma Motor Vehicle Crashes

Loo GT, Siegel JH, Dischinger PC, et al (Univ of Maryland, Baltimore, Md; Dynamic Science Inc, Annapolis, Md)

J Trauma 41:935–951, 1996 4–1

Purpose.—Various studies have estimated the number of lives expected to be saved by mandatory implementation of the frontal air bag (AB). However, there have been few detailed studies of the nature of injuries occurring with ABs, including the interaction between seat belts (Bts) and ABs. The effects of ABs on injury patterns were assessed in multiply injured patients who were in a motor vehicle crash (MVC).

Methods.—The prospective cohort study included 200 patients in MVCs admitted to 2 Level I trauma centers. All were nonejected drivers or front-seat passengers who sustained multiple trauma or severe lower extremity trauma. Detailed information was collected on each incident, including investigation by a Dynamic Science Crash Reconstruction Team. The injuries were described in standard fashion using a computer-based medical graphics program. The interaction between AB and Bt protection vs. vehicular compartment intrusion effects on injury patterns were analyzed.

Results.—For patients involved in frontal crashes, AB protection reduced Glasgow Coma Scale severity in brain injury, facial fracture, shock, and the need for extrication better than Bt protection did. The rate of lower extremity fractures was 41% with ABs vs. 66% with Bts, but there was no significant difference in the incidence of pelvic fracture. Air bags prevented brain injuries and facial fractures caused by impact contact (Fig

MOTOR VEHICLE CRASH STUDY
ASSOCIATED INJURIES
ALL FRONTAL AIRBAG VS. ALL FRONTAL NON-AIRBAG

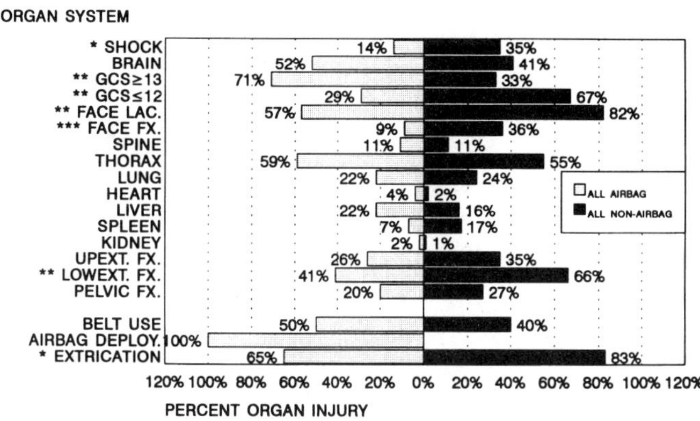

GCS FOR BRAIN INJURED PATIENTS ONLY

* P< 0.05 ** P< 0.01 *** P< 0.001
N: All Frontal Airbag=46, All Frontal Non-Airbag=92

FIGURE 7.—All frontal air bag vs. all frontal non–air bag. (Courtesy of Loo GT, Siegel JH, Dischinger PC, et al: Airbag protection versus compartment intrusion effect determines the pattern of injuries in multiple trauma motor vehicle crashes. *J Trauma* 41(6):935–951, 1996.)

7). They also lessened the incidence of such injuries caused by vehicular compartment intrusions. Patients with AB protection had less than half the magnitude of thoracoabdominal injuries resulting from steering-wheel intrusion. Air-bag protection in frontal MVCs resulted in fewer lower extremity fracture contact injuries but had no effect on lower extremity fractures caused by intrusion of the instrument panel, toepan, or floor pedals. For patients involved in lateral MVCs, Bts offered no protection against injuries to the brain, face, chest, or pelvis. Air-bag protection reduced the estimated cost of hospitalization from about $68,000 to about $37,000.

Conclusions.—Frontal ABs reduce the severity of injury for patients involved in multiple trauma MVCs. They result in less severe brain injuries and fewer facial injuries. They also reduce the incidence of lower extremity fracture contact injuries, although additional measures are needed to reduce frontal crash lower extremity injuries caused by vehicular compartment intrusions. Side ABs may offer additional protection against lateral crash injuries.

▶ This article, which will become 1 of the classical studies of motor vehicle injury patterns, clearly establishes the benefits of ABs both in reducing the severity of injury and the costs of trauma care. The amount of important material presented is so extensive that it is mandatory reading for all physicians caring for a significant number of patients injured in MVCs.

Simply stated, in frontal crashes ABs protect against shock, severe brain injuries, facial fractures, and facial lacerations and reduce the incidence of extremity fractures, although they do not protect against abdominal visceral injuries. In fact, ABs appeared to be the key factor in reducing injuries, because ABs were protective even in patients who were not wearing their Bts and the incidence and magnitude of injuries was less in unrestrained (no Bts) patients who had ABs than in restrained patients whose cars did not have ABs.

E.A. Deitch, M.D.

Trauma on the Internet: Early Experience With a World Wide Web Server Dedicated to Trauma and Critical Care

Block EFJ, Mire EJ (Louisiana State Univ, Shreveport)

J Trauma 41:265–270, 1996 4–2

Background.—The Internet is a global computer network. An interactive data/information server devoted to trauma and critical care, TraumaNET, has been created on the Internet. The use of this server for education and informational exchange was analyzed.

Findings.—During the first 6 months of usage, the numbers of files transmitted increased from an average of 80/day to 600/day. The majority of the users were American, but there were foreign users from 40 other countries. Educational institutions received 30% of all the transmitted files.

Conclusion.—TraumaNET, an interactive data/information server devoted to trauma and critical care issues, has been established on the Internet. There has been increasing interest in this site during its first 6 months of operation. Further development by other trauma centers would facilitate information exchange between care providers and help to provide educational opportunities for all interested participants.

► The use of the Internet for networking is a concept whose time has come. This article summarizes the web site put together by Dr. Block. This article was chosen for several reasons, not the least of which is that I am a subscriber and have first-hand experience with its usefulness. Anyone with an interest in trauma should subscribe. It is free and you can log on by contacting "http://www.trauma.lsumc.edu". Please do.

E.A. Deitch, M.D.

Delayed Diagnosis in a Rural Trauma Center

Aaland MO, Smith K (Univ of Illinois, Peoria)

Surgery 120:774–779, 1996 4–3

Background.—Making an expeditious diagnosis of all injuries during the primary and secondary surveys can be a challenge in trauma patients.

TABLE 1.—Predictors of Missed Injuries

Predictor	*All-patients (%)*	*Missed injury patients (%)*	*Positive predictive index*
TBI	35	65	0.65
Intoxicated	23	39	0.63
Immediate operation	7	13	0.64
Intubated	1.8	18	0.91
ISS*	11	18	

*An average.
Abbreviations: TBI, traumatic brain injury; *ISS,* injury severity score.
(Courtesy of Aaland MO, Smith K: Delayed diagnosis in a rural trauma center. *Surgery* 120:774–779, 1996.)

A rural tertiary care hospital implemented a protocol involving ongoing serial examinations throughout the course of all trauma admissions. The incidence of delayed diagnoses was determined in trauma patients between 1993 and 1995.

Methods.—Patients were evaluated by the trauma team in the emergency department and were then re-evaluated throughout their admission and within 1 week after discharge. A delayed diagnosis was defined as an injury not identified until after a stable patient was in a hospital room or until after departure from the recovery room. All delayed diagnoses prompted collection of data on the patient's age, injury severity score (ISS), mechanism of injury, time of delayed diagnosis, mental status at admission, and intubation status.

Results.—Of the 1,873 patients admitted or evaluated during the study period, 56 patients had 68 missed injuries for a 3% delayed diagnosis rate. Diagnosis of the missed injuries occurred 8 hours to 92 days after admission. Blunt trauma accounted for 97% of the mechanisms of injury in these patients. When compared with patients without delayed diagnoses, patients with delayed diagnoses tended to have a higher ISS, require more emergent operations, be intubated, and have altered mental status from traumatic brain injuries and/or alcohol intoxication (Table 1). Nonspinal closed fractures, the most commonly missed injuries, accounted for 63% of the delayed diagnoses. Other missed injuries included head and neck injuries (16%), spinal injuries (10%), pneumothoraces (4%), vascular injuries (4%), and intra-abdominal injuries (3%). Nineteen patients required surgical treatment of their missed injuries. The delay in diagnosis caused 1 death and significant morbidity in 3 patients.

Conclusions.—Delayed diagnosis is a serious concern in trauma service. To minimize the risk of delayed diagnosis, it is important to review the initial radiographs carefully, repeat any unclear studies, and perform serial examinations during the entire clinical course for each patient. Routine review and discussion of missed injuries will also help reduce this risk.

▶ The message here is very clear. Being compulsive counts. This is especially true in high-risk groups of patients and patients who are not able to communicate as a result of either their injuries, an altered sensorium, or the presence of an endotracheal tube.

E.A. Deitch, M.D.

Lowering Hospital Charges in the Trauma Intensive Care Unit While Maintaining Quality of Care by Increasing Resident and Attending Physician Awareness

Blackstone ME, Miller RS, Hodgson AJ, et al (Greenville Hosp System, South Carolina)

J Trauma: Injury Infect Crit Care 39:1041–1044, 1995 4–4

Purpose.—In the managed care era, physicians must be educated about cost containment issues. This is particularly important in the ICU, which accounts for 20% to 34% of inpatient costs but only 5% to 7% of hospital beds. Few studies have looked at the educational considerations involved in changing the way attending and resident physicians make patient care decisions. The ability of an informal bedside educational intervention to reduce trauma intensive care unit (TICU) charges was investigated.

Methods.—The prospective study was conducted in a TICU at a level I teaching hospital and included 91 consecutive patients admitted during a 6-month period. For the first 3 months of the study, no efforts were made to reduce the costs of TICU care and the residents were not even aware that a study was being conducted. In the latter 3 months, a new set of guidelines was established, including discontinuation of all standing orders and daily laboratory tests. The management changes were discussed on daily bedside rounds among residents, attending physicians, nurses, and pharmacy personnel, with an explicit emphasis on the relative costs of diagnostic and treatment procedures. The intervention sought to help the residents to use their clinical skills instead of relying on unnecessary tests. There were no changes in the makeup of the TICU staff during the study. The TICU charges incurred during the preintervention and postintervention periods were compared.

Results.—The patients in the preintervention and postintervention phases were similar in terms of median and mean age, Injury Severity Score, ICU length of stay, and male/female ratio. In the postintervention period, total median charges decreased by $818/ICU day. Medication charges decreased by $151/day, laboratory charges by $120/day, charges for chest radiographs by $61/day, respiratory therapy charges by $185/day, and miscellaneous charges by $141/day. There were no significant differences in the mortality and major complication rates from before to after the intervention.

Conclusions.—An informal bedside intervention can increase awareness of costs in the TICU setting and prompt specific efforts to achieve cost reductions. The result is a significant decline in most components of daily TICU charges, with no decrement in quality of care. The authors plan ongoing studies to determine whether the cost-effective behavior of the trauma team persists over time. It is hoped that cost-effective patient management will become a routine part of medical education for future generations of physicians.

▶ Few would argue that the high costs of medicine have led to a revolution in health care delivery that poses serious threats to medical education and the survival of urban, and to a lesser extent, rural trauma centers. The best way to improve economic trauma center survival would be to reduce costs without reducing the quality of care. Thus, the value of this educationally based and economically driven study is that it clearly documents that ICU charges can be significantly reduced (about 20%) by just changing a few bad habits. Considering that ICU medical charges, exclusive of physician fees, are about $62 billion per year, reductions in the range of $10 billion a year are possible using approaches such as described in this study. As they say in Washington DC, a billion here, a billion there, and pretty soon you are talking about real money. For this reason, I commend this article and the references it contains to you.

E.A. Deitch, M.D.

Percutaneous Dilatational Tracheostomy: A Safe, Cost-effective Bedside Procedure

Cobean R, Beals M, Moss C, et al (Maine Med Ctr, Portland)

Arch Surg 131:265–271, 1996 4–5

Background.—When performing standard tracheostomy in a critically ill patient, most surgeons prefer to do the procedure in the operating room, rather than in the ICU. Transporting these patients out of the ICU is difficult and entails some risk. Percutaneous dilatational tracheostomy (PDT) has been safely done in the ICU, yet it has not been widely adopted. The safety and cost-effectiveness of PDT were retrospectively evaluated.

Methods.—The study included 65 patients on a combined medical-surgical ICU. Over a 19-month period, all patients underwent PDT under the supervision of 1 general surgeon. All procedures were done in the ICU. The results were analyzed, and the costs were compared with those of standard operative tracheostomies done over the same time.

Results.—All attempts at PDT were successful, regardless of variations in airway anatomy, body habitus, or ventilator settings. The procedures took a mean of 14 minutes. Although intraoperative complications occurred in 22% of patients, most were minor technical problems and none had serious consequences for the patient. The postoperative complication rate was 9%: 3 patients had bleeding complications, 1 died because of premature decannulation, 1 had subcutaneous emphysema, and 1 had an air leak. At a mean follow-up of 7.5 months, there were 2 long-term airway complications. The mean charges were only $997 for PDT, compared with $2,642 for standard tracheostomy.

Conclusions.—Percutaneous dilatational tracheostomy is a quick, safe, and economical procedure. It can be done in the ICU by a surgeon with a nurse and a respiratory therapist, avoiding the need to transport a critically ill patient.

► Although as surgeons we have grown up learning the value of certain operative procedures, such as the standard tracheostomy, there are occasions when we should change. The use of PDT is 1 example. As stated in this article, PDTs are quicker and cheaper to perform than standard tracheostomies and also obviate the need to move a critically ill or unstable patient from the ICU to the operating room. Combining these considerations with the knowledge that this procedure also is as safe as a standard tracheostomy has made PDTs done at the bedside in the ICU the procedure of choice, in my mind. Furthermore, I have found that the residents whom I have supervised find PDTs easier than standard tracheostomies. I have found another advantage for PDT over a standard tracheostomy: the PDT can be done as soon as the decision is made that the patient would benefit from a tracheostomy. There is no need to await the availability of an operating room.

In summary, first there was the percutaneous endoscopic gastrostomy and now there is the PDT, and both are good. That is the message.

E.A. Deitch, M.D.

Trauma Ultrasound Workshop Improves Physician Detection of Peritoneal and Pericardial Fluid

Ali J, Rozycki GS, Campbell JP, et al (Univ of Toronto; Emory Univ, Atlanta, Ga)

J Surg Res 63:275–279, 1996 4–6

Introduction.—The reliability of ultrasound examination of the traumatized abdomen is well supported in the literature. The ability of 30 nonradiologist clinicians to detect intraperitoneal and pericardial fluid with the use of ultrasound as a diagnostic modality was assessed after attendance at a focused trauma ultrasound workshop.

Methods.—The performance of 9 trauma physicians and 21 surgical residents who attended the workshop was compared with a matched group of 30 physicians who did not attend the workshop. The workshop included discussion of ultrasound physics, demonstration of instrumentation, review of pertinent literature, videotaped demonstrations, and "hands-on" teaching of skills through the use of live patient models. The technique involved 4 placements of the ultrasound probe: right and left upper quadrants, epigastrium, and Pouch of Douglas. Acquisition of skills was tested with pre- and postworkshop performance on 12 sonograms (3 for each probe location, 6 of which were positive for fluid).

Results.—The false positive and false negative scores decreased from 12.9 and 15.0 preworkshop, respectively, to 8.9 and 5.0 postworkshop for physicians who attended the workshop. This improvement was not seen in pretests and post-tests in physicians who did not attend the workshop. The ability of workshop attendees to detect fluid was significantly improved, with no major differences noted between residents and staff.

Conclusion.—Attendance at a focused ultrasound workshop for the detection of intraperitoneal and pericardial fluid improves the performance of nonradiologists in this diagnostic approach. The workshop should be considered a crucial component of ultrasound education for trauma physicians. It should be regarded as a starting point after which supervision is needed until expertise is achieved through continued experience in the trauma setting.

▶ The message of this article is simple. You, too, can learn, but should you? I think, yes. Ultrasound is rapid, noninvasive, and it can be performed at the bedside, which avoids the risks of moving a patient from a controlled environment to the x-ray department. Plus, it appears to be accurate. However, it requires more than a course. Taking a course is an optimal way to begin, but is not sufficient to provide one with the expertise required to be a competent ultrasonographer. Competence requires experience.

E.A. Deitch, M.D.

Nonoperative Management of Blunt Splenic Injury in Adults: Age Over 55 Years as a Powerful Indicator for Failure

Godley CD, Warren RL, Sheridan RL, et al (Harvard Med School, Boston)

J Am Coll Surg 183:133–139, 1996 4–7

Introduction.—Until recently, splenectomy has been the procedure of choice for patients who have blunt splenic injuries. However, complications after surgery, such as postsplenectomy infection, have put into question the need for surgery in all cases. Nonoperative treatments have been used successfully in children, although results in adults have been less consistent. Clinical criteria, including hemodynamic stability and lack of intra-abdominal injury, have been identified for selection of patients for nonoperative treatment. Additional criteria for nonoperative treatment of blunt splenic injuries were identified retrospectively.

Methods.—Medical records of 135 patients admitted with blunt splenic injury during a 6-year period were reviewed. Laparotomy was performed on 89 patients, whereas the remaining 46 patients received nonoperative treatment. Nonoperative management consisted of bed rest, hemodynamic monitoring, serial abdominal examination, hematocrit determination, and restriction to nothing by mouth.

Results.—Abdominal CT was used to confirm splenic injury in all 46 patients. Seventeen injuries were rated in class I; 24, class II; 4, class III; and 1, class IV. Twenty-four patients were successfully treated with nonoperative management. Recurrent hemorrhage with reduced hematocrit or severe hypotension were present in the 22 patients in whom nonoperative management failed. Treatment failures were evident at a mean of 4.6 days

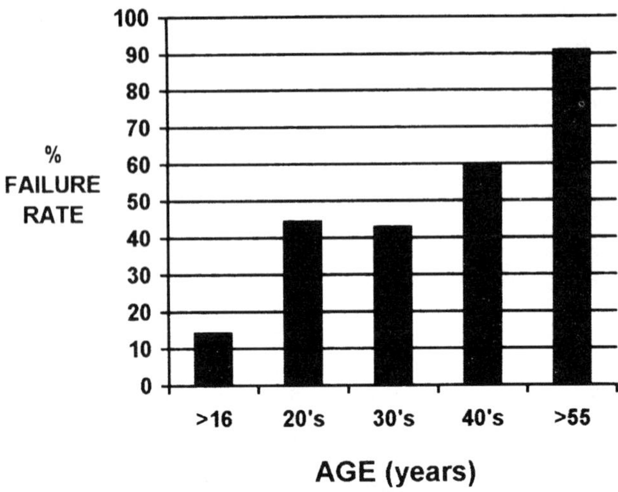

FIGURE 2.—Failure rate, by age, for patients with splenic injury who were treated nonoperatively. (Courtesy of Godley CD, Warren RL, Sheridan RL, et al: Nonoperative management of blunt splenic injury in adults: Age over 55 years as a powerful indicator for failure. *J Am Coll Surg* 183:133–139, 1996. By permission of the *Journal of the American College of Surgeons.*)

(range, 1–16 days). Splenectomy was performed in 17 patients, and splenorrhaphies were performed in 5. The failure rate of nonoperative management was significantly higher in older patients; nonoperative management failed in 10 of 11 patients aged 55 years or older, whereas such treatment failed in 12 of 35 patients younger than 55 years (Fig 2). There were no significant differences, however, in mean CT splenic injury grading or Injury Severity Scores between the 2 groups. Significantly more patients aged older than 55 years in whom nonoperative treatment failed had complications (pneumonia, sepsis, wound infection, pancreatitis), as compared with younger patients in whom nonoperative treatment failed.

Conclusion.—Nonoperative management of blunt splenic injuries was more likely to fail in elderly patients, although clinical and radiographic variables were similar to those of younger patients. Patients aged older than 55 years may be better treated with immediate laparotomy when splenic injury is diagnosed.

▶ This study, as well as others, points out the potential dangers of nonoperative therapy of splenic injuries, especially in older adults. Although the reason why nonoperative therapy for splenic injuries is more successful in children than in adults is not known with certainty, most believe that it has to do with anatomical differences between the pediatric and adult spleen. The pediatric spleen has a relatively thick capsule and contains a lot of functional smooth muscle and elastic tissue, which facilitate hemostasis and tamponade. As people age, these protective anatomical properties decrease, thereby making the adult spleen less able to tamponade bleeding. As seen in this study, 91% of patients aged 55 years or older required surgery for persistent bleeding. The failure of nonoperative management is even more remarkable when one considers that these patients all had less severe class I or II liver injuries.

In summary, the important take-home message of this study is that older patients with splenic injuries should be managed with early operative therapy, even though the risk of surgery may be higher in elderly patients than in young patients.

E.A. Deitch, M.D.

Re-engineering Ventilatory Support to Decrease Days and Improve Resource Utilization

Kirton OC, DeHaven CB, Hudson-Civetta J, et al (Univ of Miami, Fla)
Ann Surg 224:396–404, 1996 4–8

Background.—Because mechanical ventilation is expensive and can lead to serious complications, it is advisable to wean patients as soon as possible. A ventilatory strategy was developed to separate out the work of breathing masquerading as weaning failure and to facilitate weaning.

Methods.—Work of breathing (WOB), physiologic WOB, imposed WOB, and total WOB were measured 90 times prospectively in 31 patients during a period of 4 years to validate the system. Eight hundred thirty-eight additional patients were subsequently studied. Initial pressure support ventilation was adjusted to achieve an arterial pH of 7.35 or greater, a partial pressure of carbon dioxide of 45 mm Hg or less, and a spontaneous respiratory rate of 30 breaths/min or less. Oxygen saturation was maintained at 92% or greater. When pressure ventilator support could be decreased to 5 cm of water with the Hamilton-Veolar ventilator or to 8 cm of water with the Puritan-Bennett ventilator, a room air-continuous positive airway pressure of 5 cm of water was started. Extubation was attempted when arterial oxygen pressure reached 55 mm Hg or greater, $Paco_2$ 45 mm Hg or less, arterial pH 7.35 or greater, and a respiratory rate of 30 breaths/min or less. A microprocessor-based monitor allowed measurement of work of breathing through the breathing circuit.

Results.—Although blood gas measures were acceptable, respiratory rates of 27 patients ventilated for more than 2 days exceeded 30 breaths/min. Total WOB for 6 patients was less than 0.8 J/L and for the remaining 21 was 1.6 J/L including an imposed WOB of 1.1 J/L. Normal physiologic WOB is 0.5 J/L. All patients were successfully extubated, 20 immediately. When an additional 589 patients were evaluated, 18% with respiratory rates greater than 30 breaths/min were extubated. Reintubation rates were 7.6% for this group and 7.9% for patients with respiratory rates of less than 30 breaths/min. When a third group was tested, the duration of ventilation had decreased significantly from 8.8 days in the first group to 4.2 days in the third group.

Conclusion.—Using a microprocessor-based monitor to measure the WOB through the breathing circuit significantly decreased the number of days on mechanical ventilation and increased the success rate of extubation, particularly in patients previously considered weaning failures.

▶ How to wean and when to extubate remain areas of concern and controversy in trauma patients who require mechanical ventilation for more than 2 or 3 days. Even the best published studies and expert clinical judgment are associated with prolonged ventilatory support and/or a high extubation failure rate, which ranges from 20% to 50% in well-controlled studies. To circumvent this major clinical problem, the authors used a portable microprocessor to measure WOB in a large group of ventilated trauma patients. Work of breathing has 3 major components: (1) the normal physiologic WOB, (2) disease-related WOB, and (3) WOB imposed by the endotracheal tube, the ventilator, and the ventilator circuit. The WOB imposed by the ventilatory apparatus has been largely ignored in most weaning studies, yet, as shown in this study, the WOB imposed on the patient while breathing spontaneously through the breathing apparatus can in some instances be considerable.

The significance of this article is twofold. First, the authors describe a new and what appears to be more accurate method of monitoring ventilatory support and weaning (i.e., WOB). Second, the authors clearly document that in a significant number of patients in whom weaning trials appear to fail, the problem is not the patient but instead is related to the excessive imposed WOB of the ventilator system. To paraphrase the authors, in some patients the imposed WOB is masquerading as weaning failure. As this technology spreads to other centers, it should be possible to better determine its ultimate clinical utility. Nonetheless, it appears very attractive.

E.A. Deitch, M.D.

A Randomized Trial of Isonitrogenous Enteral Diets After Severe Trauma

Kudsk KA, Minard G, Croce MA, et al (Univ of Tennessee, Memphis; Regional Med Ctr, Memphis, Tenn)

Ann Surg 224:531–543, 1996 4–9

Background.—Diets containing specialty nutrients, such as arginine, glutamine, nucleotides, and omega-3 fatty acids, may decrease septic complications. This possibility was further investigated in a randomized trial.

Methods.—Thirty-five trauma victims were enrolled in the prospective, blinded, randomized trial. The patients had an Abdominal Trauma Index of 25 or greater or an Injury Severity Score of 21 or greater. All had early enteral access to an immune-enhancing diet (IED) or an isonitrogenous, isocaloric diet and Casec diet. Nineteen patients with equally severe injuries but no early enteral access composed a control group.

Findings.—Initial data on 2 patients in the treatment group who died were not included in the final analysis. Major infectious complications occurred in only 6% of the patients assigned to the IED, compared with

41% in the isonitrogenous group and 58% in the control group. Patients receiving the IED also had a significantly shorter length of stay, received significantly fewer therapeutic antibiotics, and had a significantly lower occurrence of intra-abdominal abscess than did patients in the other groups. The improved clinical outcomes in patients receiving the IED were reflected in decreased hospital costs.

Conclusions.—An IED is significantly better than an isonitrogenous diet or no early enteral nutrition in severely injured patients. The complication rate is greatest among unfed patients.

▶ This study was selected because it closes the loop and puts the last nail in the coffin of those who do not believe that the route and type of diet affect outcome in severely injured trauma patients (Injury Severity Score greater than 21). Infectious and septic complications were reduced in the group of patients who received the IED (Immuno-Aid) compared with the other 2 patient groups; their hospital stay was also shortened. Furthermore, hospital charges were lowest for the patients fed the IED and highest for the unfed controls. Thus, not only did the patients who received the IED do better clinically, but in addition their hospital charges were reduced. Therefore, the take-home message is that the early institution of a specialized enteral diet both works better than the use of a standard diet and is cost-effective.

E.A. Deitch, M.D.

Cardiopulmonary Effects of Raised Intra-abdominal Pressure Before and After Intravascular Volume Expansion

Ridings PC, Bloomfield GL, Blocher CR, et al (Virginia Commonwealth Univ, Richmond)

J Trauma 39:1071–1075, 1995 4–10

Introduction.—Critically ill patients may have acute increases in intra-abdominal pressure (IAP) caused by a variety of factors, including bowel distension, intraperitoneal or retroperitoneal bleeding, or intraperitoneal packing. There are conflicting data on how IAP affects other hemodynamic parameters. Toward a better understanding of the effects of IAP in trauma patients, the cardiopulmonary effects of acutely increased IAP were studied in pigs.

Methods.—Anesthetized, intubated, catheterized swine were subjected to an IAP of up to 25 mm Hg above baseline by intra-abdominal instillation of isotonic ethylene glycol. The effects of elevated IAP on systemic and pulmonary hemodynamic measurements were assessed. Bladder pressure, pleural pressure, and pulmonary function were evaluated as well. When IAP reached 25 mm Hg above baseline, cardiac index (CI) was restored to normal by intravascular volume expansion.

Results.—The 25 mm Hg increase in IAP resulted in a significant decrease in CI, from 3.6 to 2.2 L/min/m^2. Wedge, pulmonary, arterial, and pleural pressures increased significantly (Fig 3). There was also a non-

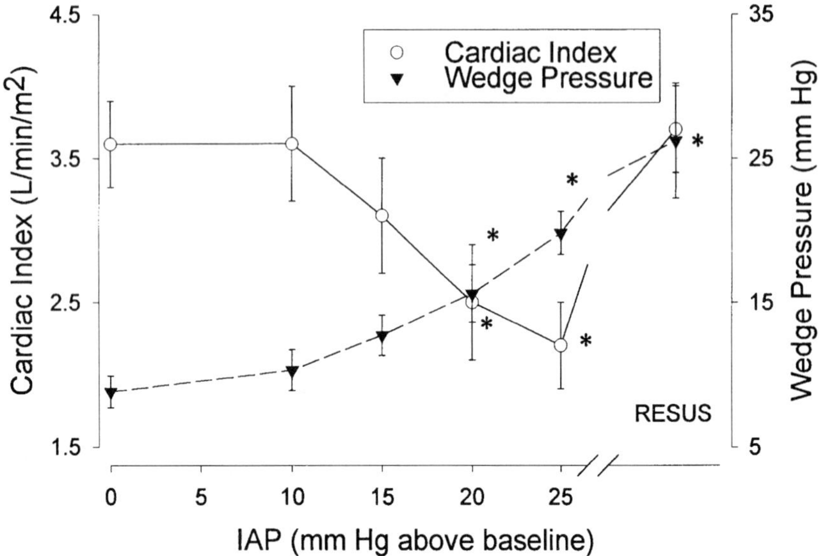

FIGURE 3.—Effects of increased intra-abdominal pressure (IAP) on cardiac index (CI) and wedge pressure (WP), and the effects of intravascular volume expansion at an IAP of 25 mm Hg above baseline (RESUS). ($P < 0.05$ vs. baseline.) (Courtesy of Ridings PC, Bloomfield GL, Blocher CR, et al: Cardiopulmonary Effects of Raised Intra-Abdominal Pressure Before and After Intravascular Volume Expansion. *J Trauma* 39:1071–1075, 1995.)

significant decrease in transarterial wedge pressure, calculated as wedge minus pleural pressure. Pulmonary function worsened as IAP rose, with a significant decline in $Pa{O_2}$ and an increase in $Pa{CO_2}$. The CI was normalized by fluid resuscitation even though wedge pressure was elevated (Fig 3).

Conclusions.—The hemodynamic changes occurring with elevated IAP are described, including a transmitted increase in pleural pressure with accompanying cardiopulmonary dysfunction. When IAP is high, increasing the intravascular volume does not appear to have any serious adverse effect on cardiopulmonary function. In patients with elevated IAP, hemodynamic data must be interpreted carefully to correctly determine the patient's intravascular fluid status.

► This physiologic study of the hemodynamic consequences of increased IAP (abdominal compartment syndrome) provides potentially useful and important clinical information. Specifically, it clearly documents that the hemodynamic profile of patients with increased IAP can mimic the hemodynamic profile of cardiac failure, i.e., the CI is decreased, the pulmonary arterial wedge pressure (PAWP) is increased, and the $Pa{O_2}$ falls. Because the renal manifestation of increased IAP is oliguria, it is all too easy for the unwary to assume that a patient with abdominal compartment syndrome has cardiac failure, and to give diuretics and inotropic agents rather than fluids and operative decompression of the abdomen. So don't be fooled. In patients at risk of having the abdominal compartment syndrome, measure the bladder pressure and check for elevated pulmonary airway pressures. I can tell you from personal experience that the early recognition and aggressive treatment of increased IAP results in the salvage of previously unsalvageable patients.

E.A. Deitch, M.D.

Effects of Increased Intra-Abdominal Pressure Upon Intracranial and Cerebral Perfusion Pressure Before and After Volume Expansion

Bloomfield GL, Ridings PC, Blocher CR, et al (Virginia Commonwealth Univ, Richmond)

J Trauma 40:936–943, 1996 4–11

Introduction.—Patients with major abdominal injuries often experience elevated intra-abdominal pressure (IAP). This complex circumstance is often made more complicated because many patients have concomitant intracranial injuries. Patients with combined moderate to severe injuries of both head and abdomen have mortality rates that are twice that of patients with moderate to severe injuries of head only or abdomen only. Recent reports have raised suspicion that the adverse effects of abdominal compartment syndrome (ACS) may extend beyond the peritoneum and thorax and into the cranial vault. A porcine model of acutely elevated IAP was used to evaluate the effects of IAP upon intracranial pressure (ICP) and cerebral perfusion pressure (CPP) before and after intravascular volume resuscitation.

Methods.—Yorkshire swine were anesthetized and an intraperitoneal balloon was placed in the abdominal cavity. The balloon was inflated until IAP was 25-mm Hg above baseline. The intravascular volume was expanded with 0.9% saline solution until the cardiac index (CT) returned to normal. Abdominal decompression was performed. Levels of arterial oxygenation ($Pa{O_2}$) and arterial carbon dioxide ($Pa{CO_2}$) were kept fairly constant by an increase in the ventilatory rate. Measurements taken at baseline and appropriate intervals included changes in ICP, and systemic and pulmonary hemodynamic parameters secondary to increased IAP. These measurements were used to determine the effect on CPP.

Results.—There were significant increases in ICP, pleural pressure (PP), and central venous pressure with elevated IAP. There was a significant decrease in CI and CPP with increased IAP. The increase in ICP was significant when IAP was 15-mm Hg above baseline. Mean arterial pressure (MAP) decreased minimally with increased IAP. The ICP, peak inspiratory pressure (PIP), and PP were significantly increased with intravascular volume expansion, whereas $Pa{CO_2}$ and MAP were slightly increased and $Pa{O_2}$ was slightly decreased. There was a nonsignificant increase in CPP with intravascular volume expansion. With abdominal decompression, PP, PIP, and CI decreased significantly; $Pa{CO_2}$ and MAP decreased; $Pa{O_2}$ increased, and ICP returned to nearly baseline.

Conclusion.—An elevation in IAP increases ICP and decreases CPP and CI. Further increases in ICP occur with volume expansion. The CPP is improved with volume expansion by its greater positive effect on MAP. Between the time of diagnosis of ACS and abdominal decompression, it is therapeutically appropriate to maintain cardiac output, MAP, and CPP through the use of volume expansion.

▶ Recognition of ACS as a clinically significant phenomenon has led a number of investigators to examine the physiologic consequences of increased IAP. This well-done experimental study examined the effects of elevated IAP on ICP and CPP. The observation that an increased IAP is associated with an increase in ICP and a decrease in CPP has important clinical implications for multitrauma patients because up to 40% of patients with major abdominal trauma have a head injury. Additionally, because the head injury is the primary determinant of outcome in patients with combined abdominal and head injuries, anything that could worsen the neurologic status of the patient (i.e., increased ICP) must be avoided. In this light, recognition that increases in IAP could cause an increase in neurologic morbidity and mortality alerts us to the need to monitor IAP and to diagnose ACS as soon as possible. What this means is that when a patient with combined abdominal and head injuries displays signs of neurologic deterioration or a rising ICP, attention must be directed to the abdomen, and intra-abdominal pressures should be checked if the abdomen appears distended or if the patient has other signs of ACS.

E.A. Deitch, M.D.

Blunt Carotid Injury: Importance of Early Diagnosis and Anticoagulant Therapy

Fabian TC, Patton JH Jr, Croce MA, et al (Univ of Tennessee, Memphis)
Ann Surg 223:513–525, 1996 4–12

Introduction.—Blunt carotid injury (BCI) is considered a rare injury, but there is suspicion that it is underdiagnosed. Diagnosis should not be delayed because patient outcome is compromised once a deficit develops. Factors that lead to diagnosis of BCI were analyzed and the efficacy of anticoagulation therapy was evaluated.

Methods.—An 11-year retrospective review was conducted of all patients with BCI identified from the registry of a level I trauma center. Patient charts were reviewed to analyze factors that led to diagnosis of BCI: demographics, data on mechanisms and associated injury patterns, brain CT findings, angiography, use of anticoagulation therapy with heparin, risk factors, and neurologic findings at admission and subsequent changes in neurologic status.

Results.—Sixty-seven patients were identified with the diagnosis of 87 BCIs. Twenty patients (30%) had bilateral injuries. Thirty-seven patients had an initial CT brain scan that was within normal limits, 18 had a mass

TABLE 4.—Comparison of the Neurologic Outcome at Discharge Death or With or Without Heparin Anticoagulation

	Neurologic Outcome		
Treatment	Good	Moderate	Bad*
Heparin	26†	7	14†
No heparin	3	1	11

*Includes deaths.
†$P < 0.01$ good vs bad outcome.
(Courtesy of Fabian TC, Patton JH Jr, Croce MA, et al: Blunt carotid injury: Importance of early diagnosis and anticoagulant therapy. *Ann Surg* 223:513–525, 1996.)

or lesion, and 5 had evidence of regional brain ischemia. Findings that prompted clinical suspicion and subsequent angiographic diagnosis for BCI included soft-tissue injury to the anterior neck in 9 patients, a neurologic examination not compatible with brain CT in 23 patients, development of a neurologic deficit subsequent to hospital admission in 29 patients, and Horner's syndrome in 6 patients. The average interval from injury to angiography for definitive diagnosis was 53 hours (range 2 to 672 hours). The initial neurologic findings that were incompatible with CT findings included 13 hemiparesis, 6 hemiplegia, 3 monoparesis, 1 monoplegia, 3 aphasia/dysphagia, and 5 Horner's syndrome. Neurologic deficits that developed after initial examination included 10 hemiparesis, 6 monoplegia, 5 depressed affect, 4 hemiplegia, 3 monoparesis, and 1 aphasia. Angiographic findings indicated 54 intimal dissections, 11 pseudoaneurysms, 17 thromboses, 4 carotid cavernous fistulas, and 1 transected internal carotid artery. Of 46 patients who survived their injuries, 63% had good neurologic outcome, 17% had moderate outcome, and 20% had bad outcome. Twenty-one patients (31%) died. Of these, 16 (76%) were directly related to strokes from BCI. Significant risk factors for mortality were coma and shock. Coma and thrombosis had significant impact of neurologic deterioration. Forty-seven patients (76%) received heparin at the time of diagnosis. Of the patients that remained, 8 received no therapy, 6 received aspirin, and 1 received surgery. Patients who received heparin had a significantly better outcome than patients who did not receive heparin (Table 4). Thirty-nine of 46 survivors with 53 arterial injuries had angiographic follow-up at a mean of 172 days after injury. Sixty-two percent of patients with dissection reverted to normal and 29% (6 patients) developed pseudoaneurysms that did not revert to normal.

Conclusion.—Blunt carotid injury is underdiagnosed. A broad-scale screening program is needed to diagnose asymptomatic lesions. Conventional angiography is not a practical approach for mass screening, so clinicians may need to rely on duplex Doppler examination or possibly magnetic resonance angiography when cost and resources are more amenable to mass screening. Until mass screening is available, it is not likely that there will be significant improvement in earlier diagnosis and subsequent outcome in patients with BCI. If started before symptom onset, heparin therapy is effective in the amelioration of neurologic deterioration.

► This article was chosen for several reasons. First, it is the largest series on BCI to date. As such, important points are illustrated about the diagnosis and natural history of this injury. For example, this clinical series points out the importance of recognizing that a patient's neurologic deficit is not explained by head CT if an early diagnosis of BCI is suspected. An early diagnosis is critical, because the authors have documented that early heparin therapy is associated with an improved neurologic outcome, and if therapy is delayed until the neurologic deficit is established, the response to therapy is worsened. Another important point in this article is that, in spite of the potential risks of heparin use in the multi-injured patient, its use was associated with an improvement in survival. In fact only 6 of their 67 patients (9%) had any complications from heparin therapy and 2 of these 6 patients subsequently developed massive strokes and died after their heparin was stopped. Finally, with their high level of awareness and aggressive diagnostic approach toward this frequently initially silent injury, they found a surprisingly high incidence of BCI in patients in motor vehicle accidents. This incidence was 1 in every 150 patients. Based on this study, it behooves all of us to consider BCI more often than we might have in the past.

E.A. Deitch, M.D.

Efficacy of an Intraperitoneal Antibiotic to Reduce the Incidence of Infection in the Trauma Patient: A Prospective, Randomized Study

Yelon JA, Green JD, Evans JT (State Univ of New York, Stony Brook)

J Am Coll Surg 182:509–514, 1996 4–13

Introduction.—The incidence of infection after penetrating abdominal trauma has been shown to decrease with the use of antibiotics. There is little information, however, regarding the use of prophylactic antibiotics after blunt abdominal trauma. The use of intraperitoneal kanamycin to reduce the incidence of infection in patients with blunt abdominal trauma was evaluated in a double-blind, prospective study.

Methods.—Sixty-nine patients who had sustained abdominal injuries that required diagnostic peritoneal lavage were included. Patients were randomly assigned to treatment with either kanamycin, 500 mg, or normal saline administered intraperitoneally after diagnostic peritoneal lavage. Patients were evaluated for infectious complications, length of hospital stay, and clinical outcome. Glasgow Coma Scale score, trauma score, and clinical status at time of admission were also recorded.

Results.—There were no significant differences in patient demographics or initial laboratory findings between the 2 groups. In 11 of 40 patients who received kanamycin, infectious complications developed during the first 3 weeks after injury, as compared with 19 of 29 patients who received normal saline (27.5% vs. 65.6%, a significant difference). Pulmonary

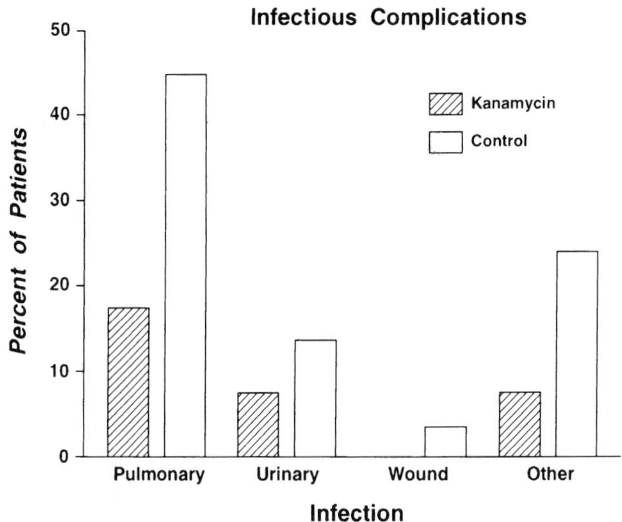

FIGURE 1.—The rate of infectious complications in patients who received kanamycin compared with controls. (Courtesy of Yelon JA, Green JD, Evans JT: Efficacy of an intraperitoneal antibiotic to reduce the incidence of infection in the trauma patient: A prospective, randomized study. *J Am Coll Surg* 182:509–514, 1996. By permission of the *Journal of the American College of Surgeons*.)

infections were the most predominant, present in 17.5% of kanamycin-treated patients and in 44.8% of normal saline–treated patients (Fig 1). The length of hospital stay was significantly shorter for patients who were treated with kanamycin, 12.3 days vs. 17.36 days for saline-treated patients. Length of ICU stay was also shorter for kanamycin-treated patients, 4.18 days vs. 6.96 days for saline-treated patients ($P = 0.047$). Use of kanamycin was not associated with any adverse effects or complications.

Conclusion.—Kanamycin, administered as a single, intraperitoneal dose, significantly reduced the incidence of infectious complications in patients who had sustained blunt abdominal trauma. The length of hospital and ICU stay were also reduced.

▶ The concept of administering antibiotics to patients who have penetrating injuries is well established, but little information is available on the role of prophylactic antibiotic administration in patients who have blunt trauma. Hence the reason the authors carried out this prospective randomized trial. Based on the results of this clinical trial, it appears that a single dose of kanamycin administered intraperitonealy reduces the incidence of infectious complications and shortens the hospital stay. Although not stated in the abstract, the 2 groups were clinically similar and had comparable Injury Severity Scale scores, Glasgow Coma Scale scores, blood loss, and mechanisms of injury. Thus, the beneficial effects of kanamycin did not appear to be related to patient selection. Nonetheless, the results almost seem too good to be true, and maybe they are. It is difficult to understand how a single dose of an antibiotic could have such a profound and long-lasting effect.

Hopefully, other groups will try to replicate this clinical trial. In the meantime, the use of a single dose of kanamycin seems harmless enough. Perhaps it is worth using.

E.A. Deitch, M.D.

Effect of Critical Injury on Plasma Antithrombin Activity: Low Antithrombin Levels Are Associated With Thromboembolic Complications
Owings JT, Bagley M, Gosselin R, et al (Univ of California, Davis)
J Trauma 41:396–406, 1996 4–14

Background.—Hemorrhage and the development of thromboembolic complications or disseminated intravascular coagulation (DIC) are risk factors in severely injured patients. Both conditions result from impaired functioning of the hemostatic process, which is down-regulated by antithrombin (AT). Results of a prospective observational study of the effect of severe injury and subsequent critical care on AT activity were presented.

Methods.—Plasma samples from 157 critically injured trauma patients (34 women), with an average age of 41 years, were drawn at arrival, at 8 and 16 hours, and on days 1 through 6 and analyzed for AT, tissue-factor pathway inhibitor, protein C, prothrombin fragment 1.2, thrombin-antithrombin complex, and D-dimer. Outcomes recorded were deep vein thrombosis (DVT), pulmonary embolus, DIC, adult respiratory distress syndrome, and death.

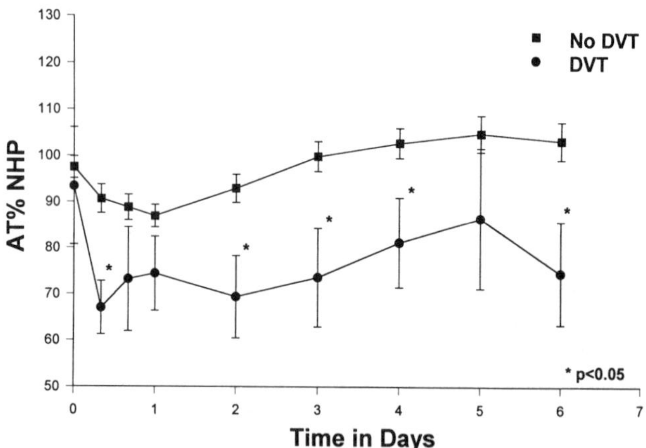

FIGURE 1.—Antithrombin (AT) activity in deep venous thrombosis (DVT). Comparison of AT levels over time in patients with (n = 5) and without (n = 59) DVT. Analysis: repeated measures analysis of variance. *Error bars* represent ± SEM. (Courtesy of Owings JT, Bagley M, Gosselin R, et al: Effect of critical injury on plasma antithrombin activity: Low antithrombin levels are associated with thromboembolic complications. *J Trauma* 41(3):396–406, 1996.)

Results.—The average injury severity score was 23. The average injury severity score in the 14 patients who died was 30. Antithrombin levels were significantly lower in 117 patients. Deep vein thrombosis developed in 9 patients. Of patients with AT levels 50% of normal, 5 died, 9 had DVT, 9 had adult respiratory distress syndrome, and 4 had DIC. Lower AT activity levels were significantly associated with an increased incidence of both DVT and DIC and related to the development of pulmonary embolism (Fig 1). Markers of thrombosis were correlated with decreased AT activity. Because heparin acts by binding to AT, the anticoagulation effects of heparin will be lessened, perhaps significantly so, in patients with decreased AT activity.

Conclusion.—Severely injured patients have decreased AT activity and are at increased risk of thromboembolic complications. Response to low-dose heparin in this group will be problematic at best.

▶ The authors' basic observation that decreased AT III activity levels were associated with DVT and DIC is important for several reasons. First, AT is the principal down-regulator of the coagulation system and is responsible for protecting the patient from the development of pathologic thrombosis. Because the incidence of pulmonary embolism in trauma patients who survive the resuscitation period ranges from at least 1% to 4% and up to 20% of patients who die have evidence of a pulmonary embolus at autopsy, pathologic clotting is a major clinical problem in the trauma patient population. Second, although the decrease in AT levels after trauma was only modest (see Figure 1), this magnitude of AT activity depression is likely to be of clinical significance, because a decrease in AT activity to 70% of normal is sufficient to cause thrombosis in patients with congenital AT activity deficiency. Last, heparin works by binding to AT, so heparin's anticoagulant effects will be impaired in patients with depressed AT activity. In fact, because heparin exerts only a weak antithrombotic effect in the absence of AT, the effectiveness of low-dose heparin for DVT prophylaxis in trauma patients becomes problematic.

Thus, to me, the take-home message of this paper is that patients with major trauma who are at the highest risk of having thromboembolic complications must be assumed to have decreased levels of AT III activity. In this circumstance, the use of low-dose heparin regimens to prevent DVT and pulmonary embolus may not be effective, and more may be needed. In my opinion, more may mean the prophylactic placement of a Greenfield IVC filter (topic discussed in last year's selections [Abstract 4–10]).

E.A. Deitch, M.D.

Posttraumatic Inflammatory Response, Secondary Operations, and Late Multiple Organ Failure

Waydhas C, Nast-Kolb D, Trupka A, et al (Ludwig-Maximilians-Univ, Munich)

J Trauma: Injury Infect Crit Care 40:624–631, 1996 4–15

Introduction.—In patients with major orthopedic injuries, secondary surgery performed after primary stabilization of major fractures can lead to increased morbidity and mortality. Because the consequences of surgical trauma are similar to those of accidental blunt trauma, the secondary operations can be viewed as additional insults to an already injured patient.

Objective.—Secondary operations were studied as inflammatory insults contributing to the development of late multiple organ dysfunction in patients with multiple trauma. The study also sought to predict the risk of organ failure after secondary operations by evaluating the specific and nonspecific indicators of the inflammatory response.

Methods.—The prospective study included 106 severely injured patients, mean Injury Severity Score 41, who underwent secondary operations more than 3 days after their trauma. The secondary surgeries included facial reconstructions and osteosynthesis procedures of the pelvic girdle, long bones, and spine, among others. Routine and specialized laboratory studies were performed daily, along with clinical and cardiopulmonary assessments. The patients' preoperative level of inflammation was assessed and compared with the sequelae of the secondary surgical trauma.

Results.—The patients were divided into 2 groups, based on their course after the secondary operation. Group 1 included the 38% of patients who had respiratory, renal, and/or hepatic failure within 2 days after the secondary procedure, or had more than 20% worsening of their pre-existing organ dysfunction. The remaining 62% of patients, comprising group 2, recovered uneventfully. Preoperative neutrophil elastase level was 92 ng/dL in group 1 vs. 61 ng/mL in group 2. Significantly greater abnormalities in C-reactive protein, 12 vs. 8 mg/dL, and platelet count, 118,000 vs. 236,000/µL were also noted in group 1. Although the PO_2/FIO_2 ratio was also reduced in group 1, there were no significant differences in blood pressure, heart rate, bilirubin, creatinine, urinary output, lactate, pH, or coagulation. An increased state of inflammation was defined on the basis of the 3 most prognostically accurate parameters, namely a neutrophil elastase level of more than 85 ng/mL, a C-reactive protein level of more than 11 mg/dL, and a platelet count of less than 180,000/µL. This definition of increased inflammation was 79% accurate in predicting organ failure after the secondary operation, with a sensitivity of 73% and specificity of 83%.

Conclusions.—Secondary operations in severely injured patients do appear to act as secondary insults. If the patient has increased posttraumatic inflammation when the secondary operation is performed, it may lead to late multiple organ dysfunction syndrome. Waiting until inflammation has subsided to perform the operation, or opting for less invasive surgical procedures, could reduce the rate of postoperative organ failure. However, any such effect will have to be demonstrated in future studies.

► It is clear that some trauma patients deteriorate after secondary elective operations performed a few days after their injury, although most do not. Why is that, and can these patients be identified preoperatively? This clinical study suggests that patients with ongoing signs of systemic inflammation are at increased risk for the development of organ dysfunction or failure as compared with patients whose systemic inflammatory response has resolved. Based on this observation, the authors propose that the presence of persistent systemic inflammation primes these patients such that a subsequent operation may result in distant organ injury. Of interest, the magnitude of the secondary procedure as well as the magnitude of the pre-existing inflammatory state appeared to influence the likelihood of the patient developing organ dysfunction. That is, the 2 factors were additive in predicting the development of organ failure. Although further clinical studies will be required to verify these results, inasmuch as surgery causes an inflammatory response, I agree with the authors that major elective operations should be delayed (to the extent possible) until the injury-induced inflammatory response has abated in patients with persistent evidence of systemic inflammation.

E.A. Deitch, M.D.

Significance of NO in Hemorrhage-Induced Hemodynamic Alterations, Organ Injury, and Mortality in Rats

Yao Y-M, Bahrami S, Leichtfried G, et al (Ludwig Boltzmann Inst, Vienna)

Am J Physiol 270:H1616–H1623, 1996 4–16

Background.—It has been suggested that the vascular impairment which occurs during circulatory shock is caused by generation of elevated levels of nitric oxide (NO), which then leads to severe hypotension and loss of vascular responsiveness and eventually, to multiple organ failure. To examine the role of NO in the pathogenesis of hemorrhagic shock, the NO synthase inhibitor, N^G-monomethyl-L-arginine (L-NMMA) was administered to rats who had received a prolonged hypovolemic insult.

Methods.—Adult rats were bled until a mean arterial pressure of 30–35 mm Hg was attained and then maintained at that level for 180 minutes. After this shock period, their blood was returned, followed by resuscitation with Ringer lactate. The animals were then given 2.0 or 20.0 mg/kg of L-NMMA or saline and monitored for 2 hours.

Results.—Rats subjected to shock had significantly increased levels of endotoxin and tumor necrosis factor. Compared with the control animals, rats that received 2.0 mg/kg of L-NMMA had less of a decrease in mean arterial pressure, a significantly increased cardiac index and stroke volume, and were protected from multiple organ damage. The 48-hour survival rate was 26.7% in controls and 68.8% in the L-NMMA group. Rats that received 20.0 mg/kg of L-NMMA had a strong blood pressure response, but had a significant reduction in cardiac index and stroke volume and an increased total peripheral resistance index, with increased organ damage, as compared with the group that received 2.0 mg/kg of L-NMMA.

Conclusion.—Hemorrhagic shock in rats is associated with increased levels of endogenous endotoxin and tumor necrosis factor, which could be involved in increased production of NO. The NO induced by hemorrhagic shock in this rat model was an important mediator of the pathophysiologic changes associated with cardiovascular abnormalities, multiple organ dysfunction, and death. Control of NO generation and inhibition may provide new avenues of treatment for hemorrhage-related conditions. The NO synthase inhibitor, L-NMMA, may be clinically useful, but further research is necessary to clarify which doses are harmful and which beneficial to patients.

► This experimental dose-response study of inhibition of NO by L-NMMA in a model of hemorrhagic shock illustrates the delicate balance between the beneficial and deleterious effects of NO inhibition. At a lower dose (2 mg/kg) L-NMMA improved survival, supported myocardial performance, and limited organ injury, whereas at a higher dose (20 mg/kg) L-NMMA exacerbated the deleterious effect of hemorrhagic shock on myocardial function and potentiated organ injury.

Well, what might these results mean and why might they be important? The answer relates to the conflicting results reported by different investigators examining the potential role of NO in hemorrhagic shock–induced organ injury and mortality; that is, some investigators have found inhibition of NO protective and others have found NO inhibition harmful. Based on the biology of NO and studies such as this one, it appears that having some NO is good and having too much is bad. The trick, however, will be to apply this approach clinically, because one cannot easily determine the appropriate therapeutic dose window in patients. Nonetheless, this study does highlight the potential dangers of excessive as well as inadequate blockade of NO activity. The next logical step will be to determine whether a therapeutic range of NO blockade can be defined in patients.

E.A. Deitch, M.D.

Mechanism of Immunosuppression in Males Following Trauma-Hemorrhage

Wichmann MW, Zellweger R, DeMaso CM, et al (Michigan State Univ, East Lansing; Brown Univ, Providence, RI; Rhode Island Hosp, Providence)

Arch Surg 131:1186–1192, 1996 4–17

Background.—Hemorrhagic shock has been shown to depress immune function. Gender differences have also shown up in studies involving animal models of susceptibility to and morbidity from sepsis. In normal males and females, the absence of immunosuppressive androgenic hormones has been shown to improve immune function. The effect of castration on cell-mediated immune functions of male mice after trauma-hemorrhagic shock and soft-tissue trauma was investigated.

Methods.—Seven-week-old male mice were castrated or sham-castrated 2 weeks before being bled through the femoral artery with and without midline laparotomy. Sham-operated animals underwent the same procedure except that they were not bled and received no soft-tissue injury. Bled mice were reinfused with their own blood. Animals were killed at the same time and bled via cardiac puncture. Plasma hormone levels were measured, splenocytes were prepared, and lymphokine release was assessed.

Results.—Splenocyte proliferation and interleukin-2 and interleukin-3 release were similar for the castrated trauma-hemorrhage and sham groups but were significantly depressed for the sham-castrated, soft-tissue trauma and hemorrhagic mice compared to the sham-operated mice. Plasma corticosteroid levels were significantly increased in castrated and sham-castrated mice after trauma-hemorrhage. Plasma testosterone levels were undetectable in castrated, trauma-hemorrhagic mice, whereas testosterone levels were similar in sham-castrated, sham-operated, and trauma-hemorrhagic mice.

Conclusion.—Androgen depletion in castrated, trauma-hemorrhagic mice appears to have a beneficial effect on impaired immune function. Use of agents inducing temporary androgen depletion may prove equally beneficial in trauma patients and may also render them less susceptible to septic infection. Additional studies are necessary to study the effects of pharmacologic depletion of testosterone in patients with soft-tissue injury and hemorrhage.

▶ Although the exact clinical relevance of this experimental study remains to be established, I found the basic observations to be very interesting—that is, although popular lore has labeled women as the weaker sex, this article suggests that after trauma, this may not be true. In truth, excess testosterone not only may account for an increased incidence of trauma but also may suppress the immune response.

E.A. Deitch, M.D.

5 Infection

Introduction

Accurate data for postoperative wound infections (preferably called surgical site infections) are becoming more difficult to obtain, as the article by Sands et al. (Abstract 5–1) demonstrates. With at least 50% of operations currently being performed on outpatients and with earlier patient discharge of hospitalized patients, the great majority of infections occur in the outpatient setting. Detecting these infections to determine accurate wound (surgical site) infection rates is difficult and extremely costly. Since the infections may not occur until patients return to their surgeons' offices, one must rely on surgeons to report postoperative infections or have the ability to perform costly surveillance. With sanctions taken against those who have wound infections (perhaps by not being given contracts with managed care organizations or being removed from panels of HMOs, etc.), it is in the surgeon's economic self-interest to try to report as few postoperative infections as possible. It is unlikely that data as good as those previously obtained when patients stayed in hospitals longer will ever be collected again.

The *New England Journal of Medicine* publication by Kurts et al. (Abstract 5–2) demonstrated that patients who are maintained as normothermic as possible have lower wound infection rates than those who become hypothermic during colorectal procedures. Anesthesiologists and surgeons should try to keep their patients as normothermic as possible, not only because it reduces wound infection rates but also because it affects a wide variety of physiologic functions.

Physicians are interested in determining how "fit" patients are in order to predict outcomes and to enable comparison with the very ill so that experimental interventions can be compared. Although many scoring systems have evolved and have similar predictability, none has the patient base behind it that the Acute Physiology and Chronic Health Evaluation (APACHE) scoring system does. Zimmermann et al. (Abstract 5–3) used a third iteration of the APACHE system to compare patients with multiorgan system failure or dysfunction. A version of this APACHE system is now commercially available, so the APACHE score of ICU patients can be compared with that of a reference group and a prediction of mortality made. While any scoring system, the APACHE III included, can predict within a broad range the likelihood of mortality, it should not be used for withholding therapy because it is still too insensitive.

Several papers are reviewed that deal with intra-abdominal infection. This is a continuing challenge to physicians in all specialties despite modern antibiotic therapy and surgical treatment. The first article by Baron et al. (Abstract 5–4) discusses endoscopic management of pancreatic necrosis. Necrotic collections were successfully drained without surgery in 9 of 11 patients. However, there were 5 patient-related complications, including 4 patients who had procedure-induced infection. Some nonsurgical groups are even beginning to treat pancreatic abscesses with antibiotics alone. While there are some suggestions of early success, the long-term effects of this therapy remain to be determined. Certainly, this most difficult of infections, infected pancreatic necrosis, should be regarded as a surgically treated disease until it is firmly established that other alternatives might be beneficial. The article by Baron et al. included only patients who were not infected at the time they were entered into this study. We should proceed cautiously with any nonoperative or endoscopic treatment of these seriously ill patients if there is any thought that the patients are infected.

The article by van der Vliet et al. (Abstract 5–6) demonstrates that bacteria can be cultured from abdominal aortic aneurysms. Although this finding has been known for quite some time, the paper was included to re-emphasize that it still remains true. While bacteria can frequently be cultured from aneurysms, they are seldom responsible for postoperative infections of prosthetic grafts.

Probably few surgeons have seen a case of abdominal tuberculosis. The resurgence of pulmonary tuberculosis is due to a large susceptible population (in such patients as those with AIDS and increased use of therapies that suppress the immune system). It is not surprising that abdominal tuberculosis should be making a resurgence. Ko et al. (Abstract 5–7) discuss the clinical findings in 7 patients with abdominal tuberculosis in Los Angeles, California. It is important that surgeons be aware of this diagnostic possibility and that it be treated promptly.

A change in trends in the treatment of hepatic abscess is discussed by Huang et al. (Abstract 5–8). There was an increase in the use of percutaneous drainage in the treatment of hepatic abscesses over the period studied. Better recognition and prompt treatment and antibiotic therapy have resulted in a sharp decrease in mortality rates, especially when multiple abscesses are present.

A most vexing problem, treating peritonitis in critically ill patients, is discussed by Anderson et al. (Abstract 5–9). Many surgeons may be reluctant to operate on extremely critically ill patients, especially those with recurrent abdominal sepsis, because of the high mortality rate. More often than not, these patients are too sick not to be operated on. Despite the adverse circumstances, 32% of the patients survived the operations and were able to leave the hospital. The effect of age on the severity of peritonitis is discussed by Watters et al. (Abstract 5–10).

Hepatitis C is more common than hepatitis B, is not prevented by vaccination, and is currently incurable, although certain cases can be treated by interferon-α. Hepatitis C can lead to chronic liver disease and may lead to cirrhosis and liver failure. The study (Abstract 5–11) investigating the use of immunoglobulin to prevent experimental hepatitis C found that hepatitis C immunoglobulin was able to prolong the incubation period but did not prevent or delay infection. Thus surgeons must be sure to adhere to universal precautions to prevent themselves from being infected with this potentially nosocomial infection.

Because of the multiple bacteria associated with intra-abdominal infections and the inability of many hospital laboratories to routinely culture all bacteria, some physicians have questioned the practice of obtaining specimens for culture at all. They maintain that all patients should be treated with broad-spectrum antibiotics. Therefore, performing cultures is unnecessary. Christou et al. (Abstract 5–12) make a strong case for obtaining intraoperative cultures.

Nosocomial infections are especially common in the ICU. Flaherty and Weinstein (Abstract 5–13) attribute inappropriate prescribing of antibiotics as a major contributor to the increase in nosocomial infections caused by antibiotic-resistant bacteria. Although increased resistance is frequently ascribed to increased use of antibiotics, there are really no data that support this claim. The article discusses means that might be used to decrease antimicrobial resistance in ICUs. Some studies demonstrate that fewer than half the hospital personnel wash their hands after examining patients in the ICU. The worst offenders are physicians. Preventive measures such as barrier precautions and hand washing can greatly decrease the spread of infections in the ICU.

Richard J. Howard, M.D., Ph.D.

Surgical Site Infections Occurring After Hospital Discharge

Sands K, Vineyard G, Platt R (Brigham and Women's Hosp, Boston; Harvard Med School, Boston; Harvard Pilgrim Health Care, Boston)

J Infect Dis 173:963–970, 1996 5–1

Introduction.—Rates of postoperative surgical site infection (SSI) are used by hospitals as a quality indicator to guide quality improvement efforts. No reliable method has been established to determine the actual rate of postoperative SSIs in patients after discharge. Most hospitals rely on responses to questionnaires mailed to either surgeons or patients. It is not known whether the reliability of these questionnaires has been rigorously tested. Little information exists regarding resource utilization for postdischarge SSIs. Records from a health information organization with automated hospital and postdischarge data was reviewed to determine utilization of postdischarge medical encounters and prescriptions and performance of mailed patient and surgeon questionnaires.

Methods.—A total of 5,572 nonobstetrical surgical procedures were screened for coded diagnoses, tests, and prescriptions. Data were gathered for all hospital and postdischarge encounters in this patient cohort. Pa-

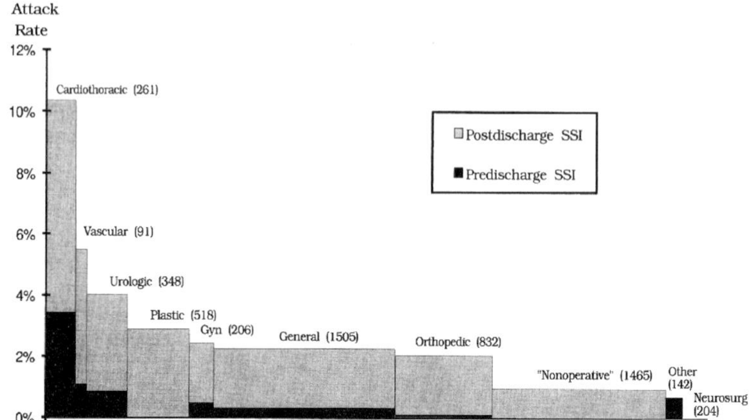

FIGURE 2.—Predischarge (*solid*) and postdischarge (*shaded*) surgical site infection (*SSI*) rates in 10 surgical procedure categories. Numbers in parentheses are total number of procedures in category; width of each column is proportional to total number of procedures. Thus, the area of each column reflects proportion of total number of SSIs occurring in that category. *Abbreviations: Gyn*, gynecology; *neurosurg*, neurosurgery. (Courtesy of Sands K, Vineyard G, Platt R: Surgical site infections occurring after hospital discharge. *J Infect Dis* 173:963–970, copyright 1996, University of Chicago.)

tients and their surgeons were mailed questionnaires about the occurrence of SSIs.

Results.—A total of 27 SSIs occurred during hospitalization, and 111 (83%) occurred after discharge (Fig 2). Seventy postdischarge infections (63%) were diagnosed and treated outside the institution at which surgery was performed. Follow-up care of the 111 postdischarge SSIs consisted of 37 visits to an emergency department, 37 hospitalizations, 202 scheduled clinical visits, 117 home care visits, and 155 nonappointment encounters. The average number of additional ambulatory and emergency department visits for patients with postdischarge SSIs was 4.6. Questionnaire response rates were 33.4% for patients and 79% for surgeons. Questionnaires had a sensitivity rate of 28% for patients and 15% for surgeons.

Conclusion.—The occurrence of SSIs after discharge is significantly greater than that of SSIs during hospitalization. Postdischarge infections are associated with considerable morbidity and resource utilization. It has been estimated that the cost of surveillance is about one fifth that of treating preventable infections. Findings indicate that mailed questionnaires are an unreliable source of information about postdischarge SSIs. Better methods of screening high-risk patients are needed.

▶ This is as good a study as one could possibly do to identify SSIs that occur after discharge. With the current emphasis on early discharge, most SSIs occur after discharge. In fact, this study found that 84% occurred after hospital discharge and that 63% were managed outside the surgical facility. The authors could do this thorough study because all hospital and outpatient records were contained on a standardized computer database consisting of records from a large HMO. Posthospital SSI surveillance is expensive. In general, 3 methods have been used: questionnaires mailed to patients and physicians, telephone calls to patients and physicians, and review of physician's records. The authors did not investigate the use of telephone calls. They did demonstrate that return of questionnaires was poor. Only 33.4% of patients returned questionnaires compared with 79% of surgeons. They also investigated various methods of detecting postdischarge SSIs for sensitivity. Reviewing the computerized database had the highest sensitivity, and reviewing questionnaires mailed to patients had the lowest. All methods had a low positive predictive value.

In the future, having a higher than expected number of SSIs may have severe consequences, such as lower referral rates or being removed from the panel of surgeons of an HMO or managed care organization. The "standard" for the expected rate of SSIs is generally derived from data provided by the Centers for Disease Control and Prevention (CDC). Surgeons reporting postdischarge SSIs may be unfairly penalized. Data provided by the CDC or gathered in other large studies generally have a low follow-up rate of posthospital discharge events. Furthermore, methods used after discharge were shown to have a low sensitivity. When you combine this with giving surgeons a real motivation for not reporting postdischarge SSIs, the quality of future data may be called into serious question.

R.J. Howard, M.D., Ph.D.

Perioperative Normothermia to Reduce the Incidence of Surgical-Wound Infection and Shorten Hospitalization

Kurz A, for the Study of Wound Infection and Temperature Group (Univ of California, San Francisco)

N Engl J Med 334:1209–1215, 1996 5–2

Background.—Perioperative hypothermia of about 2°C less than the normal core body temperature occurs commonly in patients undergoing colonic surgery. Vasoconstriction and impaired immunity can result, increasing a patient's susceptibility to perioperative wound infections. Hypothermia may increase both susceptibility to surgical-wound infection and length of hospital stay.

Methods.—Two hundred patients undergoing colorectal surgery were studied. By random assignment, half received routine intraoperative thermal care, and half received additional warming. All received cefamandole and metronidazole. Their anesthetic care was standardized.

Findings.—More transfusions of allogeneic blood were needed in the patients assigned to hypothermia. Mean final intraoperative core temperatures were 34.7°C and 36.6°C in the hypothermia and normothermia groups, respectively. Nineteen percent of patients assigned to hypothermia and 6% assigned to normothermia had surgical-wound infections (Table 2). Patients in the hypothermia group had sutures removed 1 day later than those in the normothermia group. Hospital stays were prolonged by 2.6 days (about 20%) in patients assigned to hypothermia.

TABLE 2.—Postoperative Findings in the 2 Study Groups

Variable	Normothermia (N = 104)	Hypothermia (N = 96)	P Value
All patients			
Infection—no. of patients (%)	6 (6)	18 (19)	0.009
ASEPSIS score	7 ± 10	13 ± 16	0.002
Collagen deposition — µg/cm	328 ± 135	254 ± 114	0.04
Days to first solid food	5.6 ± 2.5	6.5 ± 2.0	0.006
Days to suture removal	9.8 ± 2.9	10.9 ± 1.9	0.002
Days of hospitalization	12.1 ± 4.4	14.7 ± 6.5	0.001
Uninfected patients			
No. of patients	98	78	
Days to first solid food	5.2 ± 1.6	6.1 ± 1.6	< 0.001
Days to suture removal	9.6 ± 2.6	10.6 ± 1.6	0.003
Days of hospitalization	11.8 ± 4.1	13.5 ± 4.5	0.01

Note: Plus-minus values are means ± standard deviation.

Conclusion.—In this study, forced-air warming combined with fluid warming maintained normothermia. Unwarmed patients had core temperatures of about 2°C less than normal. Perioperative hypothermia lasted for more than 4 hours, including the period decisive for establishing an infection.

▶ Letting patients get cold during operations is bad in a variety of ways. Here is yet another way. The authors demonstrate that hypothermic patients have a higher wound infection rate after colorectal surgery than patients who are maintained at a normal temperature. There are also other benefits to avoiding hypothermia. More collagen is deposited in normothermic patients, and the time to the first solid food, suture removal, and discharge from the hospital is shorter. The latter benefits accrue to normothermic patients even if they are compared with uninfected hypothermic patients. Thus, decreased hospitalization and earlier suture removal are not found in normothermic patients solely because they are less likely to be infected.

And yet there should be a word of caution. The wound infection rate in the hypothermic patients was 19%—much higher than the predicted rate and much higher than the reported wound infection rate in colorectal surgery of 5% to 10%. The authors attribute their high wound infection rate to the method they use for defining wound infections (different from that of the United States and Great Britain) and the fact that they consider all wounds draining pus that yield a positive culture to be infected, although some may have been of minor importance (I assume that by this they mean a small amount of purulent material draining around the skin suture, something that would not be counted as a wound infection in the United States or the United Kingdom).

R.J. Howard, M.D., Ph.D.

Severity Stratification and Outcome Prediction for Multisystem Organ Failure and Dysfunction

Zimmerman JE, Knaus WA, Sun X, et al (George Washington Univ, Washington, DC)

World J Surg 20:401–405, 1996 5–3

Background.—Multiple organ system failure or dysfunction (MOSF/MODS) continues to be an important cause of death and complications in hospitalized adults. Risk factors for MODS and hospital mortality were reviewed, and recent progress in predicting outcomes for individuals with MODS or MOSF was described.

Severity Stratification and Outcome Prediction for MOSF/MODS.—Infection, injury, inflammation, poor perfusion, and hypermetabolism are commonly associated with MODS/MOSF. Other risk factors for developing MODS/MOSF are delayed or inadequate resuscitation; persistent infectious or inflammatory focus; surgical "misadventure"; hematoma; age 65 years or older; previous organ dysfunction; steroid treatment; chronic health problems, such as alcoholism, malnutrition, diabetes, or cancer; and/or a serious physiologic abnormality at ICU admission. In the 1980s, the hospital mortality rate for patients who had a single organ system failure (OSF) that lasted more than 1 day approached 40%. For those who had 2 OSFs, it was 60%. However, the mortality rate among those who had 3 or more OSFs that persisted after 3 days has been decreased from 98% to 84% between 1982 and 1990. The major determinants of survival were extent of physiologic derangement, type of associated disease or injury, increasing age, and life-threatening comorbid conditions, which were also the main determinants of risk for MOSF. Outcome prediction based on a comprehensive evaluation of patient risk factors is a more sensitive, specific, and useful method of determining MODS than a simple count of OSF number and duration. Repeated assessment of risk factors during subsequent ICU days reflects complications and treatment response; therefore, daily outcome predictions are more precise than are estimates made on admission to the ICU.

Conclusions.—Multiple organ system failure or dysfunction accounts for a large proportion of deaths among patients in the ICU. More accurate predictions of survival in such patients will improve the ability to test new treatments, assess outcome changes over time, and evaluate the efficacy of supportive treatment.

▶ The Acute Physiology and Chronic Health Evaluation (APACHE) system for scoring patients in ICUs has now progressed through its third phase and is known as APACHE III. With its extremely large database, this scoring system has substantial data behind it. Dr. Knaus has commercialized a version of this scoring system that allows one to predict the likelihood of death of a patient in the ICU. The APACHE scoring system was developed to evaluate ICU patients but has been used to evaluate patients who have a variety of illnesses. In addition, it has frequently been used to assure comparable groups of patients treated by various modalities. Many other scoring systems are equally valuable in evaluating certain groups of patients. But none of the scoring systems has the large database behind it that the APACHE system does. It is disappointing that, despite the improved care in ICUs and the tremendous knowledge that has been gained during the past decade, the mortality rate of patients who have single or double OSF has not changed. In addition, the mortality rate of patients with 3 OSFs has decreased only modestly, from 98% to 84%. This paper is one of a published symposium on MOSF in the *World Journal of Surgery*. Readers are referred to the entire series of excellent reviews of this most intractable problem in surgery by world leaders on the subject.

R.J. Howard, M.D., Ph.D.

Endoscopic Therapy for Organized Pancreatic Necrosis

Baron TH, Thaggard WG, Morgan DE, et al (Univ of Alabama, Birmingham)

Gastroenterology 111:755–764, 1996 5–4

Background.—There is debate over how to manage extensive pancreatic necrosis as a complication of severe acute pancreatitis. Some studies suggest that surgical débridement is unnecessary unless infected necrosis is present, whereas other authors maintain that the necrotic areas should be débrided if the patient continues to be ill. The use of endoscopic drainage for patients with extensive, organized pancreatic necrosis was evaluated.

Methods.—Endoscopic drainage was attempted in 11 patients with organized pancreatic necrosis after severe acute necrotizing pancreatitis. All patients were persistently ill and had persistent or progressive pancreatic collections on serial imaging studies. The pancreatic necrosis was sterile in 8 cases and infected in 3. In all patients but 1, at least 50% of the pancreas was found to be necrotic on dynamic contrast-enhanced CT. The latter 8 patients in the series were treated prospectively on a standardized protocol. This group had an intrapancreatic nasobiliary lavage catheter placed into the collection along with 10F stents.

Results.—The necrotic collections were successfully drained without surgery in 9 of the 11 patients. Five patients had procedure-related complications, including 4 with procedure-induced infected necrosis. In 1 patient, bleeding precluded entry into the pancreatic collection. The patients required a mean of 2.7 endoscopic procedures for the collections to resolve. The intrapancreatic nasobiliary lavage catheter was left in place for a mean of 19 days, and the nonoperatively managed patients were in the hospital for a mean of 9 days. The patients were studied for a mean of 12 months. A pseudocyst developed in 1 patient and was successfully drained.

Conclusions.—For some patients with organized pancreatic necrosis after an episode of acute pancreatic necrosis, endoscopic drainage may be a viable treatment option. The endoscopic approach is ideal for patients with necrosis in the accessible central area. Placement of an intrapancreatic lavage catheter is an important part of treatment. Further study of endoscopic therapy for organized pancreatic necrosis is needed before it is adopted for clinical use.

▶ This is the first report treating pancreatic necrosis (3 cases of which were infected) with endoscopic transgastric drainage or transpapillary drainage. The surgeon may shudder to think that necrotic debris would be successfully removed by the rather small (10F) catheter used. By placing a 7F catheter for irrigation, however, as the authors did in 8 patients, they successfully treated 9 of 11 patients without operation. One patient also required percutaneous drainage.

This technique may gain increasing favor for treating this most serious condition (certainly, aggressive endoscopists will find out what the limits are). Because surgeons know that the amount of necrosis and abscess is frequently greater than that suspected by imaging techniques, certainly endoscopic drainage will not be applicable to many patients. Furthermore, the authors stress that patients must have the process ongoing for at least 4 weeks so that the mass is firmly adherent to the stomach. It is frequently the retroperitoneal or peripancreatic tissues that are necrotic, not the pancreas itself. Occasionally the surgeon cannot distinguish precisely what is necrotic even by looking at the area. It is difficult to conceive that this necrotic solid tissue would be successfully removed by a catheter. It is hoped that this technique be reserved, initially at least, for only a selected group of favorable individuals (how you make that selection, of course, is unclear) and that failure is recognized promptly so that surgical drainage can be done.

R.J. Howard, M.D., Ph.D.

Emergence of Antibiotic-resistant Bacteria in Cases of Peritonitis After Intraabdominal Surgery Affects the Efficacy of Empirical Antimicrobial Therapy

Montravers P, Gauzit R, Muller C, et al (Hôpital Bichat, Paris)

Clin Infect Dis 23:486–494, 1996 5–5

Background.—Postoperative peritonitis is associated with a high mortality rate and necessitates appropriate antimicrobial therapy. The effectiveness of antimicrobial therapy in patients with nosocomial infections who are already receiving antibiotic prophylaxis is unknown. The incidence of resistant bacterial strains in patients with community-acquired peritonitis who underwent reoperation and the effect of these resistant strains on empirical antimicrobial therapy on morbidity and outcome were discussed.

Methods.—Organisms were cultured from the blood and operation site of 100 patients (39 women), average age, 59 years, operated on for peritonitis that occurred after elective surgery. The empirical antibiotic regimens selected target at least 1 pathogen (Table 5).

Results.—Before the first surgery, 86 patients had received antimicrobial therapy for an average of 6 days. Peritonitis was diagnosed an average of 10 days after surgery. There were 250 strains isolated from peritoneal fluid, and positive blood cultures were obtained from 26 patients. One hundred resistant strains were found in 70 patients. The mortality rate in this group was 45%, significantly higher than the 16% mortality rate for patients with susceptible organisms. The 37 patients with more than 1 resistant strain had a significantly longer preoperative antibiotic prophylaxis period (7 vs. 4 days) and a significantly longer wait for reoperation (12 vs. 6 days) than did other patients. Patients who received inadequate antimicrobial therapy had significantly more reoperations than did patients who received adequate therapy (103 vs. 45) and had a significantly higher mortality rate (27 vs. 12). Changing the antibiotic regimen later in the course of treatment did not affect outcome for this group.

Conclusion.—The choice of initial empirical antimicrobial therapy affected outcome in patients with postoperative peritonitis. Changing therapy later in the course of treatment for those who did not respond did not change outcome.

▶ Despite apparently adequate empirical antimicrobial therapy in all 100 patients who had community-acquired peritonitis and in whom postoperative peritonitis developed, antimicrobial-resistant pathogens were recovered from 70 patients. Fifty-four patients were considered to have inadequate empirical therapy because 1 organism was not targeted by the initial antimicrobial therapy, and these patients had a poor outcome. It is difficult to attribute the poor outcome entirely to antimicrobial therapy, because many other factors also determine outcome. The groups were not controlled for type of surgery or surgical complications (anastomotic leaks, etc.). Certainly, technical factors play an extremely important role in patients' outcomes. The adequacy of antimicrobial therapy was only known in retrospect. For instance, in some cases, combinations of imipenem and aminoglycosides or piperacillin and aminoglycosides with or without a third antimicrobial agent were determined to be inadequate because at least 1 bacterium was not targeted.

The authors do not discuss what they would consider appropriate empirical coverage. Certainly most surgeons would regard piperacillin or imipenem and aminoglycosides with or without a third antibiotic as adequate empirical therapy. Unfortunately, by the time culture results and sensitivities are obtained, usually 48 hours after operation, it may be too late to alter the course of a patient's outcome by instituting antimicrobial coverage to which these bacteria are sensitive.

R.J. Howard, M.D., Ph.D.

TABLE 5.—Empirical Antibiotics Chosen for the Initial Management of 100 Cases of Postoperative Peritonitis

Empirical therapy	No. of patients	No. of patients for whom therapy was inadequate	Pathogens not targeted
Monotherapy	5	5	
Ticarcillin/clavulanic acid	2	2	*E. faecium,* methicillin-resistant staphylococci, *E. cloacae*
Imipenem	3	3	Methicillin-resistant staphylococci (n = 3), *E. faecium, Candida* species
Two-drug combination	68	38	
Aminoglycosides + amoxicillin/clavulanic acid	48	29	Methicillin-resistant staphylococci (n = 7), *E. faecium* (n = 2), *E. coli, K. pneumoniae* (n = 2), *Acinetobacter* species, *P. aeruginosa* (n = 11), *Candida* species (n = 13)
Aminoglycosides + piperacillin	6	1	*Candida* species
Aminoglycosides + imipenem	6	2	Methicillin-resistant staphylococci, *Candida* species
Other	8	6	*E. faecalis,* methicillin-resistant staphylococci (n = 3), *K. pneumoniae* (n = 3), *P. aeruginosa* (n = 3), *X. maltophilia, Candida* species
Triple-drug therapy	27	9	
Aminoglycosides + piperacillin + ornidazole	11	5	*E faecalis, E. faecium,* methicillin-resistant staphylococci, *P. aeruginosa, Acinetobacter* species, *K. pneumoniae*
Aminoglycosides + imipenem + vancomycin	6	1	*Candida* species
Aminoglycosides + cefotaxime + ornidazole	5	2	*P. aeruginosa* (n = 2), *Candida* species
Other	5	1	*P. aeruginosa, E. faecium*

(Courtesy of Montravers P, Gauzit R, Muller C, et al: Emergence of antibiotic-resistant bacteria in cases of peritonitis after intraabdominal surgery affects the efficacy of empirical antimicrobial therapy. *Clin Infect Dis* 23:486–494, copyright 1996, University of Chicago.)

Relevance of Bacterial Cultures of Abdominal Aortic Aneurysm Contents

van der Vliet JA, Kouwenberg PPGM, Muytjens HL, et al (St Radboud Univ, Nijmegen, The Netherlands)

Surgery 119:129–132, 1996 5–6

Background.—The relationship between the presence of bacteria in abdominal aortic aneurysm contents and subsequent vascular graft infection is not completely understood. Results of a retrospective study of the relevance of intraoperative bacterial cultures of abdominal aortic aneurysms to the occurrence of prosthetic graft infection after aneurysm repair were reported.

Methods.—Between 1987 and 1991, bacterial cultures were obtained from abdominal aortic aneurysms of 216 patients (29 female), aged 44 to 87, and analyzed retrospectively. Aneurysms had ruptured in 44 patients. The remaining 172 surgeries were elective. Prophylactic antibiotics were given to 213 patients.

Results.—At 30 days, 6.5% of patients who had elective surgery and 47.5% of patients with ruptured aneurysms had died. Bacteria were cultured from aneurysm contents of one fourth of all patients and one fourth of patients with ruptured aneurysms (Table 2). Infections developed in the grafts of 4 (1.9%) patients and were significantly more common in patients with positive cultures (5.5%). The same bacterial species was isolated from aneurysm contents and vascular prostheses in 2 patients, 1 of whom subsequently died as a result of multiple organ failure after graft removal.

Conclusion.—Development of graft infection does not appear to be related to bacteria cultured from abdominal aortic aneurysm contents.

TABLE 2.—Bacteria Cultured from Aortic Aneurysm Contents of 55 Patients

	No. of isolates	
Aerobic bacteria		
Staphylococcus species		34
S. epidermidus	26	
S. saprophyticus	4	
S. coagulase negative	3	
S. aureau	1	
Corynebacterium species		6
Streptococcus viridans		2
Listeria monocytogenes		1
Streptococcus hemolyticus, group B		1
Anaerobic bacteria		
Propionibacterium acnes		10
Gram-positive rods, not further identified		4
Peptostreptococcus		1
Total		59

Note: In 4 patients, 2 different species were cultured. (Courtesy of van der Vliet JA, Kouwenberg PPGM, Muytjens HL, et al: Relevance of bacterial cultures of abdominal aortic aneurysm contents. *Surgery* 119:129–132, 1996.)

Routine intraoperative cultures are not necessary unless signs of infection are evident.

▶ The study points out what several other studies have previously shown: Bacteria can frequently be cultured from the wall of aneurysms or from aneurysmal contents. Infection of aortic graft is extremely infrequent, and if infection occurs, it is unlikely to be caused by the bacteria cultured from the aneurysms. The rate of graft infection is no higher in patients who had positive cultures than in those who had negative cultures. Furthermore, all 4 patients in whom infections developed had other infections that might have been the source of infection in the graft. In only 2 patients were the bacteria cultured from the graft cultured from the infected prosthesis. One of these had an aortic duodenal fistula with other bacteria present as well. The other had a retroperitoneal infection with spondylodiscitis.

Most surgeons do not routinely culture aneurysms or their contents. The culture results are of little predictive value and only cause the surgeon to worry. The article demonstrates again that culturing aneurysms is unnecessary and ineffective in predicting graft infections. Culturing bacteria from aneurysms should also not be used as a reason to justify prolonged prophylactic antibiotic therapy.

R.J. Howard, M.D., Ph.D.

Abdominal Tuberculosis: The Surgical Perspective

Ko CY, Schmit PJ, Petrie B, et al (Univ of California, Los Angeles)

Am Surg 62:865–868, 1996 5–7

Introduction.—With the recent resurgence of pulmonary tuberculosis (TB), an increase in TB in abdominal and other extrapulmonary sites is predicted. Abdominal TB is often unrecognized until complications occur. The surgeon's role in its treatment is uncertain. An experience with the surgical management of abdominal TB was evaluated.

Methods.—The review included all patients with TB diagnosed between 1993 and 1995 at 2 hospitals: an urban county hospital and a tertiary referral center. The diagnosis of abdominal TB was made on the basis of acid-fast bacilli on tissue stains and/or culture. The available information—including data on the incidence, presentation, and outcome of abdominal TB—was analyzed to identify factors that might aid in prompt surgical diagnosis and treatment.

Findings.—Of 407 patients who received a diagnosis of TB, 7 had abdominal TB. All 7 patients—4 men and 3 women, average age 31 years—were seen at the county hospital. Two had HIV infection. All 7 patients were Hispanic, and all but 1 were recent immigrants. All patients had abdominal pain, and most had fever and substantial weight loss. No evidence of abdominal TB was observed on preoperative imaging studies; the diagnosis was suspected preoperatively in just 1 patient. Surgery was indicated by perforated viscus in 2 patients and by acute abdomen, small-bowel obstruction, colocutaneous fistula, pelvic neoplasm, and biliary colic in 1 patient each. In 6 patients, the diagnosis of abdominal TB was either made or strongly suspected in the operating room. The surgical specimen stained positive for acid-fast bacilli, and the patients were started on antituberculous chemotherapy after surgery. Four of the 5 non–HIV-infected patients were alive and well at 1 year's follow-up.

Conclusions.—The diagnosis of abdominal TB is delayed in most cases. There are intraoperative signs of abdominal TB that can lead to the correct diagnosis, with prompt initiation of appropriate medications. These signs include peritoneal studding with whitish-yellow plaques, matting and dense adhesions of thickened bowel walls, punctate lesions of caseating granulation tissue, and peritoneal or retroperitoneal lymphadenopathy.

▶ Turberculosis has increased in the United States because of the increased number of immunosuppressed patients and patients with AIDS. Only 2 of 7 patients with abdominal TB presented by these authors had HIV, however. The diagnosis is difficult to make preoperatively. Generally physical findings, clinical symptoms, and laboratory test results are seldom typical, and patients are operated on primarily for other abdominal problems. The authors diagnosed abdominal TB based on intraoperative findings (which can also be demonstrated laparoscopically), such as the presence of peritoneal studding with whitish-yellow plaques, matting of thickened bowel walls with dense adhesions, characteristic punctate lesions of caseating granulation tissue, and peritoneal or retroperitoneal lymphadenopathy often with fluctuance and central necrosis. Surgeons certainly should be aware of these findings so they will take appropriate cultures and send tissues for appropriate diagnostic studies with a resultant minimal delay in therapy.

R.J. Howard, M.D., Ph.D.

Pyogenic Hepatic Abscess: Changing Trends Over 42 Years

Huang C-J, Pitt HA, Lipsett PA, et al (Taichung Veterans Gen Hosp, Taiwan; Johns Hopkins Med Insts, Baltimore, Md; Univ of Michigan, Ann Arbor)

Ann Surg 223:600–609, 1996 5–8

Introduction.—Pyogenic hepatic abscess is a rare and highly lethal infection. The cause, diagnosis, bacteriology, treatment, and outcome of 233 patients with pyogenic hepatic abscesses were compared. Eighty patients were treated from 1952 to 1972, and 153 patients were treated from 1973 to 1993.

Methods.—The cause of each abscess was established for both time periods and assigned to 1 of 6 categories: 1, bile ducts; 2, portal vein; 3, direct extension; 4, blunt or penetrating trauma; 5, hepatic artery; and 6, obscure origin (Fig 1). Patients' charts were also reviewed for clinical features, results of radiography, laboratory data, and microbiologic data.

Results.—Between 1973 and 1993, hospital admissions for pyogenic hepatic abscess increased from 13 to 20 per 100,000. The most dramatic

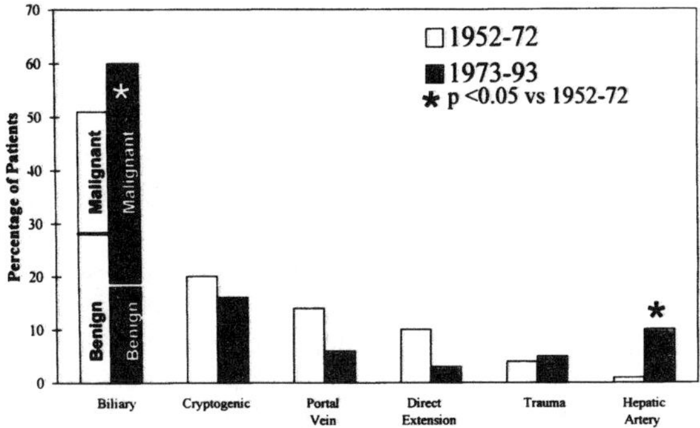

FIGURE 1.—Cause of pyogenic hepatic abscesses from 1952 to 1993. (Courtesy of Huang C-J, Pitt HA, Lipsett PA, et al: Pyogenic hepatic abscesses: Changing trends over 42 years. *Ann Surg* 223:600–609, 1996.)

change in the treatment approach between the 2 periods was the current use of percutaneous abscess drainage. This technique was not available before 1973; before that time, most patients received antibiotics alone. In the latter period, patients were more likely to have an underlying malignant condition. Most malignant conditions (81%) were hepatobiliary or pancreatic cancer. The most likely infecting organisms in the first time period were *Escherichia coli, Klebsiella*, and streptococci. In the second period, patients were significantly less likely to be infected by *E. coli* and more likely to be infected by *Klebsiella*, streptococci, fungi, and mixed bacteria. These dramatic changes may reflect the increased use of indwelling biliary stents. The appearance of fungi in abscess cultures is probably a result of the use of broad-spectrum antibiotics in patients with stents who have frequent episodes of cholangitis. In both periods, the anaerobes *Bacteroides*, clostridia, and streptococcal species were about equal. Overall mortality decreased from 65% in the first period to 31% in the second period. This reduction was greatest in patients with multiple abscesses (88% compared with 45%). Mortality for single abscesses decreased from 31% to 19%. Increased mortality in both time periods was associated with multiple abscesses, an associated malignant condition, jaundice, hypoalbuminemia, leukocytosis, bacteremia, and a significant complication. From 1952 to 1972, advanced age, biliary cause, elevated aspartate aminotransferase levels, and aerobic infection were also associated with increased mortality; these factors were not associated with increased mortality from 1973 to 1993. In the latter period, the mortality rate from surgical drainage was lower than that for percutaneous abscess drainage (14% compared with 26%).

Conclusion.—The incidence of pyogenic hepatic abscesses increased in the 1973 to 1993 period, most likely because of more aggressive approaches to the management of hepatobiliary and pancreatic neoplasms. The bacteriology of these abscesses has changed in the 2 periods, probably because of the use of biliary stents and the frequent use of broad-spectrum antibiotics. Better imaging and the development and use of percutaneous abscess and nonoperative biliary drainage have contributed to the significant reduction in mortality rates (65% compared with 31%). The mortality rate is still high and remains a diagnostic and therapeutic challenge.

▶ Hepatic abscess is an uncommon problem even at a large medical center. Fewer than 6 cases per year were seen over a 42-year period at Johns Hopkins Hospital, and only slightly more than 7 cases per year were seen over the past 21 years. It is gratifying that the rate of death from hepatic abscess has decreased, especially because these patients were more likely to have hepatic or biliary cancer as the associated disease responsible for their abscess. Also gratifying is the significant decrease in mortality in persons with several hepatic abscesses. No doubt there are numerous factors responsible for the decreased mortality rate. One might think that less use of surgery and greater use of percutaneous drainage for treating hepatic abscesses might be 1 reason for the decreased mortality rate in the recent 21-year period, and yet percutaneous drainage was associated with a higher mortality rate than was surgical treatment. The mortality rate in patients with a solitary abscess continues to be surprisingly high (20%). It may be that the underlying associated conditions are responsible for the continuing high mortality rate.

R.J. Howard, M.D., Ph.D.

Laparotomy for Abdominal Sepsis in the Critically Ill

Anderson ID, Fearon KCH, Grant IS (Western Gen Hosp, Edinburgh, Scotland)

Br J Surg 83:535–539, 1996 5–9

Introduction.—The problem of operating, sometimes repeatedly, on a patient with severe abdominal sepsis is the topic of considerable discourse, particularly in Germany, South Africa, and the United States. A recent report cited a 63% mortality rate for British patients with abdominal sepsis who required treatment in the ICU. The current surgical practice regarding further operation in patients with severe abdominal sepsis was reviewed to help determine operative outcome and evaluate the possibility of the adoption of alternative approaches.

Methods.—The medical records and surgical notes of 125 patients admitted to the ICU with severe abdominal sepsis were reviewed. Sixty patients (48%) underwent 95 laparotomies while in the ICU. The operations were classified as 1) 29 (31%) diagnostic, 2) 22 (23%) planned second look, or 3) 44 (46%) treatment.

Results.—Twenty-five patients (42%) survived laparotomy and could leave the ICU. Of these, 19 (32%) survived and could leave the hospital. Mean age of survivors and nonsurvivors was 61 and 70 years, respectively. Mean age of the 60 patients undergoing laparotomy while in the ICU was 67 years. The Acute Physiology and Chronic Health Evaluation II score at admission was 24 and was lower in survivors (21) than nonsurvivors (25).

A patient's chances of survival decreased as the number of operations after admission to the ICU increased. Patients with localized sepsis had a better outcome for all operations in the ICU and the first procedure alone than patients with generalized peritonitis (Fig 2). Eighty-one operations (85%) were considered therapeutic and resulted in drainage of pus or removal of dead tissue. The likelihood of success in sepsis clearance decreased as the number of operations in the ICU increased. Forty-one operations (43%) resulted in patient improvement within 24 to 48 hours. Patients had little chance of survival if they did not improve after their first operation. Twenty-one of 26 patients who improved after the first ICU operation left the ICU compared with only 3 of 33 patients who did not improve after the first operation. Only 2 patients with more than 2 operations while in the ICU survived to leave the hospital. Sepsis was cleared from the abdomen in 37 patients (62%). Of these, 23 (62%) survived. No patients survived to leave the hospital if sepsis could not be cleared surgically. The likelihood of surgically clearing sepsis decreased as the number of operations increased. Further surgery was needed more often in surgeries considered to be "treatment," than in those considered to be "diagnostic" or "planned second look." Pus or ischemic tissue was frequently observed during "diagnostic" and "second look" operations, suggesting that more "second look" operations should be considered. "Diagnostic" procedures were sometimes final attempts to determine a treatment approach and were associated with a worse survival compared with the other 2 types of surgeries.

Conclusion.—The need for adequate surgical treatment is crucial for survival in critically ill patients with abdominal sepsis. Survival decreased

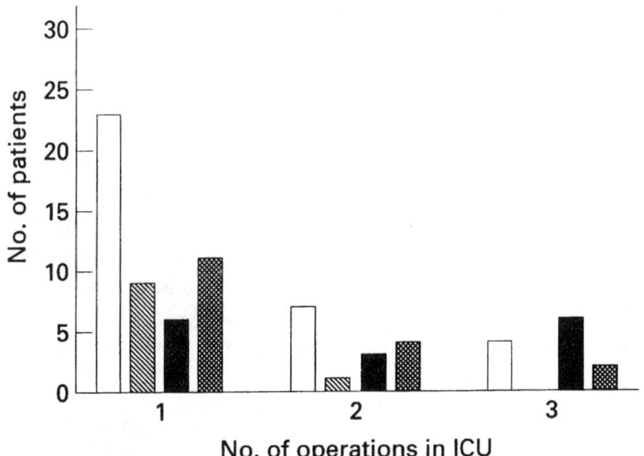

FIGURE 2.—Comparison between patients with localized and generalized sepsis at each operation and ultimate survival. Patients with localized sepsis had a better outcome overall ($P = 0.002$, Mantel-Haenszel summary test) and during the first procedure alone ($P = 0.03$, Fisher's exact test). *Cross-hatched box*, localized (alive); *solid box*, localized (dead); *Diagonal box*, generalized (alive); *empty box*, generalized (dead). (Courtesy of Anderson ID, Fearon KCH, Grant IS: Laparotomy for abdominal sepsis in the critically ill. *Br J Surg* 83:535–539, 1996.)

as the number of surgeries increased, indicating that alternative surgical strategies need to be considered.

▶ Despite improved postoperative physiologic support, better operative techniques, and effective antibiotic therapy, the mortality rate of peritonitis continues to be high, especially in older patients. This study demonstrates that many patients require repeat operations, although survival is generally highest in patients who need only 1. Because the mortality rate of recurrent peritonitis is so high, some surgeons have advocated planned laparotomy or Etappanlavage (the most ardent enthusiasts have been German) for all patients with peritonitis. Yet, subjecting all patients to relaparotomy would mean that many patients have unnecessary operations. In this series, pus was drained or dead tissue removed in 85% of reoperations. If we performed planned relaparotomy only on selected patients, what should the selection criteria be? If we wait until there are clear indications for relaparotomy, patients would frequently have multisystem organ failure or advanced recurrent peritonitis. Mortality rates are extremely high. Hopefully, this dilemma will be in part resolved during the next several years. Some surgeons have tried to organize a randomized trial. Despite the difficulty involved in coordinating such a trial, one is sorely needed.

R.J. Howard, M.D., Ph.D.

The Influence of Age on the Severity of Peritonitis

Watters JM, Blakslee JM, March RJ, et al (Univ of Ottawa, Ont, Canada)

Can J Surg 39:142–146, 1996 5–10

Background.—Mortality in all forms of surgical illness—including intra-abdominal infections—increases with advancing age. Previous studies have suggested that the local and systemic effects of peritonitis may be different in elderly vs. younger patients. The effects of age on the clinical appearance of peritonitis were evaluated in a retrospective study.

Methods.—The review included 2 groups of patients with abdominal infections seen at a university hospital: 122 patients with acute appendicitis and 100 patients with acute colonic diverticulitis that required surgery or percutaneous drainage. In addition to patient age and sex, the variables analyzed included the presence of perforation or gangrene, the extent of diverticulitis, the duration of symptoms before admission, the leukocyte count on admission, the length of hospitalization before surgery, the total length of hospital stay, and mortality.

Results.—Among the patients with appendicitis, gangrene or perforation was 3 times more frequent in those aged 65 years or older (Table 1). Similarly, generalized peritonitis was 3 times more likely for older patients with perforated diverticulitis. In both groups, the older patients were much more likely to have advanced or severe disease.

Conclusions.—Older patients with appendicitis and diverticulitis are more likely to be seen with advanced or severe disease than are younger

TABLE 1.—Data on 122 Patients With Pathologically Proved Appendicitis

Data	Age group < 65 yr, $n = 96$	≥ 65 yr, $n = 26$
Age, yr		
Mean (SD)	29 (12)	73 (6)
Range	14–63	65–93
Sex, M/F	39/57	20/6*
Gangrenous or perforated appendix, No/Yes	75/21	14/12†
Mean (SD) duration of symptoms before hospitalization, h		
All patients	25 (23)	37 (24)†
Nongangrenous, nonperforated appendix	18 (14)	26 (14)
Gangrenous and/or perforated appendix	48 (31)	49 (27)
Mean (SD) duration of hospitalization before operation, h		
All patients	8 (7)	6 (3)
Nongangrenous, nonperforated appendix	8 (6)	6 (3)
Gangrenous and/or perforated appendix	9 (10)	6 (4)
Mean (SD) leukocyte count, $\times 10^9$/L		
All patients	14.3 (4.2)	12.8 (4.1)
Nongangrenous, nonperforated appendix	13.9 (3.7)	13.8 (3.0)
Gangrenous and/or perforated appendix	15.5 (5.5)	11.8 (5.0)

*$P < 0.01$.
†$P < 0.05$ vs. age < 65 yr.
(Reprinted by permission of the publisher from Watters JM, Blakslee JM, March RJ, et al: The influence of age on the severity of peritonitis. *Can J Surg* 39:142–146, 1996.)

patients. The results support the hypothesis that the biological features of peritonitis are different in the elderly. If so, studies to find out the reasons for such a difference could lead to improved care for elderly surgical patients with abdominal infections.

▶ Many surgeons believe that virtually any pathologic process is more severe in the elderly. Other reports have indicated that appendicitis tends to be more advanced in older patients. This is 1 of few papers that directly compares younger and older patients, demonstrating that the clinical impression previously espoused is valid. There are many reasons why peritonitis in these 2 conditions may be more advanced in older patients, many of which are discussed by the authors. The clinical manifestations of the acute abdomen may be different in the elderly. Additionally, old patients may not express pain as acutely as young patients, and may allow pathologic process to progress before they seek medical attention. The authors hypothesize that anatomical changes that occur in the appendix with aging such as vascular sclerosis, diminished blood supply, narrowing of the lumen, fibrosis of the muscularis, and fatty infiltration may account for the more rapid advance from simple obstruction to gangrene and perforation. However, their data indicate that the period between onset of symptoms and surgery was prolonged in older patients, not that the rate of evolution of appendicitis was altered. They tend to discount the belief that anatomical changes contribute substantially to the more advanced presentation of appendicitis in older patients, and they do not discuss the possibility that older patients respond to initial bacterial challenge differently from younger patients. A slower progression of the inflammatory response may contribute to a less effective control of the infection with the resulting advanced presentation. If the inflammation response procedes more slowly in older patients, there may be less effective control of the infection with the resulting advanced presentation.

R.J. Howard, M.D., Ph.D.

Effect of Immune Globulin on the Prevention of Experimental Hepatitis C Virus Infection

Krawczynski K, Alter MJ, Tankersley DL, et al (Ctrs for Disease Control and Prevention, Atlanta, Ga; Food and Drug Administration, Rockville, Md; Chiron Corp, Emeryville, Calif)

J Infect Dis 173:822–828, 1996 5–11

Background.—Although several researchers have studied the value of immunoglobulin prophylaxis against post-transfusion non-A, non-B hepatitis, differences in methodology make the results difficult to interpret. The efficacy of postexposure prophylaxis against hepatitis C virus (HCV) infection was assessed in experimentally infected chimpanzees.

Methods.—Three animals were inoculated with HCV. One hour after inoculation, 2 were treated with anti-HCV–negative IV immunoglobulin (IGIV) or hepatitis C immunoglobulin (HCIG). The third chimpanzee was not treated.

Findings.—All 3 chimpanzees had HCV infection within a few days of inoculation. After levels of passively transferred anti-HCV decreased in the animals given HCIG, levels of HCV antigen–positive hepatocytes increased, followed by a reappearance of anti-HCV. Hepatitis C virus antigen disappeared as acute hepatitis developed. Acute hepatitis C developed in all chimpanzees. Liver enzyme activity peaked on day 59. In the HCIG-treated animals, however, peak liver enzyme activity was delayed until day 146.

Conclusions.—Although postexposure HCIG treatment substantially prolonged the acute hepatitis C incubation period, it did not prevent or delay HCV infection. The course of HCV infection was unaffected by IGIV.

► With an estimated 3.9 million Americans infected, HCV infection is even a greater risk to surgeons than are hepatitis B or HIV. With hepatitis B, 5% of infected individuals become chronic carriers; however, virtually all HCV-infected individuals have life-long infection. Further, HCV-infected surgeons can pass the infection to their patients and, therefore, may have their operating privileges curtailed. Yet, unlike hepatitis B infections, for which a vaccine is available and hepatitis B immunoglobulin can prevent infection after exposure, there is no hepatitis C vaccine. In addition, immunoglobulin and HCIG do not protect the individual from infection, although, as this study indicates, they can delay the onset of infection. Thus, the only way to prevent hepatitis C infection currently is by strict adherence to universal precautions and, most importantly, by avoidance of needle stick injuries.

R.J. Howard, M.D., Ph.D.

Management of Intra-abdominal Infections: The Case for Intraoperative Cultures and Comprehensive Broad-spectrum Antibiotic Coverage

Christou NV, and the Canadian Intra-Abdominal Infection Study Group (McGill Univ, Montréal; Universitè de Montréal; Univ of Toronto; et al)

Arch Surg 131:1193–1201, 1996 5–12

Background.—Intra-abdominal infections can be life threatening. When immediate antimicrobial therapy is necessary, the choice of drugs administered must be based on judgment. The results of a prospective, randomized, double-blind study of whether broad-spectrum or limited-spectrum therapy is preferable for intra-abdominal infections were reported.

Methods.—Patients from 10 centers across Canada were randomly assigned to receive either 2 g cefoxitin sodium IV every 6 hours (n= 109) or 0.5 g imipenem and 0.5 g cilastin sodium IV every 6 hours (n = 104), with either percutaneous or surgical drainage for as long as 21 days. Therapy beyond 21 days or death was considered treatment failure.

Results.—All patients had at least 1 organism cultured. Of the organisms isolated, 72% were susceptible to cefoxitin and 98% to imipenem. None of the *Pseudomonas aeruginosa* and 7% enterococci isolates were susceptible to cefoxitin, whereas 92% and 95% of those isolates were susceptible to imipenem, respectively. Only 15% of *Citrobacter* and 14% of *Enterobacter* species were susceptible to cefoxitin, whereas both of these species were susceptible to imipenem. Overall, 98% of isolates were susceptible to imipenem and 72% to cefoxitin. Treatment failures and mortality rates were similar for the 2 groups. There were 13 treatment failures in group 1; 5 were attributable to technical issues and 8 to antibiotic failure, including 12 patients who had resistant organisms at second intervention and 1 who died of imipenem- and cefoxitin-resistant *P. aeruginosa* infection. There were 9 treatment failures in group 2; 5 were attributable to technical issues and 4 to antibiotic failure, including 1 death of infections from cefoxitin-resistant *P. aeruginosa* and *Enterobacter cloacae*.

Conclusion.—Treatment failure in intra-abdominal infections is related to the presence of resistant bacteria at the site of infection. Comprehensive broad-spectrum antimicrobial therapy and routine culture are recommended.

▶ Other authors have reached the opposite conclusion: Routine operative culture of patients with peritonitis is worthless. All patients should be covered with broad-spectrum antibiotics and, therefore, culture results are irrelevant. Furthermore, many hospital laboratories cannot be expected to recover all organisms, especially anaerobes, from most cultures of patients with peritonitis. The results of this study indicate that treatment failures did not differ significantly whether limited-spectrum or broad-spectrum antibiotics were used, even though more resistant organisms were cultured from patients who had postoperative infections develop if they had received limited-spectrum antibiotics. The antibiotic spectrum did not affect the frequency of postoperative infection; it just selected whether the postoperative infections resulted from bacteria that were resistant to the limited-spectrum antibiotic. Furthermore, approximately half the patients in each group that developed treatment failures had technical problems or errors in clinical judgement that may have been as important in contributing to the postoperative infection as the spectrum of the antibiotic.

R.J. Howard, M.D., Ph.D.

Nosocomial Infection Caused by Antibiotic-resistant Organisms in the Intensive-care Unit

Flaherty JP, Weinstein RA (Univ of Chicago; Cook County Hosp, Chicago)
Infect Control Hosp Epidemiol 17:236–248, 1996 5–13

Background.—The development of resistant organisms propelled by inappropriate prescribing of antibiotics is a major contributor to the increase in nosocomial infections. Guidelines for avoiding and controlling resistance problems in ICUs are presented.

Guidelines for Prevention and Control.—Routine hospital monitoring, prospective microbiological surveillance, and susceptibility test profiles are important elements of prevention. When emerging resistance is found, infection control procedures, such as washing hands, wearing gloves, and isolation, need to be re-emphasized.

Alternative Approaches to Prevention.—Selective decontamination of ICU patients at risk of respiratory diseases, development of infection-resistant and less-invasive medical devices, and prompt removal of invasive devices can help to prevent colonization and subsequent infection. Use of noninvasive monitoring devices can also help decrease the risk of infection.

Conclusion.—Antimicrobial resistance is becoming an increasingly important problem in ICUs. Elements of an antibiotic control program are defined. Guidelines for prevention and control of antimicrobial resistance are included.

▶ The ICU is the main repository of antibiotic-resistant bacteria in any hospital. This article reviews this subject thoroughly. Some of the conclusions are not as clear as the authors might have them seem. Although antibiotic use clearly is associated with emergence of antibiotic-resistant organisms, it is not clear that the amount of antibiotics used is directly related to the emergence of resistance. It may be that underusing antibiotics (inadequate dosing) is as responsible as too much antibiotic use. Also not factored into the discussion is the low resistance of many patients in ICUs. The most susceptible hosts are generally found in ICUs. One strategy some have advocated to avoid emergence of resistant organisms is to rotate antibiotics. This approach received little attention in this article. Some centers have used antibiotic restriction, with approval required before the use of any antibiotics. Although this approach may reduce costs, there is little evidence that it leads to a decrease in resistant organisms. One step that is inexpensive and easy to do is to have more judicious attention to infection control practices. Hand washing is practiced by less than 50% of individuals in ICUs. Appropriate use of gloves and gowns also is seldom practiced appropriately in many ICUs.

R.J. Howard, M.D., Ph.D.

6 Transplantation

Introduction

This past year, authors of articles about transplantation have devoted themselves to further refinement of the field. Because of the great shortage of organs available for transplantation and the ever-expanding need, transplant surgeons have attempted to increase the use of available organs. Organs from donors previously thought not to be suitable for transplantation (expanded-criteria donors) have been successfully transplanted with good outcomes. Ratner et al. (Abstract 6–1) discuss the transplantation of kidneys from expanded-criteria donors. The use of expanded-criteria donors has allowed more kidneys to be transplanted. Perhaps the previous criteria were too conservative. Some surgeons are also using expanded-criteria donors for other organs as well, especially as liver donors. Another method to increase the supply potential is to use 1 liver for 2 donors (split liver transplantation as discussed by Rogiers et al. [Abstract 6–2]). In this technique, the left lateral segment is generally used for a pediatric recipient and the rest of the liver can be used for an adult recipient, thus allowing 2 recipients for each liver.

While modern immunosuppressive agents are very effective in preventing graft rejection and promoting long-term graft survival, they are associated with profound side effects and they are expensive. Steroids have many side effects that can frequently be debilitating and even lethal. To minimize the side effects, most transplant surgeons and physicians attempt to reduce steroid use to a minimum as early as possible. With newer immunosuppression agents, some physicians have tried to withdraw steroid treatment altogether. Two trials are reported this year: 1 in liver transplant recipients and 1 in kidney transplant recipients (Abstracts 6–3 and 6–4). Steroid withdrawal will hopefully minimize or eliminate many side effects of this agent, and the use of new immunosuppressive drugs will, we hope, not result in increased rejection or decreased graft survival.

In an attempt to improve graft survival, possibly with the decreased use of immunosuppressive drugs, physicians have been combining kidney transplants with donor bone marrow. The latter practice stems from the experimental demonstration that donor bone marrow administration can improve graft survival in experimental animals and from the demonstration of microchimerism in solid organ transplant recipients. Shipiro et al. (Abstract 6–5) demonstrate with a small group of patients that kidney transplantation combined with bone marrow transplantation does not lead to any deleterious effects. Although in a preliminary report there was no increase in graft survival, it may have been too early to demonstrate any effectiveness of bone marrow transplantation. Furthermore, the groups reported were rather small. Hopefully, subsequent studies will demonstrate efficacy of this technique.

Not so recently, portal vein thrombosis was considered a contraindication for liver transplant patients. Seu et al. (Abstract 6–6) report successful transplantation in a large number of patients who had portal vein thrombosis. While the complication rate is high and graft survival is not as good as in those who did not have thrombosis, this problem is no longer a contraindication to liver transplantation.

Gane et al. (Abstract 6–7) discuss the long-term outcome of hepatitis C infection after liver transplantation. Although the recurrence rate is extremely high, evidence of end-stage liver disease develops in only a few patients. The authors suggest that certain strains of the virus may be associated with a worse outcome. Van Twuyver et al. (Abstract 6–10) discuss changes in T-cell responses in patients with long-term kidney and renal allografts. They find certain differences in recipients of kidneys and livers, thus suggesting that patients respond differently to organ allografts.

Survival among elderly patients with end-stage renal disease is described by Schaubel et al. (Abstract 6–11). Although older patients die at a higher rate than younger patients do, the results of dialysis in this age group are continuing to improve, especially in those who are not diabetic and do not have co-morbid conditions.

Mycophenolate mofetil was used to prevent acute rejection in cadaveric renal transplant patients by the Tri-continental Mycophenolate Mofetil Renal Transplant Study Group (Abstract 6–12). It is difficult to show that a new drug will improve graft survival because current survival rates are so good. The use of mycophenolate mofetil, however, may enable other drugs, especially prednisone, to be decreased after transplantation.

Rehabilitation of patients with end-stage renal disease is a goal of transplantation. Matas et al. (Abstract 6–13) discuss employment patterns after successful kidney transplantation. It is unfortunate that the authors found, as many programs are finding, that patients are discouraged from working because of the vagaries of the payment system. If patients return to work, they frequently lose benefits so that they no longer can afford immunosuppressive drugs.

Sorof et al. (Abstract 6–14) discuss the histopathologic concordance of renal allograft biopsy specimens. The authors find a significant error between different pathologists if only 1 sample is obtained in comparison to when 2 samples are obtained. This finding confirms what has been previously suggested, that is, rejection does not necessarily occur uniformly throughout the kidney.

Richard J. Howard, M.D., Ph.D.

Transplantation of Kidneys From Expanded Criteria Donors

Ratner LE, Kraus E, Magnuson T, et al (Johns Hopkins Bayview Med Ctr, Baltimore, Md; Johns Hopkins Univ, Baltimore, Md)

Surgery 119:372–377, 1996 6–1

Introduction.—Because of the acute shortage of kidneys available for transplantation, some centers have used expanded-criteria donors (ECDs). Data on this practice is limited. A 3½ -year retrospective review of patients from a single center was conducted to compare the outcomes of patients receiving grafts from ECDs with the outcomes of patients receiving grafts from conventional cadaveric donors (CD) and live donors.

Methods.—Outcomes of 105 kidney transplantations were reviewed: 44 patients with kidneys from ECDs, 45 with kidneys from CDs, and 16 with kidneys from live donors. Patients were treated with either triple or quadruple sequential immunosuppressive therapy. High-risk recipients rarely received kidneys from ECDs.

Results.—Recipient characteristics, cold ischemic times, degree of donor–recipient human leukocyte antigen mismatching, and length of follow-up were similar for patients in the ECD and CD groups. Of 44 kidneys procured from ECDs, 16 were from donors age 5 years or younger and 17 were from donors age 55 or older. Five older donors had hypertension, and 1 had diabetes. Three donors younger than 55 had hypertension. Three donors were seropositive for hepatitis C. Five kidneys were refused by other centers because the donors had prolonged hypotension, prolonged cardiopulmonary arrest, or non-beating heart. (Fig 1). The actuarial graft survival, incidence of delayed function, length of hospital stay, and hospital charges were similar for patients in the ECD and CD groups. Four of 7 of the urinary complications occurred in recipients of pediatric kidneys. No kidneys were lost because of urinary complications. About one fourth (21.5% of all transplantations) of all cadaveric trans-

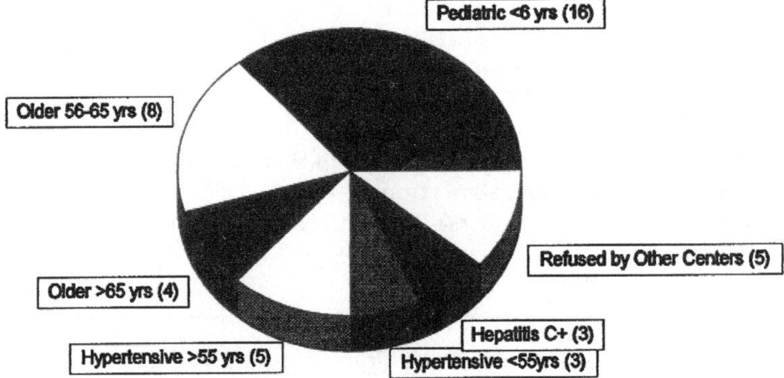

FIGURE 1.—Types of expanded-criteria donors used at Johns Hopkins Bayview Medical Center during a 3½ -year period. (Courtesy of Ratner LE, Kraus E, Magnuson T, et al: Transplantation of kidneys from expanded criteria donors. *Surgery* 119:372–377, 1996.)

plantations could not have been performed if acceptance criteria had not been liberalized.

Conclusion.—Kidneys from ECDs can be helpful in alleviating the critical shortage of kidneys needed for transplantation. The graft survival, morbidity, and cost are similar for ECDs and CDs as long as donors and recipients are properly selected. Organs from ECDs should be procured and available to centers willing to use them.

▶ The success of organ transplantation has created a tremendous shortage of cadaveric organs. Patients awaiting organ transplantation are added to the United Network of Organ Sharing waiting list at a far greater rate than the supply of cadaveric organs increases. Over the last 10 years, the number of cadaveric organs has increased only modestly. This disparity between patients awaiting transplantation and the organ supply is 1 of the main challenges currently facing the transplantation community. Many patients currently awaiting livers, hearts, and lungs will die for lack of suitable organs. Methods to alleviate this problem include recovering more of the possible cadaveric donors available (it is estimated that only one third of suitable cadaveric organs are recovered and used for transplantation), expanding the criteria of suitable donors, and using alternate donor supplies (living unrelated donors and xenografts).

This article demonstrates that organs previously thought to be unsuitable for transplantation can be successfully used and can achieve the same graft survival as "standard" donors. Because of the shortage in organs, many transplantation centers are already using expanded criteria donors. Several papers have demonstrated that use of kidneys from very young donors (< 5 years old) is associated with a reasonable graft outcome. In 1996, an article was published that showed that livers from donors older than 70 years can be safely used.[1]

R.J. Howard, M.D., Ph.D.

Reference

1. Emre S, Schwartz ME, Altaca G, et al: Safe use of hepatic allografts from donors older than 70 years. *Transplantation* 62:62–65, 1996.

One Year of Experience With Extended Application and Modified Techniques of Split Liver Transplantation

Rogiers X, Malagó M, Gawad KA, et al (Univ Hosp Eppendorf, Hamburg, Germany)

Transplantation 61:1059–1061, 1996 6–2

Background.—Current and future organ shortages pose a threat as the number of indications for organ transplantation increases. The use of split-liver transplantation (SLT) may be a reasonable strategy to optimize the use of existing donor organs. The results of SLT during a 1-year period were reported.

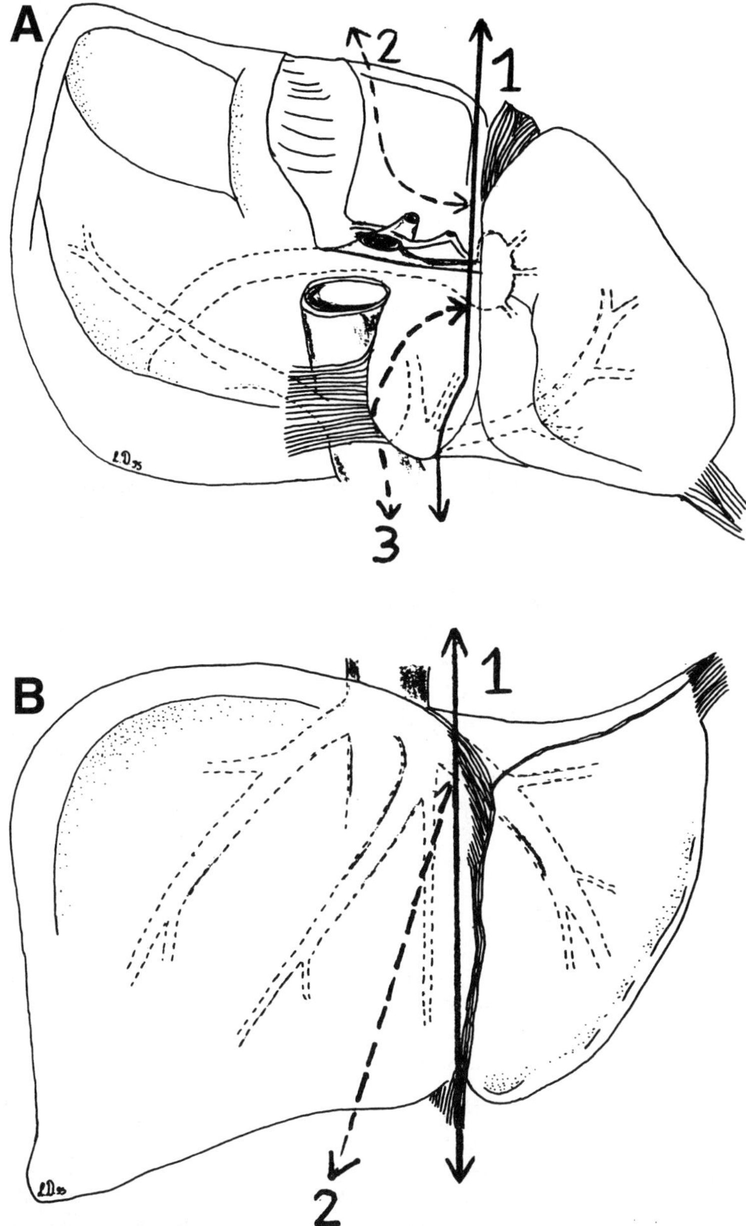

FIGURE 1.—(**A** and **B**), lines of transection in the new splitting techniques. The *numbers* show the sequence of the transections. *Transections 2* and *3* are facultative in the in situ technique. (Courtesy of Rogiers X, Malagó M, Gawad KA, et al: One year of experience with extended application and modified techniques of split liver transplantation. *Transplantation* 61(7):1059–1061, 1996.)

Methods.—During the study period, 73 cadaveric liver transplants, including 16 SLTs, were performed in 66 patients. Two new techniques were developed and used in 10 SLTs: in situ splitting (in which the liver was split while still in the donor) and second generation ex situ splitting (in which the liver was split after harvesting). Both techniques avoided dissecting the bile duct bifurcation and featured placing the primary parenchymal division at the level of the ligamentum falciforme (Fig 1).

Results.—In the patients who underwent SLT, the 3-month patient survival rate was 81.2%, and the 3-month graft survival rate was 75%. The right sides of splits resulted in a 66.6% patient survival rate and a 55.5% graft survival rate. The left sides of splits resulted in 100% patient and graft survival rates. When the new splitting techniques were used, both the graft and patient survival rates were 90%. Eight additional organ transplants were performed during the 1-year period with the systematic use of SLT with good quality organs.

Conclusions.—Split-liver transplantation can increase the usefulness of available grafts, with good graft and patient survival. The newly developed splitting techniques, particularly in situ splitting, prevent biliary complications. Further studies are needed to confirm the promising results of SLT.

▶ The critical shortage of organs, especially livers and hearts, means that many patients die while waiting for organs. Split-liver transplantation, i.e., the use of 1 liver for 2 recipients, is one of the techniques currently being used to increase the organ donor supply. (Other techniques include using living donors and extending the criteria for organ donors.) Like other recent reports, this article demonstrates that the results of SLT are comparable to those obtained with whole livers and reduced-size livers. This technique will undoubtedly be used more in the future to increase the donor supply.

R.J. Howard, M.D., Ph.D.

A Randomized Prospective Trial of Steroid Withdrawal After Liver Transplantation

McDiarmid SV, Farmer DA, Goldstein LI, et al (Univ of California, Los Angeles; Kaiser Permanente Med Group, Los Angeles)

Transplantation 60:1443–1450, 1995 6–3

Background.—Until recently, it was assumed that liver transplant recipients would have to take immunotherapy with cyclosporine and low-dose prednisone for the rest of their lives. However, because of the adverse effects of long-term steroid use, there is interest in the possibility of maintaining immunosuppression without steroids. Most studies of this issue have been performed in kidney and heart transplant recipients. A prospective, randomized trial of steroid withdrawal in liver transplant recipients was conducted.

Methods.—Sixty-four recipients of ABO-compatible orthotopic liver transplants (OLTs) were included: 42 adults and 22 children, all of whom had survived for at least 1 year after transplantation and had no episodes of rejection for more than 6 months after OLT. Those with previous graft loss after rejection, more than 2 episodes of rejection, OLT performed for autoimmune hepatitis, and inability to take azathioprine were excluded. The patients' target cyclosporine levels on high-performance liquid chromatography were in the range of 100–200 ng/mL. A mean of 3.5 years after transplantation, the patients were assigned to either steroid withdrawal (SW) or continued steroid administration. Both groups were monitored closely during follow-up, which averaged 592 days in the SW group and 527 days in the control group.

Results.—Two patients in each group had episodes of rejection, as confirmed by biopsy. The patients from the SW group were successfully treated by restarting oral prednisone. The patients from the control group required treatment with IV steroids or conversion to tacrolimus. From baseline to 12 months, the 2 groups showed no significant differences in dosage of prednisone, azathioprine, or cyclosporine; cyclosporine levels; liver function test results; or white blood cell counts. In the SW group, mean fasting serum cholesterol dropped from 194 to 175 mg/dL at 12 months. At the same time, cholesterol levels in the control group rose from 180 to 193 mg/dL. Among the children, there was no significant difference in age-adjusted height velocity over 1 year.

Conclusions.—This randomized trial demonstrates the feasibility of SW in OLT recipients. Immunosuppression can be maintained with azathioprine and cyclosporine, with no increase in the risk of rejection. The patients' lipid profiles may improve after SW. Steroid withdrawal requires close patient monitoring, and its long-term effects remain to be seen.

► Like the next article, Abstract 6–4, this study demonstrates that steroids can be withdrawn from selected recipients of orthotopic liver transplants without apparent adverse effect. Two patients in the SW group had biopsy-proved rejection, but so did 2 patients in the control group, who had steroids maintained. Perhaps significant is that only 64 of 181 liver transplant recipients asked to participate, agreed to do so. This study and the next one demonstrate that carefully selected patients can have their steroids sucessfully withdrawn. As newer immunosuppressive drugs become available, more patients may be able to have steroids successfully withdrawn.

R.J. Howard, M.D., Ph.D.

Randomised Controlled Trial of Steroid Withdrawal in Renal Transplant Recipients Receiving Triple Immunosuppression

Ratcliffe PJ, Dudley CRK, Higgins RM, et al (Churchill Hosp, Oxford, England)

Lancet 348:643–648, 1996 6–4

Background.—The combination of cyclosporine, azathioprine, and prednisolone is the most commonly used immunosuppressive regimen early after renal transplantation. However, the risks and benefits of con-

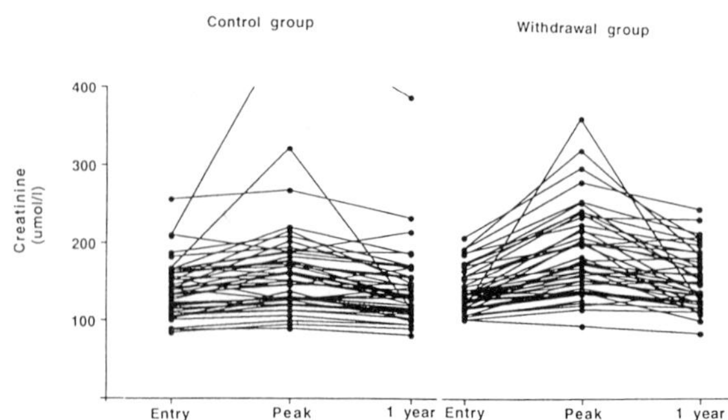

FIGURE 2.—Peak values of plasma creatinine for individual patients in the first year after randomization. (Courtesy of Ratcliffe PJ, Dudley CRK, Higgins RM, et al: Randomised controlled trial of steroid withdrawal in renal transplant recipients receiving triple immunosuppression. *Lancet* 348:643–648, copyright 1996 by The Lancet Ltd.)

tinuing steroid administration in the long term have not been well documented.

Methods and Findings.—One hundred renal transplant patients receiving triple immunosuppression were randomly assigned to prednisolone tapering to 0 over approximately 4 months or to no change in prednisolone. Complete steroid withdrawal was achieved in 86% of patients assigned to steroid withdrawal. Although these patients did not have defined acute rejection episodes, they did have insidious increases in plasma creatinine levels more often than did the patients in the control group. Ninety-seven patients were still alive 1 year after study enrollment. At some point during this first year, plasma creatinine values exceeded the baseline by more than 25% in 53% of the steroid-withdrawal group and in 18% of the control group (Fig 2). These increases were transient in some patients.

After correction for baseline value, there were significant differences between groups in both mean plasma creatinine values and mean creatinine clearance. Mean plasma creatinine values at entry, immediately after withdrawal, and at 1 year were 138, 151, and 150 µmol/L, respectively, in the steroid-withdrawal group, compared with 138, 140, and 139 µmol/L, respectively, in the control group. Patients in the steroid-withdrawal group had a further increase in mean plasma creatinine levels to 160 µmol/L at 2 years and 161 µmol/L at 3 years from study entry. Steroid withdrawal was associated with changes in several clinical and metabolic indices. Although blood pressure declined, the decrease was sustained incompletely, being more evident just after steroid withdrawal than at 1 year. Patients who underwent steroid withdrawal had a total cholesterol reduction of about 1 mmol/L. In addition, the white blood cell count and hemoglobin were reduced, and plasma phosphate and alkaline phosphatase values were increased.

Conclusion.—In most patients with stable graft function receiving triple immunosuppression, late steroid withdrawal is feasible. Although this may have beneficial metabolic effects, a substantial number of patients will have decreased graft function. Thus, caution is needed when considering long-term outcomes.

▶ Management of posttransplant immunosuppression is a constant balancing act. Too little immunosuppression and the patient rejects; too much, and the patient experiences the side effects of the medication. Prominent among the side effects are those caused by steroids. Therefore, studies have been conducted in an attempt to remove steroid therapy; these frequently have been met with acute rejection episodes and graft loss. This study from Oxford, England shows that by careful selection of patients who have maintained their grafts for at least 1 year, steroids can be slowly withdrawn without graft loss and with only a minimal risk of acute rejection. Nevertheless, steroid withdrawal was followed in this series by a modest rise in creatinine levels in a substantial number of patients.

The rise in creatinine values frequently took place insidiously over a few weeks. Such episodes of creatinine elevation were uncommon in control groups, indicating that the rise was caused by steroid withdrawal. Although in some cases, the creatinine value subsequently fell, this was not always so. It is hoped that the patients who were withdrawn from steroids will experience fewer long-term side effects of these medications without having decreased graft survival or increased rejection episodes.

It is to be hoped that the authors will present long-term follow-up data from this study so that we can assess whether the patients may pay a price in terms of graft survival over the long term. At least in the short term, steroid withdrawal seems to be safe in carefully selected patients.

R.J. Howard, M.D., Ph.D.

Combined Simultaneous Kidney/Bone Marrow Transplantation
Shapiro R, Rao AS, Fontes P, et al (Univ of Pittsburgh, Pa)
Transplantation 60:1421–1425, 1995 6–5

Introduction.—Microchimerism is present in kidney transplant recipients who have stable, long-term graft survival. Recent observations suggest that chimerism may be needed for successful long-term engraftment. The outcome of 36 patients undergoing combined kidney and bone marrow transplantation is reported.

Methods.—Six of the 36 patients received islets and 7 received a pancreas in addition to kidney and bone marrow transplantation. One patient received a kidney from a living-related donor and bone barrow (aspirated from the iliac crest) from a 1 haplotype-matched brother. Bone marrow for all other patients was recovered from the vertebral bodies of the donor. Mean recipient age was 39 years, and mean cadaveric donor age was 31.8 years. Twenty control patients underwent kidney transplantation alone. The most common reason these patients did not receive donor bone marrow was family refusal to give consent for vertebral body recovery. Three control patients also underwent pancreas transplantation. In the control group, mean recipient age was 47.9 years and mean donor age was 41.5 years. All patients received tacrolimus and steroids for immunosuppression. Induction antilymphocyte therapy, cytoreduction, and radiation therapy were not used. Before surgery and at regular intervals afterward, blood was drawn and evaluated for chimerism by fluorescent-activated cell sorter analysis and polymerase chain reaction.

Results.—The mean duration of follow-up was 11.1 months for all patients. No patients experienced graft-versus-host disease. Five (14%) and 3 (15%) patients in the kidney and bone marrow group and control group, respectively, received a diagnosis of cytomegalovirus infection; the infection responded to intravenous gancyclovir. Six (17%) patients in the kidney and bone marrow group and 4 (20%) patients in the control group experienced delayed graft function.

In the kidney and bone marrow group, all recipients were alive and 33 (92%) had functioning allografts. Three patients lost their allografts: 1 because of noncompliance, 1 because of rejection, and 1 because of polyoma (B-K) virus infection and rejection. Four patients (11%) required antilymphocyte therapy.

Eighteen (90%) patients in the control group were alive at follow-up. The 2 patients who died lost their allografts. One patient died of sepsis 2 months after surgery, and the other patient died of suspected hyperkalemia 5 months after transplantation. One patient who was alive at follow-up lost her allograft 2 weeks after transplantation because of vascular rejection. Seventeen (85%) patients had functioning allografts. Two patients (10%) needed antilymphocyte therapy.

As expected, no chimerism was detected in the pretransplantation specimen of any patient before bone marrow transplantation. Thirty-one of 33 patients were evaluable at follow-up. Thirty patients (97%) had evidence of persistent peripheral blood chimerism by 1 or more modalities at follow-up. Nine of 14 patients (64%) in the control group available at follow-up were chimeric. The level of chimerism seemed to be higher in the bone marrow–augmented group, than in the control group. Six of 29 (21%) patients in the kidney and bone marrow group and 4 of 14 (29%) patients in the control group experienced decreasing donor-specific responsiveness.

Conclusion.—Combined kidney and bone marrow transplantation provides acceptable patient and graft survival, augmentation of chimerism, and no change in the early events after transplantation. Long-term follow-up is needed.

▶ Finding that long-term recipients of organ grafts were chimeric for donor cells, the authors began to study whether they could purposely make patients chimeric by administering bone marrow from the organ donor. They were indeed able to show chimerism, which has also been shown in patients who receive blood transfusions before transplantation. These studies have an experimental backing; mice that receive bone marrow infusions before skin grafting tolerate skin from the marrow donor strain but not from third-party animals. Whether bone marrow infusion will lead to better long-term survival remains to be seen, but it may have other advantages. If chimerism is important in reducing the incidence of graft rejection, it may permit decreasing the dose of immunosuppressive drugs or withdrawing some drugs altogether, or it may decrease the likelihood of chronic rejection.

R.J. Howard, M.D., Ph.D.

Improved Results of Liver Transplantation in Patients With Portal Vein Thrombosis

Seu P, Shackleton CR, Shaked A, et al (Univ of California, Los Angeles)
Arch Surg 131:840–845, 1996 6–6

Objectives and Methods.—The operative management of pre-existing portal vein thrombosis (PVT) during liver transplantation was analyzed and outcomes between patients with and without PVT were compared. Records were reviewed for 1,423 patients who had received liver transplants over 11 years. Data were collected on the presence of PVT, surgical technique, and other parameters.

Results.—Portal vein thrombosis occurred in 70 patients (4.9%). It was an unexpected finding in 24 patients (34%). In 61 patients (87%), operative management had consisted of thrombectomy with or without endovenectomy. Nine patients had required a vein graft, the preferred method being a jump graft to the proximal superior mesenteric vein using donor iliac vein. Overall, the incidence of retransplantation was 24%, the 30-day mortality rate was 14%, and the 1-year actuarial survival rate was 74%. The 1-year survival rate for the first 35 patients was 66%, compared to 82% for the latter 35 patients. The survival rate for the latter 35 patients compares favorably with the 85% survival rate for patients without PVT who underwent transplantation during the same period.

Conclusions.—Liver transplantation can be successful in patients with PVT, and with sufficient experience survival rates can rival those for patients without PVT. Vein grafts can often be avoided if the clotted portal vein is thrombectomized and endovenectomy is conducted as necessary. In this series, imaging for PVT yielded a high false negative rate, so serial duplex studies should be considered before liver transplantation if accurate knowledge of PVT status is critical.

▶ Previously an absolute contraindication to liver transplantation, PVT does not currently provide a barrier to transplantation. With more experience and advanced techniques at endovenectomy or using a vein graft from the superior mesenteric vein to the donor portal vein, transplantation can now be successful in most patients with PVT. As with the development of most other surgical procedures, with growing experience, the results of the procedure become better and are extended to individuals previously not thought to be candidates.

R.J. Howard, M.D., Ph.D.

Long-term Outcome of Hepatitis C Infection After Liver Transplantation

Gane EJ, Portmann BC, Naoumov NV, et al (King's College School of Medicine and Dentistry, London; Innogenetics, Ghent, Belgium)

N Engl J Med 334:815–820, 1996 6–7

Background.—Liver transplantation is commonly performed because of cirrhosis related to hepatitis C virus (HCV) infection. However, persistent viremia occurs in more than 95% of patients, and HCV infection in the graft can recur within 4 weeks after transplantation. The natural history of HCV infection in liver transplant recipients was studied, including the contribution of HLA mismatches and viral genotypes to the severity of recurrent HCV disease.

Methods.—The study included 149 liver transplant recipients with HCV infection. The natural outcome of HCV infection was assessed over a median follow-up of 36 months. A group of non–HCV-infected liver transplant recipients were analyzed for comparison. Pathologic review was conducted on 528 liver biopsy specimens obtained from the HCV-infected patients, including scheduled 1-year and 5-year specimens.

Results.—The HCV-infected patients had a cumulative survival rate of 79% at 1 year, 74% at 3 years, and 70% at 5 years. These were similar to the survival rates recorded for the non–HCV-infected recipients. Among HCV-infected recipients who survived longer than 6 months, the most recent liver biopsy showed no signs of chronic hepatitis in 12%, mild chronic hepatitis in 54%, moderate chronic hepatitis in 27%, and cirrhosis

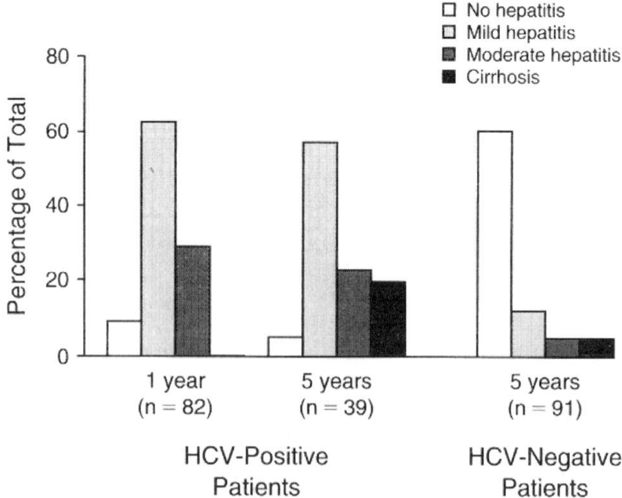

FIGURE 1.—Biopsy findings 1 and 5 years after liver transplantation in recipients with hepatitis C virus (*HCV*) infection after transplantation and in those without HCV infection. The number of patients in each group is given in parentheses. $P < 0.001$ for the comparison of each variable between the HCV-positive and HCV-negative groups at 5 years. (Reprinted by permission of *The New England Journal of Medicine* from Gane EJ, Portmann BC, Naoumov NV, et al: Long-term outcome of hepatitis C infection after liver transplantation. *N Engl J Med* 334:815–820, Copyright 1996, Massachusetts Medical Society.)

in 8% (Fig 1). Patients infected with HCV genotype 1b had more severe graft injury, whereas the immunosuppressive regimen used and the extent of donor-recipient HLA mismatching had no significant impact on the severity of recurrent disease.

Conclusion.—In patients receiving liver transplants for HCV-related cirrhosis, persistent HCV infection can cause severe graft damage, particularly in those with HCV genotype 1b. However, 5-year graft and overall survival are comparable for liver transplant recipients with and without HCV infection. Liver biopsies to assess the extent of HCV-related damage to the liver graft could help to select patients who could benefit from antiviral therapy.

▶ Liver failure caused by HCV infection is a common reason for liver transplantation at many transplant centers. This paper from London is similar to that of several others demonstrating that although the results of liver transplantation in patients with HCV are comparable to those transplanted for other reasons, the recurrence rate for HCV is very high (nearly universal). The prevalence of hepatitis and cirrhosis after liver transplantation are higher in patients transplanted for HCV than in those transplanted for other reasons. Nevertheless, graft survival through 5 years in those transplanted for HCV is comparable to those transplanted for other reasons. Thus, liver transplantation in patients with liver failure caused by HCV is justified. Yet some forms of insurance will not cover liver transplantation for patients with active viremia. With the comparability in survival demonstrated in this and other papers, this policy should now be revised.

R.J. Howard, M.D., Ph.D.

Alcohol Use Following Liver Transplantation for Alcoholic Cirrhosis

Gerhardt TC, Goldstein RM, Urschel HC, et al (Baylor Univ, Dallas)

Transplantation 62:1060–1063, 1996 6–8

Background.—Because alcohol-induced cirrhosis is the most common cause of end-stage liver disease in the United States, increasing numbers of these patients are being referred for transplantation. Yet many liver transplant programs are reluctant to accept patients with alcohol-induced cirrhosis because of the potential for recidivism and the underlying stigma surrounding alcoholism. Factors influencing recidivism after transplantation were determined in a retrospective study.

Methods.—Between December 1985 and December 1991, 67 patients with alcohol-related end-stage liver disease (ARESLD) underwent orthotopic liver transplantation (OLTX) at one institution. In all cases, transplantation was the only option for survival, and the prognosis for future sobriety was favorable. Surviving patients were contacted by phone in December 1994 to evaluate alcohol use after transplantation. Data also were obtained on pretransplant characteristics, including duration of so-

TABLE 2.—Study Results of Patients Transplanted for Alcohol-related Cirrhosis

Pretransplant abstinence	No. patients interviewed	Remained abstinent	Relapsed	Recommitted to sobriety	Abstinent at time of interview
Less than 6 months	10	3	7	2	5 (50%)
6 Months or more	31	18	13	4	22 (71%)
Total	41	21	20	6	27 (66%)

(Courtesy of Gerhardt TC, Goldstein RM, Urschel HC, et al: Alcohol use following liver transplantation for alcoholic cirrhosis. *Transplantation* 62:(8)1060–1063, 1996.)

briety immediately before the procedure. Alcohol consumption levels were classified as occasional, social, moderate, and excessive.

Results.—Survival did not differ significantly between patients who underwent transplantation for ARESLD and those who underwent transplantation for other causes, nor did survival appear to be affected by abstinence before transplantation or recurrent drinking afterward. There were 5 early deaths and 13 deaths that occurred 3 months or longer after transplantation. The deaths of 3 of these 13 patients, all women younger than 45, were related to posttransplant alcohol use and poor compliance. Another patient had resumed drinking, but his death was caused by cardiovascular failure and his survival—just short of 9 years—was the longest of all those who had died. With a mean follow-up of 47 months, 21 of 41 interviewed patients were abstinent and 20 had returned to drinking. Patients who had been abstinent for at least 6 months before transplantation were more likely to have remained abstinent than those with shorter pretransplant abstinence (Table 2), but the difference was not significant and only 2 of 41 returned to excessive drinking. Recidivism was not significantly related to other variables examined, including age, sex, educational level, participation in an alcohol treatment program, or use of a patient compliance contract.

Discussion.—About 50% of those patients with ARESLD resumed drinking after OLTX, but this did not appear to have affected their survival potential. Transplantation is appropriate in such patients, although any alcohol use involves a risk of relapse and allograft loss.

▶ Some maintain that individuals with liver failure caused by alcoholism should not undergo transplantation because they had a disease (alcoholism) for which they did not seek treatment and because of the potentially high rate of recidivism. Although this study demonstrates a rather high rate of return to alcohol consumption after liver transplantation, only 2 of 41 interviewed patients reported excessive drinking. One might question how reliable the data are because of the fact that they were gathered by telephone interview; an in-person interview by a skilled interviewer may have yielded different data (perhaps a high rate of return to drinking). In addition, 3 of 18 deaths and 3 of 13 deaths in long-term survivors were attributed to excessive alcohol consumption. Nevertheless, most studies of alcohol consumption after transplantation report a rather low rate of return to drinking. Even in this study, in which the rate of return to drinking was high, most patients reported only occasional drinking or social drinking. Thus, the authors conclude (as have virtually all others who have studied return to drinking in patients who have undergone transplantation for alcoholic liver disease) that OLTX should continue to be performed in patients who have alcohol-related end-stage liver disease.

R.J. Howard, M.D., Ph.D.

Preliminary Experience With Split Liver Transplantation

Kalayoglu M, D'Alessandro AM, Knechtle SJ, et al (Univ of Wisconsin, Madison)

J Am Coll Surg 182:381–387, 1996 6–9

Introduction.—The results of human orthotopic liver transplantation have vastly improved since the first successful transplant was performed 30 years ago. A critical problem now is the shortage of organ donors. Several techniques, including reduced-size liver transplantation, split liver transplantation (SLT), and living-related liver transplantation, have led to somewhat better organ availability. A preliminary experience with 12 SLTs was reported.

Methods.—The SLTs were performed between December 1994 and April 1995. One pediatric and 5 adult donor livers were transplanted into 12 patients—5 adults and 7 children. All donors were seronegative for hepatitis A, B, and C virus and for HIV, and donor liver function was normal. Surgeons defined the arterial and biliary anatomy, then performed the splitting procedure ex vivo on the back table of the operating room. After completion of the arterial and venous anastomoses, the liver was perfused with 500 mL of University of Wisconsin solution. The right lobe had continuity with the native hepatic artery, portal vein, bile duct, and inferior vena cava, and there were no arterial or venous anastomoses in the lobe. To reduce cold ischemia time, the 2 recipient operations were started during the splitting procedure. The adult patients received a right liver lobe and the pediatric patients received left-lobe grafts using the "piggyback" technique.

Results.—All livers functioned immediately after reperfusion. Bile leaks occurred in 1 adult and 2 children and 1 child had a hemothorax. There were 2 retransplantations, 1 in an adult with acute vanishing bile duct syndrome and 1 in a child with hepatic artery thrombosis. Another child died 2.5 months after transplantation when lymphoproliferative disease developed. The other patients were discharged with normal liver function test results. With follow-up ranging from 6 to 9 months, the patient survival rate was 91.7% and the graft survival rate was 75%.

Discussion.—Split liver transplantation has not gained wide acceptance because of the complexity of the procedure and reports of poor results. However, SLT is an acceptable option that adds to the donor pool and can be completed with acceptable morbidity and mortality. The technical problem of revascularizing the left-lobe graft can be solved with donor iliac artery and vein grafts.

▶ With the ever-increasing shortage of donor livers and the number of patients who are dying while awaiting liver transplantations, SLT offers at least some way to partially ameliorate this shortage by using 1 liver to transplant into 2 recipients. Although using split livers for transplantation is more technically demanding and not all livers are suitable for splitting, it can be done safely and with good outcomes.

R.J. Howard, M.D., Ph.D.

Comparison of T Cell Responses in Patients With a Long-term Surviving Renal Allograft Versus a Long-term Surviving Liver Allograft: It's a Different World

van Twuyver E, de Hoop J, ten Berge RJM, et al (Univ of Amsterdam; Univ Hosp Groningen, The Netherlands)

Transplantation 61:1392–1397, 1996 6–10

Background.—The ultimate goal of clinical transplantation is the induction of specific transplant tolerance, which permits lifelong graft acceptance and function without immunosuppressive therapy. The acquisition of transplantation tolerance was studied in a group of long-term surviving renal and liver allograft patients.

Study Group.—The study group consisted of 31 recipients of a first renal allograft and 9 recipients of a first orthotopic liver allograft with good graft function 2 years after transplantation. Both groups received standard maintenance immunosuppressive regimens.

Results.—Mixed lymphocyte reaction analysis was done in the 9 liver transplant recipients with peripheral blood lymphocyte samples that had been frozen before transplantation and 2 years after transplantation. Before transplantation, there were normal proliferative responses to both donor and third-party blood cells. After transplantation, the donor-specific response was absent in 8 of 9 cases, although the third-party response was unaffected. Before transplantation, there were high numbers of antidonor and anti–third party cytotoxic T-cell precursors (CTL_p). After transplantation, specific CTL nonresponsiveness had developed in 7, the CTL response was significantly reduced in 1, and the CTL response was unchanged in 1 patient. Anti–third party CTL_p was retained by all patients after transplantation. High CTL_p frequencies against donors and third parties were detected in all 31 renal allograft recipients before transplantation. After transplantation, only a minority of the recipients obtained specific CTL nonresponsiveness.

Conclusions.—In a group of kidney allograft recipients with good graft function 2 years after transplantation, only a minority had acquired specific CTL nonresponsiveness. In a group of liver transplant recipients with good graft function 2 years after transplantation, transplantation resulted in specific CTL and mixed lymphocyte reaction nonresponsiveness. This donor-specific nonresponsiveness in long-term surviving liver allograft recipients appears to reflect a state of acquired transplantation tolerance and may allow reduction of immunosuppressive therapy in these patients.

▶ It has long been appreciated that there is hierarchy among various organs in terms of the ease with which they are rejected. Whereas kidney allografts are occasionally lost from acute or chronic rejection episodes, liver allografts are rarely lost from rejection, even though acute rejection episodes are common. This investigation of T-cell responses in patients with liver and renal allografts provides laboratory documentation that patients do respond differently to these 2 organs. Because T-cell unresponsiveness is more common in liver allograft recipients, there is a greater propensity to "tolerance" in these patients. These findings are consistent with reports of circulating donor cells in long-standing liver allograft recipients.

R.J. Howard, M.D., Ph.D.

Survival Experience Among Elderly End-stage Renal Disease Patients

Schaubel D, Desmeules M, Mao Y, et al (Univ of Manitoba, Canada; Univ of Toronto)

Transplantation 60:1389–1394, 1995 6–11

Purpose.—Some elderly patients with end-stage renal disease (ESRD) are treated with renal transplantation. There have been few valid comparisons of the results of transplantation and dialysis in the elderly. The survival benefits of these 2 approaches were assessed in elderly patients with ESRD.

Methods.—The analysis included 6,400 patients aged 60 years or older who were treated for ESRD between 1987 and 1993. The data were drawn from the Canadian Organ Replacement Registry, and included information on comorbid conditions. Each transplant recipient was matched for age, underlying diagnosis, and number of comorbid conditions to 2 randomly selected patients receiving dialysis. Mortality and survival rates were compared for patients treated by transplant vs. dialysis.

Results.—About 4% of patients were treated by transplantation. Their mean age when registered was 64 years. According to Cox regression analysis, the time-dependent hazard ratio for transplantation patients compared to dialysis patients was 0.47. This meant a greater likelihood of survival for patients who received transplants, even after adjustment for other prognostic factors. On further analysis of patients who received transplants and dialysis patients matched for follow-up times, the 5-year survival rate was 81% with transplantation vs. 51% with dialysis (Fig 4). For the entire cohort of elderly patients with ESRD receiving kidney transplants, the survival rate was 93% at 1 year, 85% at 3 years, and 75% at 5 years.

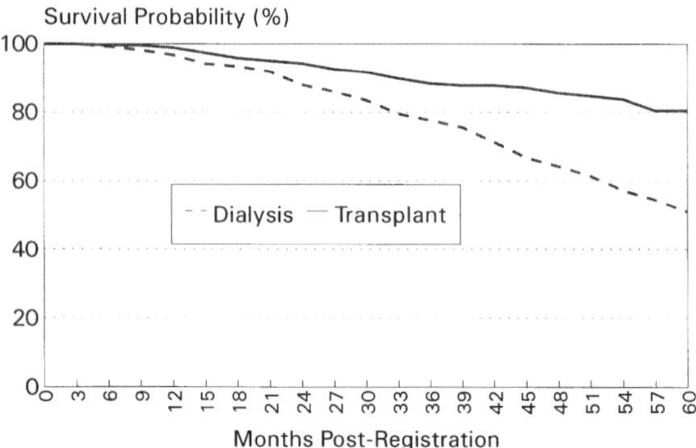

FIGURE 4.—Survival probability: patients age 60+ with end-stage renal disease—transplant vs. dialysis patients. Transplant patients were matched to dialysis patients (by age, diagnosis leading to end-stage renal disease, and number of comorbid conditions) such that each dialysis patient had follow-up time at least as great as the transplant patient's waiting time until transplant. (Courtesy of Schaubel D, Desmeules M, Mao Y, et al: Survival experience among elderly end-stage renal disease patients. *Transplantation* 60(12):1389–1394, 1995.)

Conclusions.—Compared with dialysis, renal transplantation appears to improve survival for elderly patients with ESRD. The healthier the patient, the greater the survival benefit of ESRD. Prognostic factors in elderly patients with ESRD treated by renal transplantation should be studied.

▶ The argument for transplantation over dialysis has frequently rested on the improved quality of life rather than the quantity of life. This and other studies indicate that patients treated with transplantation also enjoy greater quantity of life. A concern is the control group, that is, were the older patients who were maintained on dialysis not candidates for transplantation and therefore did they reflect a "sicker" group of patients who one might expect to die at a higher rate? The authors try to circumvent this criticism by matching transplant patients to dialysis patients by age, underlying diagnosis leading to renal disease, and number of comorbid conditions. Other studies have used as a control group patients who were accepted for transplantation but did not receive a transplant. This latter approach would more successfully obviate selection bias. It is hoped that the large number in the dialysis group (6,116) will overcome any problems with patient variability. Some individuals maintain that older (in this case, at least 60 years old) patients should not undergo transplantation because, with the limited number of kidneys available, younger patients, especially children, who have their whole life ahead of them and may likely become productive members of society, should be favored to receive the available kidneys. On the other hand, why should older patients who have contributed in the past be "punished" only because of their age and denied a kidney transplant?

R.J. Howard, M.D., Ph.D.

A Blinded, Randomized Clinical Trial of Mycophenolate Mofetil for the Prevention of Acute Rejection in Cadaveric Renal Transplantation

Keown PA, for the Tricontinental Mycophenolate Mofetil Renal Transplantation Study Group (BC Transplant Society, Vancouver, Canada)

Transplantation 61:1029–1037, 1996 6–12

Background.—Mycophenolate mofetil (MMF), which has been shown to inhibit the proliferation of T and B lymphocytes and the production of antibodies and cytotoxic T cells in in vitro studies, has effectively prevented acute renal graft rejection in animal studies. Its efficacy and toxicity were compared with those of azathioprine (AZA) in a multicenter, randomized, double-blind, controlled prospective trial of patients who underwent cadaveric renal transplantation.

Methods.—At 21 transplant centers, 503 patients were stratified by first or second cadaveric renal transplant, then randomly assigned to receive either MMF 1.5 g twice daily (MMF 3 g group), MMF 1 g twice daily (MMF 2 g group), or AZA once daily with the dosage determined by body weight (AZA group). All patients also received cyclosporine and prednisone throughout the treatment period. The patients were monitored regularly during the first year for signs of graft rejection and for adverse treatment events.

Results.—Six months after transplantation, treatment failure had occurred in 34.8% of the MMF 3 g group, 38.2% of the MMF 2 g group, and 50% of the AZA group. There was biopsy-proved acute rejection in 15.9% of patients in the MMF 3 g group, 19.7% of the MMF 2 g group, and 35.5% of the AZA group. The drug was withdrawn in 15.2% of patients in the MMF 3 g group, 13.9% of the MMF 2 g group, and 10.2% of the AZA group. A full course of treatment for acute rejection was given to 24.4% of the MMF 3 g group, 31% of the MMF 2 g group, and 47.5% of the AZA group; 6.1% of the MMF 3 g group, 14.6% of the MMF 2 g group, and 19.8% of the AZA group required at least 2 courses of treatment. There were no significant differences among groups in the mean dose of cyclosporine or prednisone. Graft function in those with surviving grafts was similar in the 3 groups. Treatment with MMF was more closely associated with leukopenia and gastrointestinal disorders, whereas AZA treatment was more closely associated with thrombocytopenia, thrombophlebitis, and metabolic disorders. There were no differences in the 1-year mortality rate in the 3 groups.

Conclusions.—Mycophenolate mofetil reduces the incidence and severity of renal graft rejection, which results in a clinically significant reduction in treatment failure, compared with AZA treatment. This benefit occurs within 6 months after transplantation. The greatest reduction in acute rejection occurs with a dose of 3 g/day. This dose, however, is associated with increased adverse events. The optimal dosing strategy may be to tailor the MMF dose to the clinical status of the individual patient.

► Mycophenolate mofetil is the newest drug to be approved for preventing rejection. This study shows that MMF can reduce the likelihood of treatment failure. Yet it did not lead to increased graft survival for the 12 months of follow-up. That finding may not be surprising. Kidney graft survival is currently so good that it is extremely difficult for any new drug or other therapy to increase outcome significantly. Is the increased cost of MMF worth it? The cost of immunosuppression is great and makes transplantation unavailable to some patients. Medicare will pay for the first 3 years of immunosuppression, but patients have to pay after that unless they have other forms of insurance. Mycophenolate mofetil and other expensive immunosuppressive drugs that are currently available or will be released in the future may find their place among selected groups of patients or may be used for certain types of organ transplants. One strategy is to use MMF or other drugs early in the course of transplantation to prevent early adverse events and then to decrease or eliminate their use (and expense).

R.J. Howard, M.D., Ph.D.

Employment Patterns After Successful Kidney Transplantation

Matas AJ, Lawson W, McHugh L, et al (Univ of Minnesota, Minneapolis)

Transplantation 61:729–733, 1996 6–13

Introduction.—No long-term investigations have determined the dynamics of kidney transplant recipients entering and leaving the workforce. Reported are employment changes over time in patients who have received kidney transplant.

Methods.—A database program with data on quality of life, employment, and rehabilitation that were entered prospectively since 1988 was reviewed. Data on patients who received transplantation from 1985 to 1988 were reviewed retrospectively. All living recipients were sent a yearly questionnaire about employment and rehabilitation. Of 822 patients contacted, 733 responded (83%). Employment data were analyzed for the following subgroups: diabetic, nondiabetic, living donor, and cadaver donor. Data were also grouped according to employment status before transplantation.

Results.—Significantly more patients receiving disability payments before transplantation continued to receive them after surgery (67% compared with 8%). In patients who worked or attended school full-time before transplantation, significantly more continued to do so compared with those receiving disability payments before surgery (83% compared with 16%). Of 273 patients with cadaver transplants, 96 (35%) were currently working or attending school full-time compared with 167 of 193 recipients (86.5%) of live donors. In both donor recipient groups, significantly more patients who worked or went to school full-time before transplantation continued to do so after surgery than did those who received disability before surgery. Of 213 diabetic recipients, 81 (38%) worked or continued to go to school full-time after surgery. In 430 recipients who were not diabetic, 220 (51%) were employed or went to school full-time. Patients undergoing preemptive transplantation dialysis (63%)

were more likely to work or attend school full-time than were those receiving pretransplantation hemodialysis (32%) or pretransplantation peritoneal dialysis (43%). Only 8% of the 33% of patients who received disability before transplantation continued to receive disability at follow-up. The most significant factors affecting employment after transplantation were diabetes and employment before transplantation. Thirty diabetic recipients dropped out of the work force: 4 because of graft failure, 2 because of death with function, 2 because of retirement, 1 because of part-time work, 6 because of a switch to being an independent homemaker, and 15 because of receipt of disability benefits. Thirty-seven nondiabetic recipients dropped out of the work force: 8 because of graft failure, 5 because of death with function, 8 because of retirement, 7 because of part-time work, 1 because of a switch to being an independent homemaker, and 8 because of receipt of disability benefits.

Conclusion.—A high percentage of patients who worked or attended school full-time before transplantation continued to do so after surgery. Employment before surgery and diabetes were the most important factors affecting employment after surgery.

▶ This is a useful paper because the purpose of transplantation is rehabilitation. A frequently cited advantage of transplantation over dialysis is better rehabilitation. Although this paper does not compare work rates among patients receiving dialysis and patients undergoing transplantation, it does show that after transplantation, a high percentage of patients are working or going to school. Not surprisingly, those who were working before work afterward, and those who were receiving disability before continue to receive disability after. The rates of returning to work or receiving disability may vary from 1 part of the country to another and even within states or cities depending on the socioeconomic status of the population in the individual transplantation program. Unfortunately, patients receiving disability are motivated to remain on disability. For many patients it may be the only way they can afford immunosuppressive drugs. If the patients return to work, the payments are cut off. These patients frequently have such low-paying jobs that their wages will not cover the cost of immunosuppression.

R.J. Howard, M.D.,Ph.D.

Histopathological Concordance of Paired Renal Allograft Biopsy Cores

Sorof JM, Vartanian RK, Olson JL, et al (Univ of California, San Francisco)
Transplantation 60:1215–1219, 1995 6–14

Background.—Because transplant rejection is the most common reason for renal allograft loss, acute rejection must be promptly diagnosed and assessed. Underrecognition of rejection results in insufficient immunosuppression, which leads to permanent graft impairment and reduced graft survival. Incorrectly diagnosed rejection results in overly aggressive immunosuppressive therapy, which leads to an increased risk of infection and

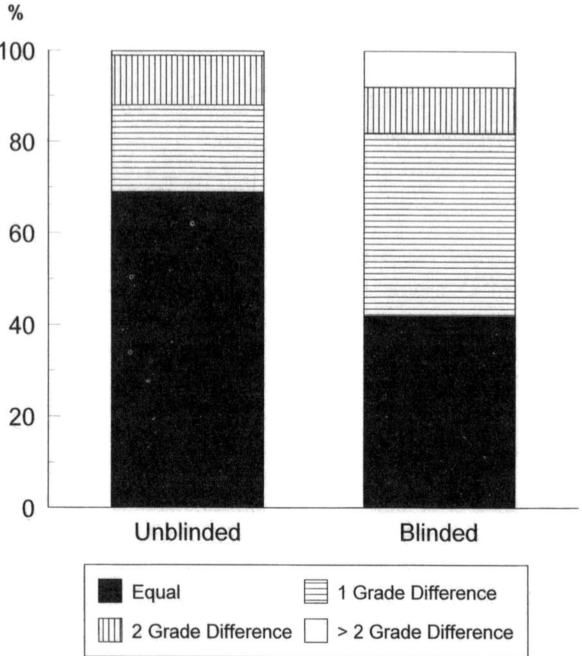

FIGURE 2.—*Stacked bars* show the relative percent agreement of the core B rejection grade diagnoses with the core A grade diagnoses for both the unblinded and blinded pathologists. (Courtesy of Sorof JM, Vartanian RK, Olson JL, et al: Histopathological concordance of paired renal allograft biopsy cores. *Transplantation* 60(11):1215–1219, 1995.)

secondary malignancy. Allograft core biopsy is the diagnostic method of choice in the evaluation of renal parenchymal disease. However, there may be a nonuniform distribution of rejection foci. The concordance of histopathologic rejection grade between 2-core biopsy samples was investigated.

Methods.—Two-core samples were obtained during 79 renal allograft biopsy procedures. The samples were processed separately and assigned an acute rejection grade with the samples side by side and with the samples randomly ordered. Each core sample was then accompanied by a set of clinical data for the determination of treatment recommendations.

Results.—Among the unblinded pathologists, the paired readings agreed exactly in 69% of samples, differed by 1 degree of rejection in 19%, and differed by at least 2 degrees of rejection in 11%. Among the blinded pathologists, readings of the paired samples agreed exactly in 42%, differed by 1 grade in 40%, and differed by at least 2 grades in 18% (Fig 2). Without 2 core samples, the diagnosis of moderate or severe acute rejection would have been missed in 9.5% of all patients and in 25.6% of patients who had moderate or severe acute rejection. Decisions regarding the choice of therapy were in exact agreement in 66%. A needed increase in antirejection therapy would not have occurred in 10.5% of patients if only 1 core sample had been obtained.

Conclusions.—Obtaining 2 renal allograft cores can provide significantly better diagnostic information, thereby leading to more appropriate therapeutic recommendations. The 2-core procedure should be used whenever possible to evaluate renal allograft status.

▶ Biopsy is used as the "gold standard" for diagnosing transplant rejection; yet, there is some tarnish. Pathologists do not necessarily agree with each other when diagnosing rejection, nor do they agree about the degree of rejection. Obtaining 2 core biopsy specimens from the same patient leads to a greater degree of reliability in diagnosing rejection. There would have been a failure to increase antirejection therapy (when rejection was diagnosed in 1 of 2 samples) in 7.5% to 10.5% of patients if only 1 core sample had been obtained. As has been known for sometime, rejection does not occur uniformly. It is therefore not surprising that the greater amount of kidney that is sampled, the more likely one will find histologic evidence of rejection.

R.J. Howard, M.D., Ph.D.

7 Endocrinology

Introduction

Many authors continue to refine the field of endocrine surgery. Fine-needle aspiration (FNA) has been used for many years to evaluate thyroid nodules. This procedure is evaluated at a teaching hospital by Borman and Hume (Abstract 7–2). They found it to be useful in the great majority of their patients, and the results of FNA biopsy altered the operation in some and avoided an operation in over half the patients. Articles dealing with anaplastic carcinoma were reviewed in the 1996 YEAR BOOK OF SURGERY, and an article by Kobayashi et al. (Abstract 7–4) recounts the authors' experience with 37 patients with large-cell anaplastic thyroid cancer. The results of treatment, even aggressive multimodality approaches, have only a marginal impact on the outcome of anaplastic thyroid cancer. Despite this finding, the authors suggest that patients can benefit from aggressive multimodality therapy.

Recurrent or persistent hyperparathyroidism can be a vexing problem for patients and surgeons alike. A standard approach to this problem is discussed by Jaskowiak et al. (Abstract 7–5). These authors were able to find most missed glands preoperatively by a combination of multiple noninvasive tests and invasive tests when the noninvasive tests failed to locate the missing gland. Bergenfelz et al. (Abstract 7–6) discussed another such set of postoperative patients with hyperparathyroidism—those who had persistent elevations of parathyroid hormone during long-term follow-up despite normal calcemia. The authors discuss the possible mechanisms and long-term effects of this problem.

Because the abnormal physiology of renal failure continues to stimulate parathyroid function, 6% to 14% of the patients who undergo subtotal parathyroidectomy or total parathyroidectomy and reimplantation require a reoperation. In a small study, Skinner and Zuckerbraun (Abstract 7–7) advocate total parathyroidectomy with reimplantation to prevent recurrent disease. Nevertheless, 11% of their patients required a reoperation. Aldosterone-secreting tumors of the adrenal gland are one of the surgically treatable causes of hypertension. Celen et al. (Abstract 7–12) analyze factors associated with the outcome of surgery for this disease. These authors show that the main determinants of surgical cure are the presence of an adenoma and preoperative responsiveness to spironolactone. Lo et al. (Abstract 7–13) also discussed the results of surgical treatment for aldosterone-secreting tumors. They note that with surgical excision of an aldosterone-secreting tumor, the hypokalemia is generally cured but mild to persistent hypertension may occur in some patients.

Cushing syndrome requiring adrenalectomy is a rather rare problem currently in the United States. A large series from Japan (Abstract 7–14) covering a 35-year period presents the clinical findings and results of surgical treatment.

Adrenocortical carcinoma has a poor prognosis. Crucitti et al. (Abstract 7–15) analyze the Italian registry for this disease. It is stressed that the optimal outcome is likely to be reached with multimodal therapy.

Laparoscopic adrenalectomy has been reviewed previously in the 1996 YEAR BOOK OF SURGERY. Another comparison of laparoscopic adrenalectomy and open adrenalectomy is presented this year by Brunt et al. (Abstract 7–1). The authors again demonstrate the safety and efficacy of laparoscopic adrenalectomy. It is associated with a shorter hospital stay and earlier return to normal activities.

Laparoscopic Adrenalectomy Compared to Open Adrenalectomy for Benign Adrenal Neoplasms

Brunt LM, Doherty GM, Norton JA, et al (Washington Univ, St Louis, Mo; St Louis VA Med Ctr, Mo)

J Am Coll Surg 183:1–10, 1996 7–1

Introduction.—Before laparoscopic adrenalectomy was first performed in 1992, adrenal tumors were usually removed by a transabdominal or posterior retroperitoneal approach. Outcomes of open adrenalectomy and laparoscopic adrenalectomy were compared in patients with small, benign adrenal neoplasms.

Methods.—Sixty-nine consecutive patients undergoing adrenalectomy were divided into 3 groups on the basis of surgical approach: group I (25 patients) underwent an open anterior transabdominal approach; group II (17 patients) underwent an open posterior retroperitoneal approach; and group III (24 patients) underwent a laparoscopic transabdominal flank approach. Data were collected from medical records, including surgical, anesthesia, and pathology reports, and physician office records. Complication rates and hospital charges were compared among the 3 groups.

Results.—The average tumor size was slightly larger in group I than in group II and group III. The mean duration of surgery for unilateral adrenalectomy was 142 minutes in group I, 136 minutes in group II, and 183 minutes in group III. The mean duration for bilateral adrenalectomies was 205 minutes in group I, 328 minutes in group II, and 422 minutes in group III. The mean intraoperative fluid requirements were higher in group I than in group II and group III. Blood loss was significantly lower for group III than for group I and group II. Five patients in group I, 3 patients in group II, and 1 patient in group III received transfusions of packed red blood cells. The patient in group III received 2 units of packed red blood cells for treatment of pheochromocytoma and baseline anemia. Compared with patients in group I and group II, patients in group III used significantly less parenteral pain medication after surgery, were able to resume a regular diet faster, had fewer postoperative complications, had a significantly shorter length of hospital stay (8.7 days for group I, 6.2 for group II, and 3.2 for group III), returned to 100% activity sooner, and, if employed, returned to work sooner. Hospital charges were higher in group I than in group II and group III.

Conclusion.—The laparoscopic approach for adrenalectomy has several advantages over open procedures. It is recommended as the preferred surgical approach in patients with small, benign adrenal neoplasms.

▶ Several articles have now demonstrated the safety of laparoscopic adrenalectomy. It leads to a shorter hospital stay, less blood loss, and reduced postoperative pain. This study now adequately shows its safety and efficacy. The authors warn that laparoscopic adrenalectomy should not be done in patients with large lesions greater than 6 cm in diameter because of the possibility of adrenal carcinoma. Adrenal surgeons will have to learn this technique to stay competitive. Several operative approaches to adrenalectomy are currently available. Open procedures can be done anteriorly, posteriorly, or laterally. You know that laparoscopic surgery has arrived when authors begin arguing about the best approach—whether it should be done transperitoneally or retroperitoneally.

R.J. Howard, M.D., Ph.D.

Credibility and Clinical Utility of Thyroid Fine-Needle Aspiration Biopsy in a Teaching Hospital

Borman KR, Hume AT (Univ of Texas, Dallas)

Am J Surg 170:638–642, 1995 7–2

Introduction.—More than 4% of adults have at least 1 palpable thyroid nodule. These nodules have a 5% to 10% malignancy rate. Because most thyroid diseases can present as nodules and because overt thyroid cancers are unusual, it is important to be able to identify the few malignant nodules. The safety, accuracy, and clinical utility of thyroid fine-needle aspiration (FNA) was evaluated at a large teaching hospital. The relationship of FNA to frozen section was analyzed.

Methods.—Thyroid FNA biopsy was done with 22- to 25-gauge needles using at least 4 passes. These procedures were performed by housestaff under faculty supervision. All FNA, frozen section, and final surgical pathology reports for 91 patients undergoing thyroid FNA were reviewed.

Results.—Three of 13 patients with inadequate FNA underwent repeat aspirations: 1 was diagnostic and 2 remained nondiagnostic. Two patients with nondiagnostic FNA underwent thyroidectomy for clinical suspicion of carcinoma. Pathologic evaluation showed goiter in 1 patient and thyroiditis in the other. The remaining reaspirations were coupled with repeat clinical examinations and imaging studies. All patients were considered to have benign disease and still did not have surgery at 2-year follow-up. In 14 of 15 (78%) patients who underwent surgery for FNA-diagnosed neoplasia, tumors were confirmed. Overall, FNA aspirates were diagnostically adequate in 78 patients (86%). Patient management, including 15 operations and observation in 48 patients, was directed by FNA biopsy in 69% of patients (63 of 91).

Conclusion.—Fine-needle aspirations were found to be safe, usually produced enough material for diagnosis, and reliably predicted neoplasm. In 69% of patients, fine-needle aspirations were the major factor in choosing whether to observe patients or perform surgery. Use of frozen section can be reduced with properly performed and analyzed FNAs.

▶ Fine-needle aspiration biopsy of the thyroid can yield reliable results that are as accurate as interpretation of frozen sections. Thus, FNA can result in fewer operations in the thyroid gland. Critical in this analysis is the skill of the cytologist who interprets the FNA biopsy specimen. In this study, from the University of Texas Southwestern Medical School, 91 FNAs were analyzed in a single year; thus, the cytologist has adequate experience. Other studies also report high accuracy rates and low false-negative and false-positive rates with interpretation of FNA biopsy specimens. These reports tend to come from large hospitals where enough FNA biopsies are done so that the cytologist gets adequate experience. It is unlikely that most pathologists in the United States who do not have the luxury of specializing in cytology will have experience with sufficient number of FNA biopsy interpretations to yield a similar accuracy rate.

R.J. Howard, M.D., Ph.D.

Nondiagnostic Fine Needle Aspiration Biopsy of the Thyroid Gland: A Diagnostic Dilemma

MacDonald L, Yazdi HM (Univ of Ottawa, Ont, Canada)

Acta Cytol 40:423–428, 1996 7–3

Introduction.—Fine-needle aspiration biopsy (FNAB) is used as a screening test to select patients with thyroid nodules for surgery. A nondiagnostic FNAB, however, poses a diagnostic dilemma. All nondiagnostic FNAB specimens with subsequent histopathologic diagnoses obtained at 1 institution from 1987 through 1992 were evaluated retrospectively and the criterion for specimen adequacy was reexamined.

Methods.—During the study period, 414 (35%) of 1,171 FNABs of the thyroid were nondiagnostic. Ninety-one patients with nondiagnostic findings had subsequent histopathologic diagnoses. Specimen adequacy was based on the presence of 8 to 10 fragments of well-preserved follicular cells on at least each of 2 smears. True cysts were defined as cysts with an epithelial lining, and thyroid aspirates with cytologic features consistent with a nodular goiter, macrofollicular adenoma, or thyroiditis were categorized as benign thyroid nodules.

Results.—Histopathologic examination of the 114 nondiagnostic aspirates from 91 patients revealed 50 nodular goiters, 23 follicular adenomas, 6 macrofollicular adenomas, 5 cases of thyroiditis, 5 true cysts, and 2 cases of malignancy. In addition to the true cysts, 33 lesions exhibited cystic changes (42% of the total). Papillary microcarcinoma was diagnosed incidentally in 9 cases. The rate of nondiagnostic aspirates varied widely among those performing the FNABs. Two general surgeons performed 681 of the 1,171 FNABs; one had 124 (36%) nondiagnostic samples and the other had 72 (22%) inadequate aspirates. The various physicians who performed the remaining 490 procedures had a combined nondiagnostic rate of 45%.

Discussion.—The overall rate of nondiagnostic thyroid aspirates was higher than that reported in previous studies and may be attributed to differences in physician experience or to the cystic nature of many of the lesions. Only 2% of the patients had malignant lesions, a finding that supports the criterion used for specimen adequacy. In both cases of malignancy, the aspirates were acellular, suggesting that repeated FNAB is advisable for acellular aspirates.

▶ The likelihood of having a nondiagnostic FNAB of the thyroid gland depends in part on the criteria used to define an adequate specimen and in part on the skill of the individual who is taking the sample. This paper had a rather high rate (35%) of nondiagnostic FNABs. The authors describe 91 patients who subsequently underwent operation and had tissue available for histologic analysis. Only 2 of these had cancer; the others had benign disease. Unfortunately, the authors do not state what happened to the remaining 323 patients. Nor do they state what should happen if a patient has a nondiagnostic FNAB. Should he or she have an operation? Should he or she have a second FNAB? Without some suggestions, the clinician is still faced with a dilemma in these cases.

R.J. Howard, M.D., Ph.D.

Treatment of 37 Patients With Anaplastic Carcinoma of the Thyroid

Kobayashi T, Asakawa H, Umeshita K, et al (Osaka Univ, Japan; Osaka Teishin Hosp, Japan; Kuma Hosp, Kobe, Japan)

Head Neck 18:36–41, 1996 7–4

Background.—Various treatment protocols have been used with patients who have anaplastic carcinoma of the thyroid, but no single treatment strategy has improved the dismal prognosis. Patients typically die within a few months after the diagnosis. The response to multimodal therapy was evaluated in a retrospective study of patients treated for anaplastic thyroid carcinoma during a 22-year period.

Methods.—The records of 37 patients who had large cell anaplastic thyroid carcinoma treated between 1971 and 1993 were reviewed. At the time of diagnosis, 13 patients had tumors smaller than 5 cm in diameter,

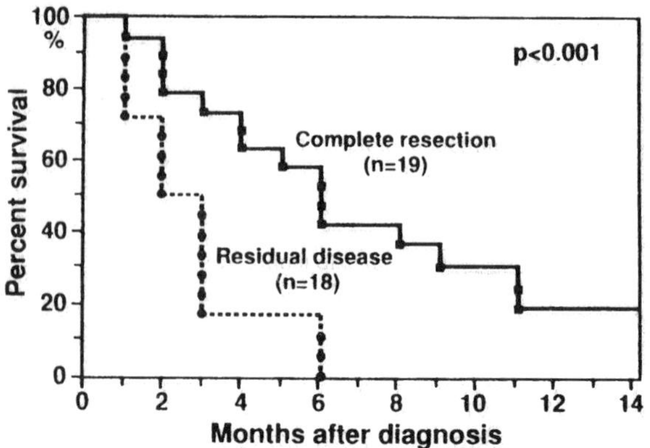

FIGURE 3.—Survival in relation to type of surgery. Complete resection improved the prognosis. (Courtesy of Kobayashi T, Asakawa H, Umeshita K, et al: Treatment of 37 patients with anaplastic carcinoma of the thyroid. *Head Neck* 18:36–41, 1996. Reprinted by permission of John Wiley & Sons, Inc.)

10 had larger tumors with mediastinal and regional tumor extension, and 9 had distant metastases. Fourteen patients were treated with multimodal therapy. Surgery plus adjuvant irradiation of the neck and upper mediastinum and chemotherapy were used in the treatment of patients who did not have distant metastases. Between 1971 and 1983, the protocol included conventional radiation therapy (consisting of 200 cGy/day for a total dose of greater than 50 Gy) plus adriamycin, mitomycin C, and cyclophosphamide. After 1983, the protocol included hyperfractionated radiation (consisting of 130 cGy twice daily) plus adriamycin and/or cisplatin. Patients who had distant metastases received hyperfractionated radiation therapy and chemotherapy.

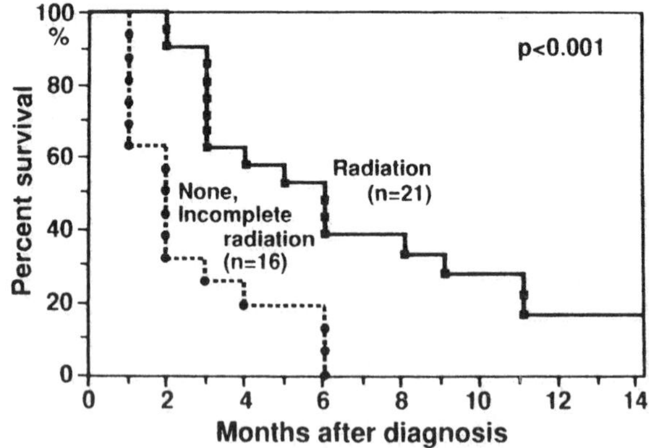

FIGURE 4.—Survival in relation to radiation therapy. Radiation improved the prognosis. (Courtesy of Kobayashi T, Asakawa H, Umeshita K, et al: Treatment of 37 patients with anaplastic carcinoma of the thyroid. *Head Neck* 18:36–41, 1996. Reprinted by permission of John Wiley & Sons, Inc.)

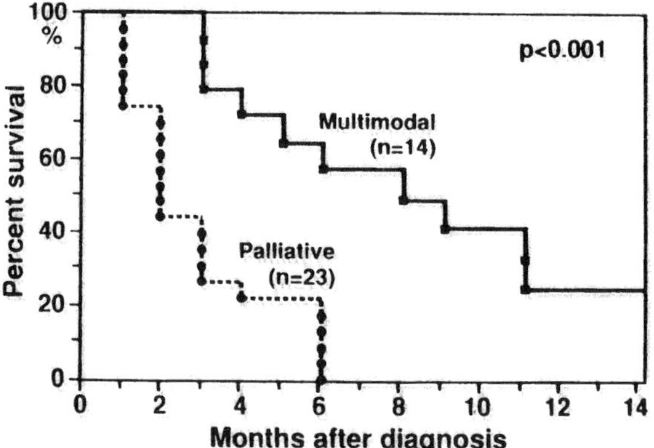

FIGURE 5.—Survival in relation to multimodal treatment. Multimodal treatment improved the prognosis when compared with palliative treatment. (Courtesy of Kobayashi T, Asakawa H, Umeshita K, et al: Treatment of 37 patients with anaplastic carcinoma of the thyroid. *Head Neck* 18:36–41, 1996. Reprinted by permission of John Wiley & Sons, Inc.)

Results.—Three patients have survived more than 3 years; all others died within 1 year of diagnosis. Prolonged survival was associated with tumors smaller than 5 cm in diameter, complete tumor resection (Fig 3), and a radiation dose of more than 30 Gy (Fig 4). Hyperfractionated radiation was effective in achieving local control. Compared with palliative treatment, multimodal treatment, including surgery, radiation therapy, and chemotherapy, significantly prolonged survival ($P < 0.001$) (Fig 5).

Conclusions.—Patients who have early-stage anaplastic thyroid cancer (those with small, resectable tumors) benefit from aggressive multimodal therapy.

► Anaplastic carcinoma of the thyroid is a rare lesion that has a dismal outlook. These authors from Osaka University Medical School accumulated the records of 37 patients who had anaplastic thyroid carcinoma during a 23-year period. Only 3 patients survived more than 1 year, despite an aggressive approach with radical surgery, radiation therapy, and chemotherapy. If any improvement in the outlook of this disease is going to be made, improved chemotherapy and radiation therapy will likely be required. In some cases of anaplastic thyroid cancer, however, very aggressive surgical treatment, including tracheal resection, can lead to long-term survival in individual patients.

R.J. Howard, M.D., Ph.D.

A Prospective Trial Evaluating a Standard Approach to Reoperation for Missed Parathyroid Adenoma

Jaskowiak N, Norton JA, Alexander HR, et al (Natl Cancer Inst, Bethesda, Md; Natl Inst of Diabetes and Digestive and Kidney Diseases, Bethesda, Md; NIH, Bethesda, Md; et al)

Ann Surg 224:308–322, 1996 7–5

Introduction.—Surgical treatment for primary hyperparathyroidism (HPT) may fail as a result of a missed parathyroid adenoma. Because of scarring, distortion of tissue planes, and possible ectopic gland location, the success rate is lower for patients who must have repeat surgery for HPT. Several techniques have been used for preoperative imaging of parathyroid adenomas. A series of patients with missed thyroid adenoma was studied to determine the results of preoperative imaging studies and the outcomes of surgical re-exploration.

Methods.—The study included 288 consecutive patients referred for treatment of persistent or recurrent HPT. All had 1 or more failed surgical procedures at other institutions. A missed single adenoma was suspected in 222 patients, who underwent a total of 228 surgeries and 227 preoperative workups. The patients went through a prespecified series of imaging studies: neck ultrasonography, nuclear medicine scanning, CT, and MRI. Surgery was performed on the basis of noninvasive studies in 27% of patients. The rest went on to invasive studies, including selective angiography in 58%, selective venous sampling for measurement of parathyroid hormone in 43%, and percutaneous aspiration of suggestive lesions in 15%.

Results.—In 209 of the 222 patients, a residual parathyroid adenoma was found at the initial surgical procedure. Adenomas were also found in 6 of 6 second procedures. Overall, these operations led to resolution of hypercalcemia in 97% of patients. Twenty-seven percent of missed adenomas were found in the tracheal-esophageal groove in the posterior superior mediastinum. The thymus was the most common site for ectopic adenomas (17%), followed by intrathyroidal adenomas (10%), undescended glands (9%), the carotid sheath (4%), and the retroesophageal space (3%). Sestamibi subtraction scanning was the most sensitive and specific noninvasive imaging study: it yielded a true positive rate of 67%, with no false positive scans. Otherwise, the noninvasive studies performed had limited sensitivity and specificity (Table 4). Even with extensive preoperative imaging studies, 14% of patients eventually underwent bilateral neck exploration. Four patients were left with permanent nerve injuries, including 3 with injuries to the recurrent laryngeal nerve.

Conclusions.—In patients with primary HPT, the initial parathyroid surgery most often fails because of a single missed parathyroid adenoma. Excellent cure rates with low morbidity can be achieved through appropriate use of preoperative imaging studies and knowledge of the most likely locations for missed adenomas. Most such lesions can be identified by the combination of sestamibi scanning and ultrasound; if the results are

TABLE 4.—Utilization of Various Imaging Tests or Procedures and Percentage True Positive and False Positive in Identifying the Abnormal Missed Parathyroid Adenoma

Test	No. Done (%)*	% True Positive	% False Positive
Nuclear medicine	194/227 (85)		
Technetium-thallium	155/187 (68)	42	8
Iodine-Sestamibi	39/40 (17)	67	0
US, neck	225/227 (99)	48	21
CT, neck/chest	218/227 (96)	52	16
MRI, neck/chest	155/227 (68)	48	14
CT or US directed FNA	35/227 (15)	69	0
Angiogram	150/227 (66)	59	9
Venous sampling for PTH	98/227 (43)	76	4

*Total 227 workups in 222 patients.
Abbreviations: US, ultrasound; *FNA,* fine needle aspiration; *PTH,* parathyroid hormone.
(Courtesy of Jaskowiak N, Norton JA, Alexander HR, et al: A prospective trial evaluating a standard approach to reoperation for missed parathyroid adenoma. *Ann Surg* 224:308–322, 1996.)

still negative, further imaging studies should be performed before surgery. Imaging studies and surgery are indicated only for patients with symptoms that are clearly related to the primary HPT.

▶ Because of tissue scarring and a loss of normal tissue planes, reoperation for missed parathyroid glands can be a daunting procedure, and the risk of injury to the recurrent laryngeal nerve is much greater than with the primary operation. As the authors demonstrate, extensive use of noninvasive and invasive localization methods can be useful in patients who had parathyroid tissue missed at the initial procedure. But even with the use of 4 noninvasive tests, the missed parathyroid tissue was localized in 2 or more of the tests in fewer than 25% of the patients. Therefore, more than 75% required invasive procedures with either aspiration, angiography, or venous sampling. Some of these patients had multiple tests. Even with invasive and noninvasive testing, 31 patients required bilateral neck exploration, demonstrating that in up to 15% of patients, it may be impossible to localize parathyroid adenoma by any amount of preoperative testing. The increased complication rate (2.6% with temporary recurrent laryngeal nerve injury, 1.3% with permanent injury, and 5.3% requiring subsequent parathyroid autografts) is a strong argument for having parathyroidectomy done correctly the first time.

R.J. Howard, M.D., Ph.D.

Persistent Elevated Serum Levels of Intact Parathyroid Hormone After Operation for Sporadic Parathyroid Adenoma: Evidence of Detrimental Effects of Severe Parathyroid Disease

Bergenfelz A, Valdemarsson S, Tibblin S (Lund Univ, Sweden)

Surgery 119:624–633, 1996 7–6

Background.—In 11% of patients operated on for primary hyperparathyroidism, parathyroid hormone (PTH) levels remain elevated 15 years later despite normocalcemia. The reason for these high PTH levels is not known. Preoperative clinical presentation and biochemical variables affecting PTH activity, renal function, and bone mineral content before and 1 year after surgery, as well as serum levels of intact PTH before and 8 weeks and 1 year after surgery were analyzed for 82 patients with sporadic parathyroid adenoma.

Methods.—Parathyroid adenomas, weighing 0.10–9.80 g, were excised from 82 consecutive patients (21 men); average age, 63 years. The mean serum calcium level was 2.74 mmol/L. Serum and urine concentrations of calcium and serum concentrations of albumin, phosphate, creatinine, urea, magnesium, and alkaline phosphatase, and bone mineral content were measured before and 1 year after surgery. Serum PTH was determined before and 8 weeks and 1 year after surgery.

Results.—Eight weeks after surgery, there was a signficant negative correlation between PTH and ionized calcium. Intact PTH levels before and 8 weeks after surgery were significantly correlated. Whereas 62 patients (group 2) had achieved normal PTH levels but had elevated bone mineral content, 20 patients (group 1) had increased levels of intact PTH (7.4 pmol/L), increased levels of creatinine, and normalized bone mineral content. Before surgery, group 1 also had higher levels of ionized calcium, intact PTH, osteocalcin, alkaline phosphatase, and larger adenomas and lower 25 hydroxy vitamin D levels compared with group 2. At 1 year, 13 patients had elevated PTH levels, including 6 patients who had achieved normalized levels at 8 weeks after surgery. Ionized calcium levels remained unchanged from 8-week levels in this group. Compared with the normal PTH group, the patients with elevated PTH levels were older, had more heart disease, had larger adenomas, and higher levels of PTH, calcium, osteocalcin, and serum urea and phosphate, but lower levels of 25 hydroxy vitamin D before surgery and normalized bone mineral content.

Conclusion.—Patients with primary hyperparathyroidism whose elevated PTH levels persist long after surgery tend to be older and have more cardiovascular disease and larger adenomas. These results underscore the necessity for early treatment of primary hyperparathyroidism.

► Parathyroid disease may not be cured in patients even after excision of a parathyroid adenoma. Twenty-four percent of patients who underwent excision of parathyroid adenoma had elevated PTH levels 8 weeks after operation, and 13 (17%) had elevated serum PTH levels 1 year after operation. Six of these patients had evidence of renal disease by virtue of an elevated serum creatinine. Because renal disease is known to lead to metabolic alterations that increase PTH activity, this may not be surprising. But the mechanism is unclear whereby the PTH level remained elevated in the other 7 patients at 1 year. The authors hypothesize an increase in the set point (that is, the calcium concentration causing half maximal inhibition of PTH release). This may be true, but we still are not clear about the cause of primary hyperparathyroidism in the first place and what leads to the alteration of the normal relationship between serum calcium levels and PTH levels. The authors hypothesize that the remaining "normal" parathyroid glands respond differently to serum calcium levels. Thus, these individuals may have increased calcium levels if they are observed long enough. Presumably, operation only interfered with the end organ (parathyroid adenoma) of the altered calcium-PTH axis. Because one does not know what led this relationship to become abnormal in the first place, the cause may still exist and may result in a continuing drive to the remaining normal parathyroid glands. Certainly this exists in patients with renal failure who have had part of 1 gland left in place or who had fragments of 1 gland reimplanted into a muscle. Continuing renal failure may cause the remaining parathyroid tissue to hypertrophy leading to recurrent hyperparathyroidism. Perhaps patients having operation for parathyroid adenomas should have prolonged follow-up to determine whether their serum calcium level remains normal.

R.J. Howard, M.D., Ph.D.

Recurrent Secondary Hyperparathyroidism: An Argument for Total Parathyroidectomy

Skinner KA, Zuckerbraun L (Univ of Southern California, Los Angeles; Univ of California, Los Angeles)

Arch Surg 131:724–727, 1996 7–7

Introduction.—Secondary hyperparathyroidism occurs in a significant number of patients with chronic renal failure. Of these, 5% to 10% require surgical intervention. Most patients undergo either subtotal parathyroidectomy or total parathyroidectomy with autotransplantation to prevent the need for long-term calcium supplementation. The experience of 9 patients treated for secondary hyperparathyroidism with total parathyroidectomy with autotransplantation was reported.

Methods.—All 9 patients had above-normal serum levels of calcium, parathyroid hormone, or both. One patient died of progressive heart failure after surgery. The other 8 patients were normocalcemic without supplementation within a few months of initial surgery. Three patients developed recurrent hypercalcemia at 18, 42, and 36 months, respectively. Two patients underwent reoperation to remove a portion of the graft. One of the 2 had a parathyroid adenoma in the autograft and was normocalcemic 4 years after surgery. The other patient had 4-gland hyperplasia with a large mass at the site of her autograft. She underwent graft excision and reautotransplantation into the contralateral side. The third patient with recurrent hypercalcemia underwent renal transplantation, and her calcium level returned to normal.

Conclusion.—Recurrent hyperparathyroidism is a substantial problem in uremic patients. It occurred in 38% of patients in this small series. Two patients (25%) required reoperation. Total parathyroidectomy without autotransplantation is suggested for patients with secondary hyperparathyroidism who are not expected to undergo renal transplantation in the near future.

► Given the large number of patients with renal failure who are maintained on dialysis in the United States, secondary hyperparathyroidism may be replacing primary hyperparathyroidism as the most common form of parathyroid disease. Surgeons are frequently asked to treat these patients because of the persistent derangement in calcium metabolism. What is the appropriate operation? Some surgeons favor total parathyroidectomy with autotransplantation, whereas others favor removing 3½ glands. Still another approach is total parathyroidectomy without autotransplantation. Patients with renal failure have a continuing drive to derangement in calcium metabolism, and recurrence is not uncommon (0% to 80% in this series). The argument favoring total parathyroidectomy and autotransplantation over subtotal parathyroidectomy is that, if recurrence does require a second operation, removing the reimplanted parathyroid tissue is much safer than reentering the neck looking for hypertrophy of the one half gland that was left behind with the possibility of injury to the recurrent laryngeal nerve. The authors' recommendation that total parathyroidectomy without autotransplantation should be favored over autotransplantation is based on only 9 patients who had a 33% recurrence rate. Three reports (total of 25 patients) of total parathyroidectomy without autotransplantation showed that most patients had detectable parathyroid hormone, yet most required calcium supplements and vitamin D. This paper represents too small an experience to make such a recommendation.

R.J. Howard, M.D., Ph.D.

Surgical Management of Hyperparathyroidism in Patients With Multiple Endocrine Neoplasia Type 2A

Herfarth KK-F, Bartsch D, Doherty GM, et al (Washington Univ, St Louis, Mo; Philipps-Univ Marburg, Germany)

Surgery 120:966–974, 1996 7–8

Introduction.—In its full expression, multiple endocrine neoplasia type 2A (MEN 2A) is characterized by the development of medullary thyroid carcinoma (MTC), pheochromocytomas, and hyperparathyroidism (HPT). The most variable manifestation is HPT, and the optimal surgical management in such cases is controversial. Thirty-five patients with MEN 2A and HPT were analyzed retrospectively to determine the long-term outcome of different operative procedures.

TABLE 3.—Surgical Outcome After First Operation for Hyperparathyroidism

Initial operation	*No. of patients*	*Persistence (%)*	*Recurrence (%)*	*Hypoparathyroid (%)*
Selective resection	21	3 (14.3)	3 (14.3)	4 (19)
Subtotal resection	8	0 (0)	2 (25)	1 (12.5)
Total PTX with AT	5	0 (0)	0 (0)	1 (20)
Total PTX without AT	1	0 (0)	0 (0)	1 (100)
Total	35	3 (8.6)	5 (14.3)	8* (23)

*Hypoparathyroidism developed in 1 additional patient after the second operation for persistent hyperparathyroidism.
Abbreviations: PTX, parathyroidectomy; *AT,* autotransplantation.
(Courtesy of Herfarth KK-F, Bartsch D, Doherty GM, et al: Surgical management of hyperparathyroidism in patients with multiple endocrine neoplasia type 2A. *Surgery* 120:966–974, 1996.)

Methods.—Using a database from the Multiple Endocrine Neoplasia Program at Washington University in St. Louis, records of 119 patients from 14 MEN 2A kindreds were analyzed for occurrence of HPT, surgical procedure, and postoperative outcome. Thirty-five patients met the strict study definition of HPT and had a minimum follow-up of 5 years. Patients underwent their primary operations in 17 different hospitals between 1963 and 1989. At the initial operation, 21 had a selective resection, 8 had a subtotal resection, 5 had total parathyroidectomy with autotransplantation, and 1 had an inadvertent total parathyroidectomy. Follow-up data were extracted from the database or by retrospective chart review. Patients were classified as cured or as having persistent HPT, recurrent HPT, or postoperative hypoparathyroidism.

Results.—The patient group had a female-to-male ratio of 1.92 to 1 and ranged in age from 7 to 64 years (mean 29.9 years) at the time of diagnosis of HPT. In 86% of patients, HPT and MTC were diagnosed at the same time. Twenty-seven patients (77%) were cured by the first operation, 5 (14.3%) had recurrent HPT, and 3 (8.6%) had persistent HPT. All those not cured by the initial procedure had undergone selective or subtotal resection (Table 3). There were 8 cases of permanent postoperative hypoparathyroidism: 6 from the selective or subtotal resection group, 1 from the total parathyroidectomy and autotransplantation group, and 1 case of inadvertent total parathyroidectomy.

Discussion.—Conclusions about the optimal surgical management of patients with MEN 2A and HPT have been hindered by the rarity and variable definition of HPT in patients with the syndrome. Because recurrent or persistent HPT tends to occur after selective or subtotal parathyroidectomy, in which glands may be missed, the recommended procedure is total parathyroidectomy and heterotopic autotransplantation.

▶ The group from Washington University in St. Louis has extensive experience in treating patients with MEN 2A. Hyperparathyroidism was seen in 29% of their patients, a rate of parathyroid disease that is much higher than is seen with this syndrome at other centers. Because of the high rate of persistent or recurrent HPT and hypoparathyroidism seen in patients after selective or subtotal resection, these authors favor parathyroid autotransplantation. This is the procedure many surgeons currently use when treating parathyroid disease in renal failure, in which hyperplasia is virtually universal. As a result, most endocrine surgeons have experience with parathyroid autotransplantation. Expanding its use to the treatment of HPT in MEN 2A seems to be a logical extension of this technique.

R.J. Howard, M.D., Ph.D.

Assessment of Patient Outcomes After Operation for Primary Hyperparathyroidism

Burney RE, Jones KR, Coon JW, et al (Univ of Michigan, Ann Arbor)
Surgery 120:1013–1019, 1996 7–9

Objective.—The value of operation in patients with mild, asymptomatic primary hyperparathyroidism (HPT) has not been studied systematically. The SF-36, a health status questionnaire that defines 8 domains of health status, was completed by patients with primary HPT to determine the effect of surgery on their overall health and quality of life.

Methods.—Study participants were 59 patients who were scheduled for operation to correct primary HPT and agreed to complete the SF-36, a questionnaire covering general health perception, physical function, physical and emotional role limitations, social function, mental health, bodily pain, and energy/fatigue or vitality. The SF-36 was administered before surgery and at 2 months and 6 months after surgery. Clinical and condition-specific data were gathered at the same time.

Results.—The patients had a mean age of 59.9 years; 73% were women. Frequently reported coexisting conditions were arthritis (50%), hypertension (48%), and back pain (30%); 45% of patients had hypercalcemia for more than 6 months. Compared with the general population, patients with primary HPT had substantially lower SF-36 scores. Many patients reported fatigue (73%), bone pain (52%), and muscle weakness (50%) at baseline. At 2 months after surgery, patients reported substantial improvement in 2 SF-36 domains: bodily pain and role limitations caused by emotional problems. Six-month outcome, available for 23 patients, showed considerable improvement in all areas except general health perception (Fig 3).

Discussion.—Routine serum calcium determinations have identified many patients with primary HPT who have no obvious clinical problems but are not entirely "asymptomatic." Removal of abnormal parathyroid tissue in such patients can improve their overall health status and well-being. In this group of patients, operation may dramatically reduce HPT-related symptoms. The SF-36 is a useful tool for assessing outcomes after operation and may be of value in preoperative screening of asymptomatic patients.

▶ Surgeons usually are concerned with normalization of the metabolic aberrations associated with HPT, and the results of parathyroidectomy for HPT usually are measured by return of parathyroid hormone and calcium

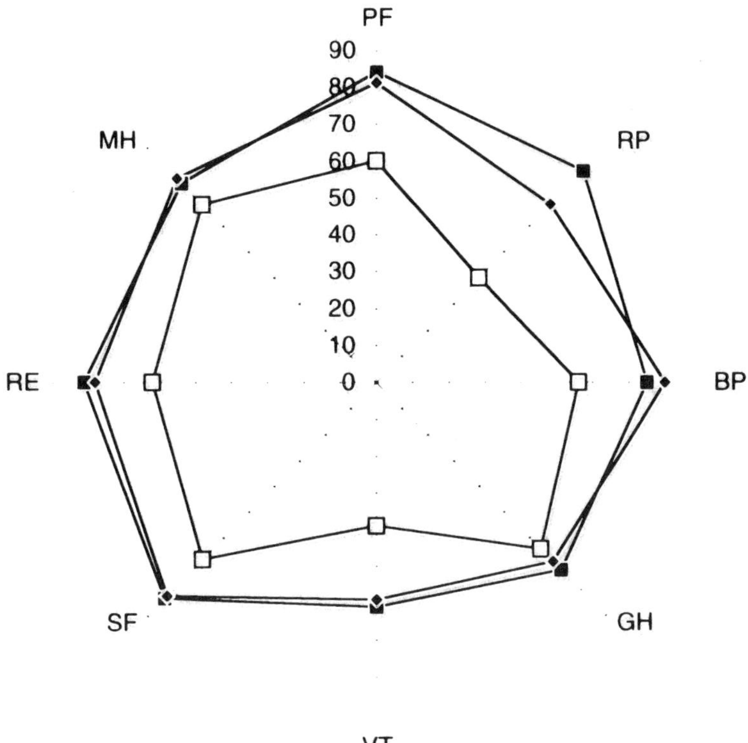

FIGURE 3.—Radar plot shows SF-36 scores for patients with HPT at baseline (n = 56) and 6 months (n = 23) compared with normal population. Scores for normal population taken from Ware and colleagues. *Abbreviations: HPT*, hyperparathyroidism; *PF*, physical function; *RP*, physical role limitations; *BP*, bodily pain; *GH*, general health perception; *VT*, vitality; *SF*, social function; *RE*, emotional role limitations; *MH*, mental health. (Courtesy of Burney RE, Jones KR, Coon JW, et al: Assessment of patient outcomes after operation for primary hyperparathyroidism. *Surgery* 120:1013–1019, 1996.)

levels to normal. Relatively little attention has been devoted to the assessment of symptoms after parathyroidectomy. Many symptoms associated with HPT, such as fatigue, weakness, confusion, moodiness, and irritability, are found frequently in patients who do not have HPT. These authors demonstrate that these subjective symptoms undergo substantial improvement by 6 months after parathyroidectomy.

R.J. Howard, M.D., Ph.D.

Intraoperative Parathyroid Hormone Monitoring as an Adjunct to Parathyroidectomy

Boggs JE, Irvin GL III, Molinari AS, et al (Univ of Miami, Fla)
Surgery 120:954–958, 1996 7–10

Introduction.—Intraoperative monitoring of intact parathyroid hormone (iPTH) allows the surgeon to determine when all hyperfunctioning tissue has been excised or when further dissection is required in patients undergoing parathyroidectomy for primary hyperparathyroidism. The sensitivity and accuracy of a non–radioisotopic iPTH assay were assessed in 89 patients, and the effect of the intraoperative monitoring on surgical judgment was evaluated.

Methods.—All patients had hypercalcemia and elevated iPTH levels before operation. Eighty-seven patients had primary hyperparathyroidism with normal renal function and 2 had multiple endocrine neoplasia type I syndrome. Levels of iPTH were reported twice before excision of the gland, 5 and 10 minutes after excision, and at other times as determined by the surgeon. A modified 2-site immunochemiluminometric assay with a turnaround time of 10 minutes was used to measure iPTH. The operation

TABLE 1.—Influence of Intraoperative PTH Monitoring on Operative Approach

Patient no.	Operative time (min)	% iPTH drop after excision	Follow-up calcium level (mg/dl)	Follow-up iPTH level (pg/ml)	Notes
1	90	82	10.4	61	MEN; previous two-gland excision; QPTH drop after one gland removed; fourth gland not explored
2	75	45, 67	9.5		MEN; two glands excised one biopsy, did not search for fourth gland
3	130	0, 84	9.3	47	Multiglandular disease; second unsuspected contralateral gland
4	65	0, 80	9.4	48	Multiglandular disease; second unsuspected contralateral gland
5	130	85	9.6	48	Previous two glands removed; localization with manipulation
6	120	21, 9, 76	8.4		Previous operation identified nonparathyroid tissue, carotid sheath
7	107	92	9.2		Unrecognized intrathyroidal parathyroid gland; thyroid lobectomy
8	97	83	9.0	78	Unrecognized intrathyroidal parathyroid gland; thyroid lobectomy
9	96	8, 0, 66	9.1	68	QPTH identified nonparathyroid in goiter; FN/FP sestamibi scan
10	75	0, 84	9.9	28	QPTH identified nonparathyroid tissue; FN/FP sestamibi scan
11	105	0, 70	9.2	46	FN/FP sestamibi scan; goiter; identified nonparathyroid tissue
12	34	60	9.6	64	Thyroiditis; no histopathologic confirmation; devascularized gland

Abbreviations: PTH, parathyroid hormone; *FN/FP,* false-negative/false positive; *MEN,* multiple endocrine neoplasia; *QPTH,* measurement of PTH during parathyroidectomy.

(Courtesy of Boggs JE, Irvin GL III, Molinari AS, et al: Intraoperative parathyroid hormone monitoring as an adjunct to parathyroidectomy. *Surgery* 120:954–958, 1996.)

was judged a success when serum calcium levels returned to the low or normal range within 24 hours and remained normal during follow-up. Patients were monitored for an average of 8 months.

Results.—Only 1 of 89 patients failed to achieve normal or low calcium levels within 24 hours after parathyroidectomy. Those with a successful outcome have maintained normal levels during follow-up. In the prediction of postoperative calcium levels, the assay had a sensitivity of 97%, a specificity of 100%, and an overall accuracy of 97%. The assay correctly predicted the operative failure and postoperative normocalcemia in the remaining patients. The average operative time was 58 minutes, and 64% of the 66 patients offered outpatient surgery did not require overnight hospitalization. Intraoperative iPTH monitoring directly aided the surgeon's operative approach in 12 patients (Table 1), including 4 with multiglandular disease and 7 with localization difficulties.

Discussion.—An experienced surgeon can achieve high cure rates in treating patients with hyperparathyroidism, but further surgery will be required when there is inadequate excision of all hypersecreting glands. The use of an intraoperative iPTH assay helps to maintain a high success rate, shortens operative time, and allows some procedures to be done on an outpatient basis.

▶ The authors presented 2 papers on intraoperative parathyroid hormone monitoring during parathyroidectomy at the annual meeting of the American Association of Endocrine Surgeons. This rapid measurement of iPTH (not yet approved by the Food and Drug Administration) takes only 10 minutes and was helpful in 13% of patients because the test results led surgeons to persist in exploring both sides of the neck for a second enlarged parathyroid gland. Because of the rapid metabolism of parathyroid hormone, this test can be helpful during the operative procedure. However, parathyroid hormone tends to degrade more slowly in elderly patients than in younger patients. In the discussion, Dr. Boggs states that they do not generally explore both sides of the neck if the iPTH level drops after the removal of 1 enlarged gland. If it does not drop after the excision of 1 parathyroid adenoma, they explore the other side and look for a second gland. Because many surgeons routinely explore both sides of the neck and attempt to identify all 4 glands, it is not clear what measuring the iPTH level adds above exploring both sides of the neck. Two of the 12 patients in whom it altered the surgical approach had intrathyroidal parathyroid glands and were treated with thyroid lobectomy. Perhaps in these patients, it truly made a difference. Although this test is not generally available and frequently is not used even when it is available, it may become so in the future.

R.J. Howard, M.D., Ph.D.

Ambulatory Parathyroidectomy for Primary Hyperparathyroidism

Irvin GL III, Sfakianakis G, Yeung L, et al (Univ of Miami, Fla; Sylvester Comprehensive Cancer Ctr, Miami, Fla)

Arch Surg 131:1074–1078, 1996 7–11

Introduction.—Although the success rate of parathyroidectomy is high when it is performed by experienced endocrine surgeons and with careful patient selection, hypercalcemia can persist when these conditions are not met. With preoperative localization and intraoperative monitoring of intact parathyroid hormone (iPTH), however, successful parathyroidectomy can be performed safely in an ambulatory setting. The methods of the procedure were described and the outcome reported for 57 patients who underwent ambulatory parathyroidectomy.

Methods.—Eighty-five consecutive patients with hypercalcemic hyperparathyroidism were referred for parathyroidectomy. Their average age was 60 years; 64 were women and 21 were men. Nineteen patients were asymptomatic, 23 had a history of renal stones, and 48 had signs of bone disease. Those selected for ambulatory surgery had no limiting medical or social problems. All patients underwent technetium Tc 99m sestamibi scintigraphy for 3-dimensional localization of abnormal parathyroid glands in the neck or mediastinum. During parathyroidectomy, monitoring of iPTH levels indicated to the surgeon that all hyperfunctioning glands were excised. The patients were sent home after postanesthetic recovery with an oral calcium supplement to be used in the event of symptoms of hypocalcemia. Samples for serum calcium determinations were obtained the morning after surgery and at regular follow-up intervals.

Results.—Technetium Tc 99m sestamibi scintiscans accurately localized all hyperfunctioning glands in 88% of patients, and monitoring of iPTH levels confirmed the excision of all hyperfunctioning glands in 98%. Parathyroidectomy was performed successfully in 84 of 95 patients. With a decreased operating time (average 52 minutes) and minimal neck dissection, 42 of 57 eligible patients could be discharged the same day. These patients had no postoperative complications and their serum calcium levels have remained normal throughout a mean follow-up period of 7 months. Eleven of the 15 eligible patients who were hospitalized overnight had prolonged operative procedures. Elevated levels of iPTH have developed in 8 (9%) patients during follow-up.

Discussion.—Localization by a preoperative parathyroid scan, confirmed at resection, and a 50% decrease in circulating iPTH levels as determined by intraoperative monitoring assures the surgeon that the operative procedure can be terminated. Operative time is decreased, and some patients need not be hospitalized overnight after parathyroidectomy.

▶ This group of experienced parathyroid surgeons used preoperative localization studies and intraoperative iPTH assays to minimize dissection in the neck and to ensure that they removed all diseased parathyroid tissue. This test combination facilitated surgery and minimized neck dissection, allowing

42 of 57 eligible patients to have their surgery as outpatients. Whether this will be proved safe and cost-effective in the long run was not established by this paper. No cost studies were done. Most experienced parathyroid surgeons believe that preoperative localization studies are not worth the expense, because such studies are less accurate than an experienced parathyroid surgeon. The use of intraoperative parathyroid hormone monitoring may find a place when the test is finally approved by the Food and Drug Administration and more surgeons begin to use it. A 50% drop in iPTH levels within 10 to 20 minutes of gland excision has been used to indicate that all diseased parathyroid tissue has been removed.

Nevertheless, concern about postoperative hypocalcemia and, especially, the dangers of neck hematoma and possible airway obstruction (which may not occur before the patient leaves the hospital if the procedure is done as same-day surgery) may leave many surgeons reluctant to perform outpatient parathyroid surgery.

R.J. Howard, M.D., Ph.D.

Factors Influencing Outcome of Surgery for Primary Aldosteronism

Celen O, O'Brien MJ, Melby JC, et al (Boston Univ)

Arch Surg 131:646–650, 1996 7–12

Introduction.—It is important to recognize the rare case of primary aldosteronism, because surgical resection of the abnormal adrenal gland can cure the patient's hypertension. Reported cure rates range from 44% to 80%. The presence of an adenoma seems to be a key predictor of complete response to surgery; other unidentified factors are probably important as well. Factors affecting the outcome of surgery for primary aldosteronism were evaluated in a retrospective study.

Methods.—The study included 42 patients (22 women and 20 men; mean age, 44.5 years) undergoing adrenalectomy for primary aldosteronism during a 23-year period. Preoperative tests—including adrenal venous sampling, postural stimulation testing, iodocholesterol I-131 scintigraphy, and CT—were done to find adrenal abnormalities. After surgery, patients whose blood pressure was normal (i.e., less than 160/96 mm Hg without medication) were considered complete responders. Patients with normal blood pressure with medication or with high blood pressure despite medication were considered incomplete responders.

Results.—The complete response rate was 60%. Adrenalectomy cured hypokalemia in all patients, and reduced the antihypertensive requirements for patients with incomplete responses. On stepwise logistic regression, a pathologic classification of adenoma, a response to spironolactone, and a duration of hypertension less than 5 years were independent factors in a predictive model. Micronodular hyperplasia on its own was linked to an incomplete response, but its presence in a patient with adenoma was not. Adrenal venous sampling was 91% accurate in the preoperative diagnosis of adenoma; CT, postural stimulation testing, and iodocholesterol scintigraphy were approximately 75% accurate.

Conclusions.—A pathologic classification of adenoma and a preoperative response to spironolactone are significantly associated with surgical cure of hypertension in patients with primary aldosteronism. Computed tomography is a reproducible and specific test for the preoperative diagnosis of adenoma. The chances of surgical cure are better for younger patients and those with a shorter duration of hypertension.

▶ Primary aldosteronism is one form of surgically treatable hypertension. Yet it only accounts for 0.05% to 2% of hypertensive patients. Therefore, most surgeons will probably never see a case. The response to surgery in these patients is gratifying. In this series 25 patients (60%) had a normal blood pressure after removal of their unilateral adenoma (24 patients) or bilateral adrenalectomy in the case of hyperplasia (1 patient). All patients who did not completely respond to this operation needed less antihypertensive therapy. With financial considerations taking on such importance in medical practice, one might be skeptical that hypertensive patients will receive a full evaluation to determine whether they have a surgically correctable form of hypertension.

R.J. Howard, M.D., Ph.D.

Primary Aldosteronism: Results of Surgical Treatment

Lo CY, Tam PC, Kung AWC, et al (Univ of Hong Kong)

Ann Surg 224:125–130, 1996 7–13

Background.—Primary hyperaldosteronism consists of hypertension and hyperkalemia associated with an adrenal adenoma. Patients with an aldosterone-producing adenoma can be cured by unilateral adrenalectomy. To describe recent experience in managing this condition and to identify risk factors for persistent hypertension after successful adrenal surgery, cases of patients who underwent adrenal surgery for primary hyperaldosteronism were retrospectively reviewed.

Study Group.—The study group consisted of 46 patients with primary hyperaldosteronism who underwent unilateral adrenalectomy from 1993 to 1994. The diagnosis was based on hypertension, hypokalemia, elevated plasma or urine aldosterone concentration, and suppressed plasma renin activity. There were 22 men and 24 women aged 28 to 71 years in the study group, with a history of hypertension of 5 months' to 15 years' duration. Localization studies included CT and adrenal venous sampling. Postural study was done when possible. Pathologic documentation of aldosterone-producing adenoma was obtained for all patients. Follow-up study was possible on 44 patients, with a 1-month to 11-year duration.

Findings.—There was no operative mortality. Complications developed in 6 patients: intraoperative hemorrhage occurred in 3, 1 required an additional anterior transabdominal incision for hemostastis, wound infection occurred in 1, and urinary tract infection occurred in 1 patient. The average postoperative hospital stay was 4 days. There was a significant decline in blood pressure on discharge, compared with the preoperative level. Of the 44 patients with follow-up available, all were normokalemic, but persistent hypertension occurred in 10 patients. This hypertension was well controlled by medical therapy. Three factors were independently associated with persistent hypertension: older age, lack of preoperative response to the blood pressure medication spironolactone, and higher blood pressure on hospital discharge.

Conclusions.—Primary aldosteronism can be accurately diagnosed and localized with the use of modern imaging technology. Unilateral adrenalectomy can be safely done in these patients with good outcome and complete control of hypokalemia. Persistent, mild, and controllable hypertension occurs in a subgroup of these patients who were older, with a poor preoperative response to spironolactone treatment and persistent elevated blood pressure after surgery.

► One of the surgically treatable forms of hypertension, a primary aldosterone-secreting tumor of the adrenal gland, can be readily removed and the disease cured by adrenalectomy. The authors stress the importance of preoperative diagnostic studies to rule out idiopathic hyperplasia because of the poor response of the latter disease to surgical treatment. The authors rely on clinical presentation consistent with an aldosterone-secreting tumor confirmed by documentation of excess aldosterone secretion and a postural study coupled with imaging with CT scan. Venous sampling was usually reserved for certain patients whose adenoma could not be localized by CT scan or who had equivocal postural studies.

As other studies have shown, the likelihood of complete relief of hypertension with adrenalectomy can be predicted by a patient's age (older patients are less likely to respond) and response to preoperative spironolactone therapy. Nevertheless, adrenalectomy should be recommended for all patients with primary aldosteronism resulting from adrenal adenoma who are otherwise surgical candidates. Although surgical excision of an aldosterone-producing adrenal adenoma cures hypokalemia, persistence of hypertension, usually of a mild degree, occurs in up to 30% of patients.

R.J. Howard, M.D., Ph.D.

Adrenalectomy for Treatment of Cushing Syndrome: Results in 122 Patients and Long-term Follow-up Studies

Imai T, Funahashi H, Tanaka Y, et al (Nagoya Univ, Japan)

World J Surg 20:781–787, 1996 7–14

Background.—Cushing's syndrome is the clinical manifestation of chronic glucocorticoid excess or hypercortisolism. Adrenalectomy is an effective treatment for Cushing's syndrome. The experience of a Japanese

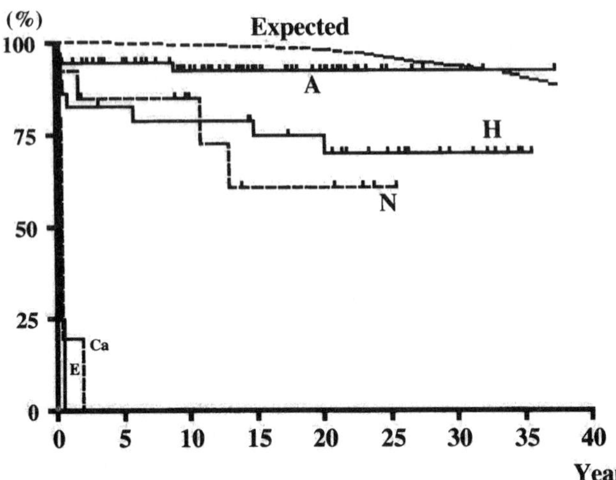

FIGURE 1.—Observed survival curves of Cushing syndrome. *Vertical bars* indicate censored observations. Expected: Expected survival curves of age-matched control population. The following comprise the pathologic subgroup: *A*: adrenocortical adenoma; *H*: Cushing's disease; *N*: nodular hyperplasia; *Ca*: adrenocortical carcinoma; *E*: ectopic ACTH syndrome. (Courtesy of Imai T, Funahashi H, Tanaka Y, et al: Adrenalectomy for treatment of Cushing syndrome: Results in 122 patients and long-term follow-up studies. *World J Surg* 20:781–787, 1996, Figure 1, Copyright 1996, Springer-Verlag.)

University Medical School in adrenalectomy for Cushing's syndrome was reviewed.

Study Group.—The study group consisted of 122 patients, with a diagnosis of Cushing's syndrome, who underwent adrenal exploration from 1957 to 1993. The average age at operation was 32.6 years; there were 23 men and 99 women. The patients were followed up until December 1994, with 2 patients lost to follow-up.

Findings.—Of the 122 patients, 70 had adrenocortical adenoma, 30, Cushing's disease; 6, primary pigmented nodular adrenocortical disease; 7, other types of primary nodular hyperplasia; 5, adrenocortical carcinoma; and 10, ectopic adrenocorticotropin (ACTH) syndrome. The survival rate of patients with adrenocortical adenoma was equal to that of the age-matched control population if postoperative complications were excluded (Fig 1). Of the 30 patients with Cushing's disease, 20 were alive at last follow-up, 63% had skin pigmentation, and 25% had Nelson's syndrome. Four patients with primary pigmented nodular adrenocortical disease and 5 with other nodular hyperplasia were alive. All patients with adrenocortical carcinoma and all those with ectopic ACTH died within 2 years of operation.

Conclusions.—Adrenalectomy is a safe and effective treatment for Cushing's syndrome if operative complications are avoided. Adrenalectomy is also the treatment of choice for adrenal adenoma, adrenocortical carcinoma, and primary aderenocortical hyperplasia, although the survival rate is lower. Total adrenalectomy remains an alternative treatment for Cushing's disease and ectopic ACTH syndrome.

▶ This study from Japan presents long-term follow-up of 120 of 122 patients who were operated on for Cushing's syndrome. The survival rate did not differ from that expected with age-matched controls if the cause of the Cushing's syndrome was adrenal adenoma. Patients with other causes of Cushing's syndrome (Cushing's disease, nodular hyperplasia, adrenal carcinoma, and ectopic ACTH syndrome) had long-term survival rates lower than those in age-matched controls. There were relatively few patients with these latter diseases, however. The late causes of death are not given, unfortunately.

The study does show that those with Cushing's syndrome resulting from adrenal cortical adenoma can enjoy long-term survival, as can patients with Cushing's disease (basophil adenoma of the pituitary gland), but they have somewhat lower survival than do age-matched controls, as might be expected. Patients with adrenal cortical cancer or ectopic ACTH-producing lesions (which are frequently neoplasms) had poor survival.

R.J. Howard, M.D., Ph.D.

The Italian Registry for Adrenal Cortical Carcinoma: Analysis of a Multiinstitutional Series of 129 Patients

Crucitti F and The ACC Italian Registry Study Group (Istituto di Clinica Chirurgica, Policlinico "A Gemelli," Rome)

Surgery 119:161–170, 1996 7–15

Background.—Adrenal cortical carcinoma carries a poor prognosis. Because this tumor is so uncommon, it is difficult to achieve reliable data on clinical manifestations, natural history, and the effects of different treatments.

Methods.—One hundred twenty-nine patients treated at 18 surgical centers were included in a retrospective analysis. The patients were 74 women and 55 men (mean age, 49 years). Endocrine symptoms were present in 45.7% of the patients at diagnosis. Surgery was performed in 124 patients for curative purposes in 91 and for palliation in 33. Sixty-three patients had local disease; 48, regional; and 43, distant.

Findings.—At 5 years, the overall survival rate was 35%. The prognosis was significantly affected by tumor stage and curative resection, but the possible influence of gender, side, age, and hormonal function was unconfirmed. Adjuvant treatment did not prolong survival. Patients undergoing reoperation had a better survival rate than patients not having reoperation, survival being a mean of 41.5 months and 15.6 months, respectively (Fig 3).

Conclusion.—Early diagnosis and complete resection may improve the poor prognosis of adrenal cortical carcinoma. Radical surgery is the only effective treatment and is especially indicated in patients with early-stage disease. Reoperation for recurrence appears to improve survival and

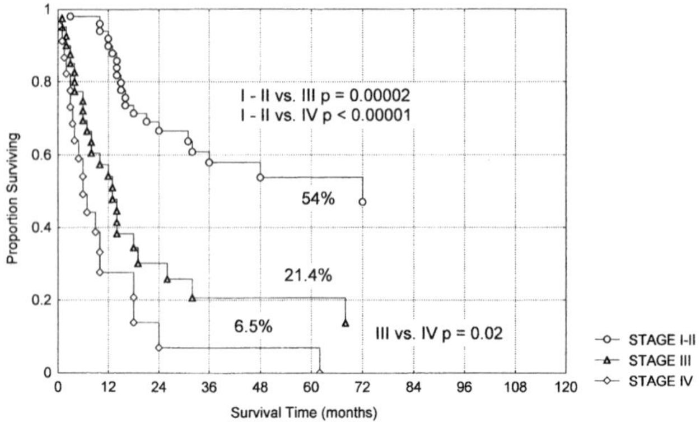

FIGURE 3.—Actuarial estimate of survival by stage. (Courtesy of Ferrante A, and The ACC Italian Registry Study Group: The Italian Registry for Adrenal Cortical Carcinoma: Analysis of a multiinstitutional series of 129 patients. *Surgery* 119:161–170, 1996.)

should be done systematically. Adjuvant treatment produced conflicting results.

▶ Adrenal cortical carcinoma is rare; it took 10 years for 18 institutions in Italy to collect 129 cases. As other studies have shown, the prognosis remains poor.

These authors found that the stage of disease at presentation was the most important predictor of survival. That is not surprising. Although more patients were being diagnosed at the earlier stages of their disease because of better diagnostic tests such as CT scans and ultrasonography, these studies were not obtained until the patient already had symptoms. Although the greater application of CT and ultrasonography for patients with signs and symptoms of carcinoma of the adrenal glands can lead to diagnosis at an earlier stage, the duration of signs and symptoms themselves reflect the stage of disease as well. The authors did not examine their series according to the duration of symptoms, something Piccirillo and Feinstein[1] have used as a major predictor of outcome in a variety of diseases.

R.J. Howard, M.D., Ph.D.

Reference

1. Piccirillo JF, Feinstein AR: Clinical symptoms and comorbidity: Significance for the prognostic classification of cancer. *Cancer* 77:834–842, 1996.

8 Nutrition and Metabolism

Introduction

Although the evolution of malnutrition during illness frequently reflects the severity of the underlying disease or toxicity associated with certain therapies, a cause-and-effect relationship between protein-calorie malnutrition and a poorer outcome has not been definitely established. Many published studies suffer from problems with experimental design, heterogeneous study populations, small sample size, or inappropriate clinical end points, or they are retrospective in nature. Some studies have included well-nourished patients, those least likely to benefit from nutrition support, thus introducing the possibility of masking efficacy. Some authors have inappropriately advocated the use of nutrition support based on transient improvements in nutritional parameters despite lack of impact on the clinical course.

Multiple and interrelated factors determine the risk of malnutrition, including pre-existing nutritional status, the disease process itself, and the magnitude and anticipated length of associated catabolic stress. Objective and biochemical measurements have been used to assess nutritional status, but no single measurement is highly sensitive and specific for identifying malnutrition. Clinical assessment (history, physical examination) of the patient is as effective a method for assessing nutritional status as are objective measurements. The cheapest and simplest way to screen for malnutrition is to ask the patient about unintentional weight loss. If reliable criteria for identifying at-risk malnourished patients were established, the value of nutritional intervention could be studied more scientifically.

Existing studies indicate that most patients do not require formal nutrition support. In the large majority of patients, short-term treatment (10 days to 2 weeks) with isotonic dextrose solutions does not have a negative impact on outcome after major elective operations or other therapies. Nutrition support should be initiated in most patients who cannot eat for longer than 10–14 days to prevent starvation-induced complications. Data in severely injured patients indicate that early aggressive enteral nutrition is superior to parenteral feedings. Despite aggressive nutrition support, it has often been difficult to make an impact on the metabolic response to illness or injury with nutrition alone, and several new strategies are under investigation, including the administration of growth hormone to promote anabolism, the provision of conditionally essential amino acids (glutamine), and the use of diets enriched with arginine, nucleotides, and ω-3 fatty acids, nutrients that can modulate immune function.

Wiley W. Souba, M.D., Sc.D.

Nutrition and Organ Function

Preoperative Total Parenteral Nutrition Is Not Associated With Mucosal Atrophy or Bacterial Translocation in Humans

Sedman PC, MacFie J, Palmer MD, et al (Scarborough District Hosp, England)

Br J Surg 82:1663–1667, 1995 8–1

Introduction.—Two recent reports suggest that adjuvant total parenteral nutrition (TPN) may have adverse effects in some surgical patients and lead to increased morbidity and death from sepsis. Animal studies support the hypothesis that mucosal atrophy in such cases predisposes to translocation of enteric organisms across the intestinal wall. A consecutive series of general surgical patients was studied for the occurrence of mucosal atrophy and gut translocation of bacteria after preoperative TPN.

Methods.—Included in the analysis were all patients who were admitted to the study unit and required elective laparotomy between January 1992 and August 1993. The TPN group, 28 patients, received preoperative parenteral nutrition for at least 10 days without any enteral nutrients. Controls were 175 patients with functional gastrointestinal tracts and the ability to tolerate oral nutrients. Bacterial translocation was determined through tissue sampling, which was performed after the peritoneal cavity was entered at laparotomy, and through simultaneously obtained peripheral venous blood samples. Mucosal atrophy was calculated by histological examination of small bowel biopsies.

Results.—The TPN and control groups were well matched for age, sex ratio, and presence of malignant disease. Because of the usual indications for parenteral feeding, the TPN group had a higher proportion of patients with inflammatory bowel disease and intestinal obstruction. There was evidence of bacterial translocation in 3 TPN and 14 control patients; not a significant difference. Only 1 of these patients had a positive blood culture. Villous height analysis of small bowel biopsies, designed to identify mucosal atrophy, showed no statistical difference between TPN and control groups. The incidence of postoperative infections did not differ significantly in TPN (4 of 28 patients) and control (15 of 175 patients) groups, nor did the rate of postoperative mortality.

Conclusion.—A short course of preoperative TPN did not increase the prevalence of bacterial translocation or lead to mucosal atrophy in patients who underwent elective laparotomy. Thus, findings do not support the hypothesis that postoperative sepsis after preoperative TPN is related to bacterial translocation, and there is no evidence that TPN has adverse effects on intestinal integrity.

▶ Several recent reports suggest that TPN may be associated with an adverse outcome in certain groups of surgical patients.[1-3] Animal models have clearly documented that TPN is associated with a higher rate of translocation of luminal bacteria to the mesenteric lymph nodes. It is unclear whether this is due directly to mucosal atrophy or to the associated reduction in villus height. In this article, Sedman and colleagues have shown that neither mucosal atrophy nor bacteria translocation was more common in parenterally fed patients than in enterally fed controls. This same group has previously shown that bacterial translocation occurs in significant numbers of surgical patients and is associated with postoperative sepsis.[4] Others have shown that TPN is associated with an increase in intestinal permeability.[5] Thus, the relationship between parenteral nutrition and intestinal barrier function in patients remains unclear. An increase in intestinal permeability may not translate into an increase in the passage of viable microbes through the gut wall.

W.W. Souba, M.D., Sc.D.

References

1. Brennan MF, Pisters PW, Posner M, et al: A prospective randomized trial of total parenteral nutrition after major pancreatic resection for malignancy. *Ann Surg* 220:436–444, 1994.
2. Kudsk KA, Croce MA, Fabian TA, et al: Enteral vs. parenteral feeding: Effects on septic morbidity following blunt and penetrating trauma. *Ann Surg* 217:503–513, 1992.
3. Moore EE, Jones TN: Benefits of immediate jejunostomy feeding after major abdominal trauma: A prospective randomized study. *J Trauma* 26:874–881, 1986.
4. Sedman PC, MacFie J, Sagar P, et al: The prevalence of gut translocation in humans. *Gastroenterology* 107:643–649, 1994.
5. Van Der Hulst R, Van Kreel BK, Von Meyenfeldt MF, et al: Glutamine and the preservation of gut integrity. *Lancet* 341:1363–1365, 1993.

Eating-Related Increase of Dopamine Concentration in the LHA With Oronasal Stimulation

Yang Z-J, Koseki M, Meguid MM, et al (State Univ of New York, Syracuse)
Am J Physiol 39:R315–R318, 1996 8–2

Intoduction.—It has been reported that dopamine release in the lateral hypothalamic area (LHA) increased significantly while eating, and there is a direct correlation between the increase and meal size. There was less of an increase in dopamine at baseline and with a much smaller meal when the smell perception was eliminated. Significantly higher levels of dopamine resulted with administration of total parenteral nutrition (TPN) alone and with eating during TPN after total liver denervation. However, dopamine levels were similar in animals after total liver denervation and

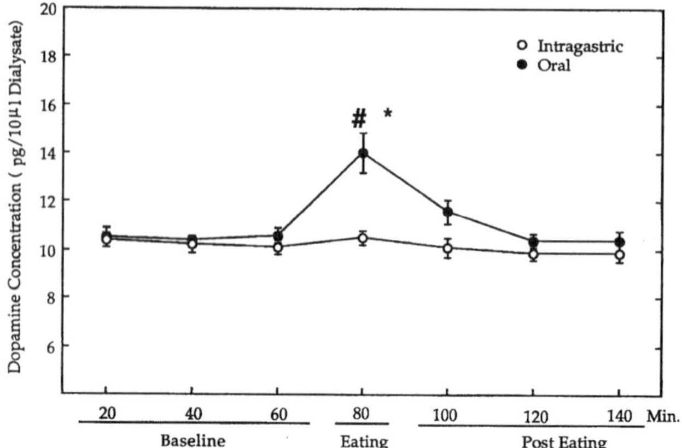

FIGURE 3.—Lateral hypothalamic area-dopamine levels at baseline, during, and after eating. Baseline dopamine level was a mean of 3 consecutive samples before eating. During eating, dopamine level was significantly greater in orally fed rats (*solid circle*) than baseline level and than intragastric-fed rats (*open circle*). There was no change in dopamine level during eating in intragastric feeding. Data are expressed as means ± SE. *$P < 0.01$ versus baseline. #$P < 0.01$ versus intragastric feeding. (Courtesy of Yang Z-J, Koseki M, Meguid MM, et al: Eating-related increase of dopamine concentration in the LHA with oronasal stimulation. *Am J Physiol* 39:R315–R318, 1996.)

sham-operation controls when food only was ingested. This indicates that the liver has a role in regulating food intake by inhibiting release of LHA-dopamine in response to food. The effect of oronasal stimulation on increases in release of LHA-dopamine that are eating-induced were studied.

Methods.—A gastrostomy tube was inserted in 12 rats. The rats were then fed a liquid diet orally or through the gastrostomy tube. Release of LHA-dopamine was compared through the use of microdialysis.

Results.—In orally fed rats, release of LHA-dopamine increased from 10.6 to 14.0 pg/10 µl dialysate within 20 minutes. There was no significant change in dopamine levels in rats fed through the gastrostomy tube (Fig 3).

Conclusions.—Oronasal stimulation results in release of LHA-dopamine. When nutrients are absorbed, the liver inhibits release of LHA-dopamine to suppress food intake. The ventromedial hypothalamus may also have a role in the suppression of food intake.

▶ The authors have previously reported that eating increases LHA-dopamine release and that the degree of dopamine release correlates with meal size. The present study nicely demonstrates that dopamine concentrations in the lateral hypothalamic area are not increased when oral nasal stimulation is bypassed. The authors suggest that the hypothalamus receives a positive feedback stimulation from oral nasal stimulation during eating, and maintains food intake by the modulation of gastric motility through a dopaminergic mechanism. When nutrients are absorbed, their presence in the blood is sensed by the liver, which in turn inhibits brain dopamine release to further suppress food intake. Whether this control is present in stressed patients, or is altered by insults such as sepsis, remains unclear.

W.W. Souba, M.D., Sc.D.

Impaired Gut Barrier Function in Malnourished Patients

Reynolds JV, O'Farrelly C, Feighery C, et al (Meath and Adelaide Hosps, Dublin; St James's Hosp, Leeds, England; Trinity College Dublin)

Br J Surg 83:1288–1291, 1996 8–3

Introduction.—Malnutrition is common in hospital patients and predisposes them to sepsis by adversely affecting the immune system. The mechanism of altered immune response and intestinal morphologic assessment for signs of malnutrition were studied in malnourished patients.

Methods.—Immunoglobulin G antibodies to wheat and milk were determined using enzyme-linked immunoabsorbent assays, and endoscopic biopsies of the second part of the duodenum were performed on 20 malnourished patients (aged 33–80 years), and 15 well-nourished controls (aged 34–78 years). Results were compared statistically.

Results.—Fifteen patients and 7 controls had cancer. No controls had antibodies to food proteins. Fifteen patients had antibodies to β-lactoglobulin, 10 had antibodies to gliadin, and 10 had antibodies to both. Gastrointestinal morphologic features were normal in both groups. The 15 patients with antibodies were compared with the 5 without antibodies. The 10 patients with 2 antibodies were compared with the 5 with 1 antibody. The number of antibodies was significantly related to the degree of malnutrition and, in the case of patients with 2 antibodies, was significantly related to the severity of malnutrition.

Conclusion.—Gut barrier function is fundamentally impaired in malnourished patients, and the degree and severity of malnutrition are correlated to the number of food antibodies present. Malnutrition rather than disease appears to be the cause of barrier breakdown. Restoration of gut barrier function is important for prevention of sepsis.

► The authors assessed gut barrier function in well-nourished and malnourished patients by evaluating antibodies to food antigens. No permeability defect was observed. A previous study[1] demonstrated that slight mucosal atrophy develops in patients who do not eat but receive total parenteral nutrition for approximately 2 weeks. With resumption of oral alimentation, brush border enzyme activities and microvillus height return toward normal values within 1 week.[2]

W.W. Souba, M.D., Sc.D.

References

1. Van der Hulst R, Van Kreel BK, Von Meyenfeldt MF, et al: Glutamine and the preservation of gut integrity. *Lancet* 341:1363–1365, 1993.

2. Guedon C, Schmitz J, Lerebours E, et al: Decreased brush border hydrolase activities without gross morphologic changes in human intestinal mucosa after prolonged total parenteral nutrition of adults. *Gastroenterology* 90:373–378, 1986.

Enteral Versus Parenteral Nutrition: Effects on Gastrointestinal Function and Metabolism

Suchner U, Senftleben U, Eckart T, et al (Ludwig Maximilians Universität, München; Abbott GmbH, Wiesbaden, Germany)
Nutrition 12:13–22, 1996 8–4

Background.—Enteral feeding is preferred over parenteral feeding for critically ill patients because the enteral approach preserves gut function better. One study, however, showed that parenteral feeding significantly increases energy and nitrogen intake. Total parenteral nutrition (TPN) and total enteral nutrition (TEN) were compared in 34 patients after neurosurgery.

Methods.—Resting energy expenditure, urea production rate, visceral proteins, liver and pancreas function, and gastrointestinal absorption were measured in 34 brain-injured patients who received either TPN or TEN for 12 days. The nutrition index was calculated as a predictor of nutritional status.

Results.—Urea production rate was similar between groups. Resting energy expenditure was at full strength between days 3 and 5 in both groups. A significant 18% increase in resting energy expenditure was

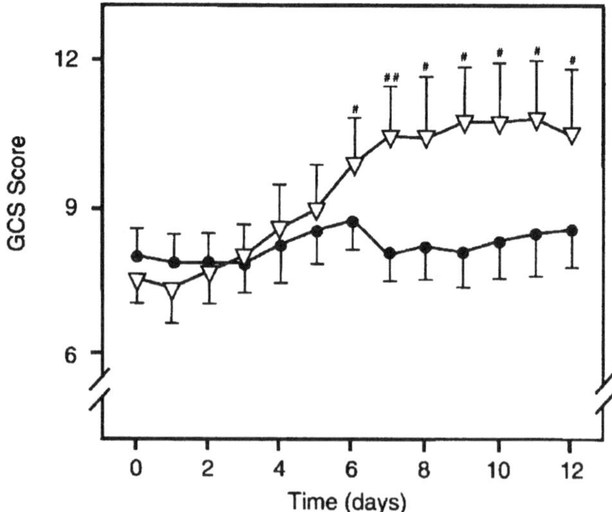

FIGURE 3.—Glasgow Coma Scale (*GCS*) scores during enteral (*triangles*) and parenteral (*circles*) nutrition; mean ± SEM, #$P < 0.05$; ##$P < 0.01$ (vs. day 0, enteral). (Reprinted by permission of the publisher from Suchner U, Senftleben U, Eckart T, et al: Enteral versus parenteral nutrition: Effects on gastrointestinal function and metabolism. *Nutrition* 12:13–22, Copyright 1996 by Elsevier Science Inc.)

observed in the TEN group but not in the TPN group between days 5 and 9. Glasgow Coma Scale score increases between days 6 and 12 were significant for the TEN group but not for the TPN group (Fig 3). Intergroup differences were not significant. Insulin demand and bilirubin, amylase, and lipase levels increased significantly in the TPN but not in the TEN group. Visceral protein synthesis increased significantly in the TEN group after 12 days. The nutrition index improved significantly in the TEN but not in the TPN group. Thrombocyte and lymphocyte counts rose mainly in the TEN group. Fat absorption was significantly reduced in the TPN group after 12 days, and xylose absorption levels remained subnormal.

Conclusion.—Total enteral nutrition appears to maintain intestinal absorption capacity and facilitate normalization of nutritional status by improving visceral protein synthesis and carbohydrate utilization.

Effect of Malnutrition After Acute Stroke on Clinical Outcome

Dávalos A, Ricart W, Gonzalez-Huix F, et al (Institut Municpal d'Investigació Mèdica de Barcelona)

Stroke 27:1028–1032, 1996 8–5

Background.—Malnutrition after acute stroke increases the risk of impaired immunity, infections and other complications, and a higher mortality rate. The prevalence of malnutrition in patients with acute stroke after 1 week of hospitalization and its relation to stress response and neurologic outcome were discussed.

Methods.—Nutritional status, glucose profile, and stress response were assessed in 104 patients (64% male) younger than 80 years who were admitted to the hospital within 24 hours of acute stroke. Cranial CT scans were obtained. Fasting glycemia, glycated hemoglobin, fructosamine, and serum albumin levels were measured on admission, and weekly thereafter. Serum cortisol levels were determined on days 1, 2, 4, and 7, and 24-hour free urinary cortisol levels were determined daily. Nutritional status was assessed by measuring triceps skinfold thickness, serum albumin concentration, and midarm muscle circumference (MAMC). Neurologic deficits were scored on a Canadian Stroke Scale, and patients were given an oral standard diet or an enteric feeding. Outcome at 1 month was rated as good for disabled or independent patients (Barthel Index greater than 50) or poor (Barthel Index less than or equal to 50, or dead).

Results.—Thirteen patients died during week 1. On admission, 16.3% were malnourished; after 1 week, 26.4% of the 91 surviving patients were malnourished; and after 2 weeks, 35% of the remaining 43 patients were malnourished. Patients who could not swallow were significantly more malnourished than those who could. After 7 days, triceps skinfold thickness decreased significantly. Serum albumin concentration was also lower. Free urinary cortisol and plasma cortisol levels, measures of stress, were significantly higher in malnourished than in nonmalnourished patients as

TABLE 4.—Clinical Outcome at 1 Month in 24 Malnourished and 67 Nonmalnourished Patients After the First Week of Hospitalization

	Malnourished		Nonmalnourished		
Score at 1 mo	No.	%	No.	%	*P*
CSS ≤5	16	66.7	15	22.4	.0001
BI					.0120
≥95	4	16.7	28	41.8	
55–90	3	12.5	15	22.4	
≤50	17	70.8	24	35.8	

Note: Canadian Stroke Scale and BI scores of 0 were assessed in dead patients.
Abbreviations: CSS, Canadian Stroke Scale; *BI,* Barthel Index.
(Reproduced with permission from Dávalos A, Ricart W, Gonzalez-Huix F, et al: Effect of malnutrition after acute stroke on clinical outcome. *Stroke* 27:1028–1032, 1996. Copyright 1996 American Heart Association.)

were the incidences of urinary or respiratory infections (50% vs. 24%) and bedsores (17% vs. 4%). At 1 month, Canadian Stroke Scale score and Barthel Index were significantly lower for malnourished patients (Table 4). Malnourished patients had a significantly higher mortality rate after week 1 and a significantly longer hospitalization. Significantly more malnourished patients than nonmalnourished patients had a poor outcome (41% vs. 14%).

Conclusion.—Malnutrition after acute stroke increases the risk of a poor outcome. Early enteric feeding during the first week of hospitalization did not prevent malnutrition. Increased stress during the first week after acute stroke resulted in a higher incidence of respiratory and urinary infection, bedsores, death, poor outcome, and longer hospital stay.

▶ Abstracts 8–4 and 8–5 collectively point out the importance of nutrition in patients with neurologic disorders that may preclude oral intake. In these individuals, malnutrition may be a risk factor, and nutritional support of the neurologically impaired patient may be indicated. The value of nutritional support in patients with head injury is also well established. In 2 earlier studies, patients with head injury receiving parenteral nutrition (vs. enteral nutrition) had a more favorable outcome, but the parenteral nutrition groups received more calories and nitrogen.[1, 2] Additional trials[3, 4] have shown that enteral nutrition is equivalent or superior to parenteral nutrition when nutrient intake is controlled. Patients with head injury are candidates for parenteral nutrition if they cannot tolerate enteral feeding (ileus or high risk of aspiration).[4] Early enteral feeding in injured patients (within 24 hours) has established benefits over feeding later in the course of the hospitalization. Feedings should be discontinued when adequate oral intake is achieved.

W.W. Souba, M.D., Sc.D.

References

1. Rapp RP, Pharm D, Young B. et al: The favorable effect of early parenteral feeding on survival in head-injured patients. *J Neurosurgery* 58:906–912, 1983.

2. Hadley MN, Graham TW, Harrington T, et al: Nutrition support and neurotrauma: A critical review of early nutrition in forty-five acute head injury patients. *Neurosurgery* 19:367–373, 1986.
3. Grahm TW, Zadrozny DB, Harrington T: The benefits of early jejunal hyperalimentation in the head-injured patient. *Neurosurgery* 25:729–735, 1989.
4. Norton JA, Ott LG, McClain C, et al: Intolerance to enteral feeding in the brain injured patient. *J Neurosurgery* 68:62–66, 1988.

High Protein Diets Are Associated With Increased Bacterial Translocation in Septic Guinea Pigs

Nelson JL, Alexander JW, Gianotti L, et al (Univ of Cincinnati, Ohio)
Nutrition 12:195–199, 1996 8–6

Background.—During sepsis, protein catabolism increases, eventually resulting in multiple organ failure. Although some studies recommend that this condition be treated with a high-protein diet, other studies demonstrate that diets low in protein improve survival. Possibly, loss of gut barrier function results in increased bacterial translocation and absorption of toxic material. Whether septic animals on a high-protein diet have increased bacterial translocation was investigated.

Methods.—Catheter gastrotomies were performed on 32 female guinea pigs, and sepsis was induced through an osmotic minipump with *Escherichia coli* and *Staphylococcus aureus*. Diets of 5% or 20% protein were

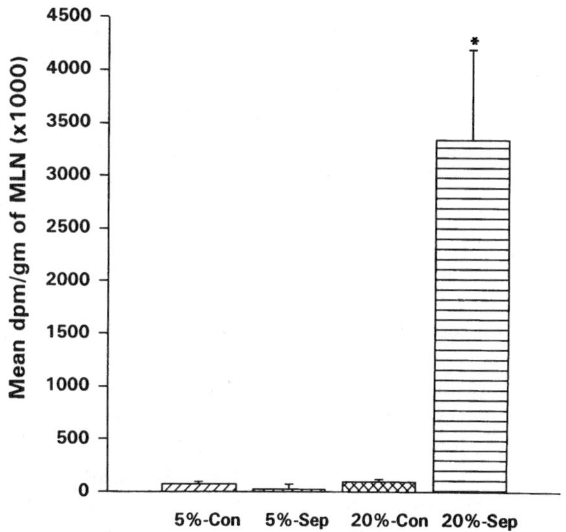

FIGURE 1.—The number of dpm per gram of mesenteric lymph node in the different dietary groups. The septic animal who received the 20% protein diet had significantly more ($P < 0.05$) dpm per gram of MLN tissue as compared to all other groups. *Abbreviations: MLN,* mesenteric lymph node; *Con,* control; *Sep,* septic. (Reprinted by permssion of the publisher from Nelson JL, Alexander JW, Gianotti L, et al: High protein diets are associated with increased bacterial translocation in septic guinea pigs. *Nutrition* 12:195–199. Copyright 1996 by Elsevier Science Inc.)

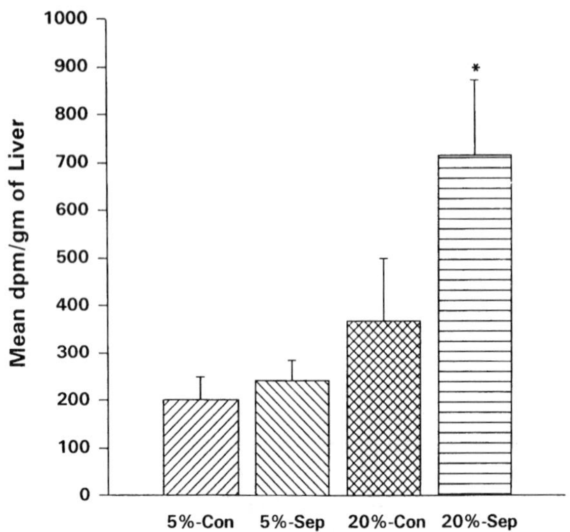

FIGURE 2.—The number of dpm per gram of liver in different dietary groups. There were significantly ($P < 0.05$) higher counts in the septic animals who received the 20% protein diet as compared to the other groups. *Abbreviations: Con,* control; *Sep,* septic. (Reprinted by permission of the publisher from Nelson JL, Alexander JW, Gianotti L, et al: High protein diets are associated with increased bacterial translocation in septic guinea pigs. *Nutrition* 12:195–199. Copyright 1996 by Elsevier Science Inc.)

fed for 4 days to infected and sham-operated control animals. All animals received 1.0 mL of ^{14}C-labeled *E. coli* and were killed 4 hours later. The amount of radioactivity was determined in selected tissues.

Results.—Septic animals on a high-protein diet had significantly more radioactivity in mesenteric lymph nodes, liver, lung, and blood, which indicated increased bacterial translocation (Figs 1–2). In the spleen, radioactivity levels were significantly different only between septic animals on a high-protein diet and septic animals on a low-protein diet.

Conclusion.—Although these results suggest that a low-protein enteral diet improves survival in septic patients because it decreases bacterial translocation, a low-protein enteral diet does not provide sufficient nourishment because of gut barrier dysfunction. Additional studies are necessary to determine the optimal therapeutic treatment for these patients.

► This is an interesting study in that previous studies from the Cincinnati group have shown that a high-protein diet improves outcome in burned children. Burned children receiving a high nitrogen enteral diet had better hepatic synthetic function, fewer days of bacteremia, and improved survival as compared with similar children who received a normal diet, but the study was small, and the former group received more nutrients intraluminally and fewer nutrients IV than did the latter group.[1]

W.W. Souba, M.D., Sc.D.

Reference

1. Alexander JW, MacMillan BG, Stinnett JD, et al: Beneficial effects of aggressive protein feeding in severely burned children. *Ann Surg* 192:505–507, 1980.

Caloric Restriction Increases the Expression of Heat Shock Protein in the Gut

Ehrenfried JA, Evers BM, Chu KU, et al (Univ of Texas, Galveston)
Ann Surg 223:592–599, 1996 8–7

Background.—Lifelong caloric restriction (CR) increases the life span of experimental animals and delays the onset of age-related diseases. Several heat shock proteins, especially *hsp*70, are induced by cellular stressors, including fasting. To evaluate whether CR induces *hsp*70 production, the effects of fasting and refeeding, and of CR on 1 heat shock protein, *hsp*70, were measured.

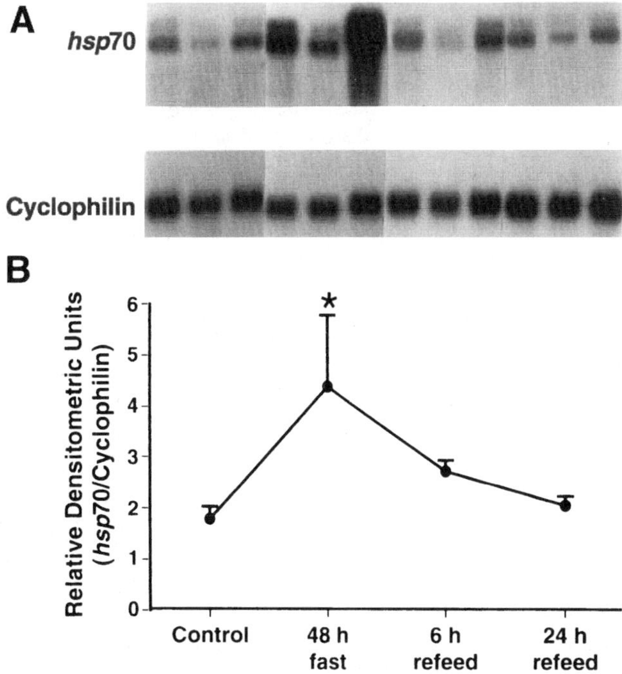

Figure 1.—**A**, representative Northern blot analysis of RNA (10 μg poly (A+) per lane) extracted from the stomach of rats either fasted for 48 hours, fasted for 48 hours and then re-fed for 6 and 24 hours, or rats fed ad libitum (control). Blots were probed with cDNA probes for *hsp*70 and cyclophilin and exposed to Kodak T-mat film (Eastman Kodak, Rochester, NY) using 2 intensifying screens at −70°C. **B**, Northern blots were quantitated using scanning densitometry and expressed as relative densitometric units after normalizing for cyclophilin expression (mean ± standard error of the mean; $^*P < 0.05$ vs control; n = 3 rats per group). (Courtesy of Ehrenfried JA, Evers BM, Chu KU, et al: Caloric restriction increases the expression of heat shock protein in the gut. *Ann Surg* 223:592–599, 1996.)

Methods.—After a 48-hour food fast, groups of 3 young adult rats were killed immediately after the fast, and at 6 and 24 hours after feeding was resumed. Northern blot analysis was used to measure the amount of messenger RNA of *hsp*70 and *hsp*27, another heat shock protein, in both gastric and ileal tissue. Next, 6 aged rats received an ad libitum diet and 6 received a CR diet for 8 weeks, after which time they were killed. Gastric and duodenal messenger RNA for *hsp*70 were measured.

Results.—After a 48-hour fast, levels of gastric *hsp*70 rose significantly, then fell to prefasting levels within 24 hours once feeding resumed (Fig 1). Levels of *hsp*27 did not rise. Ileal *hsp*70 did not increase with fasting. Caloric restriction (60% of usual intake) for 8 weeks caused a similar, though smaller, increase in gene activity in both the stomach and the duodenum.

Conclusion.—Fasting for 48 hours and, to a lesser extent, a brief CR diet both cause a significant increase in levels of specific heat shock proteins in the proximal gut of the rat.

► In response to stressful stimuli, many of the genes in the gut mucosa are turned off. The heat shock proteins, in contrast, are activated and may serve to conserve or protect vital cellular functions. A rise in heat shock proteins may be required for cells to respond or recover from an insult. If specific nutrients (e.g., fiber, nucleic acids, glutamine) can also exert protective effects on the gut during stress states, it would be interesting to study the relation between these nutrients and heat shock protein expression during catabolic states.

W.W. Souba, M.D., Sc.D.

Antioxidants Prevent the Cellular Deficit Produced in Response to Burn Injury

LaLonde C, Nayak U, Hennigan J, et al (Brigham and Women's Hosp, Boston)

J Burn Care Rehabil 17:379–383, 1996 8–8

Background.—Systemic organ dysfunction is a well-known but poorly understood complication of burn injury. Altered organ function probably results from the inability of cells to generate sufficient energy, which can be measured as the cell energy charge potential (ECP). ECP = ATP + 1/2 ADP/ATP + ADP + AMP. To study the changes in cellular energetics and organ antioxidant activity after burn injury, an animal model of burn injury was used. The effect of added antioxidants on ECP was assessed to evaluate the relation between oxidant activity and cellular energetics.

Methods.—Fifty rats were given a third-degree burn over 30% of their body area. Ten were given a sham burn treatment. Animals were fluid resuscitated and allowed access to food and water. Meperidine was administered for discomfort. Antioxidants were given beginning on the day of insult and continuing throughout the study period. The daily antioxi-

TABLE 1.—Energy Charge Potential

Organ	Control	Control plus antioxidants	Burn day 1	Burn day 3	Burn day 6	Burn day 6 plus antioxidants
Heart						
ECP	0.69 ± 0.05	0.65 ± 0.02	0.73 ± 0.03	0.73 ± 0.03	0.56 ± 0.02*	0.71 ± 0.05t
ATP μmol/gm	2.55 ± 0.37	2.59 ± 0.45	2.95 ± 0.44	2.66 ± 0.55	1.81 ± 0.13*	3.38 ± 0.68*t
TANS μmol/gm	4.71 ± 0.51	5.74 ± 0.71	5.11 ± 0.65	4.53 ± 0.96	4.79 ± 0.13	6.09 ± 0.81t
Liver						
ECP	0.46 ± 0.06	0.55 ± 0.03*	0.41 ± 0.07	0.35 ± 0.05*	0.30 ± 0.01*	0.40 ± 0.70t
ATP μmol/gm	1.02 ± 0.29	1.27 ± 0.16	1.13 ± 0.34	0.79 ± 0.21	0.52 ± 0.04*	0.82 ± 0.24t
TANS μmol/gm	3.55 ± 0.48	3.31 ± 0.04	4.61 ± 0.28*	4.44 ± 0.13*	3.84 ± 0.28	3.86 ± 0.33
Lung						
ECP	0.52 ± 0.06	0.59 ± 0.04*	0.67 ± 0.06*	0.60 ± 0.02*	0.53 ± 0.02	0.61 ± 0.03
ATP μmol/gm	0.88 ± 0.17	1.26 ± 0.04*	1.19 ± 0.11*	1.14 ± 0.10*	0.93 ± 0.10	1.02 ± 0.23
TANS μmol/gm	2.42 ± 0.39	2.89 ± 0.16*	2.28 ± 0.16	2.51 ± 0.13	2.3 ± 0.19	2.24 ± 0.55

*Significantly different from control $P < 0.05$.
t, Significantly different than day 6 after the burn injury $P < 0.05$.
(Courtesy of Lalonde C, Nayak U, Hennigan J, et al: Antioxidants prevent the cellular deficit produced in response to burn injury. *J Burn Care Rehabil* 17:379–383, 1996.)

dant dose was 1 g of reduced glutathione per kilogram, 1 g of *N*-acetylcysteine per kilogram, and 0.5 of vitamin C per kilogram. Animals were killed at 1 day, 3 days, and 6 days after injury. The enzymatic antioxidant catalase was used as a marker of endogenous cellular antioxidant activity.

Results.—The mortality rate was 0% and the animals did not appear uncomfortable with the burn injury. The ECPs of lung, liver, and heart were normal on the first day after injury. The ECP significantly decreased in the liver by day 3 and continued to decrease through day 6 in animals not treated with antioxidants. Heart ECP decreased between day 3 and day 6 (Table 1). Total adenine nucleotides were not decreased, which indicates that the ECP decrease resulted from a decrease in adenosine triphosphate. The ECP remained normal in the lung throughout the study period. Catalase was decreased in the liver and heart and remained normal in the lung. In rats that received antioxidants after burn injury, there was no decrease in the liver and heart ECPs.

Conclusions.—In the results provided by this rat model of modest burn injury, such an injury seems to cause a cellular energy deficit in the liver and heart about 3 to 6 days after injury. A decrease in antioxidants appears to precede the decrease in cellular ECP. The lungs appear to be protected from this change. Administration of antioxidants after burn injury prevented the alteration in cellular energetics, suggesting that the release of oxidants resulting from inflammation is associated with decreased antioxidant activity and altered cellular energetics.

▶ Antioxidants such as glutathione, selenium, ascorbic acid, and vitamin E may be required in increased amounts during inflammatory states. Clinical trials have shown the benefits of these compounds in selected patients. They may become routine nutritional supplements in the future.

W.W. Souba, M.D., Sc.D.

Low-Dose Enteral Feeding Is Beneficial During Total Parenteral Nutrition

Sax HC, Illig KA, Ryan CK, et al (Univ of Rochester, NY)

Am J Surg 171:587–590, 1996 8–9

Background.—Total parenteral nutrition (TPN) is accompanied by gut atrophy and immunosuppression, which lead to bacterial translocation and abnormal permeability of the bowel wall. The degree to which low-dose enteral feeding, along with TPN, might avert these problems was studied.

Methods.—Male rats, in whom IV catheters had been placed, received 1 of 4 proportions of enteral and IV alimentation: 0% enteral/100% TPN; 6% enteral/94% TPN; 12% enteral/88% TPN; or 25% enteral/75% TPN. Nitrogen balance determinations were made over 9 days of diet. The animals then received large doses of mannitol and lactulose by gavage, followed by measurement of these compounds' urine levels, to evaluate

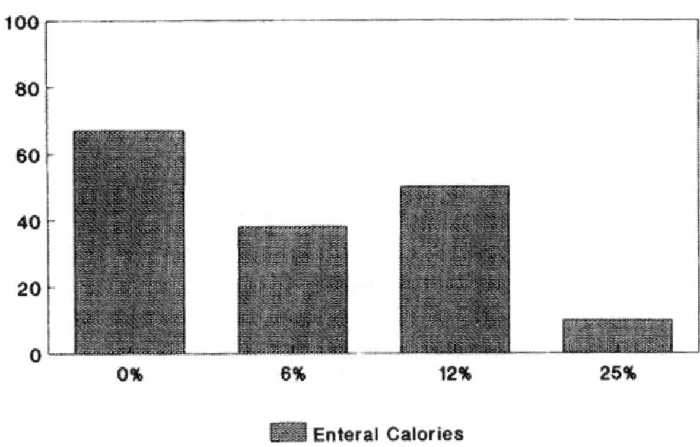

FIGURE.—There is decreasing bacterial translocation with increasing enteral support ($P < 0.03$). (Reprinted by permission of the publisher from Low-dose enteral feeding is beneficial during total parenteral nutrition, by Sax HC, Illig KA, Ryan CK, et al, *American Journal of Surgery,* vol 171, pp 2 587–590, Copyright 1996 by Excerpta Medica Inc.)

bowel wall permeability. The rats were then killed. Mesenteric lymph nodes and blood were cultured for bacteria, and jejunal, ileal, and hepatic tissues were collected.

Results.—There was no difference among groups for rates of survival or positive blood culture. The rats that received 25% enteral calories had a significantly greater mean daily nitrogen balance, and their rate of mesenteric lymph node infection was significantly lower than for those receiving 100% TPN (Fig). There was no difference in gut mucosal or villous histology among the groups, and there was no significant difference in the degree of alteration of lactulose permeability.

Conclusions.—A significant increase in positive nitrogen balance and a significant decrease in bacterial translocation was found when TPN is supported by the provision of 25% of calories enterally. Bowel permeability and morphology are not improved.

▶ The benefits of enteral nutrition are well established. All too often, we switch our patients to parenteral nutrition when they cannot tolerate complete enteral feedings because of distention or diarrhea. I fully endorse the authors' contention. Even slow rates of luminal feedings are beneficial—the patient's energy and nitrogen needs can be met by supplementing using the IV route.

W.W. Souba, M.D., Sc.D.

Complications of Nutrition Support

Pneumatosis Intestinalis and Portal Venous Air Associated With Needle Catheter Jejunostomy

North JH Jr, Nava HR (Roswell Park Cancer Inst, Buffalo, NY)
Am Surg 61:1045–1048, 1995 8–10

Introduction.—Postoperative nutritional support is especially important for patients with upper gastrointestinal malignancies. A needle catheter jejunostomy can be placed during the operative procedure and facilitate rapid resumption of enteral nutritional support. Although needle catheter jejunostomy is associated with few risks, the patient reported here shows that the complication of pneumatosis intestinalis (PI) is possible.

> *Case Report.*—Woman, 75, was treated with radical gastrectomy, subtotal pancreatectomy, and Roux-en-Y esophagojejunostomy for a T3N1M0 poorly differentiated adenocarcinoma of the gastroesophageal junction. The patient received intraperitoneal chemotherapy and had a needle catheter jejunostomy placed for postoperative nutritional support. She was treated for a controlled pancreatic fistula discovered on day 10, and 2 weeks postoperatively experienced nausea, vomiting, and abdominal distention. Abdominal radiographs, subsequently confirmed by CT, revealed a diffuse ileus, the presence of PI, and air within the portal vein. The patient then received a nasogastric tube, IV antibiotics, and parenteral nutrition. Her condition improved, and by day 17 the abdominal distention had resolved. Resolution of the PI was documented by abdominal radiographs.

Discussion.—Pneumatosis intestinalis, defined as gas within the intestinal wall, is associated with a variety of disorders and surgical conditions. The first report of PI in patients with a feeding catheter jejunostomy was published in 1982. All patients in this study were managed nonoperatively and their pneumatosis was resolved. The complication has developed as early as 3 days and as late as 14 days postoperatively. It is important to note that PI may be related to more serious underlying pathology, such as bowel obstruction and ischemic bowel, even in patients with a needle catheter jejunostomy. Mortality is high when pneumatosis occurs together with portal vein air. Both loss of mucosal integrity and raised intraluminal pressure may be involved in cases of PI secondary to needle catheter jejunostomy. When diagnosed, enteral feeding should be discontinued and broad spectrum antibiotics started.

▶ The development of PI is usually related to the loss of mucosal integrity and/or raised intraluminal pressure. Both factors are likely to be involved in patients who have PI secondary to needle catheter jejunostomy. This complication of needle catheter jejunostomy is quite rare. The jejunostomy should be implicated as a causative factor only after the absence of other explanations for the discovery of intramural air is confirmed. Intestinal obstruction and ischemic bowel are the most common causes of PI, and these are associated with a considerable morality rate. In the absence of indications for surgical intervention, a nonoperative approach can be pursued in patients who have PI from needle catheter jejunostomy.

W.W. Souba, M.D., Sc.D.

Analysis of Complications and Long Term Outcome of Trauma Patients With Needle Catheter Jejunostomy

Eddy VA, Snell JE, Morris JA Jr (Vanderbilt Univ, Nashville, Tenn)
Am Surg 62:40–44, 1996 8–11

Introduction.—Nutrition has become important in the treatment of patients who are critically ill. Enteral nutrition has been shown to reduce the risk of complications from sepsis. Needle catheter jejunostomy is associated with lower morbidity from sepsis than total parenteral nutrition. The rate and type of complications associated with needle catheter jejunostomy in patients with trauma were evaluated.

Methods.—A review was conducted of all cases of needle catheter jejunostomy during an 8-year period at a Level I trauma center. Definitions of short term complications included intraabdominal abscess, small bowel obstruction, catheter leakage, enterocutaneous fistula formation, and infection of local soft tissue or the abdominal wall. Telephone interviews were conducted to determine long-term complications.

Results.—There were 122 patients, predominantly young and male, who had needle catheter jejunostomy. There were 22 short term complications that included abscess, bowel obstruction, abdominal wall infection, leakage, local soft tissue infection, enterocutaneous fistula, blocked catheter, and tube dislodgment. Telephone interviews were conducted with 50 patients. Of these, 19 had long-term complications, including 2 operations for adhesion.

Discussion.—These findings suggest that catheter jejunostomy is associated with a significant rate of potentially dangerous complications. However, very low complication rates have been reported by previous studies (Table 3). The role of needle catheter jejunostomy as the only way to provide nutrition to patients with trauma should be reexamined. A randomized, prospective study is needed to determine the role of various modes of enteral access in these patients.

▶ The incidence of complications in this study is considerably higher than that observed by previous investigators. In previous studies, the rate of complications attributed to needle catheter jejunostomy has been less than 2%, and these trials have included both elective surgical patients and trauma patients. The authors do acknowledge the benefits of early enteral feeding over total parenteral nutrition in terms of reduction in septic morbidity, but

TABLE 3.—Comparisons of Complications Attributed to Needle Catheter Jejunostomy in Previous Series

Author	Eeftinck	Feldtman	Haun	Strickland	Heberer	Sarr	Moore	Moore	Dent	Current
Year	1983	1984	1985	1986	1987	1988	1989	1991	1993	1995
Type patients	GS	Mix	GS	Mix	GS	GS	Tr	Tr	Tr	Tr
Number pts with NCJ	210	61	55	114	42	83	29	32	30	122
Number compl (%)	4 (1.9)	0 (0)	1 (1.8)	1 (1)	0 (0)	0 (0)	0 (0)	0 (0)	0 (0)	10 (8)
Type compl	Leak	N/A	SBO	Vol	N/A	N/A	N/A	N/A	N/A	See text

Abbreviations: GS, general surgical; *Tr,* trauma; *Mix,* mixed general surgical and trauma; *Vol,* volvulus; *leak,* intraperitoneal leakage; *SBO,* small bowel obstruction.
(Courtesy of Eddy VA, Snell JE, Morris JA Jr: Analysis of complications and long term outcome of trauma patients with needle catheter jejunostomy. *Am Surg* 62:40–44, 1996.)

they suggest the use of needle catheter jejunostomy as the sole method for nutritional support in the trauma patient be reconsidered.

W.W. Souba, M.D., Sc.D.

Venopelvic Fistula: A Rare Complication of Hyperalimentation

Aihara T, Takano H, Hirata A, et al (Saitama Children's Med Ctr, Japan)
Pediatr Radiol 26:198–199, 1996 8–12

Background.—Central venous catheters are commonly used in infants and children for nutrition and venous access. A case of venopelvic fistula associated with a hyperalimentation catheter was reported.

Case Report.—Boy, 4 months, underwent surgery for a long segment of Hirschsprung's disease. A hyperalimentation catheter was placed in the inferior vena cava through the left great saphenous vein at the time of surgery. This patient's nutritional intake depended on parenteral hyperalimentation. Three months after surgery, a convulsive movement of the right eyelid developed suddenly. Moderate hypoglycemia was found, and 20 mL of 50% glucose solution was infused through the hyperalimentation catheter. Blood levels of glucose remained less than 20 mg/dL, however, and the eyelid convulsion persisted. Consecutive blood laboratory data revealed a sudden decrease in the level of glucose, which indicated that an accident had occurred. Poor blood return from the catheter strongly suggested catheter malposition. Contrast-enhanced radiography showed clear opacification of the right upper urinary tract through a venopelvic fistula. The catheter was removed immediately. The access route for hyperalimentation was transferred to the right external jugular vein, and blood levels of glucose normalized. The eye convulsions subsided, which indicated that they most likely resulted from hypoglycemia.

Conclusions.—In this infant, the prolonged placement of a hyperalimentation catheter through the left great saphenous vein resulted in an obstruction of the inferior vena cava and a venopelvic fistula. This complication may have been caused by administering hyperosmolar fluid through the catheter.

► I have never heard of this mechanical complication of parenteral nutrition. I agree with the authors' postulation that thrombosis and complete obstruction of the inferior vena cava above the renal veins probably occurred first. Continuing administration of the hypertonic solution probably led to retrograde flow through one of the small right renal vein tributaries and erosion into the renal pelvis. This would explain the high level of glucose in the urine and the concomitant hypoglycemia that occurred.

W.W. Souba, M.D., Sc.D.

Central Venous Catheter-related Infections: A Review

Adal KA, Farr BM (Univ of Virginia, Charlottesville)

Nutrition 12:208–213, 1996 8–13

Background.—Central venous catheter–related infections occur in up to 100,000 patients annually in the United States, extending each patient's hospital stay an average of 7 days. Current knowledge regarding these infections was reviewed.

Discussion.—Catheter infection can occur from bacterial colonization of the skin–catheter interface, from hub contamination because of frequent manipulation, and from seeding of the catheter by remote bacteremia. Bacterial adhesion is enhanced by host proteins that coat catheters and by adherent proteins produced by some organisms. Skin organisms are most commonly at fault, but *Corynebacterium, Enterococcus,* gram-negative rods, and fungi often infect tunneled catheters, because patients with those organisms frequently are immunocompromised. *Candida* is associated with total parenteral nutrition (TPN). Central catheters, as opposed to peripheral ones, cause 90% of catheter-related infections. Both tunneled catheters and subcutaneous ports have lower infection rates. Whether TPN increases the risk of catheter infection is no longer clear. Although duration of catheterization is a risk factor, routine catheter changes do not decrease the incidence of infection. Strict asepsis during placement, physician experience, and scrupulous catheter care are associated with fewer infections. Fever is the most common finding, and it may be the only one. Semiquantitative cultures can help diagnose infection, but qualitative techniques, especially cultures obtained through the catheter, are not helpful. Systemic signs of infection require antibiotic therapy and catheter removal. Infections in tunneled catheters usually require removal, but local exit site infections do not. Infection prevention is enhanced by chlorhexidine gluconate and povidone-iodine, but not by polymyxin-neomycin-bacitracin ointment, which increases the risk of *Candida* colonization. The risk of catheter tip colonization is significantly greater when transparent dressings are used on central catheters. Scheduled replacement of short-term catheters is not necessary.

Conclusions.—Central venous catheterization carries a significant risk of infection, which can be minimized with scrupulous attention to asepsis and catheter care.

▶ This is a very comprehensive overview of central venous catheter–related infections. Patients who receive TPN through these catheters are at higher risk of having catheter sepsis develop, in part because the high glucose infusion is an excellent nutrient source for microbes. It also has been suggested that persistent hyperglycemia may be immunosuppressive. When using a central venous catheter for parenteral nutrition, it should be a dedicated line.

W.W. Souba, M.D., Sc.D.

Severe Hypophosphataemia Due to Intraperitoneal Nutrition in a CAPD Patient

Ghattaora R, Doyle S, Farrington K (Lister Hosp, Stevenage, Herts, England)

Nephrol Dial Transplant 11:1365–1366, 1996 8–14

Background.—The malnutrition that accompanies continuous ambulatory peritoneal dialysis (CAPD) can be treated by intraperitoneal administration of nutrients. A case of intraperitoneal nutrition (IPN), complicated by severe hypophosphatemia, is reported.

> *Case Report.*—Woman, 19, with end-stage renal disease and rejection of 2 renal transplants, received IPN for very poor nutrition after resumption of CAPD. Serum phosphate levels fell progressively, reaching a low point after 6 weeks of IPN. The hypophosphatemia was corrected by the addition of phosphate to the dialysis fluid. After 12 months, CAPD failed and the patient received hemodialysis.

Conclusions.—Severe hypophosphatemia, never previously reported in patients receiving IPN, occurred in this patient with end-stage renal disease, probably as a result of her extreme malnutrition before receiving IPN. Patients who have CAPD and also receive IPN should be monitored closely for the development of hypophosphatemia.

Refeeding Hypophosphatemia in Critically Ill Patients in an Intensive Care Unit

Marik PE, Bedigian MK (Univ of Massachusetts, Worcester)

Arch Surg 131:1043–1047, 1996 8–15

Background.—Refeeding hypophosphatemia, occurring after severe malnourishment, is accompanied by potentially life-threatening cardiac, muscular, and neurologic complications. The incidence, risk factors, and clinical effects of refeeding hypophosphatemia, in a group of patients in the ICU, was studied.

Methods.—Patients in the ICU who had not received nutrition for more than 48 hours underwent nutritional and serum chemistry assessment before resumption of feeding with Jevity formula (Ross Products, Abbott Laboratories, Columbus, Ohio). Serum phosphate, electrolyte, and prealbumin levels were monitored and the clinical course was followed.

Results.—Of 62 individuals entering the study, in 21 (34%) refeeding hypophosphatemia developed, and of those, severe hypophosphatemia developed in 6; the latter was treated with IV phosphate. Serum phosphorus levels reached their lowest point 1.9 days after resumption of alimentation, returning to normal after another 1.6 days. Baseline serum prealbumin level below 110 g/L was the only significant predictor of hypophosphatemia. Patients with hypophosphatemia experienced significantly longer times of mechanical ventilation and hospital stay.

Conclusions.—Refeeding hypophosphatemia is relatively common in critically ill patients. Those whose serum prealbumin levels are below 110 g/L are at significantly greater risk of its development.

► Severe hypophosphatemia (Abstracts 8–14 and 8–15) is an uncommon complication of nutritional support, but when it occurs it can be dangerous. It is critically important to monitor the serum phosphorus level in patients receiving nutritional support, especially those receiving parenteral feedings. Phosphate is an important intracellular anion, and it can become depleted in the malnourished patient who receives aggressive nutritional support. I remember 1 patient who died of the complication of refeeding hypophosphatemia.

W.W. Souba, M.D., Sc.D.

Metabolic Derangements and Regulation in Catabolic States

Sources of Arginine for Induced Nitric Oxide Synthesis in the Isolated Perfused Liver

Pastor CM, Morris SM Jr, Billiar TR (Univ of Pittsburgh, Pa)
Am J Physiol 269:G861–G866, 1995 8–16

Background.—Arginine is the nitrogen donor for biosynthesis of nitric oxide (NO). Inducible NO synthase (iNOS) has been detected in stimulated hepatocytes. The source of the arginine for hepatic iNOS activity is unknown but may involve the urea cycle, which uses arginine as an intermediate. The hepatic iNOS arginine source was investigated in isolated, perfused rat livers.

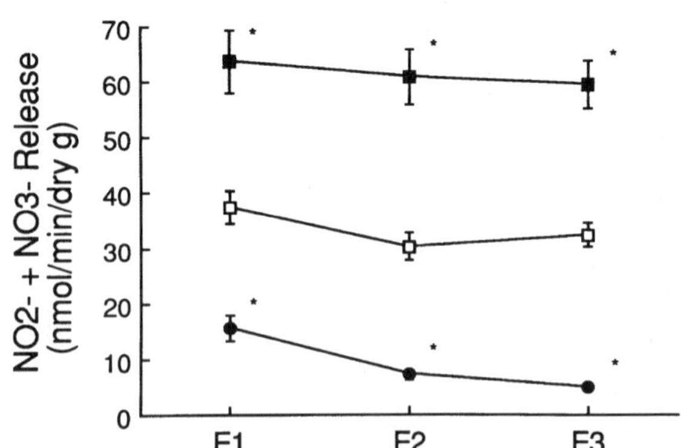

FIGURE 1.—Nitric oxide NO_2- + $(NO)_3$- release in livers perfused with Krebs-Henseleit-bicarbonate buffer (KHB, *open box, n* = 5) KHB + arginine (Arg, *solid box, n* = 5) and KHB + N_G-monomethyl-L-arginine (*solid circle,* n = 5). Rats were injected with *Corynebacterium parvum* (22 mg/kg IV), 5 days before perfusion. $P < 0.05$ vs. KHB. (Courtesy of Pastor CM, Morris Sm Jr, Billiar TR: Sources of arginine for induced nitric oxide synthesis in the isolated perfused liver. *Am J Physiol* 269:G861–G866, 1995.)

Methods.—Isolated rat livers were perfused in a recirculation model with Krebs-Henseleit-bicarbonate buffer, or buffer with arginine or precursors for urea synthesis added. To induce iNOS, rats were injected with endotoxin or with *Corynebacterium parvum*. The release of NO_2- + NO_3- and urea by the isolated, perfused rat livers was monitored.

Results.—The amount of NO released from the stimulated livers was stable in buffer alone and was doubled in the presence of exogenous arginine (Fig 1). No NO was released from unstimulated livers. When the livers were perfused with ornithine, there was no increase in NO synthesis, indicating that the urea cycle is an inefficient source of arginine for iNOS.

Conclusions.—In the intact liver, there is an endogenous source of arginine that can provide this substrate for hepatic iNOS. This endogenous arginine source is limiting, as addition of exogenous arginine can increase NO synthesis. However, arginine synthesized within the urea cycle is not an efficient source of arginine for hepatic iNOS. Further research is needed to define the intracellular and exogenous sources of arginine for hepatic NO synthesis.

▶ The observation by the authors that exogenous arginine can modulate NO biosynthesis has implications in surgical patients. Diets enriched in arginine have been proposed for specific groups of surgical patients because of the immunomodulatory effects of arginine. Previous studies have shown that hepatic arginine uptake is increased during sepsis.[1, 2] In addition, feeding a diet enriched in arginine has been shown to stimulate hepatic amino acid transport activity.[3] Thus, feeding arginine to patients with sepsis in an attempt to enhance immune function may further augment NO production in a group of patients who already display iNOS induction.

W.W. Souba, M.D., Sc.D.

References

1. Inoue Y, Bode BP, Beck D, et al: Arginine transport in human liver: Characterization and effects of nitric oxide synthase inhibitors. *Ann Surg* 218:350–362, 1993.
2. Inoue Y, Bode B, Souba WW: Hepatic Na+-independent amino acid transport in endotoxemic rats: Evidence for selective stimulation of arginine transport. *Shock* 2:164–170, 1994.
3. Espat N, Watkins K, Lind DS, et al: Dietary modulation of amino acid transport in rat in human liver. *J Surg Res.* 63:263–268, 1996.

Protection Against Lethal *Escherichia coli* Bacteremia in Baboons (*Papio anubis*) by Pretreatment With a 55-kDa TNF Receptor (CD120a)-Ig Fusion Protein, Ro 45-2081

van Zee KJ, Moldawer LL, Oldenburg HSA, et al (Univ of Florida, Gainesville; Veterinary Pathology Consultants, Nutley, NJ; École Polytechnique Fédérale, Lausanne, Switzerland; et al)

J Immunol 156:2221–2230, 1996 8–17

Background.—Despite advances in care and treatment, septic shock and systemic inflammatory response syndrome (SIRS) continue to have a high mortality associated with them. Endogenous mediators, such as TNF, a proinflammatory cytokine, contribute to septic pathology. Human plasma contains TNF binding proteins, which have been identified as the soluble extracellular domains of TNF receptors. To increase the in vivo half-lives of these circulating TNF-binding proteins, fusion proteins have been created. To determine whether these fusion proteins are effective in preventing lethal septic complications, a baboon model was used.

Methods.—Fusion proteins were created containing the complete extracellular region of the human 55-kDa TNF receptor and the hinge and downstream constant domains of human IgG1 (TNFR5-G_1) or IgG3 (TNFR5-G_3). Twenty-four baboons received 4.6, 1.0, or 0.2 mg/kg of either fusion protein before the administration of a lethal dose of live *Escherichia coli.*

Results.—Of the 8 baboons who received placebo pretreatment, 7 died or required euthanasia within 48 hours after challenge with live bacteria. Of the 16 animals who received pretreatment with either fusion protein across the entire dose range, 14 were well at day 5. Pretreatment with fusion proteins not only decreased mortality after septic challenge, but decreased hemodynamic response (Fig 1), reduced requirements for fluid, decreased systemic response by interleukins, shortened granulocytopenia, reduced the loss of cellular TNF receptors from granulocytes, reduced changes in fibrinogen concentrations, reduced increases in prothrombin and partial thromboplastin times, and decreased the rise in plasma lactate concentration. Histologic studies demonstrated protection against tissue injury by the fusion protein pretreatment.

Conclusions.—These results demonstrate the protective effect of a pretreatment with TNF receptor-immunoglobulin fusion proteins before bacterial challenge in a baboon model of lethal sepsis. The fusion protein pretreatment not only reduced mortality, but significant therapeutic benefit was observed in a broad range of functional systems, suggesting that SIRS was significantly attenuated by the pretreatment. This protective effect of the fusion proteins should be investigated for the prevention of morbidity and mortality in human sepsis.

▶ Initially, there was considerable enthusiasm for treating patients with sepsis by using strategies that targeted TNF-α and IL-1 using cytokine antibodies or receptor antagonists. Despite promising initial results in phase

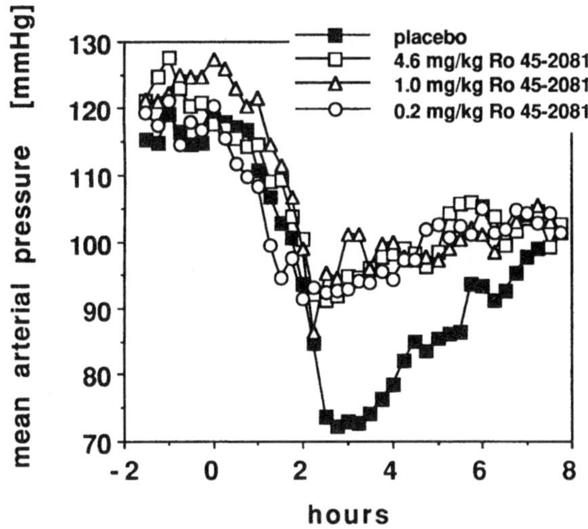

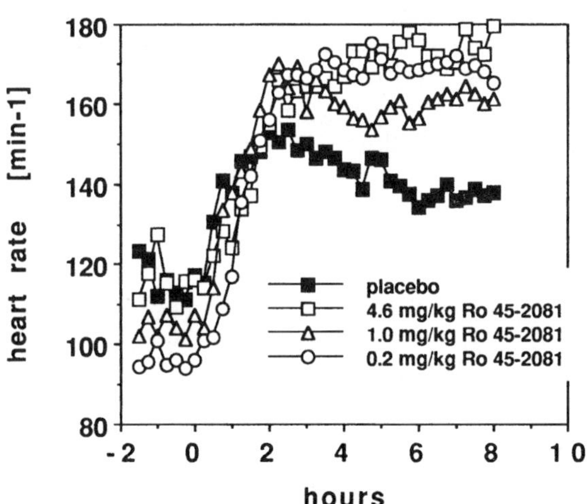

FIGURE 1.—Hemodynamic responses of baboons challenged with *Escherichia coli* and treated with 4.6, 1.0 or 0.2 mg/kg TNFR5-G_1 or placebo. Mean arterial pressure (**top**) and heart rate (**bottom**) were monitored from 2 hours before to 8 hours after bacterial challenge. In all animals, administration of *E. coli* resulted in pronounced tachycardia and hypotension. The hypotension was stabilized using crystalloid resuscitation, but the quantities of fluids required were markedly reduced by TNFR5-G_1 treatment. Data on control animals that died within the initial 8-hour study period are not included in the figure. Representative standard deviations (SD) were ± 15 to 20 mm Hg and 10 to 20 min_1. (Courtesy of van Zee KJ, Moldawer LL, Oldenburg HSA, et al: Protection against lethal *Escherichia coli* bacteremia in baboons (*Papio anubis*) by pretreatment with a 55-kDa TNF receptor (CD120a)-Ig fusion protein, Ro 45-2081. *J Immunol* 156:2221–2230, Copyright 1996. The American Association of Immunologists.)

II clinical studies, in general, it has been difficult to demonstrate convincing efficacy in larger trials. The study by Van Zee et al. uses fusion proteins of the human TNF receptor extracellular domain and human immunoglobulin heavy chain in a primate sepsis model. The beneficial effects of such treatment are compelling, and a recent phase II study in patients suggests a substantial reduction in mortality in the prospectively defined severe sepsis patient group.[1]

W.W. Souba, M.D., Sc.D.

Reference

1. Abraham E, Glausen M, Gelmont D, et al: Ro 45-2081 (TNFR55-IgG1) in the treatment of patients with severe sepsis and septic shock: Preliminary results. Presented at the International Autumnal Meeting on Sepsis, Deauville, France, 1995.

Sequential Changes in the Metabolic Response in Critically Injured Patients During the First 25 Days After Blunt Trauma

Monk DN, Plank LD, Franch-Arcas G, et al (Auckland Hosp, New Zealand)
Ann Surg 223:395–405, 1996 8–18

Background.—More than 50 years ago, Cuthbertson described various features of posttrauma metabolism. His studies and those of his colleagues showed that in patients with trauma, hypermetabolism occurs, fat and protein are consumed, and water and salt are conserved. These and other changes form the basis of critical care of injured patients, but many have not been quantified. Changes in energy expenditure and body composition were measured in critically injured patients.

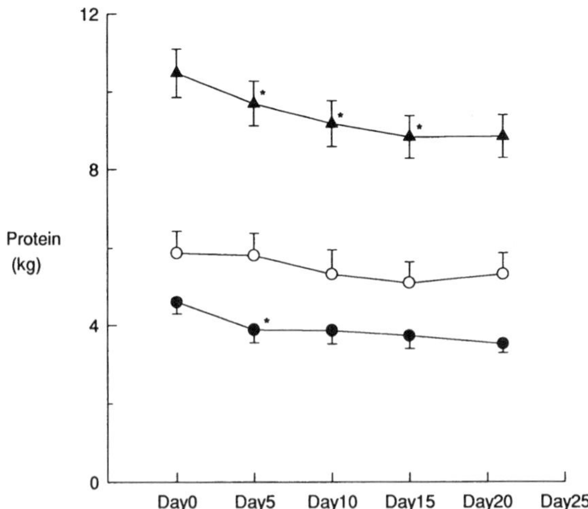

FIGURE 5.—Total body protein (*triangles*), skeletal muscle protein (*filled circles*), and nonmuscle protein (*open circles*) in 10 severely injured patients measured during a 21-day period after trauma (mean ± SEM).*, a significant ($P < 0.05$) change from previous measurement. (Courtesy of Monk DN, Plank LD, Franch-Arcas G, et al: Sequential changes in the metabolic response in critically injured patients during the first 25 days after blunt trauma. *Ann Surg* 223:395–405, 1996.)

Methods.—In 10 critically injured patients after blunt trauma, serial measurements of body composition and energy expenditure were taken after the patients became hemodynamically stable and then every 5 days for 21 days.

Results.—Measurements included total body nitrogen, fat and water, skeletal muscle mass, measured and predicted energy expenditure, energy balance, and total and activity energy expenditure. During the study period, resting energy expenditure increased 55% above predicted levels and remained elevated. Total energy expenditure was 1.32 × resting energy expenditure. When energy intake was insufficient, body fat was oxidized. Changes in body water resembled changes in body weight and were attributed to changes in extracellular water. A loss of 1.62 kg of total body protein occurred (Fig 5), of which 1.09 kg was from skeletal muscle. There were low levels of intracellular potassium, but these did not continue to decrease after patients became hemodynamically stable.

Conclusions.—Major trauma is associated with hypermetabolism, lipolysis, proteolysis, and increased extracellular water. These changes were greater and lasted longer than expected. Optimum management of patients who are critically injured with major trauma can meet energy requirements, prevent lipolysis, and prevent additional breakdown of cellular composition.

▶ This is an important paper because it demonstrates that the hypermetabolism occurring after injury lasts considerably longer than is generally thought. The patient may enter the anabolic phase of injury only after all wounds are closed and all foci of sepsis are drained. Despite adequate nutritional intake, net protein catabolism may persist for weeks and two thirds of the protein losses are from skeletal muscle. Such protein losses explain the loss of muscle strength that is observed in such individuals and suggest that methods of combating the hypercatabolism of injury may require therapies in addition to nutrition support alone. The authors did not determine the origin of the other one third of the protein losses—one might postulate that the gut and liver were the sources of loss as well.

W.W. Souba, M.D., Sc.D.

Blood Cytokine Levels Rise Even After Minor Surgical Trauma

Grzelak I, Olszewski WL, Zaleska M, et al (Polish Academy of Sciences, Warsaw, Poland; Med Academy, Warsaw, Poland; Military Hosp, Warsaw, Poland)

J Clin Immunol 16:159–164, 1996 8–19

Background.—The mechanism of postsurgical immunodepression is unclear, but the effects of anesthetics and drugs on immune cells, hormonal changes from stress, suppressor activity, suppressive serum factors, and changes in cytokine production may all have a role. There is evidence that many changes in the immune response after trauma or during infection

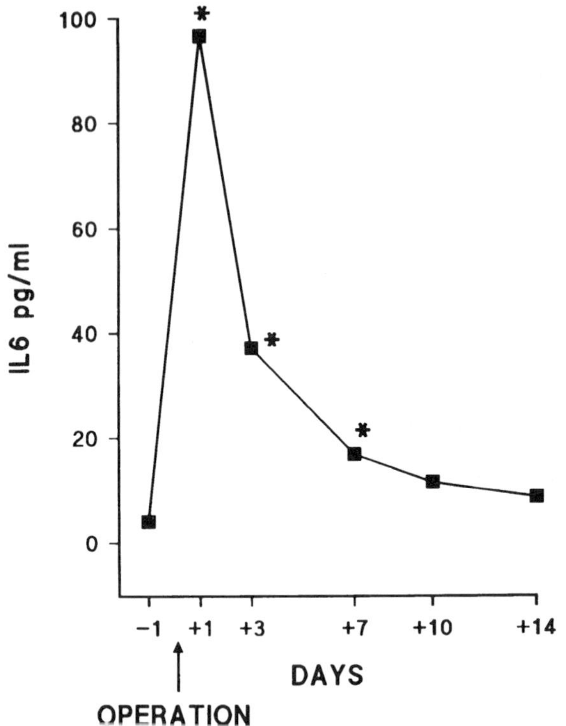

FIGURE 2.—Changes in mean plasma level of interleukin (IL)-6 (pg/mL) in patients (n = 9) after surgery.* $P < 0.05$. (Courtesy of Grzelak I, Olszewski WL, Zaleska M, et al: Blood cytokine levels rise even after minor surgical trauma. *J Clin Immunol* 16:159–164, 1996.)

result from or are affected by cytokine production. When excessive levels of cytokines are present, hemodynamic, metabolic, or inflammatory symptoms can occur after trauma and in infection, septic shock, multiple-organ failure, and wasting in cachexia. Changes in systemic production of cytokines after minor elective surgery were investigated.

Methods.—In patients scheduled for elective cholecystectomy, plasma concentrations of interleukin (IL)-1α, IL-1β, IL-1 receptor antagonist (ra), IL-6, IL-6 soluble receptor (sR), IL-8, IL-10, and interferon-γ were measured.

Results.—Levels of IL-1α and IL-1β did not change. In all patients, levels of IL-1 ra rose significantly between 1 and 14 days postoperatively. On days 1, 3, and 7 there was a significant increase in IL-6 (Fig 2). Interleukin-6 sR rose significantly on days 10 and 14. Levels of IL-8 increased significantly on days 1 and 3 postoperatively (Fig 4). An increase in IL-10 on days 1 and 3 was seen in some patients.

Conclusions.—A release of various cytokines into the blood circulation is associated with even minor surgery. Methods of downregulating systemic cytokine effects after surgery are needed in postoperative management.

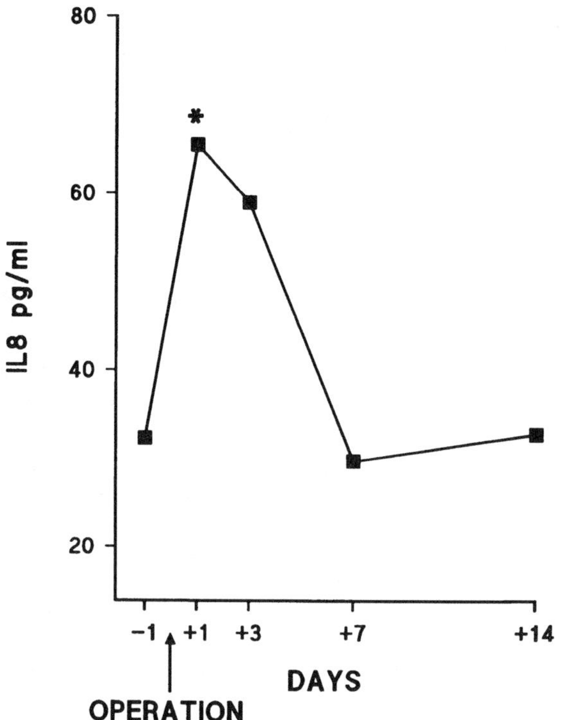

FIGURE 4.—Changes in mean plasma level of interleukin (IL)-8 (pg/mL) in patients ($n = 9$) after surgery.* $P < 0.05$. (Courtesy of Grzelak I, Olszewski WL, Zaleska M, et al: Blood cytokine levels rise even after minor surgical trauma. *J Clin Immunol* 16:159–164, 1996.)

► The authors have shown that transient elevations in IL-6, IL-8, IL-10, and IL-1ra occur after an uneventful elective cholecystectomy. They state in the abstract of the paper that these observations point to the need for identifying methods of downregulating cytokine production in the routine postoperative case. Such a statement is short-sighted and requires comment.

Cytokines exert numerous effects that are beneficial to the host after a catabolic insult. It would be inadvisable to recommend blocking this role of cytokines. There may be a role for cytokine antagonists in certain septic patients, but to date clinical trials have failed to demonstrate any consistent benefits. Exaggerated and prolonged production of cytokines after major injury or sepsis may contribute to organ dysfunction, suggesting that loss of control of the cytokine cascade may occur in some critically ill patients. In most patients, cytokine elaboration during illness must be viewed as an appropriate and adaptive response.

W.W. Souba, M.D., Sc.D.

Measurement of Muscle Protein Synthesis by Positron Emission Tomography With L-[*methyl*-^{11}C]Methionine

Hsu H, Yu YM, Babich JW, et al (Harvard Med School, Boston; Shriners Burns Inst, Boston)

Proc Natl Acad Sci USA 93:1841–1846, 1996 8–20

Objective.—The transport and metabolism of methionine in skeletal muscle of dogs is studied through the use of positron emission tomography (PET) and L-[*methyl*-^{11}C]methionine.

Background.—Currently, measurements of whole body and regional amino acid metabolism in humans are obtained with techniques that use stable isotope tracers. A noninvasive technique to obtain these measurements would be valuable. One such technique may be PET, which allows metabolic parameters to be measured in tissue as small as 1.0 cm^3. Although this technique has not been used to study amino acid metabolism in mammals in peripheral tissues, it may be used to make sequential time-dependent physiological and biochemical measurements in the same subject. L-[*methyl*-^{11}C]methionine has been shown to be useful in the evaluation of amino acid kinetics in vivo and in the detection of tumors.

Methods.—The protein synthesis rate (PSR) in paraspinal and hind limb muscles of anesthetized dogs was measured in dogs that had been injected intravenously with 25 mCi of L-[*methyl*]-^{11}C]methionine. Serial images and arterial blood samples were obtained. Data were analyzed by the placement of tissue-corrected and metabolite-corrected arterial blood time-activity curves into a 3-compartment model. The PSR was determined from fitted parameter values and plasma methionine concentrations, and the rates as measured by PET were compared to arterio-venous

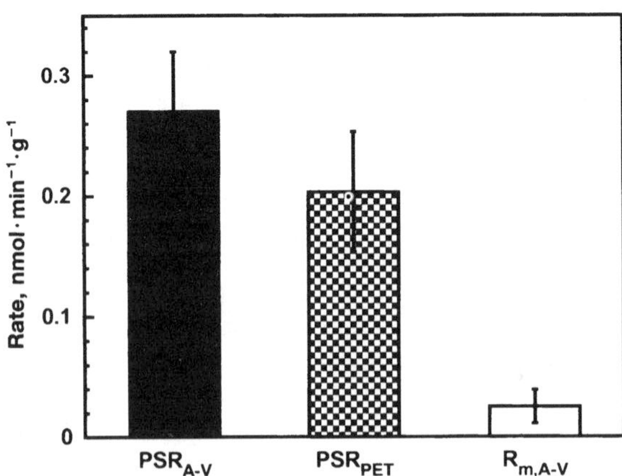

FIGURE 5.—Arterio-venous (A-V) difference measurements of PSR and transmethylation (R_m) performed by primed constant infusion of [^{13}C, $^2H_3$]methionine. The PET measurement of the PSR is reproduced for comparison. Each bar is the mean ± SD (n = 7). (Courtesy of Hsu H, Yu YM, Babich JW, et al: Measurement of muscle protein synthesis by positron emission tomography with L-[*methyl*-^{11}C]methionine. *Proc Natl Acad Sci USA* 93:1841–1846, Copyright 1996 National Academy of Sciences, U.S.A.)

difference measurements during primed constant infusion of L-[1-^{13}C, *methyl*-$^{2}H_3$]methionine.

Results.—Protein synthesis rates determined by PET were similar for paraspinal and hind limb muscles. The PSR determined by the stable isotope technique was 0.27 nmol$^{-1.-1.}$ (g of leg tissue)$^{-1}$. This indicates that transmethylation contributed about 10% to total hind limb methionine use (Fig 5). There were high levels of L-[*methyl*-^{11}C]methionine utilized by bone marrow.

Conclusions.—Positron emission tomography can effectively measure the PSR in vivo in muscle. This tecnhique may have a role in metabolic studies in humans.

▶ Positron emission tomography provides a routine, noninvasive, in vivo method for the quantitate analysis of tissue-specific biochemical processes. Positron emission tomography offers several advantages over conventional arterial venous difference techniques: (1) measurements require only a metabolite-corrected arterial input function and imaging; (2) the anatomic resolution of PET allows measurements to be performed on very small tissue volumes; and (3) repetitive studies can be performed in the same subject because of the short half lives of the tracers. Positron emission tomography appears to be a potentially useful technique for the measurement of regional amino acid metabolism. Because of the relatively noninvasive nature of the method measurements, the use of this technique on critically ill surgical patients is likely to provide new information on substrate metabolism.

W.W. Souba, M.D., Sc.D.

Biologic Control of Injury and Inflammation: Much More Than Too Little or Too Late

Guirao X, Lowry SF (Cornell Univ, New York)

World J Surg 20:437–446, 1996 8–21

Background.—When the generalized host inflammatory response is of excessive magnitude or duration, it may lead to deterioration rather than restoration of homeostasis. The factors influencing the adverse effects of excessive inflammation may be difficult to identify. Current thinking is that a cascade of endogenous proinflammatory mediators causes both the beneficial and adverse consequences of inflammation in response to infection and injury. Some of these mediators, especially tumor necrosis factor and interleukin-1, have been studied as possible targets for antagonist intervention. Preclinical and clinical studies of these anticytokine approaches were reviewed.

Discussion.—The studies have uncovered important evidence on the importance of cytokine counterregulatory mechanisms in the inflammatory process, with complex interactions between inflammatory cytokines and infection-induced antagonist proteins or counterregulatory hormones.

The most successful studies of anticytokine therapy, using models of lipopolysaccharide-induced lethal bacteremia, clearly demonstrate the failure of the counterregulatory system. However, these models do not accurately depict the balance of inflammatory events seen in clinical situations. The inflammatory process is more likely a dynamic one, in which episodes of inflammatory excess occur on top of elements of immunologic hyporesponsiveness. The balance between these 2 elements may determine the efficacy or rationale of therapy directed against inflammatory mediators. Contrary to the expectations raised by preclinical studies, blockade of either tumor necrosis factor or interleukin-1 does not significantly improve clinical outcomes. One possible explanation is that these inflammatory cytokines have independent and synergistic effects, despite sharing some efferent signaling pathways.

Summary.—The available evidence suggests that the outcomes of severe infection are influenced by an imbalance between various proinflammatory and counterregulatory influences. Progress in the clinical use of anticytokine therapy will depend on a greater understanding of the complex inflammatory response, along with patient selection issues.

Potential Strategies for Inflammatory Mediator Manipulation: Retrospect and Prospect

Fisher CJ Jr, Zheng Y (Cleveland Clinic Found, Ohio)

World J Surg 20:447–453, 1996 8–22

Introduction.—Sepsis is systemic response to infection that is characterized by alterations in regulations of body temperature, tachypnea, tachycardia, leukocytosis or leukopenia, decreased systemic vascular resistance, and evidence of organ dysfunction. Septic shock and sepsis syndrome are significant causes of mortality and morbidity. Despite considerable animal data to suggest a positive therapeutic benefit, clinical trials of novel agents to treat sepsis have failed. Recent major clinical trials on sepsis were reviewed.

Endotoxin and Tumor Necrosis Factor Blockades.—The endotoxin-induction hypothesis of gram-negative sepsis has not been proved or disproved. The possibility remains that the endotoxin-induced pathway of gram-negative sepsis is valid; however, additional clinical work is needed. Experimental evidence suggests that blocking tumor necrosis factor (TNF) may reduce mortality rates and prevent the sequelae of septic shock.

Interleukin-1 Blockade and Other Mediators.—In sepsis syndrome and septic shock, interleukin-1 is an important mediator. In experimental animals, infusion of interleukin-1 produces hypotension and functions synergistically with TNF to induce the hemodynamic features found with endotoxin-induced shock and gram-negative sepsis. The interleukin-1–mediation hypothesis of sepsis was not proved or disproved. In 1 study with platelet-activating factor, a potent phospholipid mediator involved in sepsis, the infusion of platelet-activating factor antagonist did not significantly reduce the mortality rate. Other ongoing trials include inhibition of nitric oxide, anti-TNF monoclonal antibody in patients with septic shock, and inhibition of cyclooxygenase. Antiendotoxin approaches that use more potent endotoxin binding and neutralizing drugs, granulocyte colony-stimulating factor, inhibition of coagulation, and TNF-binding protein are also being studied.

Future Directions.—The course of sepsis in human beings must be more closely approximated with animal models, which will help answer questions regarding when to introduce mediator blockade, the role of combination immunotherapy, and duration of therapy. Intrinsic differences that exist among surgical, trauma, and medical patients must be addressed. To date, there has been no new therapy to demonstrate sufficient clinical efficacy based on 28-day, intent-to-treat, all-cause mortality analysis.

▶ These 2 papers (Abstracts 8–21 and 8–22) provide a timely and comprehensive overview of the host inflammatory response after injury and infection and a review of the more recent therapeutic strategies used to manipulate the inflammatory response in critically ill patients.

W.W. Souba, M.D., Sc.D.

A Sarcoma-derived Protein Regulates Hepatocyte Metabolism via Autocrine Production of Tumor Necrosis Factor-α

Fischer CP, Bode BP, Souba WW (Harvard Med School, Boston)
Ann Surg 224:476–485, 1996 8–23

Background.—It is known that cancer cachexia is mediated in part by tumor necrosis factor-α (TNF-α). There is also evidence that this cytokine has a direct role in modulating hepatocyte metabolism. However, few tumors secrete TNF-α, and it is not known what stimulates its production in the host.

Methods.—Cultured methylcholanthrene (MCA)-induced fibrosarcoma was added to freshly isolated hepatocytes from rats. In these MCA-conditioned media and in control media, hepatocyte TNF-α production, hepatocyte albumin production, and amino acid transport were assessed.

Results.—Tumor necrosis factor-α was not present in the MCA-conditioned media alone. However, adding the MCA-conditioned media to the rat hepatocytes resulted in a 53-fold increase in TNF-α production, decreases in albumin production (reversible by addition of an antibody to TNF-α), and increases in amino acid transport, compared with the control media. The latter increases were produced via inductions of System N and System A (Fig 4). (Systems N and A are the principal carriers for the amino acids glutamine and alanine, which are important in acute-phase protein synthesis and gluconeogenesis.) Dialysis, trypsin treatment, and heat inactivation of MCA-conditioned media showed that the factor responsible for these effects must be a protein or group of proteins with a molecular weight greater than 100 kd.

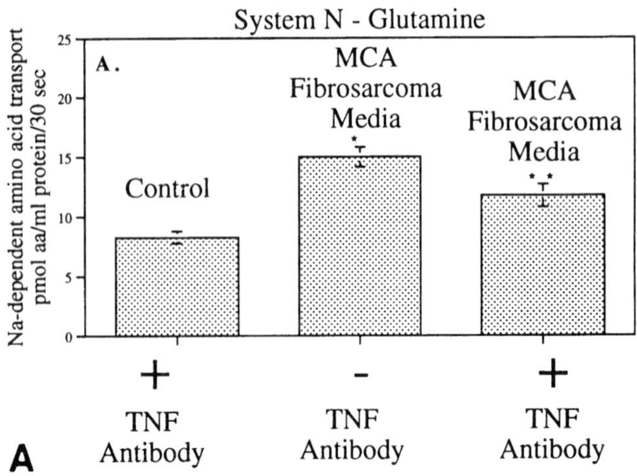

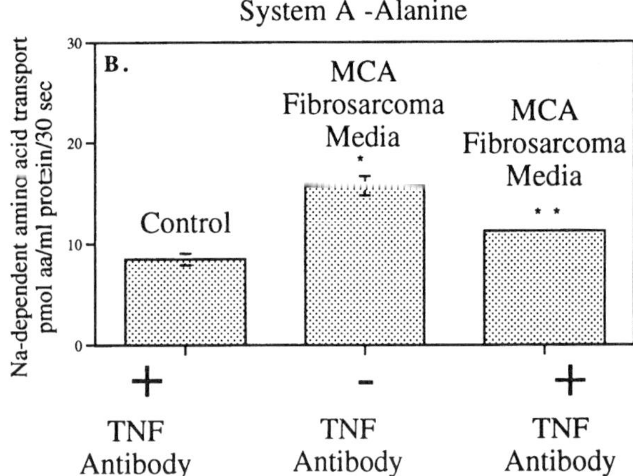

FIGURE 4.—Amino acid transport in primary rat hepatocytes in response to methylcholanthrene (*MCA*) fibrosarcoma-conditioned media. **A**, System N activity. *$P < 0.01$ MCA vs. control, **$P < 0.05$ MCA vs. MCA + tumor necrosis factor (*TNF*) antibody. Data are mean ± standard deviation of 4 separate determinations. **B**, System A activity. *$P < 0.01$ MCA vs. control, **$P < 0.01$ MCA vs. MCA + TNF antibody. Data are mean ± standard deviations of 4 separate determinations. (Courtesy of Fischer CP, Bode BP, Souba WW: A sarcoma-derived protein regulates hepatocyte metabolism via autocrine production of tumor necrosis factor-α. *Ann Surg* 224:476–485, 1996.)

Conclusions.—This study characterized a protein or group of proteins, apparently not previously described, that modulate hepatic metabolism in a tumor-bearing host. It appears that the decrease in hepatocyte albumin production and the increase in amino acid transport occur because of autocrine production of TNF-α by hepatocytes. In a paracrine manner, TNF-α then exerts its effects locally.

▶ Other tumor-derived factors that mediate cancer cachexia have been recently described. Tisdale and colleagues have isolated and sequenced a 24-kd proteoglycan that produces cachexia in vivo by inducing catabolism of skeletal muscle—the proteoglycan was derived from the murine adenocarcinoma MAC16.[1] The same 24-kd material is present in mice transplanted with the MAC16 tumor as well as in the urine of cancer patients with cachexia, but is absent from normal individuals, suggesting that cachexia in mice and humans may be produced in part by the same compound. The activity of MCA fibrosarcoma–conditioned media on muscle proteolysis has not yet been investigated—the currently isolated activity appears to induce a profile in the liver consistent with the acute-phase response, by upregulation of amino acid transport and down-regulation of albumin production.

W.W. Souba, M.D., Sc.D.

Reference

1. Todorov P, Cariuk P, McDevitt T, et al: Characterization of a cancer cachectic factor. *Nature* 379:739–742, 1996.

Clinical Aspects of Nutrition Support

Effect of Transcutaneous Electrical Muscle Stimulation on Postoperative Muscle Mass and Protein Synthesis

Vinge O, Edvardsen L, Jensen F, et al (Hvidovre Univ, Denmark; Huddinge Univ, Stockholm)

Br J Surg 83:360–363, 1996 8–24

Introduction.—Preservation of skeletal muscle protein is a major concern after surgical trauma. Even with nutritional support, immobilization during convalescence leads to loss of muscle mass and delayed recovery. Patients scheduled for elective abdominal surgery participated in an evaluation of the effect of transcutaneous electrical muscle stimulation (TEMS) on muscle protein synthesis and mass.

Patients and Methods.—Thirteen patients with a median age of 55 years took part in the study. Operative procedures included 10 colonic resections and 1 each of abdominoperineal resection, vagotomy and pyloroplasty, and gastric resection. Ambulation was started on the first postoperative day, with the goal of more than 8 hours of ambulation on day 3. On the day after surgery, each patient had TEMS applied to the quadriceps femoris on 1 leg; the other leg served as a control. A portable battery-powered stimulator provided 1-hour TEMS sessions 3 times a day for 5 days. The amplitude was adjusted to produce a visible contraction of the muscle. Both legs were examined with CT on the day before surgery and on postoperative day 6 to measure the cross-sectional area (CSA) of the quadriceps femoris muscle. Muscle biopsies were taken on the same days for ribosome analysis.

Results.—There were no postoperative complications, and all 13 patients completed the TEMS protocol with CT studies. Muscle biopsy findings were available for 10 patients. The groups of stimulated and control legs were similar in total concentration of ribosomes, percentage of polyribosomes, and CSAs of the quadriceps femoris muscle before operation. Control legs demonstrated a significant decrease in the percentage of polyribosomes in the ribosome suspension after surgery, but the TEMS-treated legs did not show this decrease. Only the legs treated with TEMS had a significant decrease in the total concentration of ribosomes. Both stimulated and control legs showed a significant decrease in CSA after surgery, but the decrease was significantly greater in control legs.

Conclusion.—Five days of TEMS led to a smaller decrease in polyribosome concentration and a smaller reduction in CSA of the quadriceps femoris muscle. This treatment may be a simple and effective way to reduce postoperative loss of muscle mass after surgery, and has potential applications in the reduction of muscle waste in other catabolic states.

▶ Previous attempts to decrease the net protein catabolism that occurs in the postoperative state and results in a loss of muscle mass have focused primarily on the use of nutrition support and anabolic agents. It is clear that muscle activity is important for muscle anabolism and that immobilization leads to a loss of muscle mass and function. The use of postoperative TEMS may increase muscle mass after abdominal surgery at a time when most patients have a decrease in activity. Whether such improvements result in an improvement in clinical outcome, an enhancement of functional capacity, or a reduced hospital stay remains to be seen.

W.W. Souba, M.D., Sc.D.

The Need for Aggressive Nutritional Intervention in the Injured Patient: The Development of a Predictive Model

Byers PM, Block EFJ, Albornoz JC, et al (Univ of Miami, Fla; Louisiana State Univ, Shreveport)

J Trauma 39:1103–1109, 1995 8–25

Introduction.—Although the benefits of early nutritional support in trauma patients are well known, these must be weighed against the invasive and expensive procedures that are usually necessary to initiate this support. A model that predicts which patients will not be able to achieve adequate oral intake within 5 days could be used to identify patients most in need of invasive procedures to ensure adequate nutritional support.

Purpose.—The purpose of this study was to develop prospective criteria that could be used to create a model to predict which patients will not be able to achieve adequate oral intake within 5 days and would therefore require early, invasive nutritional intervention.

Methods.—From April to June 1993, there were 442 consecutive admissions to Jackson Memorial Hospital/Ryder Trauma Center. Of these,

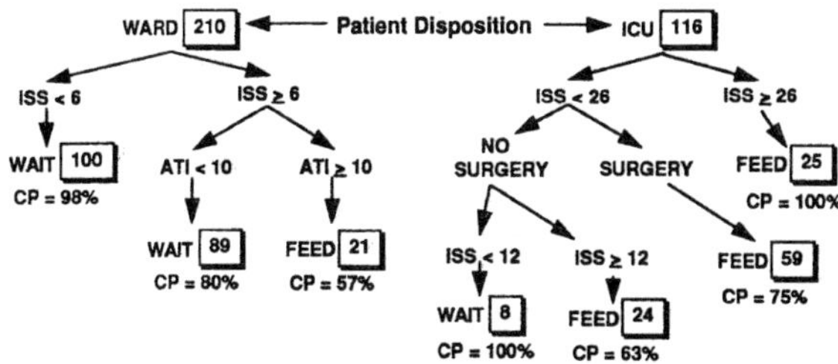

FIGURE 1.—A predictive algorithm for nutritional intervention in trauma patients. **Numbers in boxes,** number of correct predictions; **CP,** percentage of correct predictions; **FEED,** tolerance of regular diet will be delayed more than 5 days—patients in whom nutritional intervention should be initiated upon admission; **WAIT,** a regular diet should be tolerated within 5 days—wait and observe for unexpected complications to initiate nutritional support. (Courtesy of Byers PM, Block EFJ, Albornoz JC et al: The need for nutritional intervention in the injured patient: The development of a predictive model. *J Trauma* 39(6):1103–1109, 1995.)

77 were excluded from the study because of burns, age younger than 13 years, or death within the study period. The remaining study group of 365 patients was analyzed by a stepwise regression algorithm, using 21 variables, with the time to tolerance of a regular diet as the dependent variable. The predictors selected in the stepwise regression were used to develop an algorithm using the Classification and Regression Tree statistical method.

Results.—The study group consisted of 289 males and 76 females with an age range of 13–86 years. The average time until tolerance of oral diet was 8 days within this group. There was a wide range of injury severity. Of the 365 patients in the study group, 326 had complete records and were used in the development of a regression tree with 30 terminal nodes. After 10-fold cross-validation and a shrinkage algorithm, a simplified tree was produced with 4 variables: disposition, Injury Severity Score (ISS), indication for emergency surgery and Abdominal Trauma Index (ATI) (Figure 1). When this model was applied to the study population, it had a sensitivity of 83%, specificity 84% and accuracy of 84%.

Conclusions.—The final algorithm appears to be sufficiently specific and sensitive to use in the selection of trauma patients for early, invasive nutritional intervention. Further testing of this model on a large independent sample will be necessary for validation.

▶ Given the established benefits of early nutritional support in trauma patients, the authors have developed a predictive model with an accuracy of 84% that defines which trauma patients are likely to require early nutritional intervention. The model requires that the ISS and the ATI be calculated before intervention. One assumption of the paper is that patients who do not need nutritional support will not benefit from it, whereas those who need nutritional support will benefit from it.

W.W. Souba, M.D., Sc.D.

Choline Deficiency: A Cause of Hepatic Steatosis During Parenteral Nutrition That Can Be Reversed With Intravenous Choline Supplementation

Buchman AL, Dubin MD, Moukarzel AA, et al (Baylor College of Medicine, Houston; Univ of California, Los Angeles; Maimonides Med Ctr, NY; et al)
Hepatology 22:1399–1403, 1995 8–26

Introduction.—It has been demonstrated that patients receiving long-term total parenteral nutrition (TPN) have choline deficiency develop, which can lead to hepatic steatosis. To resolve this deficiency and the accompanying steatosis, 4 patients who were receiving long-term TPN were given IV choline supplementation.

Methods.—Four patients receiving long-term TPN with low plasma-free choline concentrations and hepatic steatosis were included in this study. The study group was composed of 3 women, aged 45, 50, and 72 years and 1 man, aged 43 years. These patients had received home TPN for 3.5 to 13.5 years. The patients received choline chloride IV supplementation for 6 weeks. They were examined by abdominal CT at baseline, biweekly during supplementation, and 4 weeks after supplementation was halted.

Results.—Before choline supplementation, all patients had low plasma-free choline concentrations. During the supplementation period, plasma-free choline increased to at least the normal range in all 4 patients within 1 week and this was maintained for the entire supplementation period. After discontinuation of choline supplementation, choline levels returned to their previous baseline. Abdominal CT demonstrated that hepatic steatosis resolved completely in all patients (Table 1). In 1 patient, steatosis returned 10 weeks after supplementation was discontinued.

Conclusions.—Hepatic steatosis in patients receiving long-term TPN is due to choline deficiency and can be reversed by IV choline chloride supplementation. These preliminary results suggest that choline should be considered an essential nutrient in patients who require long-term parenteral nutrition. Larger, randomized, controlled clinical trials should be performed to determine the role of choline-supplementation in the treatment and prevention of TPN-associated hepatic steatosis.

TABLE 1.—Hepatic Density as Estimated by the Liver-Spleen CT Number Difference (in Hounsfield Units)

Patient No.	Baseline	2 wk	4 wk	6 wk	4 wk After Choline
1	−47.0	−3.9	−3.8	3.3	10.6
2	−0.7	19.8	19.2	15.4	15.7
3	0.3	13.2	17.2	20.8	15.0
4	−9.4	4.5	5.6	12.8	−6.3*

*10 weeks after choline supplementation indicating return of hepatic steatosis.

(Courtesy of Buchman AL, Dubin MD, Moukarzel AA, et al: Choline Deficiency: A cause of hepatic steatosis during parenteral nutrition that can be reversed with intravenous choline supplementation *Hepatology* 22:1399–1403, 1995.)

► The authors demonstrate the value of choline supplementation in patients who require long-term TPN. They point out that lipid emulsions such as Intralipid contained some choline, primarily in the form of phosphatidylcholine, but this amount is relatively small. Although choline should be synthesized from methionine contained in TPN solutions, the intravenous delivery of nutrients bypasses the portal system such that intravenous methionine is probably not adequately converted to choline. Thus, choline may be an essential nutrient in patients with minimal oral intake or inadequate intestinal absorption.

W.W. Souba, M.D., Sc.D.

Randomised Trial of Safety and Efficacy of Immediate Postoperative Enteral Feeding in Patients Undergoing Gastrointestinal Resection

Carr CS, Ling KDE, Boulos P, et al (Univ College London)

BMJ 312:869–871, 1996 8–27

Background.—Conventional management after bowel resection involves starvation with IV fluids until flatus is passed. Although early enteral feeding has been found to improve outcomes in patients who have trauma and burns, it has not been studied thoroughly in patients undergoing bowel resection. The safety and efficacy of immediate postoperative enteral feeding in patients who had gastrointestinal resection were investigated in a pilot study.

Methods and Findings.—Twenty-eight patients were randomly assigned to receive immediate postoperative enteral feeding through a nasojejunal tube or conventional postoperative IV fluids until a normal diet could be initiated. Enteral feeding was established successfully in all 14 patients. Mean daily intake was 6.78 MJ before the reintroduction of a normal diet. Patients who were receiving IV fluids had a mean of 1.58 MJ. On the first day after surgery, urinary nitrogen balance was negative in patients receiving IV fluids but positive in all patients fed enterally. By day 5, this finding did not differ between groups. Patients fed enterally had no change in gut mucosal permeability, whereas the patients given IV fluids had a significant increase from the test ratios seen before surgery. Patients fed enterally also had fewer postoperative complications.

Conclusions.—Immediate enteral feeding is beneficial to patients who are undergoing bowel resection. Total calorie and protein intake was significantly improved, and gut mucosal permeability was significantly attenuated. The patients tolerated enteral feeding well.

► The authors do not provide information about the preoperative diagnoses of the patients, the types of operation performed, the preoperative nutritional status of the patients, or time to complete recovery (return to work or full functional capacity). Such data are important, because previously published controlled trials in patients with normal body composition or mild malnutrition who underwent major elective operations show that nutritional support produces little improvement in outcome.[1, 2] Postoperative weight loss is acceptable, because short-term undernutrition (10–12 days) does not complicate convalescence after major elective operation.[2]

Although early enteral nutrition support has been shown to be beneficial in severely injured patients,[3] the routine use of enteral nutrition in the well-nourished patient who is undergoing elective gastrointestinal surgery cannot be recommended. Weight loss is common after such surgery, but short-term undernutrition is well tolerated in most patients. Perioperative nutritional support appears to be of greatest benefit in severely malnourished patients and in patients at high risk. It therefore becomes important to determine which patients fall into these categories and to predict which patients might benefit from nutritional intervention. If reliable criteria for identifying the "at risk" patient were established, the role of nutritional intervention could be studied more scientifically.

W.W. Souba, M.D., Sc.D.

References

1. The Veterans Affairs Total Parenteral Nutrition Cooperative Study Group: Perioperative total parenteral nutrition in surgical patients. *N Engl J Med* 325:525–532, 1991.
2. Sandstrom R, Drott A, Hyltander A, et al: The effect of post operative intravenous feeding (TPN) on outcome following major surgery evaluated in a randomized study. *Ann Surg* 217:185–195, 1993.
3. Moore FA, Feliciano DV, Andrassy RJ, et al: Early enteral feeding, compared with parenteral, reduces postoperative septic complications. *Ann Surg* 216:172–173, 1992.

Loss of Upper Respiratory Tract Immunity With Parenteral Feeding

Kudsk KA, Li J, Renegar KB (Univ of Tennessee, Memphis)
Ann Surg 223:629–638, 1996 8–28

Objective.—The effect of diets that maintain or deplete gut-associated lymphoid tissue on IgA-mediated upper respiratory tract mucosal immunity was examined in mice.

Background.—Complications from infection are the most common cause of mortality in patients with trauma without severe head injuries,

TABLE 3.—Intestinal Immunoglobulin A Level

Group	Intestinal IgA (μg)
Chow	84.7 ± 8.1
IV-TPN	52.1 ± 3.3*†
IG-TPN	55.7 ± 7.1*†
Nutren (Clintec, Chicago, IL)	80.5 ± 6.8

*vs. chow, $P < 0.05$.
†vs. Nutren, $P < 0.05$.
Abbreviations: IV-TPN, IV total parenteral nutrition; *IG-TPN,* intragastric total parenteral nutrition.
(Courtesy of Kudsk KA, Li J, Renegar KB: Loss of upper respiratory tract immunity with parenteral feeding. *Ann Surg* 223:629–638, 1996.)

TABLE 4.—Viral Shedding

Group	Virus Positive
Chow	0/10*
IV-TPN	5/10
IG-TPN	0/10*
Nutren (Clintec, Chicago, IL)	0/11*

*vs. IV-TPN, $P < 0.001$.
Abbreviations: IV-TPN, IV total parenteral nutrition; *IG-TPN,* intragastric total parenteral nutrition.
(Courtesy of Kudsk KA, Li J, Renegar KB: Loss of upper respiratory tract immunity with parenteral feeding. *Ann Surg* 223:629–638, 1996.)

and commonly cause morbidity and mortality in patients who are malnourished, have surgical complications, or remain in intensive care for extended periods. Studies have reported an average of 30% mortality from sepsis. Mortality from sepsis is significantly lower in patients given enteral feeding than in those given parenteral feeding, but the reasons for this are unclear. It is hypothesized that a breakdown in the gastrointestinal barrier, permitting molecules and bacteria to enter the body, occurs when enteral feeding is not given. Immunoglobulin A is a key component in defense against mucosal infections. Gut-associated lymphoid tissue is responsible for IgA production and seems to be sensitive to the route and type of nutrition.

Methods.—Immunity was established in mice with intranasal inoculation of an influenza virus. After 3 weeks, the mice were randomly assigned to receive chow, intragastric Nutren, intragastric total parenteral nutrition, or IV total parenteral nutrition. After 5 days, an intranasal virus challenge was performed, and viral shedding from the upper respiratory tract was examined.

Results.—Body weight was similar in all mice. Animals fed with IV or intragastric total parenteral nutrition had significant atrophy in Peyer's patch cells. Levels of IgA were significantly lower in both groups of mice given total parenteral nutrition than in mice fed chow or Nutren (Table 3). No animal fed gastrointestinally had viral shedding. In 5 of 10 mice fed IV total parenteral nutrition, continued viral shedding occurred (Table 4).

Conclusions.—Normal immunity was maintained in all animals fed gastrointestinally, but not in animals fed intravenously. Upper respiratory tract immunity is influenced by route of nutrition and is not dependent on intestinal gut-associated lymphoid tissue mass.

▶ This work complements previous studies that have evaluated the effects of parenteral nutrition on gut structure and function. The effects of total parenteral nutrition (TPN) on the human gastrointestinal tract include a decrease in brush border hydrolase activity,[1] a reduction in amino acid transporter activity,[2] an increase in mucosal permeability,[3] and a slight decrease in villus height.[3] With resumption of oral alimentation, brush border enzyme activities and microvillus height return toward normal values within 1 week.[1] The splanchnic response to endotoxin appears to be exaggerated in volunteers fed parenterally compared to subjects fed enterally, suggesting that TPN may amplify the metabolic alterations that develop during sepsis.[4]

W.W. Souba, M.D., S.cD.

References

1. Guedon C, Schmitz J, Lerebours E, et al. Decreased brush border hydrolase activities without gross morphologic changes in human intestinal mucosa after prolonged total parenteral nutrition of adults. *Gastroenterology* 90:373–378, 1986.
2. Inoue Y, Espat NJ, Frohnapple DJ, et al. The effect of total parenteral nutrition on amino acid and glucose transport by the human small intestine. *Ann Surg* 217:604–614, 1993.
3. Van der Hulst R, Van Kreel BK, Von Meyenfeldt MF, et al. Glutamine and the preservation of gut integrity. *Lancet* 341:1363–1365, 1993.
4. Fong Y, Marano MA, Barber A, et al. Total parenteral nutrition and bowel rest modify the metabolic response to endotoxin in humans. *Ann Surg* 210:449–457, 1989.

Protein-sparing Therapy After Major Abdominal Surgery: Lack of Clinical Effects

Doglietto GB, Gallitelli L, Pacelli F, et al (Università Cattolica Sacro Cuore, Rome; Ospedale Niguarda, Milan, Italy; et al)

Ann Surg 223:357–362, 1996 8–29

Background.—Several researchers have demonstrated the metabolic effect of postoperative protein-sparing treatment. The clinical value of this treatment, however, has not been studied in a large prospective trial. The clinical efficacy of postoperative protein-sparing treatment was determined in a prospective, multicenter, randomized study.

Methods.—Six hundred seventy-eight patients who were undergoing major elective abdominal surgery were enrolled. The patients were randomly assigned to receive protein-sparing therapy or conventional treatment after surgery. Postoperative complications and mortality rates were analyzed.

Findings.—The 2 groups had comparable rates of major postoperative complications: 19.5% in the protein-sparing therapy group vs. 20.9% in the control group. Overall mortality rates after surgery were also comparable: 4.7% in the protein-sparing treatment group and 3.5% in the control group.

Conclusions.—Routine protein-sparing therapy nutrition for normonourished or mildly malnourished patients who are undergoing major abdominal surgery is not clinically justified. This therapy did not improve rates of postoperative complications or mortality.

▶ This paper points out that postoperative nutrition support is not justified in the vast majority of well-nourished patients who are undergoing elective abdominal surgery. Controlled trials in patients with normal body composition or mild malnutrition who are undergoing elective operations show that nutritional support produces little improvement in outcome.[1] Postoperative weight loss in these individuals is acceptable, because short-term undernutrition does not complicate convalescence after major operations. This study and others[2] indicate that postoperative nutrition in well-nourished elective surgical patients is indicted only in those who cannot eat by postoperative day 14 (these patients usually have a postoperative complication).

W.W. Souba, M.D., Sc.D.

References

1. The Veterans Affairs Total Parenteral Nutrition Cooperative Study Group: Perioperative total parenteral nutrition in surgical patients. *N Engl J Med* 325:525–532, 1991.
2. Sandstrom R, Drott A, Hyltander A, et al: The effect of post operative intravenous feeding (TPN) on outcome following major surgery evaluated in a randomized study. *Ann Surg* 217:185–195, 1993.

Effect of Nutritional Support on Routine Nutrition Assessment Parameters and Body Composition in Intensive Care Unit Patients

Phang PT, Aeberhardt LE (Univ of British Columbia, Vancouver, Canada)

Can J Surg 39:212–220, 1996 8–30

Background.—Routine measures for assessing nutrition are problematic in patients in the ICU. These assessments are technically difficult to perform, and factors other than the adequacy of nutritional support affect assessment variables. Whether routine nutrition assessment parameters and body composition change after nutritional support in ICU patients was investigated. In addition, whether such changes are associated with cumulative energy and fluid balances was determined.

Methods.—Forty-five mechanically ventilated medical and surgical patients in the ICU were included. All had received nutritional support for at least 7 days. A subgroup of 9 patients had received nutritional support for 3 weeks or more. Routine assessments of nutritional adequacy included determinations of weight, serum levels of albumin and prealbumin, and lymphocyte count and body composition, including measures of body cell mass, extracellular fluid, and body fat, which were established in bioelectric impedance analysis.

Findings.—Weight, levels of albumin and prealbumin, and extracellular mass were changed. There were no changes, however, in lymphocyte count, body cell mass, or body fat. Weight and extracellular mass changes were associated slightly with cumulative fluid balance. Changes in levels of albumin and prealbumin were uncorrelated with cumulative energy or fluid balance. The subgroup of patients who received nutritional support for 3 weeks or longer had similar findings.

Conclusions.—Fluid balance, but not energy balance, slightly affects changes in routine nutrition assessment parameters and body composition. These changes are therefore not specific indicators of the adequacy of nutritional support in ICU patients. Improved nutrition assessment parameters are needed to monitor the response to nutritional support more accurately in critically ill patients.

▶ This paper touches on the problem of and the difficulty in identifying patients who are nutritionally "at risk." Although protein-calorie malnutrition is common in hospitalized patients, and its evolution during illness frequently reflects the severity of the underlying disease or toxicity associated with certain therapies, a cause-and-effect relationship between malnutrition and a poorer outcome has not been definitely established. The identification of protein-calorie malnutrition has been based on objective measurements, including hepatic secretory proteins, anthropometry, grip strength, and cell-mediated immunity. To date, no single measurement is of value in the individual patient, and it has been shown that global clinical assessment is a more reproducible technique for evaluating nutritional status. At present, unintentional weight loss is the cheapest, simplest, and most common measurement used to screen for nutritional risk.

The magnitude of the patient's metabolic stress will also influence the amount and rate of weight loss that will negatively affect outcome. Short-term undernutrition (approximately 10 days) is well tolerated in minimally stressed postoperative patients,[1] whereas aggressive early feeding of the previously well-nourished patient who sustains a severe catabolic insult has been shown to be beneficial.[2] Thus, the factors determining nutritional risk are multiple and interrelated and include pre-existing nutritional status, the magnitude and anticipated length of associated catabolic stresses, and current nutritional therapy.

W.W. Souba, M.D., Sc.D.

References

1. Moore FA, Feliciano DV, Andrassy RJ, et al: Early enteral feeding, compared with parenteral, reduces postoperative septic complications. *Ann Surg* 216:172–173, 1992.
2. Sandstrom R, Drott A, Hyltander A, et al: The effect of post operative intravenous feeding (TPN) on outcome following major surgery evaluated in a randomized study. *Ann Surg* 217:185–195, 1993.

Ursodeoxycholic Acid for Treatment of Cholestasis in Children on Long-term total Parenteral Nutrition: A Pilot Study

Spagnuolo MI, Iorio R, Vegnente A, et al (Univ of Naples Federico II, Italy)
Gastroenterology 111:716–719, 1996 8–31

Objective.—The use of ursodeoxycholic acid (UDCA) as a treatment for cholestatic liver disease in children receiving long-term total parenteral nutrition (TPN) was investigated.

Methods.—Over a 15-month period, 7 children (4 boys; median age, 210 days) were enrolled. All were receiving TPN because of severe diar-

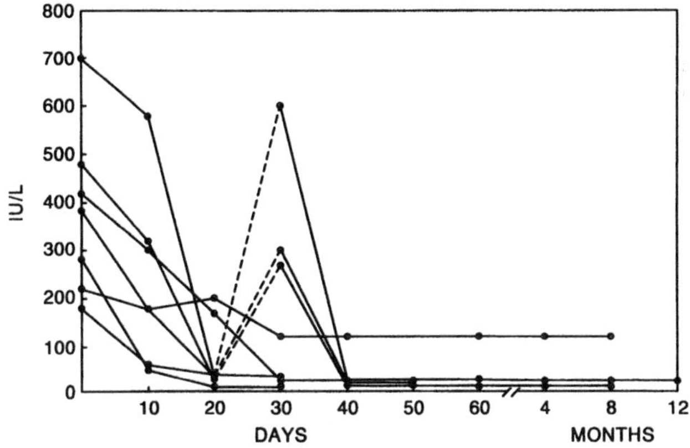

FIGURE 1.—Time course of γ-glutamyl transpeptidase serum levels in the children treated with ursodeoxycholic acid (*UDCA*). Ursodeoxycholic acid was temporarily discontinued in 3 children, and a rebound increase of γ-glutamyl transpeptidase levels was observed. *Dashed line* indicates the period of suspension of UDCA therapy. (Courtesy of Spagnuolo MI, Iorio R. Vegnente A, et al: Ursodeoxycholic acid for treatment of cholestasis in children on long-term total parenteral nutrition: A pilot study. *Gastroenterology* 111:716–719, 1996.)

rhea that was refractory to drug or dietetic therapy. Cholestatic liver disease was diagnosed on the basis of increased levels of serum γ-glutamyl transpeptidase (GGT), alkaline phosphatase, and alanine aminotransferase. The researchers ruled out liver disease, liver injury, infection, and other potential reasons for these biochemical markers to be elevated. Ursodeoxycholic acid (30 mg per kilogram body weight) was given orally 3 times a day for a median duration of 294 days (range, 48 to 575 days). No patient received other medication.

Results.—Even at this relatively high dose, UDCA did not cause adverse side effects. Clinical symptoms of liver disease resolved 1 to 2 weeks after UDCA treatment was started. Levels of GGT, alkaline phosphatase, and alanine aminotransferase were normal in 6 patients within 4 to 8 weeks. The GGT level remained elevated in the other patient, in whom the lapse between onset of cholestatic liver disease and UDCA therapy had been much longer (560 days) than in the other patients (15 to 150 days). In 3 patients, UDCA was discontinued before TPN was withdrawn, and there was a rebound increase in GGT levels 6 to 10 days later (Fig 1). Levels returned to normal 7 to 10 days after UDCA was re-instituted. When UDCA was discontinued upon TPN withdrawal, biochemical markers remained normal in all patients, which supports a cause-effect relationship between TPN and cholestatic liver disease. Six patients recovered from intestinal disease and remained well during follow-up of at least 12 months. One patient died at the age of 34 months.

Conclusion.—Patients receiving TPN should receive UDCA immediately if signs of cholestatic liver disease develop.

▶ The mechanism of action of UDCA is unknown. Several questions came to mind after reading this study: (1) is UDCA as effective in adults with

TPN-induced hepatic cholestasis as it is in children?; (2) should UDCA be provided prophylactically or only when biochemical evidence of cholestasis develops?; (3) how expensive is UDCA?; and (4) are there any long-term side effects?

W.W. Souba, M.D., Sc.D.

Aging Exaggerates the Blood Glucose Response to Total Parenteral Nutrition

Watters JM, Kirkpatrick SM, Hopbach D, et al (Univ of Ottawa, Ont, Canada)
Can J Surg 39:481–485, 1996 8–32

Objective.—Whether age affects serum glucose levels during total parenteral nutrition (TPN) was investigated.

Methods.—The participants were 78 consecutive, clinically stable patients who were hospitalized for a variety of acute conditions and received TPN with hypertonic glucose. A standardized scale was used to assess habitual level of physical activity (HAL) before hospitalization. As a measure of illness severity, an acute physiology score was calculated based on the patient's condition during the 24 hours before initial blood sampling. Immediately before TPN was initiated and again 48 to 96 hours later, blood was drawn for determination of serum glucose, serum insulin, C-peptide, and cortisol levels.

Results.—Seven patients required exogenous insulin after TPN was initiated, and their results were excluded. The other 71 patients ranged in age from 18 to 83 years. After initiation of TPN, there were increases in serum levels of glucose, insulin, and C-peptide (Table 2). Serum glucose levels increased as a function of patient age, illness severity, and the interaction of those 2 factors. Serum insulin levels declined with increasing age and increased as a function of serum glucose, rate of infusion of glucose, and HAL. The molar ratio of serum C-peptide to serum insulin did not vary with age. Serum cortisol levels increased with age and with diminished HAL.

Conclusions.—After initiation of TPN, elderly patients should be carefully monitored for hyperglycemia, even if serum glucose levels have been

TABLE 2.—Measurements of Serum Levels Before and During Total Parenteral Nutrition (Means [and Standard Deviations])

Measurement	Before TPN	During TPN
Glucose, mmol/L	5.9 (1.4)	7.5 (2.8)*
Insulin, pmol/L	80 (79)	261 (217)*
C-peptide, nmol/L	1310 (1270)	2820 (2490)*
Cortisol, nmol/L	558 (276)	518 (187)

*$P < 0.001$ vs. before total parenteral nutrition.

(Reprinted from Watters JM, Kirkpatrick SM, Hopbach D, et al: Aging exaggerates the blood glucose response to total parenteral nutrition. *Can J Surg* 39:481–485, 1996, by permission of the publisher, *CJS*, Vol. 39 No. 65 December 1996.)

normal. This is especially important for patients who are very elderly or severely ill.

▶ The insulin responses of older patients with trauma to acute glucose loading has been shown to be markedly decreased compared with those of younger individuals.[1] Because hyperglycemia occurs more frequently in older patients with trauma who are receiving parenteral nutrition, these patients should be monitored more closely. Treatment of the hyperglycemia can include both decreasing the amount of glucose infused and adding exogenous insulin.

W.W. Souba, M.D., Sc.D.

Reference

1. Watters JM, Moulton SB, Clancey SM, et al: Aging exaggerates glucose intolerance following injury. *J Trauma* 37:786–791, 1994.

In 1995 a Correlation Between Malnutrition and Poor Outcome in Critically Ill Patients Still Exists

Giner M, Laviano A, Meguid MM, et al (State Univ of New York, Syracuse)
Nutrition 12:23–29, 1996 8–33

Objectives.—The incidence and correlates of malnutrition in critically ill patients was studied, and an effort was made to determine in which clinical setting malnutrition develops.

Methods.—The participants were 129 patients who were admitted to an ICU over a 4-month period and who were discharged to the ward 24 hours to 99 days later without re-admission. Malnutrition was defined as a posthydrational serum albumin level of less than 3.5 g/dL and a weight/height ratio less than 100%. Illness severity was assessed with the Therapeutic Intervention Scoring System. Complications requiring therapeutic intervention were recorded. Nutrition data (e.g., daily caloric intake, duration of total parenteral nutrition) were collected for the 66 patients who required surgery.

Results.—Fifty-five (43%) of the patients were malnourished on admission. These patients had significantly more complications than the well-nourished group, and a significantly greater number were not discharged (they died or stayed longer than 99 days). In patients who were less severely ill (Therapeutic Intervention Scoring System groups I and II; scores less than 20), malnutrition was associated with a higher rate of nondischarge and with a longer stay. In more severely ill patients, malnutrition did not significantly affect discharge or length of stay. Of the surgery patients, 29 (44%) of the patients were malnourished. Nutrition data showed that on general wards, there had been no detection, correction, or prevention of surgery patients' nutritional deficits.

Conclusions.—Malnutrition is still a significant problem for hospitalized patients. Those whose illnesses are less severe are more likely to have adverse consequences from malnutrition. Mandatory nutrition training for surgery residents and nutritional support for all hospitalized patients, not just those who need surgery, are recommended.

▶ As stated in one of my earlier comments, malnutrition is common in hospitalized patients, and its development during illness frequently reflects the severity of the underlying disease or the toxicity associated with certain therapies. Although Giner and colleagues identify an association between malnutrition and a poor outcome, a cause-and-effect relationship has been more difficult to prove. Notwithstanding this lack of evidence, nutrition support is widely used because malnutrition is common in hospitalized patients;[1] there is an association between malnutrition and increased morbidity[2] and mortality;[3] it seems intuitive that well-nourished patients will respond most favorably to treatment; nutrition support can be administered safely to most patients; and clinical trials indicate that it is beneficial in selected patients.[4-6]

W.W. Souba, M.D., Sc.D.

References

1. Bistrian BR, Blackburn GL, Hallowell E, et al: Protein status of general surgical patients. *JAMA* 230:858–860, 1974.
2. Windsor JA, Hill GL: Risk factors of postoperative pneumonia: The importance of protein depletion. *Ann Surg* 207:290–302, 1988.
3. Hermann FR, Safran C, Levkoff SE, et al: Serum albumin level on admission as a predictor of death, length of stay, and readmission. *Arch Intern Med* 152:125–130, 1992.
4. Muller JM, Brenner U, Dienst C, et al: Preoperative parenteral feeding in patients with gastrointestinal cancer. *Lancet* 1:68–72, 1982.
5. The Veterans Affairs Total Parenteral Nutrition Cooperative Study Group: Perioperative total parenteral nutrition in surgical patients. *N Engl J Med* 325:525–532, 1991.
6. Moore FA, Feliciano DV, Andrassy RJ, et al: Early enteral feeding, compared with parenteral, reduces postoperative septic complications. *Ann Surg* 216:172–173, 1992.

9 Growth Factors and Wound Healing

Introduction

Wound healing problems continue to account for a substantial number of postoperative complications in surgical patients. Derangements in healing occur in cutaneous wounds, but they can also occur at the site of resection after extirpation of a diseased organ. Wound healing can be impaired by both local and systemic factors. Local factors include infection, hypoxia, and technical errors. Systemic factors affecting wound healing include nutritional status, age, drugs, and ischemia.

Attempts to modulate wound healing in an effort to reduce postoperative complications have led to a dearth of studies that have focused on the molecular control of wound healing. In this light, new growth factors have been discovered and purified and the genes that encode for their biosynthesis are being cloned. Despite these advances, several of which are likely to have clinical applicability, the best way to ensure "speedy" wound healing is to apply commonsense surgical care, including the use of sterile technique, judicious use of antibiotics, meticulous handling of tissues, and appropriate nutritional care.

As health care reform continues to focus on improving outcome, the institution of measures that minimize wound healing problems will greatly contribute to a reduction in length of hospital stay and lead to cost reductions. In the papers discussed in this chapter, both the clinical aspects of wound healing and some of the more important recent basic research findings are examined.

Wiley W. Souba, M.D., Sc.D.

Basic Research With Clinical Applicability

Growth Factors in Porcine Full and Partial Thickness Burn Repair: Differing Targets and Effects of Keratinocyte Growth Factor, Platelet-derived Growth Factor-BB, Epidermal Growth Factor, and neu Differentiation Factor

Danilenko DM, Ring BD, Tarpley JE, et al (Amgen Incorp, Thousand Oaks, Calif)

Am J Pathol 147:1261–1277, 1995 9–1

Introduction.—Several animal models of wound repair have demonstrated significant acceleration of healing after application of recombinant growth factors. Four of these growth factors—epidermal growth factor (rEGF), platelet-derived growth factor-BB homodimer (rPDGF-BB), keratinocyte growth factor (rKGF), and neu differentiation factor (rNDF)—were evaluated in porcine models of full and partial thickness wound repair.

Methods.—The porcine burn models were designed to be more rigorous and clinically relevant than the burn models used in previous studies. Standardized burns of reproducible depth were obtained and the burns escharectomized 4 or 5 days postburn to duplicate the standard burn treatment in humans. The 4 growth factors were then applied singly and in combination to evaluate their efficacy in burn repair. After the animals were euthanized from 12 to 18 days after recombinant growth factor treatment, the burns were harvested for assessment of reepithelialization and burn healing. Parameters of wound repair examined included extracellular matrix and granulation tissue production, percent reepithelialization, and new epithelial area.

Results.—In the group of full thickness burns only rPDGF-BB, alone and in combination with rKGF, induced significant changes in burn repair. Extracellular matrix and granulation tissue production showed a marked, significant increase after rPDGF-BB treatment, filling the burn defect within several days of escharectomy. Neither the percent of reepithelialization nor new epithelial area were significantly increased by rPDGF-BB. The rPDGF-BB/rKGF combination produced a significant increase in new epithelial area (Fig 3) and a highly significant increase in extracellular matrix and granulation tissue area. Overall, rKGF induced the most consistent changes in deep partial thickness burns. There was a trend toward increased new epithelial area in deep partial thickness burns treated with rEGF, but this growth factor had no effect on reepithelialization. No significant biological effects were observed in full or deep partial thickness burns after rNDF treatment.

Conclusion.—The most effective of the recombinant growth factors evaluated in this porcine burn model were rKGF and rPDGF-BB. Their topical application produced highly significant increases in some parameters of wound repair, but reepithelialization, the most clinically relevant

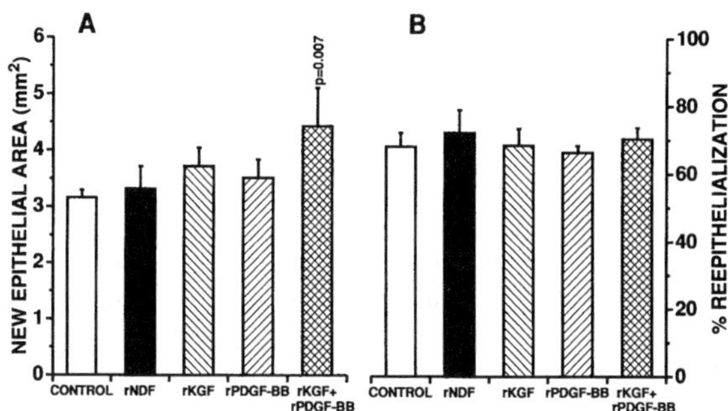

FIGURE 3.—New epithelial area and percent reepithelialization of porcine full thickness burns 18 days postburn sorted by recombinant growth factor treatment and analyzed by one way analysis of variance coupled to the Bonferroni/Dunn post-hoc test (n = 10 except pooled controls, n = 20). The keratinocyte growth factor (rKGF) and new differentiation factor (rNDF)-α_2 were both applied at 20 μg/cm² while platelet-derived growth factor-BB homodimer (rPDGF-BB) was applied at 28 μg/cm². These doses were determined to be optimal based on data from previous dose-response experiments (data not shown). There is a significant increase in new epithelial area in burns treated with the combination of rPDGF-BB and rKGF. (Courtesy of Danilenko DM, Ring BD, Tarpley JE, et al: Growth factors in porcine full and partial thickness burn repair: Differing targets and effects of keratinocyte growth factor, platelet-derived growth factor-BB, epidermal growth factor, and neu differential growth factor. *Am J Pathol* 147:1261–1277, 1995. Copyright American Society for Investigative Pathology.)

parameter, was only marginally accelerated. Additional strategies will have to be developed before these growth factors have clinical value.

▶ The authors evaluated the effects of topical application of recombinant growth factors on healing in a porcine burn model. Although application of growth factors resulted in a highly significant increase in granulation tissue production, there was only a marginal acceleration of reepithelialization, the most important clinical parameter in burn wound repair. Previous studies have also shown that epidermal growth factor fails to accelerate the rate of reepithelialization in burn patient donor graft sites[1] and that other growth factors do not significantly accelerate chronic ulcer repair[2]. Thus, additional strategies such as the use of growth factors in conjunction with extracellular matrix components may be required to accelerate wound healing in patients with large open wounds.

W.W. Souba, M.D., Sc.D.

References

1. Brown GL, Nanney LB, Griffen J, et al: Enhancement of wound healing by topical treatment with epidermal growth factor. *N Engl J Med* 321:76–79, 1989.
2. Pierce GF, Mustoe TA: Pharmacologic enhancement of wound healing. *Annu Rev Med* 46:467–481, 1995.

Basic Fibroblast Growth Factor Mediates Angiogenic Activity in Early Surgical Wounds

Nissen NN, Polverini PJ, Gamelli RL, et al (Loyola Univ, Maywood, Ill; Univ of Michigan, Ann Arbor)
Surgery 119:457–465, 1996 9–2

Introduction.—Although wound angiogenesis is thought to be initiated by the early rapid release of growth factors such as basic fibroblast growth factor (bFGF), there have been no studies of bFGF-mediated angiogenic activity in early surgical wounds. To investigate the early angiogenic environment of surgical wounds, surgical drain fluid (SDF) was collected from closed suction drains of 26 patients at periods ranging from 6 hours to 6 days postoperatively.

Methods.—Fourteen patients had undergone modified radical mastectomy and 4 had modified radical neck dissection; the remaining 8 cases were varied. None of the patients who provided SDF had received heparin, corticosteroids, or other immunosuppressive medication, and none had preoperative radiotherapy. The samples were tested for endothelial cell (EC) proliferative and chemotactic activity and for the capacity to stimulate angiogenesis in vivo in the rat corneal assay. Enzyme-linked immunosorbent assay was used to determine bFGF levels of SDF, and neutralizing antibody to bFGF to assess the contribution of bFGF to SDF activity.

Results.—A total of 78 SDF samples were collected, most by postoperative day 3. None of the wounds showed signs of infection, hematoma, or dehiscence. The EC proliferative activity was greatest (390% that of normal serum) on postoperative day 0, but fell by 41% on day 1 and subsequently to near serum levels. When implanted into rat corneas, SDF from postoperative days 0 and 1 demonstrated marked EC chemotactic activity and stimulated rapid formation of new vessels. No signs of inflammation were present. The temporal appearance of bFGF in these exudates, which peaked on postoperative day 0 and decreased 80% by day 2, exhibited a pattern similar to EC proliferative activity. The addition of neutralizing bFGF antibody to SDF before corneal implantation substantially reduced the angiogenic response of 3 of 4 samples, which indicates that bFGF is a major angiogenic mediator in early surgical wound fluids.

Conclusion.—Exudates from a variety of surgical wound types demonstrated that SDF, from the first few days after operation, stimulates endothelial cell proliferation, as well as migration in vitro and angiogenesis in vivo. Tissue or platelet stores of bFGF, which appear early in surgical wounds, may facilitate wound repair.

► Wound fluid is reflective of the proliferate environment of the wound, and the detection of angiogenic activity in wound fluid correlates with histologic examination of the wound. Nonhealing wounds such as gastric ulcers may develop in part from impaired bFGF production. The potential for the use of bFGF in the treatment of nonhealing wounds requires further study.

W.W. Souba, M.D., Sc.D.

Antimicrobial Effects of Granulocyte-Macrophage Colony-Stimulating Factor in Protein-Energy Malnutrition

Hill ADK, Naama H, Shou J, et al (New York Hosp-Cornell Med Ctr)
Arch Surg 130:1273–1278, 1995 9–3

Objectives.—The role of nitric oxide in regulating the antimicrobial activities of granulocyte-macrophage colony-stimulating factor (GM-CSF) in protein-energy malnutrition, the mechanisms of GM-CSF in improving host antimicrobial defense, and the effect of GM-CSF on T-cell cytokine patterns in protein-energy malnutrition were investigated.

Background.—There are reports of an association between protein-energy malnutrition and macrophage dysfunction, a higher risk of infection, and death. The GM-CSF encourages proliferation of bone marrow-derived progenitors of granulocytes and macrophages and regulates their development. It was hypothesized that GM-CSF would improve the host antimicrobial defense in patients with protein-energy malnutrition.

Methods.—In study 1, 60 mice were fed a protein-free diet with GM-CSF, a protein-free diet with saline, or a 24% protein diet (control group). On day 7, all mice were given *Candida albicans*. In study 2, 45 mice were fed a protein-free diet, a protein-free diet with GM-CSF, or a 24% protein diet (control group). Assays were performed to determine levels of interleukin-4, interleukin-6, interleukin-10, interferon-γ, superoxide anion, and nitric oxide.

Results.—Malnourished, infected mice treated with GM-CSF had significantly longer survival. Granulocyte-macrophage colony-stimulating factor was associated with higher levels of interleukin-6, superoxide anion, and nitric oxide in splenic macrophages, and it was also associated with lower levels of interleukin-4 in splenocytes.

Conclusions.—Granulocyte-macrophage colony-stimulating factor may have a role in malnourished hosts with a high risk of infection. Production of antimicrobial products may be increased by GM-CSF. A higher level of nitric oxide released by GM-CSF may be regulated by decreasing the inhibitory effect of interleukin-4.

▶ Granulocyte-macrophage colony-stimulating factor (GM-CSF) has been shown to stimulate bone marrow production of white blood cells and has been used for several years in patients with cancer who receive chemotherapy. The results of this preclinical study by Hill and colleagues suggest a beneficial role for GM-CSF in the non–tumor-bearing malnourished host predisposed to infection. There are no clinical trials to date.

W.W. Souba, M.D., Sc.D.

Role of Prostaglandins in Intestinal Epithelial Restitution Stimulated by Growth Factors

Zushi S, Shinomura Y, Kiyohara T, et al (Osaka Univ, Japan)

Am J Physiol 270:G757–G762, 1996 9–4

Objective.—The role of eicosanoids in regulating intestinal epithelial restitution was studied using cell lines IEC-6 and Caco-2.

Background.—The intestinal epithelial barrier recovers rapidly after superficial injury by a process called restitution, which prevents further

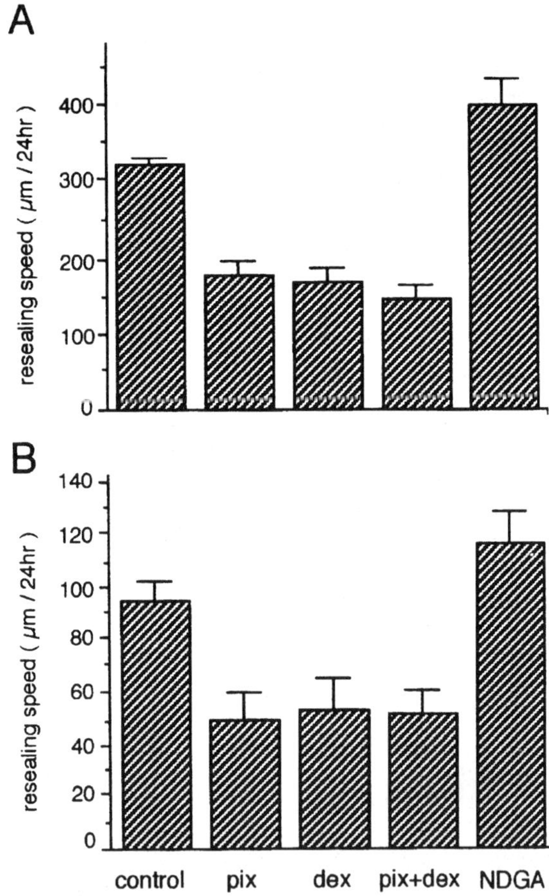

FIGURE 5.—Effect of piroxicam, dexamethasone, and nordihydroguaiaretic acid on restitution of IEC-6 (**A**) and Caco-2 (**B**) cells. Cells were exposed to mitomycin C for 2 hours to inhibit mitosis. Medium was changed to serum-deprived medium 6 hours before wounding. Each reagent was added 4 hours before wounding. Wound was created, and medium was changed to fresh medium supplemented with each reagent again. Cells were further incubated for 24 hours and resealing speed was determined. Results are expressed as means ± SE (n = 6). *Abbreviations*: *pix*, piroxicam; *dex*, dexamethasone; *NDGA*, nordihydroguaiaretic acid. (Courtesy of Zushi S, Shinomura Y, Kiyohara T, et al: Role of prostaglandins in intestinal epithelial restitution stimulated by growth factors. *Am J Physiol* 270:G757–G762, 1996.)

destructive inflammation from occurring. In epithelial restitution, epithelial cell migration reseals the wound without cell proliferation. It has been reported that fetal calf serum and other growth factors speed up intestinal epithelial restitution. It has also been reported that endogenous eicosanoids regulate intracellular mitogenic signals in response to transforming growth factor-α and 12-O-tetradecanoylphorbol 13-acetate in the intestinal cell line, RIE-1. It is unclear how endogenous eicosanoids affect intestinal epithelial restitution.

Methods.—Intestinal epithelial cell-6 and Caco-2 cells were obtained and cultured. Wounding was performed and assays were carried out to determine the effect of piroxicam, dexamethasone, and nordihydroguaiaretic acid on restitution of IEC-6 and Caco-2 cells.

Results.—Intestinal epithelial restitution was accelerated by epidermal growth factor, transforming growth factor-β, hepatocyte growth factor, and fetal calf serum. Piroxicam significantly slowed these effects, and dexamethasone mimicked the effects of piroxicam (Fig 5). There was no additive effect of piroxicam and dexamethasone. Intestinal epithelial restitution was unaffected by nordihydroguaiaretic acid. The increase in 6-ketoprostaglandin $F_{1\alpha}$ induced by fetal calf serum was eliminated by piroxicam. The slowing of restitution induced by piroxicam was reversed by adding a stable PGI_2 analogue, OP-41483.

Conclusions.—Intestinal epithelial restitution was regulated by endogenous prostaglandin. This finding may aid the development of a pharmacologic means of stimulating the restitution process to treat inflammatory bowel disease and other diseases related to epithelial barrier function.

▶ Although the damaging effects of nonsteroidal anti-inflammatory drugs on the gut mucosa have been attributed to direct mitochondrial damage during absorption[1], this study suggests that their injurious effects may also result from the inhibition of prostaglandin biosynthesis. The authors have nicely demonstrated that prostaglandins modulate intestinal epithelial restitution. A number of other growth factors including transforming growth factor-α, epidermal growth factor, and hepatocyte growth factor have been shown to accelerate enterocyte growth. Whether the use of exogenous oral prostaglandins will have clinical applicability in promoting intestinal mucosal repair is unestablished.

W.W. Souba, M.D., Sc.D.

Reference

1. Bjarnasson I, Hayllar J, Macpherson AJ, et al. Side effects of nonsteroidal anti-inflammatory drugs on the small and large intestine in humans. *Gastroenterology* 104:1832–1847, 1993.

Growth Hormone Increases the Biomechanical Strength and Collagen Deposition Rate During the Early Phase of Skin Wound Healing

Jørgensen PH, Oxlund H (Univ of Aarhus, Denmark)

Wound Rep Reg 4:40–47, 1996 9–5

Background.—The biology of wound healing is a complex process influenced by many factors. A number of growth factors that may improve wound healing are now available. Previous research has shown that growth hormone (GH), 2 mg/kg body weight/day, increases the mechanical strength of skin incisional wounds in rats after 4 days of healing, although no effect was observed after 7 and 10 days. The dose-response relationship between GH and mechanical properties in 4-day-old skin incisional wounds in rats was reported. A new method for in vivo studies of collagen deposition rate in granulation tissue of the wound cleft was also described.

Methods and Findings.—In 90-day-old female Wistar rats, biosynthetic human GH, 0.125–2 mg/kg/day, induced a marked dose-dependent increase of approximately 94% in the mechanical strength of wounds. The production of ^{3}H-hydroxy-L-proline was determined by IV injection of ^{3}H-proline into the rats with a large flooding dose of unlabeled proline. This decreases reuse of ^{3}H-proline and the effects of de novo synthesis of proline. Extractable collagens, not bound in the wound tissue and therefore not contributors to its mechanical strength, were removed from the samples. Reverse-phase, high-performance liquid chromatography with ultraviolet detection and flow scintillation counting of labeled and unlabeled proline were used simultaneously to assess these amino acids. On day 4 the collagen deposition rate in the incisional wound zone, which had

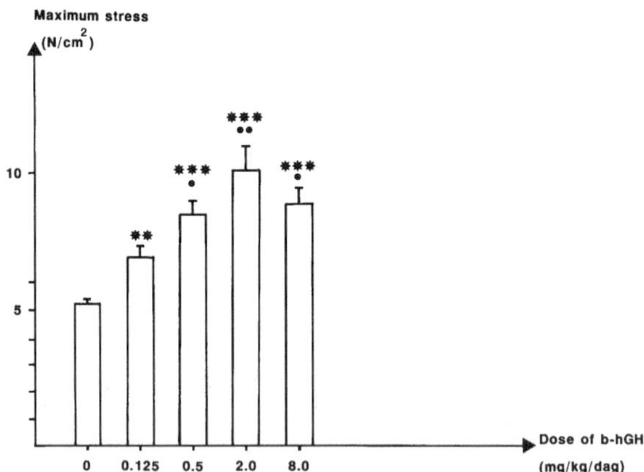

FIGURE 1.—Maximum stress of skin incisional wounds of rats determined in a materials testing machine after 4 days of healing. Each bar represents the mean value ± SEM. Statistically significant differences compared with saline solution control: 2 asterisks $P < 0.01$; *3 asterisks* $P < 0.001$. Compared with the 0.125 mg group: *filled circle,* $P < 0.05$; *2 filled circles,* $P < 0.01$. Note the x axis is logarithmic. (Courtesy of Jørgensen PH, Oxlund H: Growth hormone increases the biomechanical strength and collagen deposition rate during the early phase of skin wound healing. *Wound Rep Reg* 4:40–47, 1996.)

a width of 0.4 mm and contained the wound cleft, was 1.8% per hour of the collagen present in that zone. Compared with control group values, 2 mg/kg/day of GH increased the collagen deposition rate by 149% (Fig 1).

Conclusions.—After 4 days of healing, GH can produce a dose-dependent increase in the mechanical strength of skin incisional wounds. The increased collagen deposition rate in the wound may explain this increase. Growth hormone treatment markedly increases the collagen deposition rate in intact skin outside the wound area.

▶ This is another paper that demonstrates the ability of GH to improve wound healing. Like other studies, the key issue is whether improvements in biochemical indices translate into functional improvements. Recombinant human GH as an adjunct to nutritional support has been shown to enhance intestinal amino acid uptake[1] and nitrogen retention,[2-4] but it remains unestablished whether these biochemical changes are associated with an improvement in outcome.

W.W. Souba, M.D., Sc.D.

References

1. Inoue Y, Copeland EM, Souba WW: Growth hormone enhances amino acid transport by the human small intestine. *Ann Surg* 219:715–724, 1994.
2. Ziegler TR, Lazarus JM, Young LS, et al: Effects of recombinant human growth hormone in adults receiving maintenance hemodialysis. *J Am Soc Nephrol* 2:1130–1135, 1991.
3. Ziegler TR, Rombeau J, Young LS, et al: Administration of recombinant human growth hormone enhances the metabolic efficacy of parenteral nutrition: A double blinded, randomized, controlled study. *J Clin Endocrinol Metab* 74:865–873, 1992.
4. Voerman HJ, Van Schijndel RJ, Groeneveld AJ, et al: Effects of recombinant human growth hormone in patients with severe sepsis. *Ann Surg.* 216:648–653, 1992.

Platelet-derived Growth Factor Accelerates Gastric Epithelial Restoration in a Rabbit Cultured Cell Model

Watanabe S, Wang X, Hirose M, et al (Juntendo Univ, Tokyo)

Gastroenterology 110:775–779, 1996 9–6

Background.—Growth factors are important to gastric wound repair. The effects of platelet-derived growth factor (PDGF) BB on gastric epithelial cell restoration were investigated.

Methods.—After rabbit gastric epithelial cell wounding, 1–50 ng/mL of PDGF-BB was added to confluent cultures. Epithelial cell regrowth was monitored for 48 hours. Speed of cell migration was measured. A 5-bromodeoxyuridine staining method was used to detect cell proliferation. The labeling index for a 0.05 mm^2 area around the wound was determined.

Findings.—Lamellipodia and ruffing movements were observed in cells at the wound edge. With the addition of PDGF-BB, cell migration, cell proliferation, and gastric restoration were accelerated significantly. Migra-

TABLE 2.—Effect of Platelet-derived Growth Factor BB on Initial Migration Rates of Gastric Epithelial Cells During Restoration

	Distance from the edge of the wound		
	0 μm	200 μm	1000 μm
Migration rate (μm/h)			
Control	21.1 ± 2.5	12.5 ± 2.2	1.6 ± 0.8
PDGF (ng/mL)			
1	24.3 ± 3.6	12.9 ± 3.8	1.7 ± 0.6
10	32.3 ± 2.9	18.2 ± 1.2*	1.6 ± 0.6
50	40.5 ± 3.1"	23.7 ± 1.9*	1.8 ± 1.0

Note: Data are expressed as the mean ± SD. Each number is the average of 3 cells per experiment and 5 separate experiments.

*$P < 0.01$ compared with control.

(Courtesy of Watanabe S, Wang X, Hirose M, et al: Platelet-derived growth factor accelerates gastric epithelial restoration in a rabbit cultured cell model. *Gastroenterology* 110:775–779, 1996.)

tion speed in control cultures was 21 μm/hr; in cultures that contained 10 ng/mL of PDGF-BB, 32 μm/hr; and in cultures that contained 50 ng/mL of PDGF-BB, 40 μm/hr. The detection of 5-bromodeoxyuridine–positive cells was rare in control cultures in the first 24 hours after wounding. Maximum labeling occurred at 36 hours, with a labeling index of 3.4%. Maximum labeling in cultures that contained PDGF-BB occurred at 24 hours, with an index of 6.9% (Table 2).

Conclusions.—After wounding, the migration rate and proliferation of cultured gastric epithelial cells are accelerated by PDGF-BB in a dose-dependent fashion. Therefore, PDGF-BB may be important to gastric epithelial cell restoration during gastric mucosal lesion healing.

► Many growth factors, including epidermal growth factor, insulin, hepatocyte growth factor, and transforming growth factor α have been shown to accelerate gastric epithelial repair associated with cell migration and proliferation. Whether such compounds have clinical applicability in patients who are susceptible to gastric erosions and/or stress ulceration remains to be seen.

W.W. Souba, M.D., Sc.D.

Effect of Human Growth Hormone on Human Pancreatic Carcinoma Growth, Protein, and Cell Cycle Kinetics

Harrison LE, Blumberg D, Berman R, et al (Mem Sloan-Kettering Cancer Ctr, New York)

J Surg Res 61:317–322, 1996 9–7

Background.—The use of human growth hormone (hGH) as a nutritional adjunct for patients who have cancer is controversial because of its potential mitogenic effects on tumor growth. To date, there have been no studies of the effect of hGH on human tumor response in vivo. A cell proliferation bioassay was used to determine the in vitro effects of serum from GH-treated mice on human pancreatic carcinoma cells.

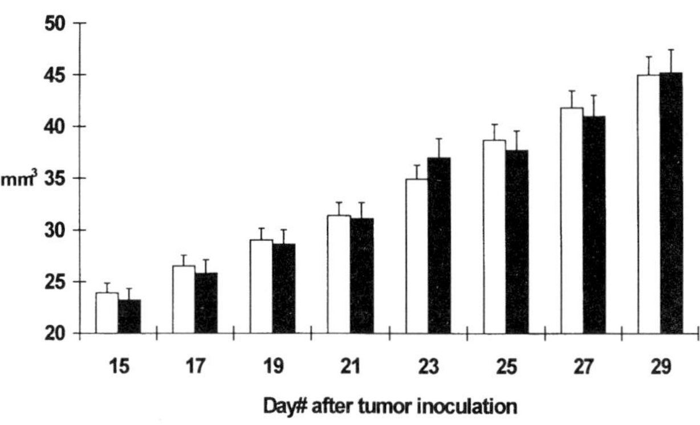

FIGURE 4.—In vivo tumor volumes during the 14 days of treatment. There was no significant difference in tumor volume during the study period. (Courtesy of Harrison LE, Blumberg D, Berman R, et al: Effect of human growth hormone on human pancreatic carcinoma growth, protein, and cell cycle kinetics. *J Surg Res* 61:317–322, 1996.)

Methods.—Fourteen days after inoculation with human pancreatic carcinoma cells, athymic mice were randomly assigned to receive hGH or saline daily. On day 29, the mice received [^{3}H]phenylalanine for tissue protein fractional synthetic rate (FSR) measurement. Tumors were then excised, and cell cycle kinetics were assessed.

Findings.—In vitro and in vivo, serum from the 14 GH-treated mice had increased levels of IgF-1 and significantly stimulated cell growth compared with serum from the 12 control mice. In vivo, GH did not significantly affect tumor growth rate, final tumor weight, DNA index, percent S phase, or tumor FSR. Serum levels of IgF-1 and liver FSR were significantly increased by GH. In vitro, serum from GH-treated mice increased human pancreatic cell growth (Fig 4).

Conclusions.—Concerns about the potential of GH to stimulate tumor growth have not been substantiated. In this mouse model, exogenous GH did not affect human pancreatic tumor growth, cell cycle kinetics, or protein synthetic rate. The liver protein synthetic rate was increased by GH. These findings indicate that exogenous GH can be safely administered to patients who have cancer.

► Growth hormone has been used in the perioperative setting and has been shown to improve nitrogen balance and the accrual of lean body mass. There has been concern about administering GH to patients who have cancer because of the possibility that tumor growth could be stimulated. Although this study did not observe any effects of GH on tumor growth in vivo, 2 previous animal studies suggest that GH may have tumor-promoting effects.[1, 2] Thus, a role for GH in cancer patients requires further study.

W.W. Souba, M.D., Sc.D.

References

1. Akaza H, Matsuki K, Matsushima H, et al: Stimulatory effects of growth hormone on rat bladder carcinogenesis. *Cancer* 68:2418–2422, 1991.
2. Ng E, Rock C, Lazarus D, et al: Impact of exogenous growth hormone on host preservation and tumor cell-cycle distribution: a rat sarcoma model. *J Surg Res* 51:99–105, 1991.

The Effects of Chronic Ketorolac Tromethamine (Toradol) on Wound Healing

Haws MJ, Kucan JO, Roth AC, et al (Southern Illinois Univ, Springfield)
Ann Plast Surg 37:147–151, 1996 9–8

Objective.—Whether a nonsteroidal anti-inflammatory drug (NSAID) affects wound healing in rats was studied.

Methods.—The NSAID chosen was ketorolac, because it can be administered by injection. Twenty rats were randomly divided into experimental and control groups. The experimental animals received injections of ketorolac, once each day beginning 7 days before wounding and continuing until all animals were killed 2 weeks after wounding. Wounding involved making a midline dorsal cut on the back of each animal in both groups. After the rats were killed, 2 strips of tissue were taken from the area of the wound and tested in blinded fashion in a tensiometer. Wound edges underwent a collagen assay.

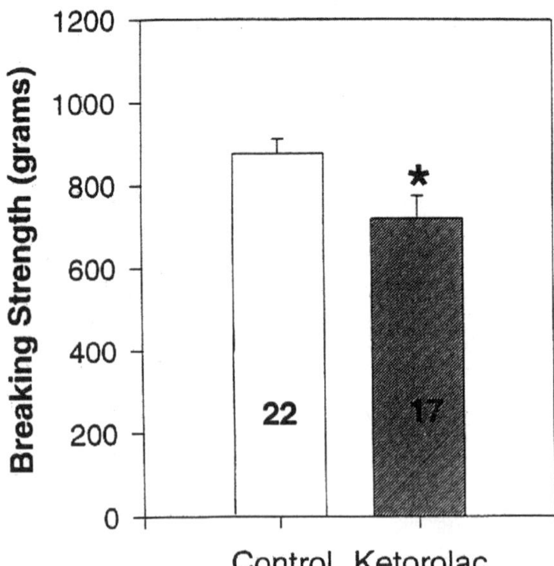

FIGURE 2.—Comparison of breaking strength of control (N = 22) and ketorolac-treated (N = 17) animals. (* = $P < 0.05$). (Courtesy of Haws MJ, Kucan JO, Roth AC, et al: The effects of chronic ketorolac tromethamine (Toradol) on wound healing. *Ann Plast Surg* 37:147–151, 1996.)

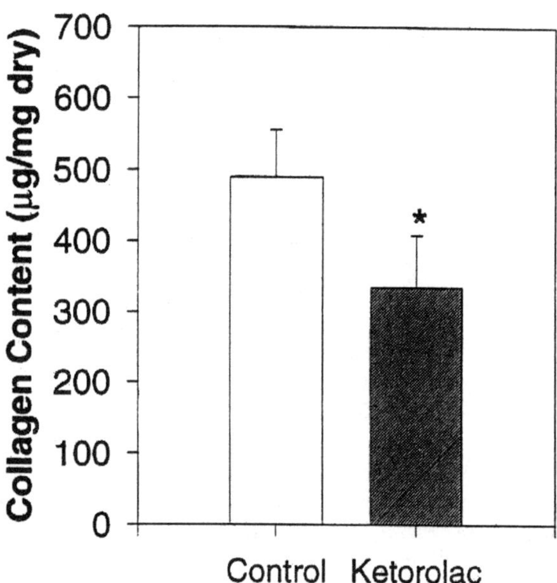

FIGURE 4.—Comparison of the collagen concentration of the wound edges of control (N = 4) and ketorolac-treated animals. Collagen concentration was measured by the Edwards and O'Brien technique (Edwards CA, O'Brien WD: Modified assay for determination of hydroxyproline in a tissue hydrolyzate. *Clin Chim Acta* 104:161–167, 1980). (* = $P < 0.05$). (Courtesy of Haws MJ, Kucan JO, Roth AC, et al: The effects of chronic ketorolac tromethamine (Toradol) on wound healing. *Ann Plast Surg* 37:147–151, 1996.)

Results.—The breaking strength of the wounds (i.e., the force required to separate them) (Fig 2) and the collagen density (Fig 4) were significantly lower in ketorolac-treated rats than in control animals.

Conclusions.—Studies should be conducted with human patients to investigate how ketorolac and other NSAIDs affect wound healing.

▶ Previous animal studies using other NSAIDs also have shown that these compounds can impair wound healing, but no clinical studies have addressed this issue. A case report of delayed wound healing in a patient undergoing head and neck reconstructive surgery has been published.[1]

W.W. Souba, M.D., Sc.D.

Reference

1. Proper SA, Fenske NA, Burnett SM, et al: Compromised wound repair caused by perioperative use of ibuprofen. *J Am Acad Dermatol* 18:1173–1179, 1988.

Nitric Oxide Regulates Wound Healing

Schäffer MR, Tantry U, Gross SS, et al (Sinai Hosp of Baltimore, Md; Johns Hopkins Med Insts, Baltimore, Md; Cornell Univ, New York)
J Surg Res 63:237–240, 1996 9–9

Introduction.—Although recent studies have shown nitric oxide to be synthesized in wounds, its source and role as a mediator of wound repair are undetermined. The effect of nitric oxide on wound healing with the use of a nitric oxide inhibitor was investigated.

Methods.—A 2.5-cm dorsal skin incision was made in anesthestized mice, and polyvinyl sponges were inserted before wound closure. A competitive inhibitor of nitric oxide synthase, *S*-methyl isothiouronium (MITU), was then administered as a continuous infusion at a dose of 10, 50, or 100 mg/kg per day. Control animals were given continuous infusions of phosphate-buffered saline. Ten days after wound healing, the animals were sacrificed, and the healing scar and the sponges were removed. Wound breaking strength was determined, as was the hydroxyproline content of the wound fluid from the sponges. Cells obtained from wound fluid were incubated with or without MITU. The nitrate and nitrite content of wound fluid was also measured.

Results.—Nitrate/nitrite content of wound fluid was found to be decreased by MITU in a dose-dependent fashion. Wound breaking strength and hydroxyproline concentration were both decreased in parallel with reductions in nitrate/nitrite concentrations. (Figs 1 and 2). Cells obtained

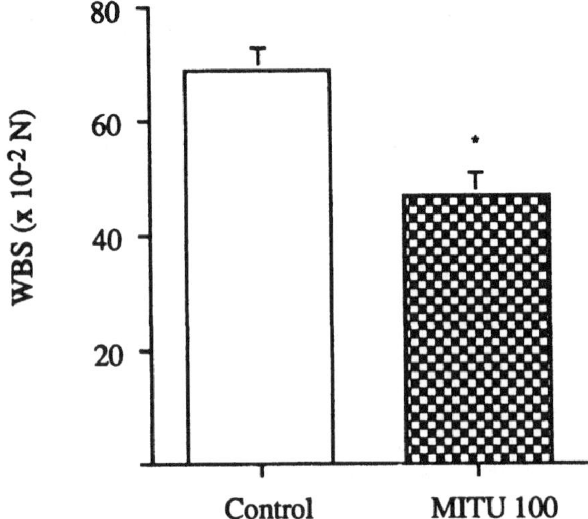

FIGURE 1.—Effect of systemic treatment with *S*-methyl isothiouronium (*MITU*) on wound-breaking strength (*WBS*) of incisional wounds 10 days post wounding. The MITU was administered at a dose of 100 mg/kg body weight per day by continuous infusion using intraperitoneally implanted miniosmotic pumps. Control animals received pumps filled with phosphate-buffered saline. Data show the means ± standard error of the mean ($N = 10$). *Asterisk* indicates $P < 0.01$ vs. control, *t* test. (Courtesy of Schäffer MR, Tantry U, Gross SS, et al: Nitric oxide regulates wound healing. *J Surg Res* 63:237–240, 1996.)

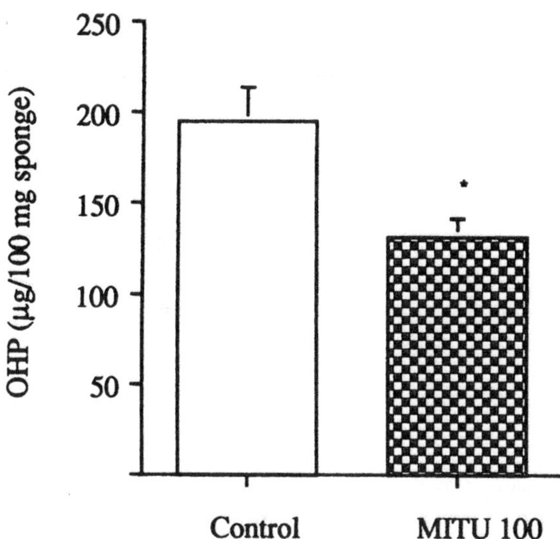

FIGURE 2.—Effect of systemic treatment with *S*-methyl isothiouronium (*MITU*) on hydroxyproline (*OHP*) content, an index of collagen accumulation, in subcutaneously implanted polyvinyl alcohol sponges 10 days post wounding. The MITU was administered at a dose of 100 mg/kg body weight per day by continuous infusion using intraperitoneally implanted miniosmotic pumps. Control animal received pumps filled with phosphate-buffered saline. Data show the means ± standard error of the mean ($N = 10$) *Asterisk* indicates $P < 0.01$ vs. control, *t* test. (Courtesy of Schäffer MR, Tantry U, Gross SS, et al. Nitric oxide regulates wound healing. *J Surg Res* 63:237–240, 1996.)

from wound fluid which were incubated without MITU showed no difference in nitric oxide synthesis as compared with controls; however, cells incubated with MITU showed nitric oxide synthesis to be inhibited by 83%.

Conclusion.—Continuous administration of MITU, a nitric oxide synthase inhibitor, resulted in a dose-dependent inhibition of wound healing. Wound breaking strength and wound collagen accumulation were both decreased in the presence of MITU.

▶ Although the authors show a correlation between nitric oxide in wounds and wound healing as measured by breaking strength and collagen deposition, no cause-and-effect relationship was shown. The role that nitric oxide plays in wound healing requires further elucidation.

W.W. Souba, M.D., Sc.D.

Expression of Secreted Platelet-derived Growth Factor-B by Recombinant Nonreplicating and Noncytopathic Vaccinia Virus

Norton JA, Peplinski GR, Tsung K (Washington Univ, St Louis)

Ann Surg 224:555–562, 1996 9–10

Background.—It has been demonstrated that platelet-derived growth factor (PDGF) and other cytokine growth factors have an important role in wound healing. However, in studies with recombinant PDGF, repeated topical applications have failed to provide high levels of PDGF in healing-impaired wounds. The feasibility of delivering PDGF to wounds via gene therapy with recombinant vaccinia virus was investigated.

Methods.—Vaccinia virus was treated with psoralen and ultraviolet radiation to make it noncytopathic and nonreplicative. Various forms of PDGF were inserted into the virus, and the biological activity of PDGF was measured.

Results.—When the full-length PDGF molecule was inserted into vaccinia, the protein became bound to cell membranes and was not secreted. When a truncated form was inserted, high levels of biologically active PDGF were secreted, as demonstrated by proliferation of a 3T3 fibroblast cell line.

Conclusion.—The results provide important preliminary evidence that healing-impaired wounds can be treated with recombinant vaccinia virus containing PDGF.

▶ Platelet-derived growth factor has been shown to improve wound healing in open nonhealing wounds in patients.[1] The use of vaccinia engineered to express growth factors may prove useful in clinical wound healing, but prospective randomized trials will be required.

W.W. Souba, M.D., Sc.D.

Reference

1. Mustoe TA, Cutler NR, Allman RM, et al: A phase II study to evaluate recombinant platelet-derived growth factor-BB in the treatment of stage 3 and 4 pressure ulcers. *Arch Surg* 129:213–219, 1994.

The Impact of Ischemia on Wound Healing Is Increased in Old Age but Can be Countered by Hyperbaric Oxygen Therapy

Quirinia A, Viidik A (Univ of Aarhus, Denmark)
Mech Aging Dev 91:131–144, 1996 9–11

Introduction.—Wound healing has been shown to decrease with aging, and previous studies have found ischemia to have a more pronounced effect on wound healing in older animals as compared to younger animals. The effects of age and treatment with hyperbaric oxygen on ischemic and normal wound healing were investigated.

Methods.—Groups of young (10 weeks) and old (102 to 104 weeks) rats were randomly divided into 6 groups each. Groups 1 and 2 had ischemic incisional wounds treated by hyperbaric oxygen for days 0–3. Groups 3 and 4 had untreated ischemic control wounds, and groups 5 and 6 had non-ischemic incisional (normal) wounds. Wounds were then evaluated for strength parameters, degree of shrinkage, and length of surface necroses.

TABLE 3.—Mean Lengths of Necroses (in cm, [95% confidence interval]) on Cranial and Caudal Flaps After 10 Days of Healing

	Cranial flap	Caudal flap
Old, control	1.4† [1.1, 1.7]	0.5* [0.3, 0.7]
Old, O_2 day 0–3	1.1 [0.8, 1.4]	0.5 [0.3, 0.7]
Young, control	2.3 [2.0, 2.6]	0.2 [0.1, 0.3]
Young, O_2 day 0–3	2.0 [1.6, 2.4]	0.3 [0.2, 0.4]

Note: Figures are given in centimeters with 95% confidence interval in brackets.
Comparison between old and young controls: *indicates $P < 0.01$; †indicates $P < 0.001$.
(Courtesy of Quirinia A, Viidik A. The impact of ischemia on wound healing is increased in old age but can be countered by hyperbaric oxygen therapy. *Mech Aging Dev* 91:131–144, 1996.)

Results.—In comparison with younger animals, older animals had a reduction in all wound strength parameters by 30% to 40% in normal wounds after 10 days of healing. Reductions of 40% to 51% were seen in ischemic wounds of the older animals compared with the younger with a decrease by 22% to 28% in strain parameters. After 20 days of healing, strength parameters of normal wounds were decreased by 29% to 37% and breaking strain by 11% in older animals. All the corresponding strength parameters in ischemic wounds in older animals were decreased by 46% to 58% and strain parameters by 22% to 28% as compared with younger animals. After 10 days of healing, hyperbaric oxygen treatment resulted in an increase in strength parameters in ischemic wounds in both young and old animals as compared with untreated animals. Hyperbaric oxygen treatment also increased all strength parameters of ischemic wounds in older animals as compared with older untreated animals after 20 days of treatment. In cranially based flaps, the length of necroses was significantly shorter in the older untreated animals as compared with younger untreated animals. However, for caudally based flaps, the length of necroses was significantly longer in the older untreated animals (Table 3).

Conclusion.—Ischemia was found to amplify the decreases in wound strength and strain parameters in older animals, whereas hyperbaric oxygen treatment had a greater effect on ischemic wounds in older animals. Both age and ischemic diseases may be factors in impairment of wound healing observed in older patients.

► The selective benefits of hyperbaric oxygen in patients have been reported.[1, 2] In the study by Quirinia, it was unclear to me why hyperbaric oxygen therapy was more beneficial to older rats with ischemic wounds.

W.W. Souba, M.D., Sc.D.

References

1. Perrins DJ: Influence of hyperbaric oxygen on the survival of split thickness skin grafts. *Lancet* 1:868–871, 1967.
2. Hammarlund C, Sundberg T: Hyperbaric oxygen reduced size of chronic leg ulcers: A randomized double-blind study. *Plast Reconstr Surg* 93:829–833, 1994.

Wound Healing and Growth Factors in Clinical Practice

Transcutaneous Oxygen ($TcPO_2$) Estimates Probability of Healing in the Ischemic Extremity

Padberg FT Jr, Back TL, Thompson PN, et al (East Orange VA Med Ctr, NJ Univ of Medicine and Dentistry, Newark, New Jersey)

J Surg Res 60:365–369, 1996 9–12

Introduction.—The ability of extremity wounds to heal is related to the severity of arterial ischemia. Assessment of an individual patient's risk would aid in the clinical management of the ischemic extremity. A method of assessment proposed here uses a probability approach based on the laboratory measurement of transcutaneous oxygen tension ($TcPO_2$) in the ischemic lower extremity wound site.

Methods.—Wounds evaluated in the study were 126 amputations and 78 gangrenous ulcerations of the foot or toes. All patients had critically ischemic lower extremities, and 63% of the wound sites had diabetes mellitus as a coexisting condition. The wounds were assessed by $TcPO_2$, arterial segment pressure (ASP), and arterial segment indices (ASI). These 3 techniques were compared for their ability to predict the probability of healing, defined as complete wound closure with epithelialization of the wound surface or a healed suture line.

Results.—A total of 112 wounds healed. Of the 92 failures, 45 required arterial reconstruction and 47 required proximal amputation. The best of the 3 noninvasive examinations for determining the likelihood of healing or failure was $TcPO_2$, which was the only test to meet the $P < 0.05$ entry criteria for selection in stepwise multiple logistic regression. This technique was equally accurate in patients with diabetes mellitus, in those with chronic renal failure, and where neither medical condition was present. Techniques that used pressures or indices did not discriminate between healing and failure in patients with diabetes or chronic renal failure.

Conclusion.—Of the 3 noninvasive tests evaluated here, only $TcPO_2$ was found to be sufficient for objective risk stratification of ischemic extremity wounds. Many patients at risk for failure of wound healing in the extremity have diabetes mellitus or chronic renal sufficiency, and ASP and ASI can yield inaccurate or deceptive findings in such cases.

▶ This simple but well done study suggests that $TcPO_2$ is a reliable method of assessing the probability of healing of an ischemic extremity. The $TcPO_2$ may be more accurate than ASP or ASI. Such information is likely to play an important role in surgical decision.

W.W. Souba, M.D., Sc.D.

Anabolic and Cardiovascular Effects of Recombinant Human Growth Hormone in Surgical Patients With Sepsis

Koea JB, Breier BH, Douglas RG, et al (Auckland Hosp, New Zealand)

Br J Surg 83:196–202, 1996 9–13

Background.—Treatment with (TPN) and (rhGH) may diminish loss of protein and improve the clinical course of patients with protein catabolism. There is no documentation of improved clinical course or outcome in catabolic patients that can be attributed to rhGH. Recombinant human

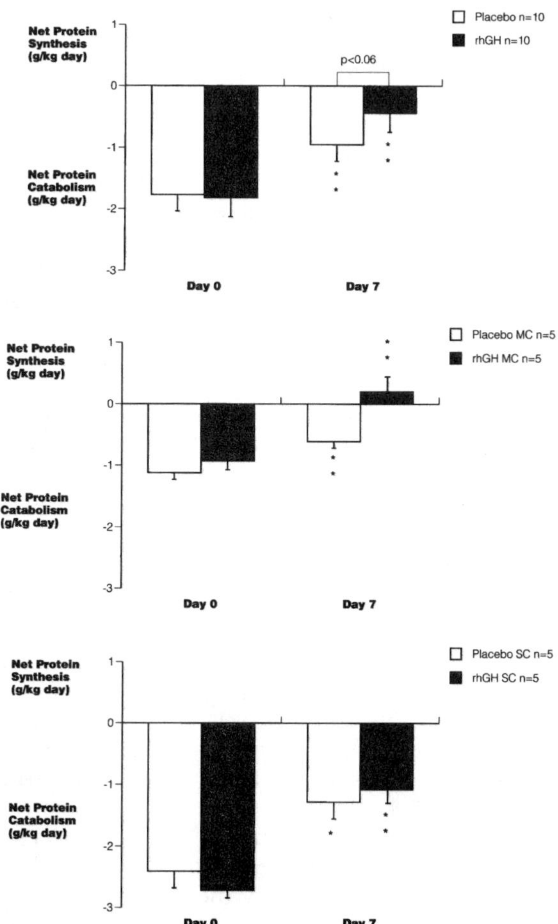

FIGURE 1.—Net protein catabolism at baseline and on day 7 in patients receiving total parenteral nutrition with placebo *open bars* or human growth hormone *solid bars*. **A**, for all patients (n = 10 in each group); **B**, for moderately catabolic patients (n = 5 in each group); **C**, for severely catabolic patients (n = 5 in each group). Values are mean (S.E.M.). $^*P < 0.001$. †$P < 0.01$ versus baseline value (Student's t test. ‡$P < 0.06$ (analysis of variance). (Courtesy of Koea JB, Breier BH, Douglas RG, et al: Anabolic and cardiovascular effects of recombinant human growth hormone in surgical patients with sepsis. *Br J Surg* 83:196–202, 1996.)

growth hormone may have a role in the treatment patients who are severely stressed, catabolic, hemodynamically stable, and in need of strong nutritional support. The metabolic and clinical effects of (rhGH) and TPN in patients with protein catabolism that resulted from severe sepsis were studied.

Methods.—In a randomized, double-blind, placebo-controlled trial, 20 surgical patients received 7 days of TPN and injections of rhGH or placebo. The rate of net protein catabolism was determined.

Results.—In patients with a mean net protein catabolism rate of 1.5 g/kg/day or less at baseline, treatment with rhGH resulted in a decrease in net protein catabolism from 0.93 to −0.20 g/kg/day in 5 patients (Fig 1). Treatment with TPN alone resulted in a decrease from 1.12 to 0.61 g/kg/day in 5 patients. In patients with a mean net protein catabolism rate of more than 1.5 g/kg/day at baseline, treatment with rhGH resulted in a decrease in net protein catabolism from 2.72 to 1.08 g/kg/day in 5 patients. Treatment with TPN alone resulted in a decrease from 2.41 to 1.28 g/kg/day in 5 patients. There were no adverse effects. Clinical course was not improved, but mean systolic and diastolic pressure decreased.

Conclusions.—In these patients, 7 days of treatment with rhGH combined with TPN was safe and well tolerated. Recombinant human growth hormone is a useful anabolic agent and may improve myocardial and cardiovascular function in patients with catabolism and sepsis.

Lack of Effects of Recombinant Growth Hormone on Muscle Function in Patients Requiring Prolonged Mechanical Ventilation: A Prospective, Randomized, Controlled Study

Pichard C, Kyle U, Chevrolet J-C, et al (Univ Hosp, Geneva and Lousanne, Switzerland)

Crit Care Med 24:403–413, 1996 9–14

Introduction.—Approximately 24% of patients receiving mechanical ventilation in ICUs have been found to be protein-calorie malnourished. This malnourished state can result in reductions in maximal muscle strength and relaxation rate and increases in muscle fatigability. Recombinant growth hormone has been shown to reduce amino acid loss and promote positive nitrogen balance in malnourished and stressed patients, with improvement in skeletal muscle function in postoperative patients. The effects of recombinant growth hormone on muscle function in patients undergoing prolonged mechanical ventilation were investigated.

Methods.—Twenty patients receiving mechanical ventilation were randomly assigned to treatment with either recombinant growth hormone, 0.43 IU/kg body weight per day or saline given subcutaneously for 12 days. Patients also received enteral nutrition at a constant rate, with caloric needs determined by indirect calorimetry. Nitrogen balance, energy requirements, and peripheral muscle function (as determined by thumb muscle function) were determined.

Results.—Patients treated with recombinant growth hormone had a significant increase in body cell mass as compared with untreated patients. Recombinant growth hormone resulted in increases in plasma growth hormone, insulin-like growth factor–1, and insulin. Patients receiving recombinant growth hormone also had a positive cumulative nitrogen balance throughout the study period. Both groups of patients had decreases in muscle performance throughout the study, with no significant differences seen between the groups for any parameters assessed. No significant differences in duration of mechanical ventilation were found between the groups; there were no significant differences in blood gases.

Conclusion.—Use of recombinant growth hormone in patients undergoing prolonged mechanical ventilation was not found to improve muscle performance or alter the need for mechanical ventilation. However, improvements were found in nitrogen balance.

▶ In the Koea study, the authors demonstrated that recombinant human growth hormone decreased the rate of net protein catabolism in septic surgical patients. However, significant improvements in physiologic function or clinical outcome were not observed. Treatment with growth hormone was shown to decrease the mean systolic and diastolic blood pressures, suggesting that growth hormone may improve myocardial and cardiovascular function in some septic patients. The Pichard study noted an improvement in nitrogen balance in critically ill patients receiving mechanical ventilation, but this was not accompanied by improvements in muscle strength or a shorter duration of ventilatory support. These studies are similar to other studies showing that administration of recombinant human growth hormone as an adjunct to nutritional support enhances intestinal amino acid uptake[1] and nitrogen retention,[2-4] but whether these biochemical changes are associated with an improvement in outcome is not well established.

W.W. Souba, M.D., Sc.D.

References

1. Inoue Y, Copeland EM, Souba WW: Growth hormone enhances amino acid transport by the human small intestine. *Ann Surg*, 219:715–724, 1994.
2. Ziegler TR, Lazarus JM, Young LS, et al: Effects of recombinant human growth hormone in adults receiving maintenance hemodialysis. *J Am Soc Nephrol* 2:1130–1135, 1991.
3. Suchner U, Rothkop, MM, Stanislaus G, et al: Growth hormone and pulmonary disease: Metabolic effects in patients receiving parenteral nutrition. *Arch Intern Med*,150:1225–1230, 1990.
4. Ziegler TR, Rombeau J, Young LS, et al: Administration of recombinant human growth hormone enhances the metabolic efficacy of parenteral nutrition: A double blinded, randomized, controlled study. *J Clin Endocrinol Metab*, 74:865–873, 1992.

Advanced Age Alone Does Not Suppress Anastomotic Healing in the Intestine

Stoop M-J, Dirksen R, Hendriks T (Univ Hosp Nijmegen, The Netherlands)
Surgery 119:15–19, 1996 9–15

Introduction.—Leakage of anastomoses in the intestine is associated with high morbidity and mortality. Surgeons may forgo construction of anastomoses if certain complicating factors are present. It is generally believed that advanced age significantly increases the risk of dehiscence in anastomotic repair. There is conflicting evidence on the association between age and anastomotic leakage. There are no reports of intestinal healing in animals. The effect of age on anastomotic healing in rats was studied.

Methods.—Two groups of healthy rats were used. The age of rats was 2 to 3 months in one group and 27 to 30 months in the other. Each group contained 31 rats. Ileal and colonic anastomoses were constructed, and healing was evaluated at 3 and 7 days. Anastomotic strength, anastomotic hydroxyproline, and collagen synthetic capacity in anastomotic explants were determined. Morphometry was also performed.

Results.—Anastomotic strength was similar in young and old rats. For bursting pressure (Fig 1) and breaking strength, anastomotic strength increased from day 3 to day 7 and was never lower in older rats. In older animals, collagen production capacity was suppressed, especially in the ileum, but synthesis of noncollagenous protein was unchanged. This did not result in decreased accumulation of collagen around the anastomoses. There was no change in anastomotic hydroxyproline content or volume percentage of collagen around the wound. There were no premature deaths.

Conclusions.—Anastomotic healing in the intestine is not suppressed by advanced age alone. Illness or disease must be considered in any study on the direct correlation between age and healing in surgical patients. Further research is needed to determine if certain conditions affect healing differently in young and old patients.

▶ This study in rats suggests that advanced age per se does not adversely impact the strength or deposition of collagen in the early repair of an intestinal anastomosis. The authors suggest that, in the absence of detrimental factors, anastamotic repair will essentially be unimpaired in older patients. In these studies, the animals were well nourished; it would be of interest to examine anastomotic healing in young and old rats that were nutritionally depleted.

W.W. Souba, M.D., Sc.D.

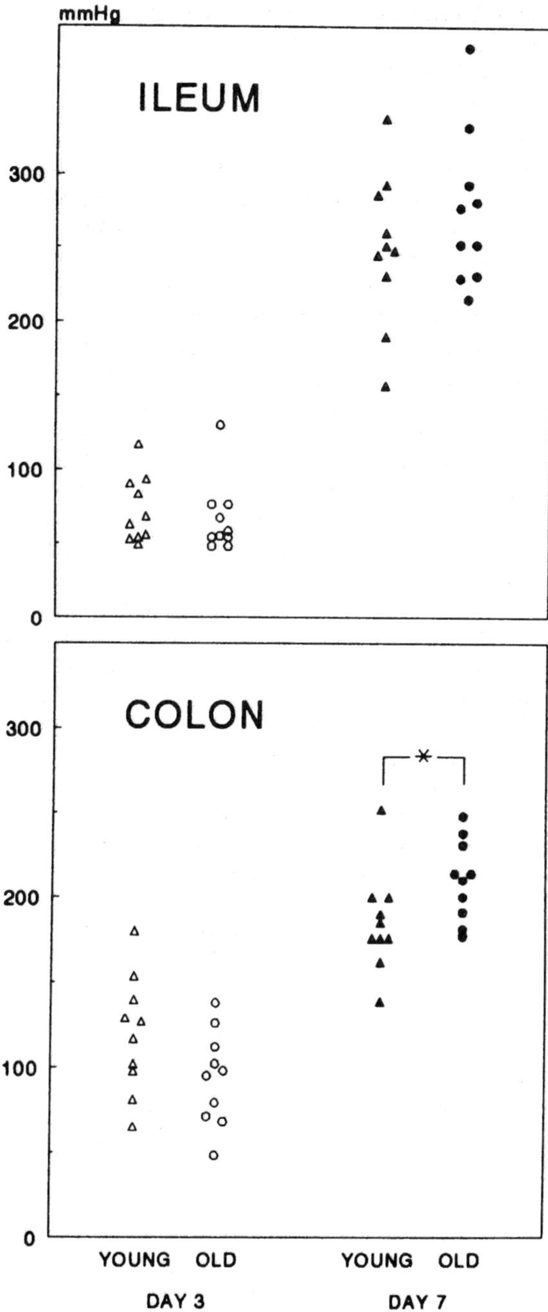

FIGURE 1.—Anastomotic bursting pressures in individual rats. *Triangles*, young animals; *circles*, old animals; *open symbols*, bursting sites within the anastomotic area; *filled symbols*, bursting sites outside the anastomotic area. *$P < 0.05$ (Wilcoxon). (Courtesy of Stoop M-J, Dirksen R, Hendriks T: Advanced age alone does not suppress anastomotic healing in the intestine. *Surgery* 119: 15–19, 1996.)

The Tension-Free Hernioplasty in a Randomized Trial

Friis E, Lindahl F (Univ of Copenhagen)

Am J Surg 172:315–319, 1996 9–16

Introduction.—Since its first use, many variations of the Bassini operation for hernia repair have been proposed. However, one persistent problem has been the creation of a solid repair of the abdominal wall without the creation of tension on the surrounding tissue. A tension-free hernioplasty that uses an implanted prosthetic mesh was evaluated.

Methods.—Patients requiring hernioplasty were randomly assigned to surgery with one of two approaches: the tension-free approach with implantation of a prolene mesh vs. the Cooper ligament repair in direct hernias or the abdominal ring repair in indirect hernias. The two surgical groups were compared for recurrence rates, postoperative complications, and time off from work. The effect of the surgeon's experience on the recurrence rate was also evaluated.

Results.—One hundred two tension-free hernioplasties, 53 Cooper ligament repairs, and 53 abdominal repairs were performed. The overall recurrence rate was 10%, with significantly fewer recurrences with the tension-free technique. For 171 primary hernia repairs, the overall recurrence rate was 10%; with 3 (3.6%) recurring with the tension-free technique and 14 (16%) recurring with the Cooper repair (Table 2). The differences in recurrence rates for secondary hernias were not significant. For all herniotomies, complication rates were similar. Time off from work after surgery did not differ significantly between the groups. There was no effect of the surgeon's experience on recurrence rates.

Conclusion.—The tension-free hernioplasty was associated with a lower rate of recurrence as compared with a traditional herniotomy. No additional complications were found with the tension-free approach, nor was there more time lost from work by patients.

► I thought the recurrence rate for the hernias repaired by the Cooper ligament method was very high. Nonetheless, there is no question that wound tension is a risk factor for healing problems.

W.W. Souba, M.D., Sc.D.

TABLE 2.—Primary Hernias: Recurrence Rate

Type of Hernia	Operation	n	Recurrences (%)	Chi-Square
Indirect	Tension-free	38	0 (0)	$P = 1.0$
	Annulorrhaphia	46	1 (2.2)	
Direct, femoral and combined	Tension-free	44	3 (6.8)	$P = 0.0081$
	McVay repair	43	13 (30.2)	
Total		171	17 (9.9)	

(Reprinted by permission of the publisher from Friis E, Lindahl F: The tension-free hernioplasty in a randomized trial. *Am J Surg* 172:315–319, Copyright 1996 by Excerpta Medica Inc.)

Computer-assisted Documentation and Analysis of Wound Healing of the Nasal and Oesophageal Mucosa

Weber R, Keerl R, Jaspersen D, et al (Univ of Marburg, Fulda, Germany)
J Laryngol Otol 110:1017–1021, 1996 9–17

Purpose.—It can be difficult to analyze physiologic and pathologic processes that change over time. Continuous measurements done over a period of days or weeks are often impractical. Endoscopy is an established technique for assessing the nasal and esophageal mucosa. Computer-assisted "morphing" of endoscopic images obtained over time was used to analyze the dynamics of mucosal healing.

Methods.—The morphing software can smoothly and continuously transform one image into a chronologically discrete image, thus showing the natural dynamics of a process over time. This technology was used to illustrate changes in the nasal and esophageal mucosa during wound healing. Twelve patients were studied for 6 months after endonasal sinus surgery, with periodic videoendoscope images "morphed" into continuous computer animations. The healing process of esophagitis with omeprazole treatment was tracked over 3 weeks.

Findings.—The images showed 4 overlapping and meshing phases of wound healing after sinus surgery. The duration of each phase varied between patients. Blood crusts covered the wound for a week or two, then were replaced by granulation. There was increasing edema from 3 to 5 weeks, which then decreased from 7 to 12 weeks. The mucosa was macroscopically normal in most cases by 12 to 18 weeks. Long-term packing prevented the formation of blood crusts; topical budesonide therapy reduced the length of each phase of wound healing. The esophageal mucosa healed symmetrically, from the wound edges to the center, at a constant velocity. Healing was complete within 20 days.

Discussion.—Computer-assisted "morphing" of endoscopic images permits dynamic analysis of mucosal healing. This technique can be applied only with the use of a valid imaging technique that generates congruent images. The process being studied must follow a steady course, without sudden leaps, and the individual measurement procedures must be appropriately timed. The morphing technique provides some valuable insights into the course of mucosal healing.

▶ I thought this was a nifty technique that is likely to have applicability to the assessment of healing of wounds that are otherwise difficult to visualize.

W.W. Souba, M.D., Sc.D.

10 Gastrointestinal

Introduction

The period 1996–1997 has been an innovative year for clinical and basic science contributions to gastrointestinal surgery. With the hundreds of published manuscripts reviewed for the 1997 YEAR BOOK OF SURGERY, the editors have sought to include signal contributions by various clinics and universities throughout the world. Understandably, not every clinical or basic research manuscript can be included in the 1997 edition of the YEAR BOOK. Rather, the editors continue to select contributions that have major impact on the daily management of benign and malignant diseases of the gastrointestinal tract. This editor has also sought to review contributions that have an impact on technical, anatomical, and pathophysiologic issues, whereas other articles represent basic science contributions that will have sustained impact for the future practice of surgery. Other selections include clinical trials for benign or malignant diseases of the gastrointestinal tract that may influence practice patterns and the outcome of surgery.

Kirby I. Bland, M.D.

Esophagus and Stomach

INTRODUCTION

The first successful therapy for disorders of the esophagus was the management of achalasia, credited to Thomas Willis in 1674. Ordinary esophageal bougienage was used to forcibly treat physiologic obstruction of the organ. Although treatments for diseases of the esophagus and stomach were undoubtedly attempted in the 250-year interim, Browne and McHardy in 1939 gained international acclaim by successfully treating achalasia by disruption of the lower esophageal sphincter with pneumatic dilatation. The successful application of hydrostatic dilators by Olsen and Harrington, in 1951, improved the results and allowed better selection of patients. However, we must give credit to Heller, who in 1913 revised the physiologic concepts of esophagomyotomy for the treatment of achalasia. Zaaijer modified this approach in 1923 to a single esophageal incision. Recently, Ellis and colleagues developed the transthoracic esophagomyotomy for the treatment of this benign disorder.

The modern era of surgical therapy for esophageal and gastric diseases began in the mid to late 1940s with the application of pathophysiologic concepts to applied research; this pioneering effort to apply physiologic principles to therapy was led by the late Lester R. Dragstedt of the University of Chicago. Several of his surgical students, including the late Edward R. Woodward, applied these approaches in the management of benign (fistula, ulceration, obstruction, hemorrhage, achalasia) and malignant disorders. Although the pathophysiology of gastroesophageal reflux is multifactorial, the basic tenet of surgical therapy is focused principally on enhancing the function (strength) of the lower esophageal sphincter.

New studies have examined other principal factors that influence the outcome of gastroesophageal reflux surgery. Concerns regarding the open or laparoscopic antireflux approaches have included the subsequent (and frequent) appearance of troublesome postoperative dysphagia. Since the first report in 1991 of the laparoscopic Nissen fundoplication, there has been a surge in popularity of this technique as the principal reatment for gastroesophageal reflux disorders. Unequivocally, postoperative side effects occur with both the open and laparoscopic Nissen fundoplication approaches. From the accumulated data of the past 5 years, persistent troublesome solid food dysphagia is more common after the laparoscopic Nissen fundoplication approach (range, 4% to 24%) than is evident after the open "floppy" Nissen technique (<3%). The typical Rosetti-Nissen laparoscopic fundoplication more commonly creates dysphagia than its antecedent laparoscopic technique (Toupet), Nissen fundoplication with greater curvature mobilization. As a consequence, the Toupet fundoplication has been typically adopted by the majority of international surgeons who use laparoscopic approaches. Abstracts 10–1 and 10–2 each address the minimally invasive surgical approach to gastroesophageal reflux and outcomes regarding early and persistent dysphagia. Hunter and associates (Abstract 10–1) of the Emory University departments of surgery and gastroenterology, Atlanta, Georgia, and the Department of Surgery, Oregon Health Sciences University, Portland, Oregon, found that laparoscopic Rosetti-Nissen fundoplication resulted in a higher rate of early (and persistent) dysphagia in the postoperative period than either the Nissen or Toupet fundoplication approaches. Patti and associates (Abstract 10–2) of the University of California–San Francisco evaluate preoperative gastroesophageal reflux disease with the objective of tailoring the operation to the preoperative findings. These authors conclude that minimally invasive surgery for this benign disorder has good to excellent outcomes, even for patients in whom abnormal esophageal body manometric dysfunction is evident. These outcomes reflect adherence to the tenet that the operation is tailored to the individual patient based on the results of these preoperative tests. In no patients having the Nissen or Guarner technique did postoperative persistent dysphagia or the "gas-bloat" syndrome develop. In contradistinction, the Rosetti fundoplication caused dysphagia or "gas-bloat" in 27% of the operated patients. The UCSF series has therefore prompted a switch to the Nissen or the Guarner fundoplication incorporating takedown of the short gastric vessels. Moreover, careful preoperative evaluation to characterize gastroesophageal reflux in the individual patient is an important recommendation of this paper.

These surgical techniques may result in pneumothorax in some patients during laparoscopy—particularly during laparoscopic fundoplication. The development of this complication in the left parietal pleura as a result of dissection is emphasized by Joris et al. (Abstract 10–3) of the Department of Anesthesiology and Intensive Care Medicine, University Hospital of Liège, Belgium. Although pneumothorax is most commonly observed during laparoscopic fundoplication, it also occurs spontaneously during any laparoscopic approach that requires dissection of the peritoneopleural ducts, which exist as embryonic remnants. These authors conclude that this is a common event in laparoscopic fundoplication and that early diagnosis is essential, and possible, by simultaneously monitoring the end-tidal CO_2, total lung-thoracic compliance, as well as airway pressures. Moreover, the authors emphasize that not all patients require therapy with chest tube placement; treatment with positive end-expiratory pressure provides an alternative when pneumothorax occurs from the passage of peritoneal CO_2 into the interpleural space. An additional complication of laparoscopic Nissen fundoplication is gastric and esophageal perforations. Schauer and associates (Abstract 10–4) of the departments of surgery at Duke University Medical Center, Durham, North Carolina, and University of Texas Health Science Center at San Antonio, Texas, identified 3 mechanisms of perforation in 17 gastric and laparoscopic Nissen procedures: improper retroesophageal dissection, passage of the bougie dilator or the nasogastric tube, or surgery secondary to suture pullthrough. Further, these serious and potentially lethal complications are specific to the laparoscopic technique, and prevention requires a comprehensive understanding of detailed anatomy and the application of physiologic principles to the gastroesophageal region at the time of the procedure.

Replacement of normal squamous epithelium of the distal portion of the esophagus with metaplastic columnar epithelium continuous with the gastric mucosa was described independently by Barrett and Lortat-Jacob in 1957. Retention of the term "Barrett's esophagus," which is specific for the anatomical transformation of squamous to metaplastic columnar epithelium, recognizes the importance of the link between adenocarcinoma and ectopic gastric mucosa, an association identified in 1952 before Barrett's classic description. Mameeteman and associates estimate the incidence of adenocarcinoma in the esophagus to be 1 in 52 patient-years—a 125-fold enhancement in the risk of carcinoma when compared with the general population. Ortiz and associates (Abstract 10–5) of the University Hospital V, Arrixaca, El Palmar, Spain, evaluated a long-term prospective study to compare the results of conservative treatment and antireflux surgery in the treatment of patients with Barrett's esophagus. In this prospectively randomized study of significant duration (range, 1–11 years; median follow-up, 4 years), severe dysplasia was detected with equal frequency in the medical treatment vs. the surgical therapy groups. Patients in whom antireflux surgery proved effective showed no dysplastic changes or progression to adenocarcinoma. The authors therefore question the systematic conservative approach to the initial management of patients with Barrett's esophagus. However, performance of these antireflux operations would not obviate the requirement for lifelong endoscopic surveillance of patients who have had Barrett's esophagus—this follow-up modality is essential despite the evidence that surgical antireflux procedures appear to be superior to conservative medical therapy.

Carcinoma of the esophagus represents 1% to 2% of all cancers in the United States and accounts for approximately 99% of all esophageal neoplasms. Although squamous carcinoma has been considered the most common variant of esophageal neoplasms, the frequency of adenocarcinoma arising in Barrett's mucosa continues to increase and may now surpass that of squamous carcinoma. The primary modality for the treatment of localized esophageal carcinoma continues to be resection. Alternatives to resection have included radiation and/or chemotherapy, whereas locally advanced esophageal carcinoma is most commonly approached with preoperative neoadjuvant chemoradiation followed by potentially curative resection methods. Stahl and associates (Abstract 10–6) of Essen University Medical School, Technical University Munchen, and St. Johannes Hospital, all in Germany, describe an intensive program with preoperative chemoradiation to evaluate curative resection rates, pathologic response, and survival of patients with locally advanced carcinoma of the esophagus. This noteworthy interim analysis of a phase II trial demonstrates the high efficacy rates of preoperative chemoradiation for locally advanced esophageal carcinoma.

The importance of benign gastric disorders in our society is evident, although the frequency of gastroduodenal ulceration continues to diminish in industrialized societies. Notwithstanding, infantile hypertrophic pyloric stenosis continues to occur in 3 of every 1,000 live births and is a common etiology of emesis in infants. Theories regarding the pathogenesis of this disorder include abnormalities of hormonal influence on the gastric pylorus, reduction in nitric oxide, axonal degeneration in the myenteric plexus, and loss of peptide-containing nerve filaments in nerve fibers. The signal paper by Yamataka and associates (Abstract 10–7) of the departments of pediatric surgery at Dokkyo University, Tochigi, Japan, and Juntendo University School of Medicine, Tokyo, emphasizes the important role that the proto-oncogene c-*kit* plays in the development of a component of the pacemaker system required for the generation of autonomic gut motility. Moreover, the c-*kit* gene protein product (C-KIT)-positive cells in the mammalian gut appear to be responsible for intestinal pacemaker activity. These authors suggest that absence of C-KIT expression in the hypertrophic pyloric smooth musculature appears to be an important etiologic factor in the pathogenesis of infantile hypertrophic pyloric stenosis. These important molecular pathologic data are deserving of further study but do not appear to indicate that the effect of pyloric stenosis occurs as a consequence of the absence of this molecular biological expression. However, the importance of the application of molecular biology to outcomes in translational research will have an increasing effect on progress in clinical medicine.

Reproducible fetal models to study anatomical, pathophysiologic, and cellular events are investigated by Diez-Pardo and associates (Abstract

10–8) in the Department of Pediatric Surgery, Hospital La Paz, Universidad Autonoma, Madrid, and the Department of Pathology, Hospital do Meixoeiro, Vigo, Spain. These authors describe a reproducible fetal model to evaluate esophageal atresia and tracheoesophageal fistula (TEF) in a rodent model. This new rodent model has great potential for clarification of the pathophysiologic mechanism of tracheoesophageal cleavage and its progression to interruption of the upper digestive tract with fistulization to the trachea. This experimental construct may also provide better clarification of the structural abnormalities and anomalies of nerve plexuses, muscles, and mucosa that permanently impair function of the esophagus in human TEF survivors.

With the original introduction of vagotomy as definitive therapy for duodenal ulcers by Dragstedt in 1945, antrectomy with truncal or selective vagotomy emerged as the superior therapeutic approaches because of the low recurrence rates (2% to 5%). Alternatives to gastric resection have included conservation approaches with antral retention and duodenal preservation to lessen postgastrectomy syndromes. Parietal cell vagotomy and proximal gastric vagotomy continue to have a low frequency of operative mortality and morbidity and are associated with the fewest intestinal sequelae postvagotomy. Nonetheless, these procedures are technically demanding, time-consuming, and exacting to obtain proper results for diminution of ulcer recurrence. Brullet and associates (Abstract 10–9) of the Endoscopy Unit at Consorci Hospitalari Parc Taulí, Sabadell, Spain, assessed factors that are thought to cause failure of endoscopic injection for bleeding in patients with duodenal ulcers. The authors evaluated 120 patients with active bleeding duodenal ulcers and confirmed arterial hemorrhage or a visible nonbleeding vessel. Technical measures precluded endoscopic injection in 11.6% of the patients because of inaccessible massive hemorrhage. Thus the remaining 106 patients underwent therapy by injection of adrenaline and polidocanol, and endoscopic therapy was successful in achieving bleeding control in 83% (88/106). This important analysis confirmed that failure of injection was related to age, the presence of shock, ulcer size (>2 cm), and the hemoglobin level. Extension of this analysis to multivariate technique confirmed that ulcer size greater than 2 cm and the presence of shock were the principal factors that predicted endoscopic treatment failures. Moreover, poor physiologic status (measured by the American Society of Anesthesiology classification) and failure to achieve hemostasis were significantly related to mortality. Thus Brullet et al. conclude that the severity of hemorrhage and ulcer size are predictive of endoscopic injection failures in patients with actively bleeding, high-risk duodenal ulcers. Long-term results and cost-effective outcome data are essential to confirm the validity of all these reports.

Kirby I. Bland, M.D.

Dysphagia After Laparoscopic Antireflux Surgery: The Impact of Operative Technique

Hunter JG, Swanstrom L, Waring JP (Emory Univ, Atlanta, Ga; Oregon Health Sciences Univ, Portland)

Ann Surg 224:51–57, 1996 10–1

Introduction.—Recent studies suggest that persistent solid food dysphagia occurs more often after Nissen fundoplication than after open "floppy" fundoplication, and after laparoscopic Rosetti-Nissen fundoplication compared with laparoscopic Nissen fundoplication. A prospective study compared the results of 3 laparoscopic operations for gastroesophageal reflux disease, all performed at a single institution.

Methods.—Between October 1991 and November 1995, 184 patients underwent surgery for medically refractory gastroesophageal disease. Toupet fundoplication was done in 83 cases, Nissen fundoplication in 46, and Rosetti-Nissen fundoplication in 55. The choice of procedure was based on the anatomy of the gastroesophageal junction. Excluded from operation during the study period were patients with extremely poor esophageal motility.

Postoperative care was similar in all cases. Patients were seen for follow-up at 4 weeks and at 3 months after operation; those with postoperative difficulties were seen more frequently. Endoscopy and esophageal dilatation was offered those reporting severe dysphagia at the first postoperative visit or moderate to severe dysphagia at the second visit.

Results.—The incidence of new-onset food dysphagia in the first month after surgery was 54% in the Rosetti-Nissen group, 16% in the Toupet group, and 16% in the Nissen group. At 3 months, dysphagia persisted in 11% of patients in the Rosetti-Nissen group, 2% in the Toupet group, and 2% in the Nissen group. Dysphagia improved in all 6 patients who underwent dilatation, but 4 (all in the Rosetti-Nissen group) have residual dysphagia to meats and bread. Patients undergoing Nissen fundoplication experienced no additional morbidity related to division of short gastric vessels.

Discussion.—Patients treated with laparoscopic Rosetti-Nissen fundoplication have significantly higher rates of early and persistent postoperative dysphagia than those undergoing laparoscopic Nissen or Toupet procedures. Of the latter 2 techniques, Toupet fundoplication takes 15 to 30 minutes longer to perform and may provide less durable protection from reflux. Postoperative dysphagia may be minimized by mobilizing the fundus of the stomach and performing a short (1–2 cm) fundoplication over a large dilator (5F–60F).

Minimally Invasive Surgery for Gastroesophageal Reflux Disease
Patti MG, Arcerito M, Pellegrini CA, et al (Univ of California, San Francisco)
Am J Surg 170:614–618, 1995 10–2

Objective.—To determine whether surgical outcome can be improved, a group of 68 patients who underwent laparoscopic fundoplication for gastroesophageal reflux disease (GERD) was assessed. The pathophysiology of the disease in each patient was characterized, the operative technique was tailored to the results of preoperative esophageal function tests.

Methods.—The patients were 40 men and 28 women with a mean age of 50 years. All had GERD that was refractory to medical treatment. The average duration of symptoms was 158 months; the most frequently reported symptom was heartburn, followed by chest pain and regurgitation. Preoperative evaluation showed a hiatal hernia in 62% of patients and a distal esophageal stricture in 13%. Grade III or IV esophagitis was present in 47%, and 63% had an incompetent lower esophageal sphincter (LES). Patients were divided into 3 groups on the basis of amplitude, duration, velocity, and morphology of peristaltic contractions. Thus, 26 (38%) had normal peristalsis, 31 (46%) had mild impairment of peristalsis, and 11 (16%) had severe impairment.

Results.—Twenty-two patients had a Rosetti fundoplication, 35 had a Nissen fundoplication, and 11 with severe impairment of peristalsis had a Guarner fundoplication. No patient who had Nissen or Guarner procedures experienced postoperative persistent dysphagia or gas bloat, but these symptoms developed postoperatively in 27% of those who had a Rosetti fundoplication. With a mean follow-up of 12 months, 91% of patients in the Nissen group and 82% of patients in the Guarner group are asymptomatic. The 3 procedures were similar in average operating time and in postoperative improvement in LES pressure and total and abdominal length of the LES.

Discussion.—By tailoring laparoscopic fundoplication to the individual patient on the basis of preoperative esophageal function tests, minimally invasive surgery for GERD can yield good to excellent results. And with individualized planning and adherence to technical principles, dysfunction of the esophageal body or stomach is not a contraindication for surgery. Use of the Nissen or Guarner methods rather than a Rosetti fundoplication prevents the development of postoperative dysphagia and gas bloat.

▶ Patti and associates are to be commended for utilization of a careful preoperative workup to characterize gastroesophageal reflux disease for individual patients. These results occurred with tailoring of the operative approach to the results of the preoperative functional tests. The authors emphasize that the Rosetti fundoplication had significant postoperative sequelae inasmuch as "gasbloat" syndrome and dysphagia developed in 27% of the patients. Although the majority are asymptomatic (91%), an additional fundoplication using the Guarner technique was necessary to achieve relief of symptoms in 82% of these patients. Moreover, in none of the patients in whom the Nissen or Guarner technique was applied did postoperative persistent dysphagia or "gas-bloat" symptoms develop. Despite the presence of abnormal esophageal body function by manometric techniques, minimally invasive approaches for gastroesophageal reflux disease provide good to excellent results in the majority of these patients. This important paper emphasizes that the operation can best be tailored to the individual patient based on the results of preoperative function tests and that these approaches should be emphasized in the preoperative discussion of techniques with the patient to predict outcomes.

K.I. Bland, M.D.

Pneumothorax During Laparoscopic Fundoplication: Diagnosis and Treatment With Positive End-expiratory Pressure

Joris JL, Chiche J-D, Lamy ML (Univ Hosp of Liège, Belgium)

Anesth Analg 81:993–1000, 1995 10–3

Introduction.—Pneumothorax may occur during laparoscopy, particularly during laparoscopic fundoplication because the left parietal pleura is exposed and may be torn during dissection in the diaphragmatic hiatus. Tears may allow passage of intra-abdominal CO_2 under pressure into the pleural cavity and can cause pneumothorax. Pathophysiologic changes may include mild to moderate reduction in oxygen saturation (SpO_2), increases in airway pressures, and observation by laparoscope of abnormal motion of the hemidiaphragm. When this happens, the pneumothorax usually disappears within 1 hour after surgery. Patients undergoing laparoscopic fundoplication were extensively monitored to document pathophysiologic changes caused by pneumothorax, and the benefit of intraoperative positive end-expiratory pressure (PEEP) in the treatment of pneumothorax was evaluated.

Methods.—Patients undergoing laparoscopic fundoplication were extensively monitored intraoperatively for heart rate, mean arterial pressure, end-tidal CO_2 ($PETCO_2$), SpO_2, minute ventilation, tidal volume, dynamic total lung thorax compliance, and airway pressures. Oxygen uptake, CO_2 elimination, and arterial blood gases were also measured in 25 patients.

Results.—Seven of 46 patients (15.2%) experienced pneumothorax. Pathophysiologic changes included decrease in total lung thorax compliance, increase in airway pressures, and increase in CO_2 absorption. The $PaCO_2$ and $PETCO_2$ also increased, but SpO_2 remained normal. Drainage was not needed for any of the pneumothoraces. All pneumothoraces were diagnosed by auscultation of decreased breath sounds over the entire left lung. The intensity of breath sounds was decreased compared with the contralateral side and compared to breath sounds heard over the left lung 10 minutes after beginning of pneumoperitoneum. These changes were corrected using PEEP.

Conclusion.—Pneumothorax occurred in 15.2% of patients undergoing laparoscopic fundoplication. Early diagnosis can be made with simultaneous monitoring of P_{ETCO_2}, total lung thorax compliance, and airway pressures. Treatment with PEEP can be an alternative to chest tube placement when pneumothorax is secondary to passage of peritoneal CO_2 into the interpleural space. The high incidence of pneumothorax in this report compared with others is probably best explained by the fact that pneumothorax may be underdiagnosed. In this series, the condition of 6 or 7 patients would not have been diagnosed without close monitoring. Positive end-expiratory pressure was used to decrease the pressure gradient between the abdominal and pleural cavities during both inspiration and expiration to subsequently inflate the lung. When the gradient pressure is reduced or reversed, CO_2 should leave the pleural space. This noninvasive treatment approach was effective in treating pneumothorax and its pathophysiologic consequences and prevented the need for thoracentesis.

▶ Joris and colleagues present an important discussion of a common intraoperative complication during laparascopic Nissen fundoplication, capnothorax. Much of the controversy and confusion in the management of this problem results from the nomenclature that has been used, namely "pneumothorax." The use of this term implies the need for a chest tube. As pointed out by the authors by the term CO_2 pneumothorax, the chest cavity is filled with CO_2 that has entered the chest through a hole in the left parietal pleura. Once insufflation of CO_2 stops, the CO_2 present will be rapidly absorbed, usually within 1 hour.

Not stressed by the authors is the means to prevent this complication. It usually results from dissection high in the hiatus during mobilization. To avoid the injury, the surgeon should work low in the hiatus after complete visualization of the left leg of the right crus. The authors note that most if not all patients respond to intraoperative PEEP without the need for chest tube. In addition, the intra-abdominal insufflation pressure should be reduced if possible.

Finally, this complication generally has no postoperative sequelae. However, pleuritis can result and resolves following treatment with nonsteroidal anti-inflammatory drugs.

J.F. Amaral, M.D.

Mechanisms of Gastric and Esophageal Perforations During Laparoscopic Nissen Fundoplication

Schauer PR, Meyers WC, Eubanks S, et al (Duke Univ, Durham, NC; Univ of Texas, San Antonio)

Ann Surg 223:43–52, 1996 10–4

Background.—Gastroesophageal reflux disease occurs in 10% to 40% of the population in the United States. Laparoscopic Nissen fundoplication can effectively treat severe gastroesophageal reflux disease and provides advantages similar to those of laparoscopic cholecystectomy. Gastric or esophageal perforation is associated with high morbidity and mortality and is a serious complication of open antireflux procedures. The mechanisms of gastric and esophageal perforation during laparoscopic Nissen fundoplication were determined to develop effective prevention methods.

Methods.—Details of 17 cases of gastric or esophageal perforation during or after laparoscopic Nissen fundoplication were obtained. The information related to mechanism of injury, diagnosis of injury, contributing factors, surgeon's experience, treatment, and short-term outcome.

Results.—Three mechanisms of injury accounted for all 17 perforations. The majority of these perforations occurred during the first 10 laparoscopic Nissen fundoplication procedures performed by the surgeon. Ten perforations occurred after injuries related to improper retroesophageal dissection, 5 occurred during passage of the bougie dilator, and 2 occurred postoperatively secondary to suture pull-through. A delayed diagnosis negatively affected outcome in 6 patients. The majority of perforations were successfully treated by primary closure and wrap to include the repair. When perforations were recognized late, morbidity was substantially higher. One death resulting from sepsis was associated with delayed diagnosis.

Conclusions.—Gastric or esophageal perforation during laparoscopic Nissen fundoplication chiefly occurs during retroesophageal dissection or incorrect passage of the bougie. Perforation is generally preventable. Knowledge of the detailed anatomy of the gastroesophageal region and awareness of specific mechanisms of injury are important. Early diagnosis is also important; unusual postoperative pain may indicate a perforation.

▶ Schauer and colleagues discuss an important problem that has arisen from laparoscopic Nissen fundoplication, namely, esophagogastric perforation. They identify 3 factors, all technical, responsible for these injuries: improper dissection, bougie passage, and suture pull-through. Although the first 2 are indisputable causes, the last factor is debatable. My experience with these injuries suggests that delayed postoperative perforations result from unrecognized gastric trauma from the babcock and graspers used during the operation to place the stomach on traction. The use of these instruments can result in a thinned area of stomach, which may blow out if there is any postoperative gastric ileus. Although suture pull-through can certainly account for the injuries, this seems rather unlikely to occur if there is no tension on the wrap when the sutures are placed and, furthermore, they would result in only a tiny perforation. On this basis, my preference is to always inspect the areas where the stomach has been grasped and to reinforce with Lembert sutures when there is any question. Furthermore, we limit grasping the stomach during the procedure because adequate tension can often be achieved without grasping the stomach, even to take down short gastric blood vessels.

J.F. Amaral, M.D.

Conservative Treatment Versus Antireflux Surgery in Barrett's Oesophagus: Long-term Results of a Prospective Study

Ortiz A, Martinez de Haro LF, Parrilla P, et al (Univ Hosp V, Arrixaca, El Palmar, Murcia, Spain)

Br J Surg 83:274–278, 1996 10–5

Background.—Authorities disagree on the best treatment for Barrett's esophagus. Most authors report treating it as they do gastroesophageal reflux disease, starting with conservative treatment and reserving antireflux surgery for patients in whom symptoms are not controlled. The long-term outcomes of conservative treatment and antireflux surgery in patients who had Barrett's esophagus were compared.

Methods.—Fifty-nine patients who had Barrett's esophagus were randomly assigned to receive medical therapy or antireflux surgery. The status of 27 patients who were treated medically was followed for a median of 4 years, and the status of 32 who were treated surgically was followed for 5 years.

Findings.—Symptomatic control was excellent or good in 24 medically treated and 29 surgically treated patients. Fifty-four percent of patients had persistent inflammatory lesions, and 47% had recurrent stenosis after medical treatment, compared with 5% and 15%, respectively, after surgery. These differences were significant. Eight patients who underwent antireflux surgery and only 2 who underwent medical therapy had a reduction in the length of the segment of columnar mucosa. The medically treated group more frequently had an upward progression of the columnar lining. Five patients, all of whom were treated medically, had mild dysplasia. Two patients had severe dysplasia (1 in each group), both of whom underwent esophageal resection with verification of a carcinoma in situ. No dysplastic changes or progression to adenocarcinoma was observed in patients who responded well to antireflux surgery.

Conclusions.—Conservative and surgical therapy appear to be equally effective in controlling the symptoms of Barrett's esophagus. Antireflux surgery should be offered especially to young patients, who would otherwise need a lifetime of medication and in whom surgery is more effective.

▶ The treatment for Barrett's esophagus, a premalignant condition that carries an approximate 40% increase in the incidence of adenocarcinoma, remains controversial. The role of antireflux surgery in preventing the progression of Barrett's metaplasia to dysplasia is unknown. This article represents one of the few prospective studies in which patients have been randomized to receive conservative medical therapy vs. early surgical antireflux intervention. Of note, the median follow-up was approximately 5 years and ranged from 1 to 11 years. Although the numbers were small, progression to dysplasia was documented in 6 of the conservatively treated patients and in only 1 surgically treated patient. Notably, this patient had a failed antireflux procedure. Whether this decrease in progression to dysplasia is durable remains to be proved. Long-term control of reflux symptoms in combination with a decreased risk of cancer would make surgical antireflux procedures superior to conservative medical therapy. One note of caution: In the report from the Mayo Clinic of 112 survivors of antireflux procedures among patients with Barrett's esophagus, 3 patients subsequently had adenocarcinoma of the esophagus at 13, 25, and 39 months after surgery. The performance of an antireflux procedure would therefore not obviate the requirement for life-long endoscopic surveillance.

W.G. Cioffi, M.D.

Combined Preoperative Chemotherapy and Radiotherapy in Patients With Locally Advanced Esophageal Cancer: Interim Analysis of a Phase II Trial

Stahl M, Wilke H, Fink U, et al (Essen Univ, Germany; Technical Univ München: St Johannes-Hosp, Germany; et al)

J Clin Oncol 14:829–837, 1996 10–6

Background.—Esophageal cancer (EC) continues to be fatal in a high proportion of patients. Recently, improved surgical techniques and perioperative management have significantly increased the resection rate and reduced the operative mortality rate. Long-term survival rates, however, remain low. Only 10% of patients are still alive at 5 years, partly because disease is usually advanced at the time of diagnosis and partly because, even in earlier stages, anatomical features lead to early lymphatic and hematogenous dissemination. A trial of intensive preoperative chemotherapy and subsequent chemoradiotherapy was reported in operable patients who had locally advanced EC (LAEC).

Methods.—Before surgery, 90 patients who had LAEC received chemotherapy, which consisted of 3 courses of fluorouracil, leucovorin, etoposide, and cisplatin (FLEP), followed by concurrent chemoradiotherapy, which consisted of 1 course of cisplatin plus etoposide combined with 40 Gy of radiation. Four weeks after the end of radiation, transthoracic esophagectomy was done.

Findings.—Of the 90 patients, 72 had a follow-up of 12 months or more and were included in the final analysis. Sixty-one percent of these patients had a complete tumor resection. Twenty-two percent had no tumor in the resected specimen. The operative mortality rate was 15%. Twenty-three patients did not undergo surgery. At a median follow-up of 22 months, the median survival among all 72 patients was 17 months. Calculated 3-year survival rates were 42% among those who had complete resection, 68% among pathologic complete responders, and 33% overall.

Conclusions.—Preoperative chemotherapy with FLEP, followed by concurrent chemoradiotherapy, is active against LAEC. In this series, the pathologic complete response rate was 33% among patients who underwent surgery. These outcomes appear better than those associated with surgery alone, approximately doubling the 3-year survival rate. The efficacy of preoperative chemoradiation in LAEC warrants assessment of the role of surgery in this disease.

► The dismal outcome of patients who have EC has been partly related to the presence of advanced local disease at the time of diagnosis and therapy. This article provides strong support for a prospective randomized evaluation of preoperative chemoradiation in patients who have LAEC. The surprising 3-year survival rate of 33% in all patients remains to be validated. This multimodality, multidisciplinary approach to EC is in keeping with trends in cancer therapy, in which significant improvement in disease-free and long-term survival have been achieved in other tumors. Because long-term survival rates are only 10% at 5 years for patients undergoing surgical resection alone, support for such trials should be overwhelming.

W.G. Cioffi, M.D.

Lack of Intestinal Pacemaker (C-KIT-Positive) Cells in Infantile Hypertrophic Pyloric Stenosis

Yamataka A, Fujiwara T, Kato Y, et al (Dokkyo Univ, Tochigi, Japan; Juntendo Univ, Tokyo)

J Pediatr Surg 31:96–99, 1996 10–7

Introduction.—The pathogenesis of infantile hypertrophic pyloric stenosis (IHPS) is not clearly understood. Theories include abnormality of hormonal control of the pylorus, loss of peptide-containing nerve fibers, marked reduction of nitric oxide, and axonal degeneration in the myenteric plexus. The proto-oncogene *c-kit* is known to encode a transmembrane tyrosine kinase receptor. The ligand for the *c-kit* receptor is the *S1* factor. It has been shown in mice that *c-kit* is important in the development of a component of the pacemaker system required for the generation of autonomic gut motility. It has also been shown that the *c-kit* gene protein product (C-KIT) positive cells in the mammalian gut are responsible for intestinal pacemaker activity. Full-thickness muscle-biopsy specimens were obtained during pyloromyotomy in 16 babies treated for IHPS to determine if C-KIT–positive (C-KIT+) cells were present in the smooth muscles of the pylorus.

Methods.—In addition to the aforementioned biopsies, control samples of pyloric tissues were taken from neonatal, infantile, and adult sources at autopsy. All specimens were imbedded in O.C.T. compound and stored until cut into 4-μ-thick cryostat sections. Half were stained with hematoxylin and eosin, and the remaining sections underwent immunohistochemical analysis to visualize C-KIT+ cells in the pyloric tissues. Three investigators evaluated the number of C-KIT+ cells semiquantitatively and graded them on a scale of "−" (no C-KIT+ cells visible) to "+++" (many C-KIT+ cells).

Results.—Many C-KIT+ cells were seen in the muscle layers in the normal pyloric tissue from normal neonatal, infantile, and adult controls.

The C-KIT+ cells were either absent or markedly reduced in the pyloric muscles of patients with IHPS. There were also no C-KIT+ cells observed around the myenteric plexuses.

Conclusion.—Many C-KIT+ cells were observed in normal pyloric muscle tissue. The expression of *c-kit* was greatly reduced in the pyloric smooth muscle from patients with IHPS. It is possible that C-KIT+ cells are needed for the development or maintenance of normal gut motility and that a significant reduction in the expression of *c-kit* in the pyloric muscle may allow the smooth muscle cells to escape from this regulatory mechanism in patients with IHPS. This may cause the pylorospasms that result in hypertrophy. Further investigation is needed to support these findings.

▶ Little has changed in the treatment of pyloric stenosis since Fredet and Ramstedt described their lifesaving operation,[1, 2] but the etiology of this entity is still largely unknown and is the object of many a research project. Here, the authors demonstrate that expression of a proto-oncogene responsible for gut motility may be missing in the pylorus of affected children. Unfortunately, they do not tell us whether this defect is present elsewhere in the intestinal tract of patients with pyloric stenosis (this disease is usually *not* associated with other motility disorders), or whether it is still present in the pylorus later in life (pyloric stenosis is a self-limiting disease and supposedly leaves no sequelae). Although the finding is certainly interesting and merits further study, it does not establish a cause-and-effect relationship between lack of C-KIT expression and pyloric stenosis.

F.I. Luks, M.D.

References

1. Fredet P: La Cure de la Sténose hypertrophique du pylore chez les nourrissons par la pyloromyotomic extra-muqueuse. *J Chir* 29:604, 1927.
2. Ramstedt C: Zur Operation der angeborenen Rylorusstenose. *Med Klin* 8:1702, 1912.

A New Rodent Experimental Model of Esophageal Atresia and Tracheoesophageal Fistula: Preliminary Report

Diez-Pardo JA, Baoquan Q, Navarro C, et al (Universidad Autónoma, Madrid; Hospital do Meixoeiro, Vigo, Spain)

J Pediatr Surg 31:498–502, 1996 10–8

Background.—Much progress has been made in the treatment of esophageal atresia (EA) and tracheoesophageal fistula (TEF) in infants. However, no experimental models of these conditions are available. Preliminary experiments have shown that prenatal exposure of fetal rats to doxorubicin results in a variety of tracheoesophageal and related malformations anatomically identical to those in humans.

Methods.—Time-mated Wistar rats were injected intraperitoneally with 1.5, 1.75, or 2 mg/kg of doxorubicin on days 6 to 9 of gestation. The fetuses were harvested carefully by cesarean section on day 21, examined for external abnormalities, then dissected under a microsurgical binocular microscope. Some fetuses selected randomly from each dose group were prepared and examined histologically.

Findings.—Fetuses exposed to doxorubicin weighed significantly less and had significantly larger amounts of amniotic fluid than control fetuses. More amniotic fluid was noted in the fetuses with EA and TEF than in those without malformations. Twenty-eight percent of the fetuses in the low-dose group, 45.5% in the medium-dose group, and 41.6% in the high-dose group had EA with TEF. None of the control fetuses had this anomaly. All but 1 esophageal anomaly corresponded to Gross type C[1]. The exception was consistent with human H-type fistula. Defect anatomy was very similar to that seen in human newborns. The upper esophagus ended in a cone-shaped blind pouch just below the larynx, approximately at the level of the cricoid ring. Fetuses with EA and TEF had small stomachs with thicker-than-normal walls. Those with duodenal atresia had large stomachs distended by bile-stained fluid. There was a high incidence of related digestive and urinary tract malformations in all treatment groups. Duodenal and jejunoileal atresia were common.

Conclusion.—The anatomy and histologic findings of the malformations created in these mice are strikingly similar to those in humans. Associated anomalies are also very similar, although their incidence and severity are more extreme. This new animal model may be useful for clarifying how and why abnormal tracheoesophageal cleavage results in upper digestive tract interruption with distal fistulization to the trachea. It may also be useful for increasing understanding of the structural anomalies of the muscle, nerve plexuses, and mucosa in survivors of TEF and of the undernutrition in affected fetuses.

▶ Over the years, Dr. Tovar and the rest of the group in the study reported here have developed or described many excellent small animal models of surgical conditions, such as congenital diaphragmatic hernia (CDH), gastroschisis, open neural tube defects, and now EA and TEF. These teratogenically induced models complement the more "simplistic," surgically created anomalies in larger animals (of which diaphragmatic hernia in the fetal lamb is the most publicized example).

Whereas the large animal models are necessary for developing fetal and neonatal surgical procedures, the doxorubicin (EA/TEF) or nitrofen (CDH) rat model allow a more rapid and reproducible creation of large numbers of abnormal fetuses available for pathophysiologic research. They may help us understand aberrant embryonal or fetal development and time the occurence of certain defects. This is particluarly true when a single stimulus creates disorders in multiple organ systems. Indeed, a number of fetuses in the present model exhibited vertebral, anorectal, renal, and limb anomalies in addition to EA/TEF—i.e., the VATER syndrome...

F.I. Luks, M.D.

Factors Predicting Failure of Endoscopic Injection Therapy in Bleeding Duodenal Ulcer

Brullet E, Calvet X, Campo R, et al (Consorci Hospitalari Parc Taulí, Sabadell, Spain)

Gastrointest Endosc 43:111–116, 1996 10–9

Background.—Because endoscopic injection therapy (EIT) has a low cost and needs minimal equipment, it is the first treatment approach in patients who have a bleeding peptic ulcer in many centers. The factors that cause endoscopic injection failure in such patients were investigated.

Methods and Findings.—One hundred twenty patients were hospitalized with active arterial hemorrhage associated with a bleeding duodenal ulcer or a nonbleeding visible vessel. Endoscopic injection was possible in 106 patients. Definitive hemostasis was obtained in 88 patients (83%), although 3 of these patients needed a second injection. In 18 patients (17%), EIT failed. Four of these patients underwent emergency surgery for persistent bleeding, 10 underwent semi-elective surgery, and 4 were treated conservatively because of preterminal status. In a multivariate analysis, shock and ulcer size exceeding 2 cm were independent prognostic factors for EIT failure. Failure of EIT and poor clinical status were associated with significantly increased mortality in a multivariate analysis.

Conclusions.—In patients who have bleeding, high-risk duodenal ulcers, ulcer size and hemorrhage severity predict EIT failure. Clinical status and related diseases are determinants of survival.

▶ The evolution of endoscopic techniques has revolutionized the care of patients who have upper gastrointestinal hemorrhage. Success of EIT has considerably decreased the requirement for operative intervention. This success, however, has led to repeated endoscopic attempts at controlling hemorrhage and subsequent delay in surgical intervention in some patients, perhaps because the predictors of endoscopic failure are not understood. This appropriately analyzed study found, via multivariate analysis, that ulcer size and the presence of shock predicted endoscopic failure. Of note, these factors tripled the failure rate from approximately 12% to 36%. The take-home message would be that when patients are in shock with large ulcers, an endoscopic failure should result in surgical intervention, at a point when the patient is in a better physiologic state, not after repeated endoscopic attempts.

W.G. Cioffi, M.D.

Hepatobiliary, Pancreas, and Spleen

Introduction

With the introduction in 1987 of laparoscopic cholecystectomy, it remains the standard therapy for symptomatic cholelithiasis. Although many studies have confirmed the efficacy and cost-effectiveness of the procedure, acute cholecystitis still develops in approximately one fifth of the patients. The safety of laparoscopic cholecystectomy in this setting and the timing of the operation have been reviewed by Koo and Thirlby (**Abstract 10–10**) of the Department of Surgery, Virginia Mason Medical Center, Seattle. Surgery in the "golden interval" within 24 hours of the onset of symptoms allows surgeons to achieve planes that permit safe and expedient dissection. However, the optimal timing for laparoscopic cholecystectomy in this acute setting has not been precisely determined because of the absence of retrospective or prospective studies that identify and confirm the optimal interval for this approach. Koo and Thirlby retrospectively reviewed the results of laparoscopic cholecystectomy in this acute setting, with attention to the interval from the onset of symptoms to the timing of the operative approach. Although the procedure can be performed safely in the majority of patients with acute manifestations of cholelithiasis, these authors confirm that the length of duration of symptoms before the procedure affects the following outcomes: hospital costs, conversion rates, and duration of convalescence. The authors note that convalescence time is increased for patients having symptoms for more than 72 hours before exploration. These authors suggest that interval cholecystectomy may be superior when this 72-hour delay before onset of symptoms is exceeded.

The frequency and safety of the application of laparoscopic cholecystectomy to neoplasia diseases of the gallbladder have not previously been evaluated. The prevalence of incidental carcinoma of the gallbladder ranges from 1% to 2% of all open cholecystectomies. The Southern Surgeons Club recently completed a prospective analysis of 1,518 laparoscopic cholecystectomies that required conversion to the open conventional approach owing to the incidental finding of carcinoma of the gallbladder in 0.1%. Yamaguchi and associates (Abstract 10–11) from the Department of Surgery I, Kyushu University Faculty of Medicine, Hamanomachi Hospital, Sada Hospital, National Kokura Hospital, Kosei Nennkin Hospital, and Kyushu Rosai Hospital, Kitakyushu, Japan, reviewed the experience in 2,616 laparoscopic cholecystectomies performed over a 4-year period in which 24 gallbladder carcinomas were treated laparoscopically. These authors confirmed that a pTis or pT1 stage of carcinoma of an organ removed laparoscopically requires no further operative intervention. In this small series with a short follow-up (mean of 11 months), the authors cannot claim conclusive results regarding the timing and necessity for additional maneuvers after laparoscopic cholecystectomy. However, these authors advocate opening the gallbladder in the operating room, with frozen section analysis when carcinoma is suspected. If stage pT2 or pT3 disease is found, these cases should be converted to more extensive (perhaps open) procedures, depending on the depth of neoplastic invasion and the findings at the time of laparoscopic visualization of the gallbladder, gallbladder fossa, and porta hepatis. The authors also recommend excision of all port sites for advanced carcinoma.

The next abstract addresses primary gallbladder carcinoma. Wibbenmeyer and associates (Abstract 10–12) from the departments of surgery and pathology, St. Mary's Health Center and Saint Louis University, define a population of patients at risk for carcinoma of the gallbladder. These authors illustrate the effect of laparoscopy on the disease course and review strategies for definitive management when the gallbladder is excised at laparoscopic cholecystectomy. The authors of Abstracts 10–11 and 10–12 conclude that laparoscopic cholecystectomy appears sufficient when the disease is confined to the mucosa of the gallbladder and the organ is excised intact, without spillage of bile. In contradistinction, transmural injury to the gallbladder with spillage of bile in patients with invasive tumors requires laparotomy and local re-excision. The latter procedure may entail wedging of the gallbladder fossa and regional node dissection for invasive lesions with tumor fixation; the procedure is best converted to an open technique to enhance regional resection and improve cure of disease.

The formation of supersaturated bile and the subsequent formation of gallstone crystals are dependent on the supersaturation of biliary cholesterol and the pronucleating effects of gallbladder mucin and inflammation. Kam and associates (Abstract 10–13) from Michigan State Univesity and Butterworth Hospital, Grand Rapids, Michigan, evaluated the effects of aspirin and a 5-lipoxygenase activating protein inhibitor (FLAP) on the precipitation of cholesterol and on leukotriene levels in a gallstone formation animal model. Certain factors among proinflammatory amino acid metabolites may modulate pronucleating responses in the gallbladder. This important manuscript outlines the initial cellular events for the use of FLAPI to prevent cholesterol gallstone formation in the prairie dog cholelithiasis model. This study is the first to use a novel leukotriene inhibitor at high doses that resulted in a significant diminution in the rate of formation of cholesterol stones.

Endoscopic stenting of the biliary tree remains a viable option to surgery for the initial management of cholangitis and jaundice in patients with chronic pancreatitis in whom biliary stricture develops. The morbidity and mortality rates associated with biliary stent placement remain low; however, dysfunction of the stent and subsequent recrudescence of cholangitis and jaundice remain frequent complications that often require stent exchanges. Smits and associates (Abstract 10–14) of the departments of gastroenterology, hepatology, and surgery at the University of Amsterdam evaluated whether the endoscopic approach or surgical drainage is preferred for long-term management. In this study of the long-term effects of polyethylene stenting of the biliary tree in 58 patients with benign stricture secondary to chronic pancreatitis, the authors used surgical bypass in 16 of 58 patients with persistent biliary stricture. The authors conclude that endoscopic stenting and surgery are effective modalities in these patients; endoscopic stenting was associated with fewer early complications. Nonetheless, late complications related to stent placement remain major sources of morbidity while offering definitive therapy in over one quarter of these patients. Preferably, surgical drainage should be performed as the treatment of choice in young patients with persistent stricture, after a short interval (6–12 months) of preoperative stenting.

The late John H.C. Ranson of New York University is credited with documentation of the severity of disease and the risk of mortality for patients with acute pancreatitis; Ranson's criteria have been established as the reference standard for evaluation and management of this disorder. Ranson's criteria are measurable and applicable to the first 48 hours after the onset of pancreatitis and may alert the physician and surgeon to whether severe pancreatitis is present. Malcynski and associates (Abstract 10–15) of the Department of Surgery, Dartmouth-Hitchcock Medical Center, Lebanon, New Hampshire, emphasize that severe pancreatitis is a life-threatening alteration with characteristic peaks at 2 different time intervals. In the first interval after onset of the disorder, cardiopulmonary malfunction is the greatest threat for mortality. Subsequently, inflammatory and infectious complications that initiate multisystem organ failure are the predominant causes of mortality. These authors evaluated 27 patients transferred from other institutions and observed various criteria to allow documentation of the determinants of mortality. Only older age, the use of ionotropic agents and/or vasopressor support, and evidence of renal malfunction were associated with death. These authors emphasize the importance of early recognition of severe pancreatitis, especially in the aged, and the application of aggressive hemodynamic management and/or early transfer to centers that can manage these disorders. These measures are essential to diminish the incidence of renal failure and mortality in progressive severe pancreatitis. Of interest, this small series indicates that early renal failure is a marker of severe pancreatitis that cannot be altered by more aggressive intervention with early circulatory resuscitation. Although the majority of pancreatitis cases are mild, the identification of any patient with severe pancreatitis necessitates prompt transfer to tertiary care centers experienced in the management of this life-threatening disorder.

New gene-based therapies in clinical practice range from therapy for single-gene defects in cystic fibrosis to gene replacement therapy for multiple genetic abnormalities associated with neoplastic disorders. After a recent report on the feasibility of liver-directed ex vivo gene therapy for homozygous familial hypercholesterolemia, Raper and associates (Abstract 10–16) from The Institute of Human Gene Therapy and the department of molecular and cellular engineering, medicine, and surgery, University of Pennsylvania Medical Center, and the Wistar Institute, departments of internal medicine, biological chemistry, and pediatrics at the University of Michigan Medical Center, and the Division of Pediatric Cardiology at the Children's Hospital of Philadelphia selected 5 patients with homozygous familial hypercholesterolemia for a trial of liver-directed ex vivo gene therapy. The patients thereafter underwent partial hepatic resection and placement of a portal venous catheter. Hepatic tissue grown ex vivo produced primary hepatocyte cultures that were then transduced with recombinant retrovirus to encode the gene for the human low-density lipoprotein receptor. Genetically modified cells were subsequently transplanted into the liver via the portal venous catheter. The authors observed transient elevations in portal pressure during cell infusion. No major perioperative morbidity occurred with this protocol. Although these procedures and programs are likely to be limited by technical and physiologic considerations, this novel approach may be used for future therapy for familial hypercholesterolemia and other genetically related metabolic and neoplastic diseases.

The report of long-term results with the Kasai procedure for biliary atresia by Karrer and associates (Abstract 10–17) from the department of surgery and pediatrics of the University of Colorado School of Medicine and The Children's Hospital, Denver, emphasized the treatment of this disorder in a consecutive series of 104 infants. The long-term outcome for children after this portoenterostomy procedure remains uncertain. This study was undertaken to investigate 10-year outcome results after the treatment of infants with biliary atresia. The authors conclude that surgical correction offers the best long-term survival for approximately one quarter of the patients. Moreover, portoenterostomy provides palliation until hepatic transplantation is essential. These investigators conclude that the outlook is good to excellent for children who survive more than 10 years and justifies technical approaches that initiate and enhance biliary flow in infants with biliary atresia. The authors emphasize that primary transplantation for all infants with biliary atresia is important to avoid because a significant percentage will be long-term survivors with portoenterostomy. Moreover, a successful Kasai procedure may delay the inevitable transplantation until organ availability is ensured.

The important manuscript by Winde and associates (Abstract 10–18) of the departments of surgery, medicine, and laboratory medicine, the Gerhard Domagk Institute of Pathology and The Institute of Medical Statistics at the Westfalische Wilhelms-University of Muenster, Germany, emphasizes the role of splenectomy for the management of idiopathic thrombocytopenic purpura (ITP). This prospective trial was designed to clarify the rate of complete remission after splenectomy, the morbidity and mortality rates of the procedure, and the influence of the postoperative rise in platelet counts in response to preoperative medical therapy, and assess to the significance of megakaryocytopoiesis. Early postoperative morbidity and mortality rates were low (3% each). Splenectomy allowed complete remission in 72%, partial remission in 15%, partial remission affording further medical support in 6%, and no remission in 4%. Correlation of megakaryocytopoiesis and the site of thrombocytolysis to the stages of remission was significant. Hyperplasia of splenic follicles was a pathologic finding in patients who had significantly higher platelet counts 2 years after the procedure than in those with absence of these follicles. Winde and associates conclude that this low-morbidity, low-mortality procedure is the treatment of choice following relapse after immunosuppressive courses. The authors further determined that postoperative outcomes were best correlated with hyperplasia of megakaryocytopoiesis and with splenic follicles and isolated splenic thrombocytolysis. These factors are considered to be prognostic factors for the postoperative course in ITP. It is essential that other studies evaluate and support these findings to allow a reduction in postoperative patients' immunosuppressive drugs.

Kirby I. Bland, M.D.

Laparoscopic Cholecystectomy in Acute Cholecystitis: What Is the Optimal Timing for Operation?

Koo KP, Thirlby RC (Virginia Mason Med Ctr, Seattle)

Arch Surg 131:540–545, 1996 10–10

Introduction.—Reports indicate that open cholecystectomy should be performed within the first 72 hours after the onset of symptoms of acute cholecystitis. An optimal timing for performing laparoscopic cholecystectomy (LC) in patients with acute cholecystitis has not been determined. Results of patients who underwent LC for acute cholecystitis were retrospectively reviewed, with attention to the interval from onset of symptoms to operation.

Methods.—Sixty of 446 patients who underwent LC had acute cholecystitis. Records of these 60 patients were reviewed for medical history, laboratory findings, ultrasound findings, timing of operation from the onset of symptoms, length of surgery, surgical findings, gallbladder histologic features, surgical outcome, postoperative mortality and morbidity, postoperative length of stay, cost of operative procedure and hospitalization, and number of days before the patient could return to normal daily activities. Patients were divided into 3 groups: group 1 (16 patients) had LC within 72 hours after onset of symptoms; group 2 (19 patients) had LC between the 4th and 7th day after onset of symptoms; and group 3 (25 patients) had symptoms for more that 7 days before surgery was performed.

Results.—The average duration of symptoms before cholecystectomy was 9 days. All patients had acute inflammation of the gallbladder. The inflammation was severe in 32 patients. Technical difficulty in dissection was noted for 5 (30%) group 1 patients, 10 (52%) group 2 patients, and 10 (40%) group 3 patients. The frequency of hemorrhagic or necrotizing cholecystitis was 6% for group 1, 26% for group 2, and 20% for group 3. Of the 60 patients, 15 (25%) underwent conversion to open laparotomy and conventional cholecystectomy. Thirteen of these patients had extensive adhesions, inflammation, or gangrenous changes precluding a safe dissection of the cystic duct and common duct junction. The average patient age in the LC group was 50 years. In the converted group, it was 56 years. One (8%) of 12 patients who had surgery within 48 hours of symptoms needed conversion to an open procedure, compared with 14 (27%) of 52 patients who underwent surgery more than 48 hours after symptom onset. The highest conversion rates (38%) occurred in patients who underwent LC 4 to 8 days after onset of symptoms. Patients whose operation took place more than 8 days after onset of symptoms had a conversion rate of 20%. Laparoscopic procedures were converted to open procedures in 2 (12.5%), 6 (32%), and 7 (28%) group 1, 2, and 3 patients, respectively. None of the laboratory tests reliably predicted which patients would need open cholecystectomy. There were no bile duct injuries nor mortalities in this cohort.

Conclusion.—The LC procedure could be safely performed in most patients with acute cholecystitis. The duration of symptoms before the patient underwent LC affected the surgical outcome. The conversion rates, and, thus, hospital costs and convalescence times, were increased in patients with symptoms lasting for more than 72 hours before LC. It is unknown whether a conservative approach to treatment with antibiotics and elective LC 6 to 8 weeks after acute inflammation subsides would result in safer, less costly outcomes.

▶ This large retrospective study evaluated the critical issue of timing in patients with acute cholecystitis and LC. Four hundred forty-six patients were evaluated over a 2-year period. Laparosocopic cholecystectomy was attempted in 16 patients within 72 hours of the onset of symptoms, in 19 patients with symptoms for 4–7 days, and in 25 patients with symptoms lasting more than 7 days. The authors demonstrated that LC done within 72 hours of the onset of symptoms had lower rates of conversion to open procedures, less difficult operations, shorter operative times, and shorter convalescences. The conversion rates in patients operated within and after the 72 hours were 12% and 30%, respectively. There were no bile duct injuries or mortalities in this group of patients.

The authors have concluded that LC for acute cholecystitis should optimally be performed within 72 hours of the onset of symptoms. We concur with these findings and commend the authors on a series of patients who had LC for acute cholecystitis without any bile duct injuries. I think this points to the increasing safety of this operation, even in an acute setting. We concur that LC for acute cholecystitis performed within the first 20 hours is generally easier, as the patient's pathologic condition remains within the edematous phase, and fibrosis and increased blood vessel proliferation have not yet occurred. After 72 hours, the procedure tends to be more sanguinous and is more difficult to perform.

H.H. Simms, M.D.

Gallbladder Carcinoma in the Era of Laparoscopic Cholecystectomy

Yamaguchi K, Chijiwa K, Ichimiya H, et al (Kyushu Univ, Fukuoka, Japan; Hamanomachi Hosp, Fukuoka, Japan; Sada Hosp, Fukuoka, Japan)

Arch Surg 131:981–984, 1996 10–11

Introduction.—Few reports have addressed the role laparoscopic cholecystectomy plays in the treatment of gallbladder carcinoma. The long-term effects of initial laparoscopic cholecystectomy on the prognosis of gallbladder carcinoma are not known. The usefulness of laparoscopic cholecystectomy was evaluated in 2,616 patients with suspected and unsuspected gallbladder carcinoma (10 and 14 patients, respectively).

Methods.—Twenty-four of 2,616 patients (0.9%) who underwent laparoscopic cholecystectomy had gallbladder carcinoma. Records were retrospectively reviewed for data on clinical findings, imaging findings, use of radiotherapy and chemotherapy, histolopathologic results, and patient outcome.

Results.—Patients' clinical courses depended on the histopathologic depth of gallbladder carcinoma invasion. Six patients with pathologic tumor (pT) stage in situ (pTis) and 2 patients with pT1 gallbladder carcinoma had no evidence of invasion to lymphatic, venous, or perineural spaces. At a mean follow-up of 11 months after surgery, all patients were doing well. There were 16 patients with pT2 or pT3 gallbladder carcinoma that invaded the subserosal layer or liver. Five of these patients died of liver dysfunction, abdominal wall recurrence, or liver metastasis at 5 days and 7, 12, 15, and 18 months, respectively, after surgery. Three of 16 patients with pT2 or pT3 gallbladder carcinoma had abdominal wall recurrence without distant metastasis secondary to inoculation of cancer cells in the abdominal stab wound where the gallbladder or laparoscope were removed.

Conclusion.—No other treatment is required for gallbladder carcinoma at the pTis or pT1 stage removed laparoscopically. For patients with pT2 or pT3 carcinoma undergoing laparoscopic cholecystectomy, it is recommended that the gallbladder be removed by vinyl bag and that port sites be excised or washed with normal saline to prevent port recurrence. Laparoscopic cholecystectomy is recommended only for patients with pTis and pT1 gallbladder limited within the muscle coat. More extensive surgery should be performed by laparotomy in patients with pT2 or pT3 invasive gallbladder carcinoma infiltrating the subserosal layer or liver. Earlier reports indicate that solitary sessile polypoid lesions more than 1 cm in diameter on ultrasonographic examination are highly suggestive of malignancy. Gallbladders removed though a trocar site should be removed using a vinyl bag, and all ports should be excised or cleaned by normal saline to eliminate abdominal wall infiltration or spillage of cancer cells.

► Gallbladder carcinoma is a rare, but unfortunately aggressive, gastrointestinal tract malignancy that has been the focus of controversy with regard to treatment in the laparoscopic era. Numerous isolated case reports have noted recurrence of gallbladder carcinoma not only at the surgical site but also at any of the port sites, including the umbilical port. Unfortunately, these isolated reports have been used to make recommendations on the management of gallbladder carcinoma. This has resulted in near-universal condemnation of the laparoscopic approach to initial management of suspected gallbladder carcinoma.

We now have the first large series of gallbladder carcinomas reported in the laparoscopic era by Yamaguchi and colleagues. Interestingly, their review of 2,616 laparoscopic cholecystectomies, of which 24 identified carcinomas, led them to conclude that a laparoscopic approach was adequate and did not seem to result in any greater risk for recurrence than the open technique for pTis or pT1 stage cancers. For early cancers, the bottom line is good technique, no spillage of bile, and no spillage of tumor. In addition, the gallbladder should be removed in a bag to obviate spreading at port sites. In context, pT2 and pT3 stage gallbladder cancers should be converted to an open procedure for more radical resection. These findings are consistent with the recommendations for management of gallbladder cancer by the open technique.

J.F. Amaral, M.D.

Laparoscopic Cholecystectomy Can Disseminate *in Situ* Carcinoma of the Gallbladder

Wibbenmeyer LA, Wade TP, Chen RC, et al (St Louis Univ, Mo)
J Am Coll Surg 181:504–510, 1995 10–12

Introduction.—Primary gallbladder carcinoma (GBC) is the fifth most common carcinoma of the gastrointestinal tract. The site of recurrence of GBC after open resection seems to be local with intraoperitoneal spread by direct extension. After laparoscopic cholecystectomy (LC), recurrence is observed more frequently at the port sites, with diffuse peritoneal implantation. Because the LC procedure introduces a greater risk for gallbladder rupture, this approach should be abandoned and converted to open cholecystectomy when carcinoma is suspected or dissection is difficult. The experience of GBC after LC is reported.

Methods.—Medical records were retrospectively reviewed, and pertinent patient, operative, histologic, and outcome data were collected. Findings were compared with those from a series of 24 patients who underwent LC for benign disease.

Results.—Of 928 cholecystectomies performed in a 30-month period, 699 were done with laparoscopy and 229 were done with laparotomy. Seven of 9 patients had gallbladder neoplasms that were discovered after LC. The overall incidence of GBC in this cohort was 0.97%. There was no suspicion of GBC in any patients before laparoscopy. Patients with GBC were significantly more likely to be older, have thicker gallbladder walls, and have more abnormalities detected intraoperatively than patients without GBC. After LC, GBC recurred more rapidly and in diffuse peritoneal and port sites compared with recurrence patterns after open cholecystectomy.

Conclusion.—This is the first known report on successful management of early GBC with LC. The appropriate treatment when GBC is detected after LC has not been determined. It may be that patients whose gallbladders are removed without bile spillage and are found to have early carcinoma can be adequately followed with simple observation or laparoscopic re-exploration. Laparoscopy allows a more thorough tactile and visual examination of the sites of operation and instrumentation. Enough evidence exists to recommend prompt, wide port-site and hepatic bed excision with portal lymphadenectomy when locally advanced GBC is detected after LC.

▶ Wibbenmeyer and colleagues have provided us with a very small series of patients with gallbladder carcinoma from which they make rather strong recommendations regarding the management of gallbladder carcinoma. In this article, they go so far as to suggest that conversion should be considered in patients with "increased gallbladder adhesions or inflammation." Does this make sense? That is, should 25%–30% of patients who have gallbladder adhesions or inflammation be converted to an open cholecystectomy to try to help the less than 1% of cholecystectomy patients who have gallbladder cancer and the even smaller percentage of patients who may benefit from this more aggressive approach for a disease with such a dismal prognosis. I think not.

The important point to take home from this article in my opinion is that conversion to an open cholecystectomy should not be used as an excuse for a lack of meticulous operative technique. The latter appears more at issue in the data the authors provide us than the method used. In some regards, a "universal precautions" type of mindset should be used in dealing with cholecystectomy: that is, consider all patients undergoing cholecystectomy to potentially harbor gallbladder cancer. Make every possible effort not to tear the gallbladder, spill stones, or spill bile. If there is any question, remove the gallbladder in a bag. Finally, if there is spillage, aggressively wash the abdominal cavity and excise the port sites.

J.F. Amaral, M.D.

A Novel 5-Lipoxygenase Inhibitor Prevents Gallstone Formation in a Lithogenic Prairie Dog Model

Kam DM, Webb PA, Sandman G, et al (Michigan State Univ, Grand Rapids)
Am Surg 62:551–556, 1996 10–13

Background.—The formation of gallstones results from biliary cholesterol supersaturation, the pronucleating effects of gallbladder mucin, and inflammation. There is conflicting evidence regarding the role of prostaglandins and prostaglandin inhibitors in gallstone formation. Leukotrienes are produced by the lipoxygenase pathway of arachidonic acid metabolism. Adjusting the production of leukotrienes by lipoxygenase inhibition may clarify the role of the leukotriene pathway in the formation of gallstones. The effect of aspirin and a 5-lipoxygenase inhibitor on formation of gallstones and levels of leukotriene was evaluated in prairie dogs.

Methods.—Male prairie dogs were fed 4 different diets: a 1.2% cholesterol diet, a 1.2% cholesterol diet plus aspirin at 100 mg/kg/24hr, a 1.2% cholesterol diet plus a 5-lipoxygenase activating protein inhibitor at 100 mg/kg/12hr, or a normal diet. Cholecystectomy was performed at 3 weeks. The common duct was cannulated for bile sampling, and cholesterol precipitation, lithogenic indices, and leukotriene content were assessed.

Results.—Cholesterol crystals were not present in animals fed the 5-lipoxygenase activating protein inhibitor but were present in animals fed aspirin. Lithogenic indices were significantly higher in animals fed cholesterol compared with control animals. In animals fed the 5-lipoxygenase activating protein inhibitor, there was a significant and paradoxical increase in levels of leukotriene TB4.

Conclusion.—High doses of a leukotriene inhibitor significantly decreased the incidence of gallstone formation in these animals, despite a high cholesterol diet. There was a paradoxical increase, however, in levels of leukotriene. The paradoxical high levels of leukotriene TB4 in bile and tissue may either mean that leukotriene TB4 is an antinucleating factor in this model, or that unidentified antinucleation factors are influenced by the 5-lipoxygenase activating protein inhibitor.

▶ In this study, the authors evaluated the effect of aspirin and a 5-lipoxygenase inhibitor on cholesterol precipitation and levels of leukotriene in an animal model of cholesterol gallstone formation. The common bile ducts of male prairie dogs were cannulated for bile sampling. The authors further analyzed cholesterol precipitation with lithogenic indices and leukotriene content. The animals that received a cholesterol-enhanced diet with aspirin showed significantly more cholesterol precipitation than those who received a 5-lipoxygenase inhibitor. All the cholesterol-fed animals showed a significant increase in lithogenic indices compared with controls. To the best of my knowledge, this is the first study that has demonstrated a significant decrease in the rate of cholesterol stone formation through the use of a novel leukotriene inhibitor at high doses, even though the animals had a high cholesterol diet. Although 5-lipoxygenase inhibition has not yet come into clinical practice, studies such as this one provide insight into the process of cholesterol gallstone formation in patients at risk.

H.H. Simms, M.D.

Long-term Results of Endoscopic Stenting and Surgical Drainage for Biliary Stricture Due to Chronic Pancreatitis

Smits ME, Rauws EAJ, van Gulik TM, et al (Univ of Amsterdam)

Br J Surg 83:764–768, 1996 10–14

Background.—Jaundice from obstruction of the intrapancreatic segment of the common bile duct reportedly occurs in 3% to 46% of patients who have chronic pancreatitis. Authorities continue to disagree on whether endoscopic treament or surgical drainage is the best long-term treatment. The long-term outcomes of polyethylene biliary stenting were investigated in patients who had benign biliary stricture from chronic pancreatitis.

Methods and Outcomes.—Fifty-eight patients, aged 19–76 years, were treated; their status was followed for a median of 49 months. Insertion of an endoscopic stent immediately relieved jaundice and cholestasis in all patients. Complications occurred in 9% of patients after therapeutic endoscopic retrograde cholangiopancreatography. Sixty-four percent had late stent-related complications, requiring stent exchange. None of the patients died. In 28% of patients, biliary stricture regressed, and stents were removed permanently. In 42 patients, biliary stricture persisted. Twenty-six patients had continued stenting, and 16 underwent surgery. Six patients had early morbidity after surgery, but no one died. Fifteen patients had relief of jaundice after surgery.

Conclusions.—Endoscopic stenting and surgery are both effective for alleviating biliary stricture in patients who have chronic pancreatitis. Endoscopic stenting provides definitive treatment in more than one fourth of patients. Although fewer early complications occur with endoscopic stenting than with surgery, the occurrence of stent-related complications is a major limiting factor.

► The advent of endoscopic and transcutaneous methods for biliary stenting has significantly altered our approach to patients who have benign biliary obstruction. Unfortunately, few studies have evaluated the long-term success of nonoperative drainage. The long-term results of endoscopic biliary stenting in these 58 patients provide some data by which rational treatment decisions may be made. Sixteen patients avoided surgery. However, if after 3–6 months the endoscopic stent could not be removed, many patients required surgical intervention. The long-term success rate of endoscopic drainage did not approach that of surgical drainage. In patients who are deemed surgical candidates, surgery should occur after 3–6 months, if the benign stricture has not resolved.

W.G. Cioffi, M.D.

Severe Pancreatitis: Determinants of Mortality in a Tertiary Referral Center

Malcynski JT, Iwanow IC, Burchard KW (Dartmouth Hitchcock Med Ctr, Lebanon, NH)

Arch Surg 131:242–246, 1996 10–15

Introduction.—The severity and mortality criteria of Ranson et al., published in 1974, have long been used in the evaluation and management of acute pancreatitis. Using data readily available in the first 48 hours, the criteria help the clinician to decide whether the patient has severe pancreatitis. However, referral centers often see patients with severe pancreatitis several days after onset, when the criteria of Ranson et al. may not be as useful. A series of patients with severe pancreatitis treated in a tertiary referral center ICU was analyzed to identify factors associated with mortality.

Findings.—The analysis included 30 patients with pancreatitis, 27 of whom were transferred from other institutions. Thirty percent of the patients died, and the survivors stayed in the ICU a mean of 53 days. The mean age was 64 years in the patients who died vs. 47 years in survivors. The mean serum creatinine concentration was 410 and 150 μmol/L, respectively. Patients who received inotropic and/or vasopressor support and/or had renal failure—defined as a creatinine concentration greater than 170 μmol/L—were more likely to die.

Conclusions.—Factors associated with death in patients with pancreatitis referred to a tertiary care center are advanced age, use of inotropic and/or vasopressor support, and signs of renal malfunction. The best way to reduce the incidence of renal failure and death in patients with severe pancreatitis is to recognize the condition, particularly in older patients. Aggressive hemodynamic management and earlier referral may be important as well.

▶ This manuscript deals with 30 patients admitted to a tertiary care ICU from 1986 to 1995 with a primary diagnosis of acute pancreatitis. Twenty-seven patients were transferred from another institution. The patients who died during this study were older on admission, and their serum creatinine levels were higher. Death was associated with use of inotropic and/or vasopressor support and renal failure any time during ICU stay. Importantly, mortality was not associated with respiratory failure, insulin use, positive blood cultures, positive pancreatic cultures, and abdominal surgery for pancreatitis and infected pancreatic necrosis. Peritoneal lavage was used in 9 of the 27 patients. The authors conclude that prompt recognition of severe pancreatitis, especially in older patients, aggressive hemodynamic management, and/or earlier transfer to a tertiary care center may diminish the incidence of renal failure and mortality in severe pancreatitis. Our experience at this institution tends to confirm the report of these investigators, in that age does appear to be an independent risk factor for mortality after severe pancreatitis. However, because of the limited number of patients who underwent pancreatic lavage, an interesting and important question that remains unanswered is, Would the earlier use of peritoneal lavage reduce mortality in critically ill elderly patients with acute pancreatitis?

H.H. Simms, M.D.

Safety and Feasibility of Liver-directed Ex Vivo Gene Therapy for Homozygous Familial Hypercholesterolemia

Raper SE, Grossman M, Rader DJ, et al (Univ of Pennsylvania, Philadelphia; Univ of Michigan, Ann Arbor)

Ann Surg 223:116–126, 1996 10–16

Background.—In familial hypercholesterolemia (FH), an autosomal dominant disease, the gene encoding the low-density lipoprotein receptor is defective. Levels of cholesterol are extraordinarily high in patients homozygous for this mutation, which results in accelerated atherosclerosis and premature death from myocardial infarction. The safety and efficacy of liver-directed ex vivo gene therapy for patients with homozygous FH are reported.

Methods and Outcomes.—Five patients, aged 7–41 years, underwent left lateral lobectomy and portal venous catheter placement. Primary hepatocyte cultures were prepared from resected liver, then transduced with a recombinant retrovirus encoding the human low-density lipoprotein receptor gene. These genetically modified cells were transplanted into the liver through the portal venous catheter. The patients had increased hepatic transaminases and leukocyte counts and decreased hematocrit counts. Portal pressure increased during cell infusion. There were no instances of myocardial infarction, perioperative bleeding, or portal vein thrombosis. None of the patients died.

Conclusions.—The intraportal transplantation of many genetically modified autologous hepatocytes is feasible, without short-term complications. The inferior mesenteric vein seems well suited for catheter placement. Routine fluoroscopic confirmation is needed. The left gastric vein is not recommended for catheter placement. A suitable tributary of the middle colic or other portal tributary should be used when there is no inferior mesenteric vein. The use of ex vivo gene therapy in selected patients will depend largely on the likelihood that incomplete genetic reconstitution will result in clinically significant metabolic correction.

▶ Advances in gene-based therapy have led to the initiation of human trials. Raper and colleagues have presented data concerning the technical considerations for 1 type of ex vivo liver-directed gene therapy in a trial for the treatment of FH. The initiation of such programs will likely be fraught with technical limitations and complications. The general surgeon will be called to make contributions toward these problems, so that the full benefit of gene-based therapies may be realized.

W.G. Cioffi, M.D.

Long-term Results With the Kasai Operation for Biliary Atresia

Karrer FM, Price MR, Bensard DD, et al (Univ of Colorado, Denver)

Arch Surg 131:493–496, 1996 10–17

Introduction.—The Kasai portoenterostomy operation is the accepted treatment for biliary atresia worldwide. Surgical outcomes of this procedure are unclear. The outcome of treatment of infants with biliary atresia was investigated after 10 years of follow-up.

Methods.—Between 1973 and 1985, 104 consecutive infants in whom biliary atresia was diagnosed were enrolled. Diagnosis was based on findings of preoperative assessment, surgical findings, intraoperative cholangiography, and histologic evaluation of the liver and biliary remnants. Ninety-eight infants underwent surgical reconstruction and 6 had exploration only. The types of reconstruction were 74 Roux-en-Y with exteriorization, 6 simple Roux-en-Y, 11 portocholecystostomy ("gallbladder Kasai") in infants with patent gallbladder and distal common bile duct, and 7 other modifications. Records were retrospectively reviewed for information on survival, liver function, complications, and growth and development. Some data were gathered via telephone interview.

Results.—Thirty-five children were still alive a mean of 14.8 years after reconstructive surgery for biliary atresia. Of these, 12 required liver transplantation. Twenty-three children (24%) survived a decade or more after portoenterostomy without transplantation. There were no long-term survivors among infants who were older than 90 days at the time of operation. The best long-term outcome was achieved in children who underwent surgery before 60 days of age. Ten-year survival rates for types of reconstructive surgery were 36% for gallbladder Kasai and 26% for Roux-en-Y with exteriorization. There were no long-term survivors among children with other types of reconstruction. Five of the 6 children who did not undergo any type of Kasai operation died before age 1 year; the other child died at age 18 months. Despite biliary reconstruction, 63 children died: 43 before age 2 years and 19 between ages 2–10 years. Of 22 children who had liver transplantation, 4 had surgery in the second decade of life; the remaining procedures were performed at ages 10, 11, 12, and 16 years, respectively. Ten children who underwent liver transplantation died. The remaining children were still alive at a mean age of 15.1 years. Among survivors of transplantation; 2 developed lymphomas; 2 had portal vein thrombosis; and 1 had chronic rejection, pancreatitis, and diabetes mellitus. Two thirds of long-term survivors had 1 or more episodes of cholangitis. Complications of portal hypertension were common and were manifested by variceal bleeding, hypersplenism, and symptomatic ascites. Twenty-five of 30 children in whom growth and development data were available were within the range of expected height for their age. Five children were below the 10th percentile for height.

Conclusion.—Of 98 children who underwent portoenterostomy, 26% achieved 10-year survival. With Kasai portoenterostomy and transplantation combined, 35 of 98 children achieved long-term survival. Two thirds of survivors developed complications of portal hypertension. The success rate of transplantation is constantly improving, and some suggest that it should be considered the primary treatment for infants with biliary atresia. Others advocate the Kasai procedure as primary treatment, with transplantation reserved for those who do not establish bile flow or who progress to end-stage liver disease.

► The message is clear and has been stated in various forms many times before: despite the impressive advances of liver transplantation (and the authors acknowledge that their dismal 55% survival after transplantation partially refers to the precyclosporine era), Kasai portoenterostomy still has a place in the treatment of this otherwise fatal disease. Twenty-five percent of children who undergo a portoenterostomy will be "cured" and will not need a new liver. In addition, liver transplantation in infants younger than 1 year is still fraught with too many complications and graft failures, often requiring retransplantation (even though recent reports, such as from Johns Hopkins Hospital,[1] have shown much improved results). Primary transplantation for all infants with biliary atresia would therefore waste many livers.

Thus, a successful Kasai operation is one that allows the child, if not to live free of disease, to at least outgrow infancy before transplantation.

F.I. Luks, M.D.

Reference

1. Colombani PM, Cigarroa FG, Schwarz K, et al: Liver transplantation in infants younger than 1 year of age. *Ann Surg* 238:658–664, 1996.

Results and Prognostic Factors of Splenectomy in Idiopathic Thrombocytopenic Purpura

Winde G, Schmid KW, Lügering N, et al (Westfälische Wilhelms Univ of Muenster, Germany)

J Am Coll Surg 183:565–574, 1996 10–18

Introduction.—For patients with idiopathic thrombocytopenic purpura (ITP), the treatment of choice is immunosuppressive therapy. For patients who relapse after immunosuppressive therapy, splenectomy offers a 50% to 85% chance of complete remission. The results of splenectomy were prospectively examined in 72 patients with ITP.

Findings.—In this series, splenectomy had an early postoperative mortality rate of 3% and morbidity rate of 3%. Seventy-two percent of patients achieved complete remission, and 15% had partial remission. Six percent of patients had partial remission that permitted further medical support, and 4% had no remission. The degree of remission was significantly correlated with megakaryocytopoiesis and the site of thrombocytopoiesis. At 2 years' follow-up, platelet counts were significantly higher in patients with hyperplasia of the splenic follicles.

Conclusions.—Splenectomy gives good results in patients with relapsing ITP after immunosuppressive therapy. The results may be best in patients with isolated splenic thrombolysis, hyperplasia of megakaryocytopoiesis, and hyperplasia of the splenic follicles.

► This prospective clinical study was undertaken to evaluate the complete remission in ITP after splenectomy. Seventy-two patients who had undergone splenectomy were examined. The early postoperative mortality and morbidity rates were 3% each. The following degrees of remission were achieved in this study: complete remission, 72%; partial remission, 15%; partial remission that afforded further medical support, 6%; and no remission, 4%. The correlation of megakaryocytopoiesis and the site of thrombocytolysis to the degree of remission was significant. Patients with hyperplasia of splenic follicles had significantly higher platelet counts 2 years after operation than did those without hyperplatic splenic follicles. The authors therefore stated that splenectomy appears to be the treatment of choice for relapse after immunosuppressive courses. An examination of results at our institution would support the concept that splenectomy remains the procedure of choice for patients with ITP. The major advancement in this manuscript appears to be that megakaryocytopoiesis and hyperplasia of splenic follicles could serve as possible prognostic factors for the postoperative course in ITP. If these factors are supported by other studies, it might be possible to reduce or change patients' postoperative immunosuppression.

H.H. Simms, M.D.

Abdomen and Small Bowel

Introduction

The surgeon of the 1990s must be well advised of the increasing role of minimally invasive (laparoscopic) surgery in clinical practice. In the past few years, the use of minimal access has embraced a multitude of operative procedures in general surgery. Laparoscopic cholecystectomy remains the only operative procedure in general surgery in which a clear advantage for application of the minimal-access technique has been confirmed. Wright and associates (Abstract 10–19) of the West Glasgow Hospitals University NHS Trust, the Glasgow Royal Infirmary University NHS Trust, and Southern General Hospital NHS Trust, Glasgow and Aberdeen, Scotland, compared open tension-free hernioplasty with totally extraperitoneal endoscopic tension-free hernioplasty in a randomized, controlled clinical trial. Wound complications occurred significantly more often with the open technique. No difference was found in pulmonary function or metabolic response to trauma as evaluated by interleukin-6, C-reactive protein, glucose, or albumin levels between these 2 randomized groups. The authors concluded that there is significant short-term advantage for the endoscopic tension-free approach over the open method. As in any randomized study, however, the authors and the editors of the YEAR BOOK advise that larger studies with longer follow-up be completed to establish the relative merits of both procedures for the management of inguinal hernia.

Abstracts 10–20 through 10–23 evaluate congenital abdominal wall defects, diaphragmatic hernias, and the sequelae that these events have on infant morbidity and mortality. Abstracts 10–20 and 10–21 evaluate long-term gastrointestinal and pulmonary sequelae for survivors of congenital diaphragmatic defects. Children who survive diaphragmatic defects usually do well in the long term but have a reduction in lung capacity in adult life. Vanamo et al. (Abstract 10–20) from Children's Hospital, Laboratory of Clinical Physiology, Meilahti Hospital and Hospital for Allergic Disorders, University of Helsinki, evaluate lung volumes, ventilatory capacity, and lung function in adults who had previously undergone diaphragmatic repair in childhood. These authors indicate that long-term follow-up in these cohorts defined obstructive and restrictive ventilatory capacity impairment in over half of the adult patients who had undergone surgery as children. Both events are evident in one quarter of the patients. The prevalence of bronchial hyperreactivity and asthma was higher in these patients as well. Despite these abnormal functions, few had clinical symptoms, a reflection of the reserve capacity of the lung. Abstract 10–21, also by Vanamo and associates, evaluates the results of a survey of adults to determine gastrointestinal morbidity after repair of congenital diaphragmatic defects. Gastroesophageal reflux was evident in the first year of life in 20% to 84% of these patients with diaphragmatic hernias. More than 50% have evidence of esophagitis by endoscopic or histologic criteria. Although the incidence of esophagitis is only 2% in the general population and 50% in patients with ulcer symptoms, this study suggests substantial long-term gastrointestinal morbidity arising principally from esophagitis and late intestinal obstruction. The authors therefore enumerate the appropriate concerns of progressive esophagitis and Barrett's esophagus in these individuals. The appropriate recommendation for careful follow-up of patients with congenital diaphragmatic defects is the thrust of this paper, and follow-up should include routine examination for the sequelae expected.

The surgeon of the 1990s has become versed in the use of diagnostic imaging for a variety of benign and malignant diseases. Recent advances in fetal and adult US commonly allow noninvasive diagnostic approaches that facilitate management and enhance quality outcomes in adults and children. Advances in US of the fetus and infant allow early detection of abdominal wall defects, which may be crucial to prenatal care and infant morbidity and mortality. Additional anomalies in fetuses with abdominal wall defects diminish quality outcomes. To determine whether associated anatomical features are useful in fetal prognosis was reviewed by Kamata and associates (Abstract 10–22) of the Department of Pediatric Surgery, Osaka University, Japan. These authors caution against a simplistic view after the prenatal diagnosis of these defects because only ruptured omphalocele in the presence of scoliosis was associated with a high mortality. Of interest, outcomes for other forms of abdominal defects such as omphalocele and gastroschisis were more favorable. We would advise future parents to obtain information about the true nature of the defect to place in proper perspective the importance of detectable associated anomalies as predictors of the quality of survival. Similarly, Dommergues and associates (Abstract 10–23) of Maternité Port Royal-Baudeloque, the Institut de Puériculture, and The Service de Chirurgie Infantile, Hôpital Necker Enfants Malades, Paris, evaluated severe oligohydramnios associated with fetal gastroschisis that was treated in utero by serial transabdominal amnioinfusions of saline. This important contribution to the pediatric surgical literature suggests that serial amnioinfusion is a feasible therapeutic approach for severe third-trimester oligohydramnios when associated with gastroschisis.

Inflammatory bowel disease (IBD) in the pediatric and adult population continues to increase. Crohn's disease, an idiopathic, chronic, panintestinal disorder, tends to progress despite surgical or medical management and at present has no known cure. Moreover, approximately half of the patients managed medically will eventually require some form of surgical intervention. Quite simply stated, surgical intervention is designed to alleviate symptoms uncontrolled by medical therapy or to correct complications initiated by Crohn's IBD. Although resection remains the operation of choice for long-term cure, the 10-year reoperative rates for recurrent disease have been static at one third to one half of the patients so managed. The important long-term analysis by Ozuner and associates (Abstract 10–24) of the Department of Colorectal Surgery, the Cleveland Clinic Foundation, Cleveland, Ohio, determined reoperative rates after strictureplasty. These authors analyzed the frequency of recurrence or complications at a previous strictureplasty site rather than recrudescence of disease at other anatomical sites. For patients treated by strictureplasty alone, the cumulative reoperative rate at 5 years was 31%, and for patients with concomitant bowel resection, this rate was 27%. There was no statistical difference between the 2 groups. The authors correctly concluded that strictureplasty is an effective and safe method for the management of Crohn's disease in selected patients. The reoperative rates in this study were comparable with those for resective surgery; most recurrences appear at new anatomical sites. The technique is a very safe procedure and should be considered an excellent alternative to bowel resection for suitable patients.

To further address the long-term results of the management of Crohn's disease, Sagar and associates (Abstract 10–25) of the Division of Colon and Rectal Surgery, Mayo Clinic and Mayo Foundation, Rochester, Minnesota, evaluated the long-term results of ileal pouch–anal anastomosis (IPAA) for patients with Crohn's IBD. The objective of this analysis was to determine the long-term outcome for patients who had undergone mucosectomy with hand-sewn IPAA. Complex fistulas (pouch-cutaneous, pouch-vaginal, or pouch-vesicle) developed in 11 of 37 patients. In this long-term analysis (range, 3–14 years), the pouch remained in situ in 20 of 37 patients in whom the frequency of bowel movements was 7 times per day. The IPAA was excised in 10 patients and made defunctional in 7 patients—a failure rate of 45%. Therefore the authors concluded that inadvertent IPAA performed incorrectly for Crohn's disease is associated with a high rate of failure but was noted to have an acceptable long-term functional result when the pouch can be maintained in its functional in situ state. The inappropriate and ill-advised creation of an IPAA in patients with Crohn's disease should diminish as the importance of pathologic distinction of Crohn's disease from ulcerative colitis is emphasized in the initial medical management of patients with IBD.

The confirmation of intestinal atresia as a consequence of an in utero vascular accident is credited to Leuw and Bernard in 1955. However, intussusception is an extremely uncommon physiologic state among premature infants. The symptoms of intussusception are quite difficult to recognize because they share symptoms common to both entities: vomiting, abdominal distension, and gastrointestinal hemorrhage. Moreover, the distinction between necrotizing enterocolitis, sepsis, and intussusception in premature infants is difficult and may cause a delay in diagnosis. Puvabanditsin and associates (Abstract 10–26) of the departments of pediatrics and surgery, University of Medicine and Dentistry of New Jersey, Newark, and the Department of Pediatrics, Jersey City Medical Center, New Jersey, report the presence of postnatal intussusception in a premature infant of 26 weeks' gestation. This appears to be the first case in which a postnatal vascular accident initiated an atretic intestinal segment.

Recurrent abdominal pain in infants and children can be perplexing and obfuscate a definitive diagnosis. Moreover, extensive radiologic evaluation of these children with recurrent pain is rarely diagnostic and only infrequently cost-effective. Stylianos and associates (**Abstract 10–27**) from the Division of Pediatric Surgery, Babies and Childrens Hospital of New York, Department of Surgery at Columbia University College of Physicians and Surgeons, New York City, sought to define the role of laparoscopy for the evaluation of children with recurrent abdominal pain. The authors emphasize that laparoscopy is an accurate technique for the evaluation and treatment of children with the disorder. Early laparoscopic intervention may provide economic benefit by the elimination of inappropriate, cost-ineffective, and low-yield studies initiated with radiologic imaging. It is highly probable that minimally invasive approaches in children will gain increasing application and efficacy as the technique is used more frequently.

The final abstract in this section is included as an important contribution to the understanding and prevention of postsurgical adhesion formation; the contributions of laboratories to advance techniques to inhibit serosal tissue damage with ultimate progression to fibroblast accumulation and adhesions are emphasized. **Abstract 10–28** by Burns et al. of the Biopolymers Department, Genzyme Corporation, Cambridge, Massachusetts, the Tufts School of Veterinary Medicine, Boston, and the Biomedical Engineering Center, University of Florida, Gainesville, examined the effects of hyaluronic acid (HA) on tissue precoating to prevent adhesions in a rat cecal abrasion model. The authors conducted an efficacy study at 3 independent study sites with 3 identical HA concentrations. In addition, tissue precoating with the solution was investigated by histologic parameters before gauze abrasion and desiccation. The HA solutions significantly inhibited serosal tissue damage and ameliorated the inflammatory response to abrasion and desiccation. Tissue precoating with dilute solutions of hyaluronic acid diminished damage to serosal tissue during surgery, thereby limiting the formation and progression of adhesions in the postsurgical state. These important concepts have recently been introduced into prospectively randomized clinical trials, the results of which are forthcoming.

Kirby I. Bland, M.D.

Early Outcome After Open Versus Extraperitoneal Endoscopic Tension-free Hernioplasty: A Randomized Clinical Trial

Wright DM, Kennedy A, Baxter JN, et al (Univ of Aberdeen, Scotland; Glasgow Royal Infirmary Univ NHS Trust, Scotland; Southern Gen Hosp NHS Trust, Glasgow, Scotland)

Surgery 119:552–557, 1996 10–19

Background.—Minimal access surgery is now used in most general surgical procedures. Cholecystectomy is still the only operation, however, for which minimal access has been shown to have clear advantages over open surgery. The use of minimal access surgery in patients who have inguinal hernias is controversial. Endoscopic tension-free hernia repair (preperitoneal approach) was compared with open tension-free hernia repair.

Methods.—One hundred twenty patients were enrolled by 3 Glasgow hospitals in the randomized clinical trial. Four surgeons performed the operations during 1 year. Intention to treat analysis was applied to determine early outcome measures.

Findings.—Patients who underwent endoscopic hernia repair had significantly lower median postoperative pain scores and analgesia requirements than did those who underwent open hernia repair. Those who had endoscopic hernia repair also had a significantly shorter hospital stay. Patients who underwent open hernia repair had wound complications significantly more often. There were no between-group differences in pulmonary function or metabolic responses to trauma.

Conclusions.—Postoperative pain and morbidity were significantly reduced by extraperitoneal endoscopic tension-free hernia repair compared with the open procedure. Larger trials are currently being conducted to assess recurrence rates after both procedures.

► Minimal access surgery has expanded to encompass most procedures performed by general surgeons. Laparoscopic cholecystectomy has been well accepted. Numerous reports on laparoscopic hernia repair, appendectomy, pancreatectomy, aortic surgery, gastrectomy, and splenectomy have been published in the past year. Prospective evaluation of these procedures, however, is lacking. The authors have compared open vs. endoscopic tension-free hernioplasty in a group of 120 patients. The strength of the paper is that similar repairs (i.e., tension-free) were used. Previous reports have usually compared endoscopic tension-free with open "tension" repairs. Although the short-term advantages of decreased pain and a decrease in wound complications are desirable, no data are provided concerning return to work and resumption of normal activities. Most importantly, longer follow-up studies will be required to establish the relative merits of endoscopic tension-free hernioplasty, especially concerning recurrence rates.

W.G. Cioffi, M.D.

Long-term Pulmonary Sequelae in Survivors of Congenital Diaphragmatic Defects

Vanamo K, Rintala R, Sovijärvi A, et al (Meilahti Hosp, Helsinki; Univ of Helsinki)

J Pediatr Surg 31:1096–1100, 1996 10–20

Introduction.—Reports indicate that children who survive congenital diaphragmatic defect usually do well but may have reduced lung capacity as adults. Lung volumes, ventilatory and diffusing capacity, and regional lung function were assessed in adults who had undergone diaphragmatic defect repair during childhood.

Methods.—Of 164 children with congenital diaphragmatic hernia or eventration who underwent repair between 1948 and 1980, 107 survived. Questionnaires were mailed to 98 survivors who could be located and 60 were evaluated for long-term follow-up. Mean patient age at follow-up was 29.6 years (range, 14–49 years). Twenty-one patients with diaphragmatic defects with areas devoid of muscle and consisting of fibrous tissue only were considered to have eventrations. Thirty-five patients who had defects with well-defined borders and 4 patients with only a thin peritoneum-like covering were considered to have hernias. All patients underwent a detailed medical history, physical examination, anteroposterior and lateral chest radiographs, spirometry, diffusing capacity measurement, and diffusing capacity for carbon monoxide measurement. A more detailed pulmonary evaluation with body plethysmography, radiospirometry, and testing for bronchial hyperreactivity was performed in 27 patients.

Results.—Eighty-three percent of patients considered themselves healthy and 70% were engaged in sports. Seven patients (12%) had asthma, 4 (7%) had more than 1 respiratory infection every 6 months, 7 (12%) had occasional pain in the region of the incision during lifting, bending, and similar activities. Twenty-nine patients (48%) had a clinically asymmetric chest, 11 had a pectus excavatum deformity, and 1 patient had a pectus carinatum deformity. There was a radiolucent area on chest radiograph in 26 patients (43%), and it was more common on the side of the defect (19 patients—32%). Sixteen patients (27%) had significant radiologic scoliosis. Twenty-nine patients (48%) had normal spirometric and diffusing capacity. Abnormal findings included the following: 9 (15%) obstructive ventilatory impairment, 7 (12%) restrictive impairment, and 15 (25%) had both. Restrictive ventilatory impairment was more common in patients with eventration, those who underwent transthoracic diaphragmatic repair, and those with a diaphragmatic defect large enough to include the liver in the defect. Restrictive findings increased with age. Patients with large diaphragmatic defects and postoperative complications and pneumothorax were more likely to have combined ventilatory impairment. Patients with eventration were more likely to have restrictive findings and patients with hernia were more likely to have obstructive findings (Table 2). Nine of 26 patients (35%) tested had bronchial hyperreactivity, which was mild in 7, moderate in 1, and severe in 1. One of 9 patients with bronchial hyperreactivity had

TABLE 2.—Spirometric and Diffusing Capacity Results for 60 Survivors of Congenital Diaphragmatic Defects

	No. of Patients (%)		
	Hernia	Eventration	All Patients
Normal	19 (49)	10 (48)	29 (48)
Obstructive	8 (21)	1 (5)	9 (15)
Restrictive	1 (3)	6 (29)	7 (12)
Obstructive and restrictive	11 (28)	4 (19)	15 (25)
Total	39	21	60

(Courtesy of Vanamo K, Rintala R, Sovijärvi A: Long-term pulmonary sequelae in survivors of congenital diaphragmatic defects. *J Pediatr Surg* 31:1096–1100, 1996.)

previously diagnosed asthma. Bronchial hyperreactivity was significantly more frequent in children considered high risk. In 12 (44%) and 15 (58%) patients, respectively, ventilation and perfusion on the ipsilateral lung was below the −2-SD limit. Reduced perfusion of the ipsilateral lung was correlated with the presence of prenatal risk factors. The mean perfusion and ventilation of the ipsilateral lung was markedly lower in patients with left-sided defects, compared to patients with right-sided defects, whose findings were normal (Table 3).

Discussion/Conclusion.—Long-term follow-up in this cohort of patients followed from childhood to adulthood indicated obstructive or restrictive ventilatory impairment in 52%. Both obstructive and restrictive impairment was found in 25% of patients. Findings correlated with later pulmonary dysfunction and not disturbance in gas exchange at the level of the alveolar membrane. It may be that these patients experienced persistently reduced lung parenchyma and air trapping in the small airways with secondary airway obstruction. The finding of bronchial hyperreactivity was not expected. There was a slightly higher prevalence of asthma in this cohort, compared to the general population (6% vs. 12%). Few patients with abnormal lung function had clinical symptoms, reflecting the reserve

TABLE 3.—Percentage Share (Mean ± SD) of Ventilation (n = 27), Perfusion (n = 26), and Lung Volumes (n = 27) of the Ipsilateral Lung Assessed With ^{133}Xe Radiospirometry in Survivors of Congenital Diaphragmatic Defects

	Side of Defect		
	Right	Left	All
Ventilation (%)	53.5 ± 2.2	43.3 ± 4.4*	44.8 ± 5.7
Perfusion (%)	49.7 ± 2.8	40.3 ± 5.2*	41.8 ± 5.9*
Vital capacity (%)	48.5 ± 4.1	45.1 ± 2.7	45.8 ± 3.1
Total lung capacity (%)	51.6 ± 3.4	45.8 ± 2.8	46.7 ± 3.5
Ventilation: Perfusion ratio	1.077 ± 0.087	1.087 ± 0.152	1.081 ± 0.143

*Mean value > 2 SD below predicted value.

(Courtesy of Vanamo K, Rintala R, Sovijärvi A: Long-term pulmonary sequelae in survivors of congenital diaphragmatic defects. *J Pediatr Surg* 31:1096–1100, 1996.)

capacity of the lung. The increasing incidence of restrictive impairment with age and the high prevalence of bronchial hyperreactivity suggest a possibly progressive problem that warrants ongoing evaluation in patients who have undergone congenital diaphragmatic repair.

Long-term Gastrointestinal Morbidity in Patients With Congenital Diaphragmatic Defects

Vanamo K, Rintala RJ, Lindahl H, et al (Univ of Helsinki)

J Pediatr Surg 31:551–554, 1996 10–21

Background.—Because pulmonary hypoplasia is an important indicator of survival in patients with congenital diaphragmatic defects, many long-term studies have focused on lung function. There has been a recent report of a patient with high-risk congenital diaphragmatic hernia who experienced severe gastrointestinal morbidity related to esophageal dilatation and early gastroesophageal reflux. Gastrointestinal morbidity in adults after repair of congenital diaphragmatic defects was investigated.

Methods.—A questionnaire was mailed to 60 patients who had undergone surgery for congenital diaphragmatic hernia. A follow-up examination was conducted. The mean patient age at follow-up was 29.6 years. The information obtained included medical history and current symptoms. Symptoms that indicated gastroesophageal reflux were classified as typical, atypical, or alarm symptoms. Gastrointestinal endoscopy was performed in 41 patients. Biopsy specimens were obtained from the duodenum, the antrum and corpus of the stomach, and the esophagus. Histologic esophagitis, duodenitis, and gastritis were graded from 0 to 3. Assays of *Helicobacter pylori* were performed on biopsy specimens from the stomach.

Results.—Patient characteristics were tabulated (Table 1). Early postoperative gastroesophageal reflux was recorded in 11 of the 60 patients. The diagnosis was based on history and current symptoms in 7 patients, radiology in 2 patients, and endoscopy in 2 patients. Patients with respiratory distress and who were symptomatic within 6 hours after birth had a higher rate of gastroesophageal reflux. Patients with symptomatic gastroesophageal reflux also had longer ventilatory support, postoperative intolerance to enteral feeding, and hospital stay. Twelve patients had intestinal obstruction and were hospitalized. Ten of the 12 patients had prior transabdominal repair of the diaphragmatic defect, and 2 had prior transthoracic repair. In 8 of the 12 patients, the obstruction was treated surgically from 1 month to 20 years after initial operation. At follow-up, 38 patients had symptoms indicative of gastroesophageal reflux. Twelve of the 41 patients who had endoscopy had macroscopic esophageal pathologic conditions (Table 3): 8 had grade 1 esophagitis, 4 had Barrett's esophagus. Also, 30 patients had a hiatal hernia. Ten patients had grade 1 histologic esophagitis, 2 patients had grade 2, and 1 patient had grade 3. Gastric metaplasia was found in 2 patients, and metaplasia and grade 1 esophagitis were found in 1 patient. The overall prevalence of esophagitis

TABLE 1.—Patient Characteristics

	Available for Study	Patients With Endoscopy	All Survivors
Patients	60	41	107
Diaphragmatic hernia (%)	39 (65)	28 (68)	70 (65)
Eventration (%)	21 (35)	13 (32)	37 (35)
Males (%)	31 (52)	20 (49)	59 (55)
Duration of pregnancy wk ± SD	39.3 ± 2.3	39.2 ± 2.5	39.5 ± 2.1
Birth weight (g) ± SD	3341 ± 542	3400 ± 562	3324 ± 588
Mean Apgar at 1 min ± SD	6.8 ± 2.6	6.25 ± 3.0	7.3 ± 2.4
Associated anamolies (%)	16 (27)	12 (30)	26 (24)
Symptomatic at <6 h of age (%)	27 (45)	21 (51)	48 (45)
Left-sided defect (%)	48 (80)	32 (78)	84 (79)
Large defect (intrathoracic liver) (%)	14 (23)	10 (24)	25 (23)

(Courtesy of Vanamo K, Rintala RJ, Lindahl H, et al: Long-term gastrointestinal morbidity in patients with congenital diaphragmatic defects. *J Pediatr Surg* 31:551–554, 1996.)

was 54%. There was poor correlation between current symptoms and esophagitis. Histologic examination revealed gastritis in 14 of the 41 patients, and all 14 were positive for *H. pylori.*

Discussion.—Gastroesophageal reflux occurs in the first year of life in 20% to 84% of patients with congenital diaphragmatic hernia. High-risk patients with congenital diaphragmatic hernia have the highest rate of gastroesophageal reflux. Gastroesophageal reflux is often associated with esophageal dilatation seen in many high-risk patients with congenital diaphragmatic hernia. Many of the patients in this study reported symptoms indicative of gastroesophageal reflux, but these symptoms had poor predictive value for esophagitis. More than 50% of patients had evidence of esophagitis revealed by endoscopy or histology. The estimated incidence is only 2% in the general population and 56% in patients with ulcer symptoms. There is substantial long-term gastrointestinal morbidity in

TABLE 3.—Endoscopic and Histologic Findings in 41 Patients Who Had Upper Gastrointestinal Endoscopy

	No. of Patients (%)
Hiatus hernia	30 (73)
Esophageal pathology	22 (54)
Esophagitis	17 (41)
Barrett's esophagus	5 (13)
Gastritis	14 (34)*
Duodenitis	4 (10)
No esophageal pathology	19 (46)
No esophageal, gastric, or duodenal pathology	11 (27)

*All were positive for *Helicobacter pylori.*

(Courtesy of Vanamo K, Rintala RJ, Lindahl H, et al: Long-term gastrointestinal morbidity in patients with congenital diaphragmatic defects. *J Pediatr Surg* 31:551–554, 1996.)

patients with congenital diaphragmatic defects, largely arising from chronic esophagitis and late intestinal obstruction. Because of the high rate of esophagitis and Barrett's esophagus seen in these patients, it is recommended that follow up studies of patients with congenital diaphragmatic defects include routine examination for gastroesophageal reflux.

▶ Many years ago, Michael Harrison[1] coined the term "hidden mortality" to describe the overly enthusiastic prognosis of diaphragmatic hernia: infants who died before they reached the pediatric surgeon never made it into those statistics. By analogy, "hidden morbidity" of congenital diaphragmatic hernia was later described as well, contradicting the common belief that, if a child with diaphragmatic hernia survived infancy, the child was otherwise completely normal. According to the darkest view, these children were looking at a miserable life of pulmonary and other sequelae and complications. Here, now, is a well-designed, long-term, follow-up study giving a slightly more optimistic, and one hopes, realistic view. This is one of the first such studies available, since routine survival of infants with diaphragmatic hernia is less than 50 years old.

The authors are to be congratulated for obtaining an 85% response rate 30 years later, and convincing 60% of the patients to undergo follow-up studies (including upper endoscopy)! In addition, Drs. Lindahl and Louhima and their group have documented that the responders do not differ from the overall group in terms of perinatal parameters, justifying the extrapolation of their conclusions to all their patients. Their results are reassuring, in a way. The vast majority of patients felt healthy, and a good number of them engaged in sports. Surprisingly, 35% of them had bronchial hyperreactivity (a few had frank asthma), and 12% had restrictive airway disease, which seemed to worsen with age. Not surprisingly, a large hernia, immediate postnatal distress, and a complicated course were all associated with poorer pulmonary function. Symptoms of gastroesophageal reflux were reported by 63% of the respondents; however, a similar prevalence was found among the normal Finnish population. More alarming was the fact that, regardless of the presence or absence of symptoms, 54% of the patients who agreed to undergo endoscopy had esophagitis, and 4 (of 41, or 10%!) had Barrett's esophagus. The authors conclude, correctly, that surveillance in adult life is important to identify occult esophageal and pulmonary sequelae with potentially far-reaching implications.

F.I. Luks, M.D.

Reference

1. Harrison MR, Bjordal RI, Landmark, et al: Congenital diaphragmatic hernia: The hidden mortality. *J Pediatr Surg* 13:227–231, 1979.

Prenatal Diagnosis of Abdominal Wall Defects and Their Prognosis
Kamata S, Ishikawa S, Usui N, et al (Osaka Univ, Japan)
J Pediatr Surg 31:267–271, 1996 10–22

Introduction.—The outcome for fetuses with abdominal wall defects appears to be worse when associated anomalies are present. Records of 43 fetuses who were evaluated with ultrasound were reviewed to determine whether associated anatomic features are of value in predicting fetal prognosis.

Methods.—The 43 cases studied had undergone prenatal evaluation from 1982 through 1994. Excluded were cases associated with conjoined twins, severe brain damage, hypoplastic left heart syndrome, obstructive uropathy, and severe chromosomal abnormality. Infants with an exposed liver underwent staged repair immediately after delivery by cesarean section at 36 or 37 weeks' gestation. Those without liver herniation (small omphalocele and gastroschisis) underwent vaginal delivery and direct repair. Since 1987, high-frequency oscillatory ventilation has been used in patients with an $AaDO_2$ of more than 500 mm Hg.

Results.—Thirty-one fetuses had omphalocele and 12 had gastroschisis. Of those with omphalocele detected at US, 12 had giant omphalocele, 12 had small omphalocele, and 7 had ruptured omphalocele. Initial diagnosis of abdominal wall defects had been made at a mean of 29.9 weeks' gestation. Thirty of the fetuses survived and 13 died; included among the deaths was one stillborn case and one with fetal death. There were 15 cases of uncontrolled preterm labor. Birth weight was significantly lower among infants with ruptured omphalocele compared with those with giant or small omphalocele, and only 1 fetus with ruptured omphalocele survived. Associated anomalies were present in 24 infants; 10 did not survive (Table 6). Severe neonatal complications occurred in 9 patients, and 7 of these infants died. The infants with ruptured omphalocele died of pulmonary hypoplasia and respiratory insufficiency; 3 had polyhydramnios, 4 had scoliosis, and 1 had no covering membrane.

Discussion.—Although most infants with abdominal wall defects now survive, spine deformity and the rupture or absence of a covering mem-

TABLE 6.—Associated Anomalies and Prognoses

Diagnosis	Isolated (Death)	Associated Anomalies (Death)
Omphalocele		
Ruptured	2 (1)	5 (5*)
Giant	6 (1)	6 (1)
Small	2 (0)	10 (3)
Gastroschisis	10 (1)	2 (1†)
Total	20 (3)	23 (10*†‡)

*A stillborn case was included.
†A case with fetal death was included.
‡$P < 0.05$ compared with the values for isolated cases.
(Courtesy of Kamata S, Ishikawa S, Usui N, et al: Prenatal diagnosis of abdominal wall defects and their prognosis. *J Pediatr Surg* 31:267–271, 1996.)

brane with an exposed liver are associated with poor prognosis because of pulmonary hypoplasia. Despite advanced respiratory care, few fetuses with ruptured omphalocele will survive. Anomalies found at autopsy in these cases of ruptured omphalocele included scoliosis, diaphragmatic defects, vesicointestinal fissure, unilateral renal agenesis, and spina bifida.

▶ Although an abdominal wall defect is 1 of the most commonly diagnosed surgical anomalies of the fetus, it is still not clear whether advance knowledge of the condition has helped the management and outcome of babies so afflicted. Current controversies over antenatal intervention center around the benefit of early delivery for gastroschisis and ruptured omphalocele (to reduce the caustic effect of amniotic fluid on the exposed viscera) and the termination of pregnancy if omphalocele, rather than gastroschisis, is suspected, because the former is more often associated with other anomalies. The present review cautions against such a simplistic view, only ruptured omphalocele in the presence of severe scoliosis (all 4 of which were picked up antenatally) was associated with a high mortality. Outcome for all other forms of abdominal wall defects, gastroschisis and omphalocele alike, was more favorable. When future parents are counseled, the true nature of the abdominal wall defect seems therefore less important than the presence of detectable associated anomalies.

F.I. Luks, M.D.

Serial Transabdominal Amnioinfusion in the Management of Gastroschisis With Severe Oligohydramnios

Dommergues M, Ansker Y, Aubry MC, et al (Hôpital Necker Enfants Malades, Paris)

J Pediatr Surg 31:1297–1299, 1996 10–23

Introduction.—Oligohydramnios complicates gastroschisis in about 25% of pregnancies. The oligohydramnios can be severe enough to put the fetus at risk for pulmonary hypoplasia, limb deformities, and fetal distress secondary to cord compression. Two patients with severe oligohydramnios associated with gastroschisis were treated via serial transabdominal amnioinfusions of saline.

Case Report 1.—Woman, 19, gravida 1, was referred at 19 weeks after gastroschisis was detected on routine ultrasonography. At 27 weeks' gestation, the intra-abdominal and extra-abdominal bowel loops were moderately dilated. There was no mural thickness or modification of the bowel content. Oligohydramnios was moderate at this time. Follow-up ultrasound examination at 30.5 weeks revealed severe oligohydramnios. Under ultrasound guidance, the patient received a transabdominal amnioinfusion of 500 mL of warm saline. This was repeated at weeks 34 and 35 with 350 mL, as weekly sonograms revealed a progressive decrease in amniotic fluid volume. The amniotic fluid volume was normal at 36 weeks' gestation. The membranes ruptured prematurely at 36 weeks and a 2,450-g girl was delivered by cesarean section 2 days later. The baby's exterior bowel was normal morphologically and there was no bowel thickening or fibrous peel. A primary closure was performed on day 1 and the postoperative course was uneventful.

Case Report 2.—Woman 23, primigravida, was referred at 19 weeks' gestation because of fetal gastroschisis. The amniotic fluid was normal at this time. There was moderate oligohydramnios at 27.5 weeks. Severe oligohydramnios was diagnosed at 31.5 weeks. A transabdominal amnioinfusion of 400 mL of warm saline was administered at 32 weeks and repeated whenever severe oligohydramnios was detected. A total of 3,400 mL of saline was infused from weeks 32 to 36. The membranes ruptured prematurely at 36.5 weeks and a 2,360-g boy was delivered by cesarean section. There was no bowel thickening and a very moderate fibrous peel, and primary closure was performed on day 1.

Discussion/Conclusion.—Even in the presence of prenatal diagnosis of gastroschisis and immediate appropriate neonatal care, serious postoperative morbidity can occur, possibly subsequent to bowel damage in utero. Although oligohydramnios occurs in nearly 25% of pregnancies, there are no adverse consequences when it is moderate. It is potentially harmful when it is severe, even during the third trimester. Serial transabdominal amnioinfusions are feasible and allow pregnancy to be prolonged to 36 weeks' gestation. Neither neonate experienced adverse consequences of prolonged oligohydramnios exposure, suggesting the efficacy of serial amnioinfusion. It may be that the amnioinfusions precipitated premature labor, but this has to be weighed against the possible benefit of premature cesarean section providing a positive effect on the neonatal bowel. If the theory is that prolonged exposure of the gastroschisis to amniotic fluid is detrimental, then the lack of natural amniotic fluid and its replacement with saline would be a favorable approach. At this time, the experience with serial transabdominal amnioinfusion as treatment for gastroschisis with severe oligohydramnios is too limited to reach conclusions, but this approach may be beneficial in selected patients.

► An ever-increasing percentage of infants with abdominal wall defects are diagnosed antenatally, raising the possibility of intervention in utero. However, more than a decade of animal and clinical research has not changed the notion that these conditions are best treated after birth. Awareness of the condition has allowed a more planned delivery, preferably, close to a tertiary pediatric surgery/neonatology center, to minimize infant transport. Yet mode of delivery (vaginal or by cesarean section) has not influenced outcome, and, contrary to what the authors suggest here, neither has the timing of delivery. It was once believed that early induction of labor (as soon as the fetal lungs were mature enough, i.e., around 35–36 weeks) would prevent the prolonged contact of exposed bowel to the causticity of late-gestational amniotic fluid. More recent experience (both in animals and in human beings) has failed to substantiate that claim, and we have seen infants with gastroschisis born at 40 and 42 weeks with completely normal-appearing intestines. In view of this, the authors' speculation that "exchange" amnioinfusion to dilute amniotic fluid may decrease the risk of intestinal damage, seems unfounded. Still, this group has had a long-standing interest and expertise in antenatal intervention and is to be commended for their results in these 2 patients. After all, the goal of fetal "surgery" is rarely to cure the patient, but to optimize him or her for definitive, postnatal treatment.

F.I. Luks, M.D.

Reoperative Rates for Crohn's Disease Following Strictureplasty: Long-term Analysis

Ozuner G, Fazio VW, Lavery IC, et al (Cleveland Clinic Found, Ohio)
Dis Colon Rectum 39:1199–1203, 1996 10–24

Background.—More than half of patients with Crohn's disease will require surgery to resect gross disease. Moreover, the 10-year reoperative recurrence rate is 30% to 53%. The reoperative rates after strictureplasty, an alternative to intestinal resection, is unknown. A report of resection rates at 1 institution after strictureplasty and a comparison of reoperative rates in patients with strictureplasty alone vs. patients with resective procedures in addition to strictureplasty are presented.

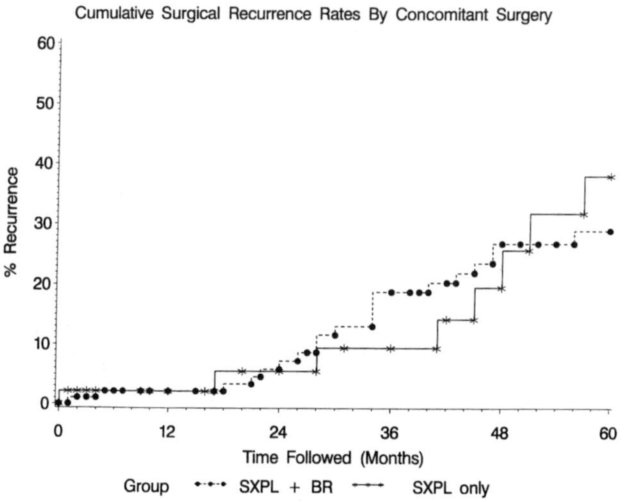

FIGURE 2.—Cumulative surgical recurrence rates by concomitant surgery. *Abbreviations, SXPL*, stricture; *BR*, bowel resection. (Courtesy of Ozuner G, Fazio VW, Lavery IC, et al: Reoperative rates for Crohn's disease following strictureplasty. *Dis Colon Rectum* 39(11):1199–1203, 1996.)

Methods.—A retrospective analysis was performed on 162 patients (87 men), average age, 36 years, with Crohn's disease who had 698 strictureplasties between June 1984 and July 1994. There were 52 patients with strictureplasty alone (group A) and 110 with strictureplasty plus resection (group B). Reoperative rates were compared statistically.

Results.—Patients had an average of 3 strictureplasties, and average duration of disease was 13 years. There were no deaths. The median hospital stay was 8 days. Eight patients had septic complications. Patients were studied for an average of 42 months. Surgery relieved obstructive symptoms in 159 patients. After 6 months, 136 patients rated their symptomatic relief as significant or marked, 23 as moderate, 2 as minimum or unchanged, and 1 as worsened. The reoperation rate for all patients at 5 years was 22%, for patients with strictureplasty only, 20.4%; for patients with additional resection, 24.3%. Most recurrences were at new sites. The cumulative 5-year recurrence was highest in group A, although there was no statistical difference between groups (Fig 2).

Conclusion.—Reoperative rates after strictureplasty for Crohn's disease are similar to those after resection and strictures usually occur at new sites. Strictureplasty is a safe and effective operation in selected patients and has a low complication rate.

► This report is a comprehensive review of the 10-year experience in strictureplasty for Crohn's disease from the institution that has the greatest experience in this area. Several important points can be made from the data presented in this paper. Obviously, strictureplasty has obviated the need for extensive small bowel resections and thereby decreased the incidence of short gut syndrome in patients with Crohn's disease. The issue of negative resection margins for Crohn's is obviously a debate of the past, inasmuch as the excellent success rate for strictureplasty has demonstrated the healing ability of macroscopically involved tissue.

The complication rate (leak, fistula, abscess) was limited to 5% in these 162 patients who underwent a total of 698 strictureplasties. This result demonstrates a minimal tendency to fistula formation, even in the presence of suture-line disease in the small intestine. Of further interest is the finding that the addition of bowel resection to strictureplasty did not increase the need for reoperative surgery over strictureplasty alone, at a minimum of 5-year follow-up, as demonstrated in Figure 2.

Strictureplasty can definitely be considered a very safe procedure and represents an excellent alternative to bowel resection for suitable Crohn's disease lesions of the small bowel. The incidence of recurrent symptomatic disease may also be affected by maintenance medical management, which, unfortunately, was not addressed in this review.

V.E. Pricolo, M.D.

Long-term Results of Ileal Pouch-Anal Anastomosis in Patients With Crohn's Disease

Sagar PM, Dozois RR, Wolff BG (Mayo Clinic and Mayo Found, Rochester, Minn)

Dis Colon Rectum 39:893–898, 1996 10–25

Introduction.—Ileal pouch-anal anastomosis (IPAA) is widely accepted as the surgical gold standard for most patients with chronic ulcerative colitis. The IPAA procedure is contraindicated in patients with Crohn's disease because of the risk of recurrence of disease within the ileal reservoir and subsequent fistulas, stricture, suture line failure, and abscess formation. Even with the entire specimen of colon and rectum, the pathologist may have difficulty distinguishing between chronic ulcerative colitis and Crohn's disease. Thus, some patients with Crohn's disease inadvertently undergo IPAA. Reported are clinical and functional outcomes of IPAA in 37 such patients.

Methods.—Of 1,705 patients who underwent IPAA at Mayo Clinic from 1981 through October 1995, 1,509 had inflammatory bowel disease. Thirty-seven patients (2.5% of patients with inflammatory bowel disease) eventually received a diagnosis of Crohn's disease. Clinical suspicion of Crohn's disease was not sufficient for diagnosis. Histologic examination was necessary for confirmation of disease. All 37 patients with Crohn's disease underwent mucosectomy with handsewn IPAA. Of those, 35 were J-pouch procedures and 1 each was a W-pouch and an S-pouch.

Results.—Eleven patients with Crohn's disease who underwent IPAA had complex fistulas at a median of 29 months after surgery. Six fistulas were pouch-cutaneous, 4 were pouch-vaginal, and 1 was pouch-vesical. The sites of recurrent Crohn's disease in these patients were: 20 in the pouch, 4 in the anal canal alone, 10 in both pouch and anal canal, 2 in small bowel proximal to the pouch, and 1 in the duodenum. At 10 years, the pouch remained in situ in 20 patients (55%), but defunctionalized in 7 patients. It was excised in 10 patients. The overall failure rate was 45% in this cohort.

Conclusion.—The rate of failure of the pouch after IPAA in patients with unsuspected Crohn's disease at the time of operation was 45%. The functional result in patients who retained the pouch was acceptable.

▶ This interesting review, from the institution that has performed the largest number of ileal pouch-anal anastomoses in the world, addresses the complex issue of performing such a procedure in patients with Crohn's disease. The results can prompt the reviewer to look at the glass as either half full or half empty. In fact, the pouch failure rate in IPAA procedures inadvertently performed for Crohn's disease is as high as 45%. However, in more than 50% of the patients, the pelvic pouch can be kept in place with acceptable long-term results.

Although most surgeons agree that these results in procedures that were inadvertently performed are interesting, the real question is, "Should patients with known Crohn's disease limited to the large intestine be considered for restorative proctocolectomy with ileal-pouch-anal anastomosis?" It has been postulated by some centers that in a certain percentage of cases, the disease may be limited to the large intestine and the risk of recurrence of Crohn's disease in the small intestine (and, therefore, in the pelvic pouch) should be rather limited, provided that the patients had only large intestinal disease for more than 10 years. Alternatively, the patient may choose to accept a 45% to 50% risk of losing the pelvic pouch and ending up with a permanent ileostomy, if a medically intractable Crohn's pouchitis were to develop, in exchange for a few years of ileostomy-free, improved quality of life with acceptable fecal continence.

The implication of this study may be that restorative proctocolectomy may be considered in highly selected patients with Crohn's disease if the patients are willing to accept such a high failure rate.

V.E. Pricolo, M.D.

Postnatal Intussusception in a Premature Infant, Causing Jejunal Atresia

Puvabanditsin S, Garrow E, Samransamraujkit R, et al (Univ of Medicine and Dentistry of New Jersey, Newark; Jersey City Med Ctr, NJ)
J Pediatr Surg 31:711–712, 1996 10–26

Introduction.—Intussusception is uncommon in the neonatal period and is even rarer in preterm infants. Intussusception in preterm infants is usually associated with a meconium plug and necrotizing enterocolitis (NEC). Ileal atresia has been reported in association with in utero intussusception, but jejunal atresia secondary to intussusception has not yet been reported. Thus, the first known case of jejunal atresia caused by postnatal intussusception is reported in a premature infant.

Case Report.—Male infant, born at 26 weeks' gestation and weighing 690 g, began gavage feedings on the fifth day of life. He had 3 stools daily. On the eighteenth day of life, his feeding was stopped because of increased gastric residual and bilious gastric aspirates. One week later, sepsis developed and he was treated with vancomycin. After treatment for sepsis, a dark brown mucoid plug, then greenish black stool was noted. Radiographs performed at 5 weeks of age indicated intestinal obstruction. An exploratory laparotomy was performed and a proximal jejunal atresia was observed. There was a 10-cm intussusception distal to the atresia and a 1-cm gap in the mesentery of the jejunum. No significant adhesions were identified that could be associated with NEC. The patient did well after surgery and gavage feedings were well tolerated 5 days after surgery. Pathologic examination revealed an intussusceptum segment within the distal jejunum. There was a blind end on the proximal atretic jejunum.

Discussion/Conclusion.—Historically, it was suspected that intestinal atresia may be secondary to prolonged bowel ischemia in utero and that was confirmed in 1955 by Louw and Barnard. They were able to produce intestinal atresia in utero in 2 puppies by ligating the mesenteric vessels that supplied a bowel segment. Surgical and pathologic findings are presented here in the first known case of postnatal intussusception that caused jejunal atresia in an infant born at 26 weeks' gestation.

▶ Ever since Hendrik Louw and Christian Barnard[1] reproduced intestinal atresia by causing an in utero vascular accident, it has been well recognized that the fetus has the ability to completely, and scarlessly, reabsorb necrotic tissue. In fact, at least some cases of small bowel atresia are believed to have been caused by antenatal intussusception and subsequent necrosis of the intussusceptum. A 26-week-gestation premature infant is, in some ways, still a fetus, and may exhibit the wound-healing properties of a (late gestational) fetus. This is a well-recognized phenomenon, as any pediatric surgeon may attest. The present case appears to be the first instance in which a postnatal vascular accident caused intestinal atresia—acquired intestinal atresia, as it were.

F.I. Luks, M.D.

Reference

1. Louw JH, Barnard C: Congenital atresia, *Lancet* 2:1065–1067, 1955.

Laparoscopy for Diagnosis and Treatment of Recurrent Abdominal Pain in Children

Stylianos S, Stein JE, Flanigan LM, et al (Babies & Children's Hosp of New York; Columbia Univ, New York)

J Pediatr Surg 31:1158–1160, 1996 10–27

Introduction.—Recurrent abdominal pain (RAP) can be perplexing to diagnose in children. Children with RAP usually undergo extensive radiographic evaluation, which often is not diagnostic or cost-effective. The possible role of laparoscopy in children with RAP as a tool to expedite evaluation and therapy was explored.

Methods.—Fifteen children with RAP were referred for surgical consultation. The mean age of 13 females and 2 males was 12 years. The mean duration of symptoms was 11 months. The abdominal pain was localized to the right lower quadrant in 9 children and was midabdominal in 6 children. All patients had normal white blood cell counts and temperatures. These patients underwent 38 imaging studies (excluding plain films) before laparoscopy: 19 abdominal sonograms, 9 upper gastrointestinal (GI) series, 4 abdominal CT scans, 3 barium enemas, 2 isotope scans, and 1 MRI of the head. Two of these studies (5%) provided a definitive diagnosis: 1 Meckel's diverticulum was detected on upper GI series with small bowel follow-through, and a urachal cyst was suggested on ultrasonographic examination. All patients were evaluated and treated by laparoscopy.

Results.—Thirteen patients underwent laparoscopic appendectomy. The remaining 2 patients had already undergone open appendectomy. Eleven of 15 patients (87%) had positive findings that were diagnosed by laparoscopy: 8 appendiceal abnormalities in 6 children (4 lymphoid hyperplasia, 2 chronic inflammation, and 2 inspissated fecaliths), 3 Meckel's diverticula, 1 inguinal hernia, and 1 adhesion from a previous appendectomy stump. The mean follow-up was 14 months. Symptoms were immediately resolved subsequent to laparoscopy in 8 of 11 children (73%). Symptoms resolved in 3 of 4 children with normal laparoscopic and histologic findings.

Discussion/Conclusion.—Because the natural history of RAP suggests symptoms remit spontaneously in 30% to 50% of children within 6 weeks of evaluation, the initial management of RAP may need to be conservative: dietary manipulations, antacids, antispasmodics, and reassurance of the family. The surgical treatment of RAP has historically been limited to open appendectomy, using right lower quadrant incisions after multiple imaging studies fail to indicate a cause. Schisgall reported inspissated casts in 73% of 70 children who underwent appendectomy for RAP and theorized that appendiceal "colic" resulting from inspissated fecal material leads to intermittent obstruction and distention of the appendix, thus an important cause of RAP. This theory has met resistance. Laparoscopic examination for RAP allows visualization of abdominal and pelvic structures that is superior to imaging and standard open appendectomy incision. In this patient cohort, positive findings were detected in 73% of laparoscopic procedures and 5% of imaging studies. Early use of laparoscopy in selected patients may provide economic benefit by eliminating the need for low-yield imaging studies and may minimize lost time from school.

► It is difficult to support the notion that laparoscopic appendectomy for acute appendicitis is easier, faster, cosmetically superior, and cheaper than the standard open procedure. In certain circumstances, however, the global view through a laparoscope may offer an advantage over a limited, right lower quadrant exploration. Hence, laparoscopy has been advocated in those special circumstances where diagnosis is uncertain, particularly in postpubertal girls. Unfortunately, other diagnostic modalities, such as ultrasonography, are even less invasive and often more helpful.

What, then, is the place of laparoscopy in suspected appendicitis? The authors of this paper argue that recurrent abdominal pain, once all other causes have been eliminated, responds well to laparoscopic exploration and appendectomy. Indeed, unexplained recurrent abdominal pain (particularly when localized to the right lower quadrant) is caused by appendiceal pathology unless, and sometimes even *when*, proved otherwise. And so the authors performed an appendectomy in all their patients, even when a Meckel's diverticulum or a urachal cyst was the likely cause of chronic symptoms. Their results prove them right: even when the appendix turned out to be normal, symptoms resolved, a finding that we all have experienced first-hand.

F.I. Luks, M.D.

Prevention of Tissue Injury and Postsurgical Adhesions by Precoating Tissues With Hyaluronic Acid Solutions

Burns JW, Skinner K, Colt J, et al (Genzyme Corp, Cambridge, Mass; Tufts School of Veterinary Medicine, Boston; Univ of Florida, Gainesville)

J Surg Res 59:644–652, 1995 10–28

Introduction.—Tissue precoating with hydrophilic polymeric solutions of polyvinylpyrrolidone and carboxymethylcellulose has been used in experimental models to limit pericardial and peritoneal adhesions. Dilute solutions of the naturally occurring hydrophilic polymer hyaluronic acid (or sodium hyaluronate) (HA) has been successfully used for tissue precoating in surgical adhesion models. An efficacy investigation was conducted at 3 independent study sites to analyze the effect of HA solution concentration on tissue precoating to prevent adhesions in a rat cecal abrasion model.

Methods.—Three-hundred seventy-five adult female Sprague-Dawley rats (125 at each treatment site) were assigned to 1 of 5 treatment groups: 0.1% HA, 0.25% HA, 0.4% HA, phosphate-buffered saline solution (PBS), or no solution. The peritoneal cavity of rats in each treatment group was accessed by a midline incision and 4 mL of test solution, in all but the no-solution group, was used to precoat the abdominal cavity. A constant force, constant area rotary cecal abrasion device was used to deliver a consistent degree of tissue trauma. Animals were sacrificed at 1 week after surgery and the cecal adhesions were scored on a scale of 0 to 4. A separate histologic investigation with 150 rats was conducted to determine the effect of tissue precoating with HA solutions on tissue injury generated by abrasion and desiccation. A protocol similar to that of the first experiment

TABLE 1.—Adhesions Summary for 3-Center Independent Study.

Group	n	% Animals with no adhesions	Mean incidence of adhesions ± (SEM)	% Animals with adhesions ≥ 2
No coating	70	12	1.7 ± 0.13	79
PBS	72	11	1.6 ± 0.11	79
0.10% HA	75	21	1.0 ± 0.09	47
0.25% HA	74	38	1.0 ± 0.09	41
0.40% HA	74	50	0.7 ± 0.09	25

Note: Data shown are pooled totals of the 3 study sites. Statistical analysis showed no difference in trends between sites.

Abbreviations: SEM, standard error of the mean; *HA,* hyaluronic acid; *PBS,* phosphate-buffered saline solution.

(Courtesy of Burns JW, Skinner K, Colt J, et al: Prevention of tissue injury and postsurgical adhesions by precoating with hyaluronic acid solution. *J Surg Res* 59:644–652, 1995.)

was used for the histologic investigation. Rats were sacrificed at 2 days after cecal abrasion to allow time for an inflammatory response.

Results.—Data were pooled because there was no statistical differences in the trends among the 3 sites. The PBS and no–tissue-precoating treatment groups had a similar and significantly higher incidence of cecal adhesions than the HA groups (Table 1). The mean incidence of cecal adhesions diminished in a concentration-dependent manner from 1.6 to 0.7 as the HA concentration in the precoating solution increased. The percentage of animals with no adhesions increased from 11% in the PBS group to 50% in the group treated with 0.4% HA solution. In the histologic investigation, HA solutions significantly inhibited serosal tissue damage and eliminated the inflammatory response to abrasion and desiccation, compared with the no-coating and PBS groups.

Conclusion.—Findings indicate that tissue precoating with dilute HA solutions decreases damage to serosal tissues during abdominal surgery. Tissue precoating solutions used during surgery can help prevent the formation of adhesions caused by normal surgical manipulations and desiccation of tissue.

▶ Postsurgical adhesions result in a significant complication rate and are common after surgery. It is estimated that small-bowel obstruction caused by adhesion occurs in 5% of all general surgical procedures. In a rat model of cecal abrasion, the authors have used different concentrations of HA to reduce adhesion formation. The results are striking, and as HA concentrations in a precoating solution increased from 0% to 0.4%, the incidence of cecal adhesions declined significantly. Further, in separate histologic studies involving 150 rats, HA solution significantly inhibited serosal tissue damage and ameliorated the inflammatory response caused by abrasion and desiccation, compared with no coating or precoating with buffered saline. As can be seen from the abstracted data from Table 1 which combined the results of 3 independent studies centers, the effect of HA was statistically significant.

Parenthetically, the Food and Drug Administration has recently approved the first polyvinylpyrrolidone and carboxymethylcellulose substances for use in humans to prevent adhesion formation after gynecological surgery. Methods to reduce postoperative adhesion formation will gain increasing acceptance. It is my impression that research in the area of postsurgical adhesion prevention will continue and that an increasing number of modalities will become available to the clinician in the attempt to reduce postoperative adhesion formation.

H.H. Simms, M.D.

Colorectum and Anus

INTRODUCTION

Laparoscopic-assisted colectomy is undergoing intense evaluation to determine its cost-effectiveness and efficacy. Although technically feasible and well tolerated, the procedure remains controversial relative to its merits vs. open colectomy. The recent reports of early tumor recurrence at trocar sites after laparoscopic colectomy has stimulated investigators to hypothesize that pneumoperitoneum initiates detrimental consequences of tumor embolization and implantation at these sites. Moreover, surgeons have grave concerns that manipulation of tissues may increase tumor spillage and encourage subsequent recurrence. Jones and associates (Abstract 10–29) of the Division of Colorectal Surgery and Department of Surgery, Washington University School of Medicine, St. Louis, Missouri, and Ethicon Endosurgery Inc., Cincinnati, Ohio, studied whether pneumoperitoneum alone could enhance the incidence of tumor at trocar sites during laparoscopic colectomy. This important manuscript emphasizes that pneumoperitoneum may increase tumor implantation of the human colon cancer GW-39 in hamsters in the cecal mesentery and the midline incision. The authors suggest that there is a trebled implantation frequency with the addition of pneumoperitoneum and recommend that laparoscopic colectomy for patients with colon cancer be initiated and completed only within a protocol setting to evaluate the effect of pneumoperitoneum on therapy for colon cancer. Similarly, Reissman and associates (Abstract 10–30) of the Department of Colorectal Surgery, Cleveland Clinic, Fort Lauderdale, Florida, found that the morbidity associated with laparoscopic colorectal surgery correlates with a steep learning curve and the type of colorectal procedure. The authors emphasize that total abdominal colectomy has high complication rates when performed laparoscopically. The laparoscopic procedure should not be undertaken routinely and should only be performed within the confines of a prospectively randomized trial.

Modern-day immunosuppressive agents have been incorporated into therapy for inflammatory bowel disease (IBD). Cyclosporine has been reported to be variably successful in the treatment of IBD. The recently completed, prospective randomized studies of cyclosporine as therapy for severe active ulcerative colitis by Lichtiger and Present have determined that its application can rapidly improve severely ill, chronic ulcerative colitis patients who were refractory to conventional medical management and would otherwise be considered for colectomy. Of great interest, approximately half of the patients treated with cyclosporine have a sustained remission after discontinuance of this immunosuppressive agent. Furthermore, the recent placebo-controlled, prospectively randomized trial by Lichtiger and Present demonstrated the clear efficacy of this agent in the treatment of precolectomy ulcerative colitis patients. However, the impact of these prospective trials on the practice patterns of community gastroenterologists remains unclear. The important paper by Kozarek and associates (Abstract 10–31) of the Pacific Northwest Gastroenterology Society surveyed members of the state of Washington gastroenterologic community about their practice patterns regarding the use of cyclosporine in precolectomy ulcerative colitis patients. The multitude of potential reasons that preclude the use of cyclosporine by the gastroenterologic community includes deficits of knowledge about the therapy and results of these trials, skepticism, treatment philosophies, and fear of medication side effects.

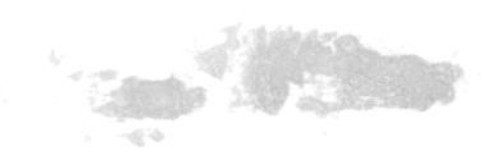

Physicians' skepticism and philosophies will change after the positive long-term effects of cyclosporine are definitively known. Before cyclosporine can be universally adopted, durable responses must be ensured because it has potential serious long-term effects, including high cost and nephrotoxicity. Restorative proctocolectomy as a safe, cost-effective, low-morbidity procedure still remains the standard of therapy against which all other medical therapies will be evaluated.

Rintala and Lindahl (Abstract 10–32) of the Children's Hospital, University of Helsinki, and the Department of Pediatric Surgery, Alder Hey Children's Hospital, Liverpool, England, compared the surgical complications and functional outcomes of children with ulcerative colitis who had proctocolectomy and straight ileoanal anastomosis (IAA) with those of children who had proctocolectomy with IAA and a J-pouch procedure. The authors observed no significant differences in early or late surgical complications between the 2 groups. Endoscopy revealed symptomatic pouchitis during the first postoperative year in 36% of the patients with the straight IAA and in 18% of the patients with the IAA completed with a J-pouch (P=NS). The early and long-term functional results were determined by the authors to be superior in the IAA J-pouch technique. Because the complications are similar between the 2 techniques, the authors conclude that the J-pouch methodology is the preferred technique for continence-pereserving surgery in children impaired with ulcerative colitis.

To evaluate the long-term results and complications of operative therapy for Hirschsprung's disease, Fortuna and associates (Abstract 10–33) of the Division of Pediatric Surgery, St. Louis University School of Medicine, and Cardinal Glennon Children's Hospital, St. Louis, Missouri, completed a retrospective study in 82 infants and children. Aganglionosis was limited to the retrosigmoid area in 81%; 55 Soave (endorectal) and 27 Duhamel retrorectal primary pullthroughs were completed. The most common operations for Hirschsprung's disease (Soave and Duhamel) resulted in uneventful recovery in only 60% to 67% of the patients. This important paper suggests that complications after Soave pullthrough operations require more subsequent procedures than their Duhamel counterparts. The authors emphasize that further refinements in these operative techniques and close follow-up are warranted because short-term total continence rates are less than 50%.

Catto-Smith and associates (Abstract 10–34) of the departments of gastroenterology and surgery, Royal Children's Hospital, Parkville, Australia, and the Clinical Epidemiology and Biostatistics Unit, University of Melbourne, Australia, found results similar to those of the group at St. Louis with the examination of 60 children after surgical therapy for Hirschsprung's disease to determine the extent of fecal incontinence. Fifty-three percent of these children had significant fecal soilage, and 27% had less severe incontinence. These authors report that the prevalence of incontinence did not diminish with increasing age (follow-up, 5.3–16.6 years). They found minimal evidence that fecal incontinence tends to resolve with time after surgery, nor was it improved with timing of definitive surgery in the neonatal period or the length of the residual colonic mucosa preserved. This report also suggests that the frequency of incontinence is markedly underreported and occurs in a surprisingly high proportion of patients who properly complete questionnaires in long-term follow-up. This report further emphasizes the importance of enhancing surgical techniques to improve fecal continence after therapy for Hirschsprung's disease. The importance of Hirschsprung's disease in the pediatric surgical literature is emphasized in the paper by Kobayashi and associates (Abstract 10–35) of the Children's Research Center, Our Lady's Hospital for Sick Children, Dublin. Because the cellular and molecular biology of Hirschsprung's disease is not fully understood, these authors studied expression of intercellular adhesion molecule type 1 (ICAM-1) and the major histocompatibility complex (MHC) of class II antigens in the resected bowel segments of patients with Hirschsprung's disease. These patients had no evidence of IBD. Strong expression of ICAM-1 and MHC class II antigens on hypertrophic nerve trunks was evident in both the submucous and myenteric plexuses of the aganglionic colon. Because no staining of the ganglia or nerve fibers in the submucosa and myenteric plexus of colons was found in controls or in the ganglionic colon from patients with Hirschsprung's disease, these results suggest the presence of an immunologic response in the pathogenesis of this disorder. Confirmation of this important work and its application to clinical practice must be evaluated.

Managing infants born with a high imperforate anus remains a major therapeutic challenge for the surgeon. Sigalet and associates (Abstract 10–36) of the Division of Pediatric Surgery, Montreal Children's Hospital, describe the anterosagittal approach to the management of a high imperforate anus with a modification of the Mollard anteroperineal method. This technique dramatically improves the posterior sagittal anorectoplasty described by DeVries and Pena in 1982. It is highly probable that this new technique described by the authors will be embraced as a method to create a shorter anal canal lined with specialized anoderm that will enhance the anatomical and short-term functional results.

The perplexing dilemma of differentiating other abdominal disorders from appendicitis in children and adults continues to challenge the general surgeon. Recent application of high-frequency compression sonography in children and adults with acute abdominal pain has enhanced both diagnostic accuracy and outcomes of therapy. Only rarely is the appendix visible on routine abdominal sonography. Moreover, active acute appendicitis cannot be conclusively identified without high-frequency linear transducers and careful graded compression. The report by Patriquin and associates (Abstract 10–37) of the departments of radiology, surgery, and pathology, Hôpital Sainte-Justine, Hôpital St. Luc, and the University of Montreal, compared arterial Doppler signals in normal appendix as with those in acutely inflamed appendixes. Furthermore, the authors evaluated the effect of necrosis of the appendix on the Doppler pattern and the flow pattern of sonography in recurrent and chronic appendicitis. In the presence of inflammatory hypervascularity of the appendix, an increased number of color signals and high diastolic Doppler shifts were evident when compared with normal appendixes. No Doppler shifts were evident in areas of appendiceal ischemia. Ultrasound may therefore become most useful in precisely the cases that are most difficult to diagnose clinically. Its future application in the diagnosis and management of acute/chronic appendicitis awaits the results of prospective randomized trials.

Wang and associates (Abstract 10–38) of the Children's Research Centre, Our Lady's Hospital for Sick Children, Dublin, also investigated methods to enhance diagnosis of inflammation of the appendix. These authors examined appendicular specimens for the expression of abnormal amounts of cytokines, an indicator of the inflammatory response. Tumor necrosis factor α (TNF-α) and interleukin-2 were measured in acute appendicitis specimens, in normal appendix specimens, and in specimens removed from patients with the clinical diagnosis of appendicitis in whom the appendix was found to be histologically normal. The authors conclude that acutely inflamed appendixes demonstrate intense cellular TNF-α in germinal centers and moderate levels of expression through the mucosa. Interleukin-2 mRNA was strongly expressed in the lamina propria but less so in germinal centers. Normal appendixes lacked these cytokine responses, as was evident in the majority of histologically confirmed normal appendixes removed from patients who had a clinical diagnosis of appendicitis. Thus these molecular markers may be a sensitive technique for the identification of appendicular inflammation. Its application in clinical medicine, although of interest, is best relegated to the physiologic consequences of inflammation rather than to its diagnosis. Nonetheless, it may be used in postoperative patients to differentiate definitive inflammatory states from normal appendixes, which suggests nonappendicular septic events that occur in the presence of a normal appendix.

Lejus and associates (Abstract 10–39) of Service d'Anésthesie et de Réanimation Chirurgicale, Bloc opérataire de Chirurgie Pediatrique, Nantes, France, conducted a randomized, single-blinded trial of laparoscopic vs. open cholecystectomy in children to determine the effects of postoperative analgesia. Appendectomy is the most frequent application for laparoscopy in children, whereas cholecystectomy is the most frequently used laparoscopic technique for adults. Both are thought to decrease hospital length of stay, pain and ileus, analgesic requirement, and convalescence and improve outcomes. However, appendectomy for children via laparoscopic approaches has not been comprehensively evaluated for its effects on postoperative analgesia. This study compared the quality of the postoperative period during the first 3 days postlaparoscopy vs. open appendectomy in children aged 8–15 years. In this well-matched group of 63 children, no differences were noted in demographic data for the laparoscopic vs. the open technique. Operative time was longer in the laparoscopic group. The authors conclude that laparoscopy does not improve analgesia or enhance postoperative recovery in children. Specifically, a delay in eating and walking was not evident in the open technique when compared with the laparoscopic method. The authors conclude that improvement in the postoperative period for these children is not a valid argument in the decision to use the minimally invasive technique.

Kirby I. Bland, M.D.

Impact of Pneumoperitoneum on Trocar Site Implantation of Colon Cancer in Hamster Model

Jones DB, Guo L-W, Reinhard MK, et al (Washington Univ, St Louis; Ethicon Endosurgery Inc, Cincinnati, Ohio)

Dis Colon Rectum 38:1182–1188, 1995 10–29

Introduction.—Laparoscopic-assisted colectomy has been associated with tumor recurrence at trocar sites, the result of excessive manipulation of tissues and tumor spillage into the abdominal cavity. To determine whether the incidence of tumor at trocar sites is increased by pneumoperitoneum, a hamster model of trocar implant and pneumoperitoneum was developed.

Methods.—A midline laparotomy, insertion of 4 5-mm trocars, injection of viable GW-39 human colon cancer cells into the mesentery of the cecum, and free peritoneal cavity was done in 2 groups of hamsters. Forty-one controls did not receive a pneumoperitoneum, and a comparison group of 50 animals underwent CO_2 pneumoperitoneum for 10 minutes at an insufflation pressure of 10 mm Hg. After 6 weeks, the animals were sacrificed and tissue samples prepared for staining. A veterinary pathologist blinded to the operation reviewed sections of trocar wounds, midline wound, small intestine, cecum, liver, and lung for the presence or absence of tumor.

Results.—Although pneumoperitoneum increased tumor implantation in the cecal mesentery and the midline incision, the procedure had no effect on recurrence in the liver, lung, or jejunum. The addition of pneumoperitoneum significantly increased trocar site implantation, from 26% to 75%. Overall, 98% of hamsters with pneumoperitoneum and 56% of animals without pneumoperitoneum had tumor implantation in at least 1 trocar site.

Discussion.—The use of pneumoperitoneum in this animal model increased the implantation of free intra-abdominal cells at wound sites on the abdominal wall or within the abdominal cavity. The gas-pressure gradient required for creating pneumoperitoneum appears to disseminate colon cancer cells, and the ports and instruments may become contaminated with tumor cells. In a potentially curative operation, the advantages of laparoscopic-assisted colectomy do not justify compromise of outcome by tumor spillage.

▶ Jones and co-workers provide us with an important piece of information in the ongoing search to determine the relation between laparoscopy and tumor implantation. This study convincingly shows that the presence of a pneumoperitoneum leads to a significant and marked increase in tumor implantation at the sites of surgical injury, whether they be trocar sites or laparotomy incisions. More important, there was a definite dose-relationship between trocar implantation and the number of cells inoculated into the peritoneal cavity. This implies that careful and meticulous technique that avoids tumor spillage is likely to be associated with less tumor spillage. In this regard, the use of a pneumoperitoneum appears to magnify the importance of meticulous operative technique with minimal tumor manipulation that is already held as a tenet of oncologic surgery. Because it is difficult to "palpate" the tumor laparoscopically and more traumatic manipulation is required laparoscopically because of the use of graspers rather than soft fingers, one wonders whether a laparoscopic approach to colon cancer is a good idea at all. In addition, it adds strength to the concept of "handoscopy," in which a hand is inserted into the abdomen via a large port.

J.F. Amaral, M.D.

Laparoscopic Colorectal Surgery: Ascending the Learning Curve

Reissman P, Cohen S, Weiss EG, et al (Cleveland Clinic Florida, Fort Lauderdale)

World J Surg 20:277–282, 1996 10–30

Objective.—The use of laparoscopy in colorectal surgery is expanding rapidly, despite the lack of prospective, randomized trials demonstrating the benefits of this technique. A substantial learning curve would be expected with laparoscopic colorectal surgery, given the unfamiliarity of the technique and the new instrumentation involved. The results of 100 laparoscopic and laparoscopy-assisted colorectal procedures were prospectively assessed.

Methods.—The study evaluated the first 100 laparoscopic colorectal surgical procedures performed in 1 institution by 1 surgical team from 1991 to 1994. Variables analyzed included the type and length of the procedure, intraoperative and postoperative complications, the need for

TABLE 3.—Results of Laparoscopic Colorectal Surgery According to Procedure

Parameter	TAC (*n* = 36)	Segmental resections (*n* = 47)	Nonresection procedures (*n* = 17)	Total (*n* = 100)
Overall complications	15 (42%)	9 (19%)*	2 (12%)*	26
Length of procedure (hours), mean and range	4 (2.5–6.5)	2.5 (1.5–5.5)	1.6 (1.0–2.5)*	2.8 (1.0–6.5)
Length of ileus (days), mean and range	3.5 (2–7)	3 (2–7)	2 (1–4)	3 (1–7)
Hospitalization (days), mean and range	8.4 (5–40)	7 (4–12)	6.8 (2–11)	7.3 (2–40)

*P < 0.01.

Abbreviations: TAC, total abdominal colectomy.

(Courtesy of Reissman P, Cohen S, Weiss EG, et al: Laparoscopic colorectal surgery: Ascending the learning curve. *World J Surg* 20:277–282, copyright 1996, Springer-Verlag.)

conversion to open surgery, the duration of postoperative ileus, and hospitalization.

Findings.—The patients were 60 males and 40 females (mean age, 49 years). Inflammatory bowel disease was the most frequent indication for surgery (34 patients) followed by cancer (15 patients). The experience included 36 total abdominal colectomies (TAC), most involving creation of an ileoanal reservoir; 39 segmental resections of the colon and small bowel; 8 rectal resections; 7 diverting stomas; 7 reversals of Hartmann's procedure; and 3 miscellaneous procedures. Seven patients required conversion to open surgery. There were 26 complications in 22 patients including 5 cases of enterotomy; 6 of hemorrhage; 4 of intra-abdominal abscess; 4 of prolonged ileus; 2 wound infections; and 1 case each of anastomotic leakage, aspiration, cardiac arrhythmia, upper gastrointestinal bleeding, and postoperative small bowel obstruction (Table 3). None of the patients died in the postoperative period.

The complication rate declined from 42% in the early part of the experience to 27% in the middle part and 12% in the late part. The decline in complication rate was associated with a declining number of TAC procedures performed. The overall complication rate in TAC procedures was 42%, compared with 9% in segmental resections and 12% in nonresectional procedures. The mean operating times were 4.0, 2.5, and 1.6 hours, respectively, and the mean durations of ileus were 3.5, 3.0, and 2.0 days, respectively. Patients undergoing TAC procedures stayed in the hospital a mean of 8.4 days, compared with 7.0 days for those undergoing segmental resections and 6.8 days for those undergoing nonresectional procedures.

Conclusion.—Laparoscopic colorectal surgery has been established as a feasible technique. The complication rate declines as experience is gained. However, morbidity is also affected by the type of procedure performed, with TAC procedures having a higher complication rate than other types of procedures. Laparoscopic colorectal surgery is safe for use in selected cases of benign disease or for palliative purposes in patients with malignancies. It should be used for curative resections in cancer patients only as part of prospective, randomized trials.

► This review documents the steep learning curve associated with laparoscopic or laparoscopy-assisted colorectal procedures. Given the significant complication rate and the lack of a quantifiable benefit, one can only agree with the authors' conclusion that such procedures should be undertaken only within the confines of a prospective randomized trial. The feasibility of performing such laparoscopic colorectal procedures should not lead to widespread acceptance until benefit can be proven.

W.G. Cioffi, M.D.

Cyclosporin Use in the Precolectomy Chronic Ulcerative Colitis Patient: A Community Experience and Its Relationship to Prospective and Controlled Clinical Trials

Kozarek R, and Members of the Pacific Northwest Gastroenterology Society (Virginia Mason Med Ctr, Seattle)

Am J Gastroenterol 90:2093–2096, 1995 10–31

Background.—Rapid improvement has been reported in severely ill patients with chronic ulcerative colitis (CUC) being considered for colectomy who were treated with either bolus or continuous infusion of cyclosporin in recent clinical trials. The effect of such seminal studies on gastroenterologic practice patterns are uncertain and were therefore investigated in a survey of a group of gastroenterologists.

Methods.—A questionnaire regarding the use of cyclosporin in hospitalized patients with CUC who had not responded to high-dose steroid infusion was mailed to all 155 members of the Pacific Northwest Gastroenterology Society. All physicians who reported using cyclosporin were then interviewed directly or by telephone.

Results.—Of the 155 members, 81 (52%) completed the questionnaire and 17 of the respondents (21%) reported using cyclosporin to treat 30 patients with CUC before colectomy. The 30 patients had a mean disease duration of 1.8 years. Twenty-eight patients had failed to respond to 5 to 7 days of treatment with high-dose prednisolone. Of the 30 patients treated with cyclosporin, 16 received a continuous infusion of 4 mg of cyclosporin per kilogram per day, and 14 received a bolus infusion of 5–7 of the drug per kilogram per day. The duration of therapy was more than 7 days in 9 patients, 6 to 7 days in 18 patients, and less than 5 days in 1 patient. Eight patients had side effects, including paresthesias, hypertension, elevated creatinine levels, arthralgias, severe malaise, herpetic esophagitis, and colon perforation. Among the patients with side effects, 4 were treated with continuous infusion and 4 were treated with bolus infusion. Acute colectomy was required for 4 patients receiving bolus infusion and 9 patients receiving continuous infusion. Of the 17 responders, 9 subsequently required colectomy at a mean of 6 months after discharge. The acute colectomy rate was 43%, and the overall colectomy rate was 73%.

Conclusions.—The mode of infusion did not affect the side effect profile or rate. The rate of acute colectomy was significantly higher than that in the controlled trials. However, the total rate of colectomies was similar to that of controlled trials of high-dose corticosteroids. The reasons for the discrepant findings may include inadequate treatment duration, the learning curve associated with the use of a new medication, or patient or physician philosophies or both.

► Surgeons consulted for acutely ill patients with ulcerative colitis who are not responding to maximal medical management (IV antibiotics, IV steroids, total parenteral nutrition) often are involved in a decision-making process between restorative proctocolectomy and use of cyclosporin. It is well known that most patients who are hospitalized for a severe exacerbation of the disease (80%-85%) will require colectomy within a 6-month period.

The most interesting piece of information in this cooperative article from the Pacific Northwest Gastroenterology Society is that even in patients who chose cyclosporin therapy, subsequent colectomy was required within a 6-month follow-up period in approximately 73% of patients. This observation raises significant questions about the enthusiasm reported by other gastroenterologists on the use of cyclosporin in acutely ill patients with ulcerative colitis. The drug may have significant side effects (especially nephrotoxicity), and it appears to only postpone the inevitability of surgery in most cases. The availability of restorative proctocolectomy as a procedure that can cure the disease with an acceptable morbidity rate and restore a very acceptable quality of life should be offered to patients early on, and it should be weighed against the option of immunosuppressive therapy to temporarily control a disease otherwise incurable by medical means.

V.E. Pricolo, M.D.

Restorative Proctocolectomy for Ulcerative Colitis in Children: Is the J-Pouch Better Than Straight Pull-through

Rintala RJ, Lindahl H (Univ of Helsinki; Alder Hey Children's Hosp, Liverpool, England)

J Pediatr Surg 31:530–533, 1996 10–32

Background.—Surgical resection of the colon can cure ulcerative colitis, a chronic inflammatory disease of the colonic mucosa with unknown etiology. The preferred surgical treatment in children is a restorative proctocolectomy and ileo-anal anastomosis (IAA). The complications and functional outcome of children with ulcerative colitis was compared between those undergoing proctocolectomy and straight IAA and those undergoing proctocolectomy and IAA with a J-pouch.

Methods.—A series of 22 children with intractable ulcerative colitis who underwent restorative proctocolectomy with ileo-anal anastomosis between 1985 and 1994 were studied. The first 11 patients underwent a straight pull-through (SIAA) procedure; the other 11 patients underwent a J-pouch ileal reservoir (JIAA) procedure. The patients in the SIAA group were followed up for a median period of 4 years, and the patients in the JIAA group were followed up for a median period of 2.3 years. Functional outcome, as defined by the total number of defecations over 24 hours, the number of defecations during the day and during the night, soiling during the day and night, and pouchitis symptoms, was evaluated at 3, 6, and 12 months postoperatively and at the last follow-up visit. Complications were recorded.

Results.—No patients died. There were no statistically significant differences between the SIAA group and the JIAA group in the rates of early complications (27% vs. 45%), late complications (55% vs. 27%), or overall complications (72% vs. 55%). Pouchitis was confirmed with endoscopy during the first postoperative year in 4 patients with SIAA (36%) and 2 patients with JIAA (18%), a nonsignificant difference.

At 3 months, there was a mean stool frequency over 24 hours of 8.4 in the SIAA group and 5.3 in the JIAA group. This improved to 7.1 at 6 months, 6.1 at 1 year, and 6.1 at final follow-up in the SIAA group and to 5.0 at 6 months, 3.5 at 1 year, and 3.3 at final follow-up in the JIAA group. At 3 months, nighttime bowel evacuations were recorded for all patients with SIAA but only 6 patients with JIAA. In the SIAA group, 4 patients had both daytime and nighttime soiling and 3 had only nighttime soiling. In the JIAA group, only 1 patient had soiling during both daytime and nighttime and 3 had only nighttime soiling. At 1 year, nighttime bowel evacuation was recorded for all but 2 patients in the SIAA group but none of the patients in the JIAA group. All of the patients had normal daytime continence, but 3 in the SIAA group and 2 in the JIAA group had nighttime soiling. At the last follow-up, 6 of the patients with SIAA and none of the patients with JIAA still had bowel evacuations during sleep.

Conclusions.—The JIAA produces significantly better short- and long-term functional results than does SIAA. The 2 methods are associated with similar incidences of complications and pouchitis, contrary to common wisdom. Therefore, JIAA is recommended as the preferred technique for treating ulcerative colitis in children.

▶ Proctocolectomy and ileoanal anastomosis, with or without an ileal pouch, is the preferred method for the surgical treatment of ulcerative colitis in children. The authors compared the surgical complications and functional outcome for patients with ulcerative colitis who had proctocolectomy and IAA with a J-pouch. Twenty-two children (aged 7 to 15 years) with intractable ulcerative colitis had an IAA, 11 by SIAA and 11 with a JIAA. The median clinical and endoscopic follow-up period for patients with SIAA was 4 years (range, 3.0 to 6.5 years); for patients with JIAA it was 2 years (range, 1 to 3 years).

The frequency of daytime and nighttime defecation was significantly higher ($P < 0.03$) for patients with SIAA at 3, 6, and 12 months postoperatively. At the last follow-up visit, the mean frequency of defecation for patients with SIAA was 6.1 ± 2.5/day; that for patients with JIAA was 3.3 ± 0.5/day ($P < 0.03$). Six of 10 patients with SIAA but none with JIAA had nighttime bowel evacuations. None of the patients had daytime soiling; 3 with SIAA and 2 with JIAA had slight soiling during sleep. There was no significant difference in the incidence of early (SIAA 27% vs. JIAA 45%) and late (SIAA 54% vs. JIAA 27%) surgical complications between the 2 groups. Endoscopically confirmed symptomatic pouchitis during the first postoperative year was found in 4 of the 11 (36%) patients with SIAA and in 2 of the 11 (18%) with JIAA (difference not significant). The early and long-term functional results of JIAA are superior to those of SIAA. There is no difference in the incidence of surgical complications and pouchitis between patients who have JIAA and those who have SIAA.

This cooperative effort between a Finnish and an English institution addresses an issue that is still debated in the pediatric surgical literature. Does the adaptive ability of the terminal ileum of very young children obviate the need for performing an ileo-anal pouch and does a straight ileo-anal pouch prevent pouchitis? In this comparative study, even young children (aged 7 to 15 years) had a better functional result when a J-pouch was constructed. More interesting is the observation that through a moderately long follow-up period, there was no difference in the incidence of pouchitis between patients with straight IAA and ileal pouch-anal anastomosis. In 1 of 4 children at least a transient episode of pouchitis develops, which is comparable to other series, especially in patients with ulcerative colitis. Even in small children, therefore, ileo-anal anastomosis should be done with a pelvic pouch.

V.E. Pricolo, M.D.

Critical Analysis of the Operative Treatment of Hirschsprung's Disease

Fortuna RS, Weber TR, Tracy TF Jr, et al (St Louis Univ, Mo; Cardinal Glennon Children's Hosp, St Louis, Mo)

Arch Surg 131:520–525, 1996 10–33

Introduction.—Hirschsprung's disease (HD) is characterized by congenital absence of ganglion cells in nerve plexuses of the gastrointestinal tract. It is limited to the retrosigmoid in most patients. The Soave and Duhamel pull-through operations are 2 of the most common procedures used to resect the aganglionic bowel and restore bowel continuity. Short- and long-term results of these procedures are controversial. Postoperative complications and long-term bowel function associated with the surgical treatment of HD was evaluated in 1 pediatric surgical center.

Methods.—The medical records of 82 infants and children treated for HD between 1975 and 1994 were retrospectively reviewed. Telephone interviews were conducted to ascertain information on current bowel habits, medications, and dietary restrictions.

Results.—Age at diagnosis was younger than 30 days in 47 children, 30 days–1 year in 22 children, and older than 1 year in 13 children. Six children had positive family history. In 66 patients, aganglionosis was limited to the rectosigmoid. The remaining children had more extensive disease. Children were first seen for HD with initial symptoms of intestinal obstruction (66 patients), chronic constipation (11 patients), acute abdomen (3 patients), and persistent diarrhea (2 patients). A total of 55 Soave and 27 Duhamel primary pull-through operations were performed. Eighteen (67%) children undergoing the Duhamel surgery and 33 children (60%) undergoing the Soave operation recovered uneventfully. Most other children had complications that required reoperation. Complications of the Duhamel operation included 5 cases of enterocolitis, 4 cases of rectal achalasia, and 2 cases of persistent rectal septum. Seven patients required reoperation. One patient required more than 1 operation. Complications of the Soave operation included 15 cases of enterocolitis, 12 cases of rectal stenosis, 4 cases of anastomotic leak, 3 cases of late perirectal fistula, 1 case of rectal prolapse, and 1 case of recurrent severe constipation. Sixteen patients who underwent the Soave procedure required reoperation. Approximately 2 reoperative procedures were required for each patient. Telephone interview was conducted at a mean of 89.3 months in 61 patients. Thirteen patients used daily medications. Only 1 of 4 patients older then age 5 years was totally continent. By 15 years after surgery, all patients were totally continent. Most patients had no dietary restrictions. Interview results were similar for patients who underwent either surgical procedure.

Conclusion.—Recovery was uneventful in 60% and 67% of children with HD who underwent the Soave and Duhamel procedures, respectively. Some surgeons advocate the Swenson procedure, but the Duhamel and Soave pull-through operations are more commonly practiced. Complication and reoperation rates were similar for the Soave and Duhamel procedures. The most common postoperative complication for both procedures was enterocolitis.

► The good news is that long-term outcome after definitive treatment of HD is encouraging; most children will be free of constipation, enterocolitis, or incontinence; and it does not really matter which operation one chooses (it is unfortunate that the authors chose to ignore the third common operation, the Swenson procedure). The bad news is that a very significant minority of patients (up to 40%) will have problems. Whether caused by associated intestinal neuronal dysplasia, stenosis, rectal achalasia, or "acquired" (ischemic?) aganglionosis, these complications will often lead to reoperation. The high number of diversions in this series attests to the fact that, despite sphincterotomy, myectomy, or salvage pull-through operation, many of these children cannot be cured.

F.I. Luks, M.D.

Fecal Incontinence After the Surgical Treatment of Hirschsprung Disease

Catto-Smith AG, Coffey CMM, Nolan TM, et al (Royal Children's Hosp, Parkville, Australia; Univ of Melbourne, Australia)

J Pediatr 127:954–957, 1995 10–34

Objective.—Sixty children who underwent surgical treatment of Hirschsprung disease were followed for a mean period of 2.6 years to determine the rate of fecal incontinence. Previous studies of postoperative fecal incontinence have had conflicting results because of their reliance on retrospective chart reviews.

Methods.—Eighty-seven patients who were treated for Hirschsprung disease at the study institution were eligible for the study; those with permanent bowel stomata were excluded. Data were obtained through a review of medical charts, interviews with the surgeons, and a structured questionnaire that was completed at interview by the parents of 60 children. The mean age of these patients was 10.1 years; 83% were male.

TABLE 1.—Clinical Parameters and Summary Results of CBCL for Children Who Claimed on Questionnaire Significant Soiling as Defined for the Study Compared to Those Who Did Not Soil

Clinical parameters	Soiling (n = 32)	Not soiling (n = 28)	*p*
Age at definitive surgery (yr)	0.9 ± 0.9	1.4 ± 3.1	0.39
3 Mo or younger	4 (13%)	2 (7%)	0.68
6 Mo or younger	11 (34%)	9 (32%)	0.86
Interval since surgery (yrs)	8.7 ± 2.5	9.1 ± 2.7	0.56
Extent of aganglionosis			
Rectosigmoid	23 (72%)	24 (86%)	—
More extensive	9 (28%)	4 (14%)	0.19
Type of surgery			
Soave	29 (91%)	23 (82%)	0.58†
Duhamel	2 (6%)	4 (14%)	—
Swenson	1 (3%)	0	—
Sphincterotomy	0	1 (3%)	—
Early postoperative complications	8 (26%)	10 (36%)	0.37
Late postoperative complications	28 (90%)	21 (75%)	0.17
Developmental delay (inc. Down syndrome)	2 (6%)	2 (7%)	1.00
SES (low Daniel score >3)	22 (69%)	13 (48%)	0.11
Maladjustment by CBCL	5 (19%)	4 (20%)	0.90

Note: Child Behavior Check List adjusted by removal of all soiling-related items.
**P* values are for 2-sided tests.
†Soave vs other types of surgery.
Abbreviations: SES, socoeconomic status; *CBCL,* Child Behavior Check List.
(Courtesy of Catto-Smith AG, Coffey CMM, Nolan TM, et al: Fecal incontinence after the surgical treatment of Hirschprung disease. *J Pediatr* 127:954–957, 1995.)

Questionnaires sought detailed information on bowel habits, soiling accidents, use of continence aids, enuresis, treatments, and diet. Thirty-nine of the 60 patients completed 4-week home diaries.

Results.—Over half of the children (57%) had an urge to pass stool before a bowel movement occurred, but 20% of the children experienced the urge only sometimes and 18% rarely or never. Diaries and questionnaires indicated that fecal soiling occurred in 80% of children. In contrast, medical records suggested that soiling was a problem in only 44% of patients. The 4-week diaries showed significant fecal soiling in 20 of 39 children. Children who soiled were more likely to have loose stools and a history of anal dilation, but they did not differ from those who did not soil in age at surgery or at stoma closure, sex, type of surgery, extent of aganglionosis, the presence of complications or developmental delay, or time elapsed since surgery (Table 1).

Conclusion.—Even when fecal streaking, defined as a small amount of stool on underclothing, was excluded, over half of the patients who underwent surgery for Hirschsprung disease were reported to have fecal soiling. Soiling indicative of fecal incontinence appears to be underreported on medical charts, and time after surgery does not lead to improvement. Emotional disturbance was not associated with an increased incidence of fecal soiling.

▶ The optimism and partisanship of many reports in previous decades notwithstanding, the definitive treatment of Hirschsprung disease does not produce excellent results; and the type of operation (Duhamel, Swenson, Soave, or any variant thereof) probably does not much matter. Catto-Smith and colleagues are here to remind us again that, if follow-up studies are carried out more carefully, a substantial number of patients will have less than perfect long-term results that range from constipation to soiling and incontinence. These authors did not see any improvement over time; this is in contrast to several other recent reports that suggest the percentage of short- and medium-term complications (30% to 60%) decreases at 10 years follow-up. It is hoped that the sequel to the present study will show a similar trend.

F.I. Luks, M.D.

Overexpression of Intercellular Adhesion Molecule-1 (ICAM-1) and MHC Class II Antigen on Hypertrophic Nerve Trunks Suggests an Immunopathologic Response in Hirschsprung's Disease

Kobayashi H, Hirakawa H, Puri P (Our Lady's Hosp for Sick Children, Dublin)

J Pediatr Surg 30:1680–1683, 1995 10–35

Introduction.—The pathogenesis of Hirschsprung's disease (HD) is not well understood. A recent report indicates that there is marked elevation of major histocompatibility complex (MHC) class II antigens throughout the intestinal wall of aganglionic colon, with abnormal localization in the mucosa, lamina propria, and hypertrophic nerve trunks. It is possible that ectopic expression of class II antigens indicates that an underlying immunologic mechanism is responsible for causing HD. The intercellular adhesion molecule (ICAM-1) seems to have an important role in the process of leukocyte adhesion and regulation of leukocyte extravasation and infiltration into inflammatory tissues. This cell-surface molecule facilitates interaction between leukocytes and recruitment of leukocytes at sites of inflammation. The expression of ICAM-1 and MHC class II antigens were investigated in bowel specimens after Swenson's pull-through operation in patients with HD to determine whether immunologic mechanisms are important in the pathogenesis of HD.

Methods.—Full-thickness strips of colon from the entire resected specimens of colon of 18 patients with HD were removed and fixed in periodatelysine paraformaldehyde solution. Control specimens were collected at the time of closure of colostomy in 3 patients with imperforate anus and during bladder augmentation in 5 additional patients. Frozen sections were serially cut to 10-µm thickness and underwent immunohistochemical analysis. The sections were incubated with mouse anti-ICAM-1 monoclonal antibody and mouse anti-HLA class II monoclonal antibody.

Results.—Very few ICAM-1–positive cells were observed in the lamina propria and muscle in the control bowel or the ganglionic bowel from patients with HD. Strong ICAM-1 expression was observed in the abnormal small ganglia in the hypoganglionic transition zone. A marked increase in ICAM-1–positive cells was seen throughout the intestinal wall of the aganglionic segment in all patients. The most remarkable finding was the increased number of ICAM-1–positive cells around and within the hypertrophic nerve trunks in the submucosal and myenteric plexuses. In patients over age 2 years, colon specimens exhibited very markedly increased ICAM-1 expression in the hypertrophic nerve trunks. The staining and distribution patterns of MHC class II antigen observed in tissues from controls and patients with HD were identical to those of I-CAM-1. In patients over age 2 years, the hypertrophic nerve trunks in the aganglionic colon segment showed very strong MHC class II expression.

Discussion.—The ICAM-1 is a cell-surface glycoprotein. It is a known ligand for lymphocyte function-associated antigens. Together, these 2 are involved in the leukocyte recruitment processes into inflammatory sites. The ICAM-1 is expressed on tissue macrophages, mitogen-stimulated T-lymphocyte blasts, vascular endothelial cells, certain epithelial cells, and fibroblasts. The MHC class II antigen is also a cell-surface glycoprotein. It is involved in the immune recognition of foreign tissue and the regulation of the immune response. The finding of aberrant expression of MHC class II antigens may signify altered local immune reactions in different types of disease, particularly those of autoimmune or viral origin. Other reports indicate that ICAM-1 antigens are not expressed in the central or peripheral nervous systems.

Conclusion.—Strong expression of ICAM-1 and MHC class II antigens was observed in the hypertrophic nerve trunks in the submucosal and myenteric plexuses of aganglionic colon and in small ganglia of the myenteric and submucosal plexuses in the transition zone. There was no histologic evidence of inflammation. It is possible that the antigen-presenting cell function of the hypertrophic nerve trunk and abnormal transitional ganglia may be partly mediated through the expression of both antigens. This points to an immunologic response in the pathogenesis of HD.

► Dr. Puri and his group continue to explore HD at the cellular and molecular levels and elegantly demonstrate upregulation of adhesion molecule ICAM-1 in aganglionic segments. As in similar research in other surgical diseases of the intestinal tract (such as pyloric stenosis), however, the finding that certain functional proteins are overexpressed or underexpressed in the diseased tissues does not establish their role in the disease's pathophysiology. Indeed, the fact that ICAM-1 expression in hypertrophic nerve trunks is higher in older children—whereas HD is present at birth—could suggest a reactive, rather than a causative, effect.

F.I. Luks, M.D.

The Anterior Sagittal Approach for High Imperforate Anus: A Simplification of the Mollard Approach

Sigalet DL, Laberge J-M, Adolph VR, et al (Montreal Children's Hosp)
J Pediatr Surg 31:625–629, 1996 10–36

Introduction.—The embryology and anatomy of imperforate anus is understood, but its management remains a challenge. A modified Mollard's approach is described for male patients that creates a shorter anal canal lined with specialized anoderm instead of perineal skin.

> *Technique.*—With the patient in the lithotomy position and placement of a urinary catheter, the rectourethral fistula is identified and controlled through a transversed suprapubic incision. This approach allows precise identification and closure of the fistula and preserves the entire internal sphincter. With dissection starting at the level of the peritoneal reflection, extensive mobilization of the rectosigmoid is not needed. A circumferential dissection of the rectal pouch is completed right against the rectal wall, then continued until it tapers into the rectourethral fistula. The fistula is divided and the rectal side of the fistula is dilated gently using mosquito forceps to preserve the internal sphincter fibers present around the fistula site. An anterior sagittal incision is used to approach the peritoneum. The posterior limit of the incision is just beyond the center of the external sphincter complex and is identified via muscle stimulation and visible anoderm. After the external sphincter and striated muscle complex are divided anteriorly and tagged with sutures, the dissection is completed in the midline. The striated muscle complex is followed with electric stimulation. The posterior urethra is then identified by palpation and inspection. It is followed until the puborectalis sling is seen. A 1-inch Penrose drain is passed and the space between the urethra and the muscle sling is dilated up to no. 10 or 12 Hegar, depending on the patient's size. The previously mobilized rectum is brought down using stay sutures. It may take some tension to do so, but it is brought to the level of the puborectalis without tapering since stretching the pouch tapers it effectively.

Sharp dissection is used to dissect the anoderm off the underlying muscle and subcutaneous tissue. The anoderm is sutured to the rectal wall at the puborectalis level. When the repair is completed, the anorectal angle is normal and the anal canal is short and is lined with anoderm and transitional epithelium.

Results.—Five patients have undergone this procedure, with follow-up of 8–40 months. All patients received proximal sigmoid colostomies in the neonatal period. A pull-through procedure was performed at 6–16 weeks of age. One patient had a small skin dehiscence at the peritoneum, but there were no further surgical complications or recurrent fistulas. Two patients also had esophageal atresia and tracheoesophageal fistula. The 2 patients with longest follow-up at 36 and 40 months of age, respectively, had good results. They were toilet-trained, had 3–5 stools daily, and were not soiling themselves. The younger patients were not old enough to evaluate with respect to continence but had normal anal appearance with normal length and function of the anus and anal canal. There was no problem with prolapse or ectropion.

Discussion/Conclusion.—The technique described here has many advantages over the posterior sagittal approach. It allows the normal processes of continence to function, decreases the risk of damage to the urethra, minimizes dissection of the puborectalis, minimizes damage to the posterior nervi erigentes while it allows adequate exposure, and preserves the internal sphincter so that normal rectoanal reflexes remain intact. Preservation of the external sphincter allows it to be used as the landmark of positioning the opening of the anal canal. This approach eliminates problems of the posterior saggital approach: (1) the long tube below the puborectalis increases risk of mucosal prolapse and soiling, (2) use of skin flaps causes difficulty with retained stool between the puborectalis and external sphincter, and (3) use of skin flaps doesn't allow much use of the anoderm with its specialized sensory role. The anterior sagittal approach attempts to solve these problems. With a shorter anal canal lined with proctodeal skin with its specialized sensory fibers, this approach makes maximal use of native tissues with minimal dissection and optimal reconstruction of this complex deformity. With modifications, this approach may be used in female patients.

▶ When DeVries and Peña[1] introduced the concept of posterior sagittal anorectoplasty for the treatment of imperforate anus in the early 1980s, it was embraced almost unanimously by the surgical community. A decade later, it has become a gold standard of sorts, and one tends to forget that alternative methods were available before, and have been used successfully since. The main advantages of the midline posterior approach are the impunity with which one can divide the different muscle layers, the predictability of finding the rectal pouch, and the organized fashion in which the reconstruction can occur. That this is all very didactic, and can be easily taught to fellows and residents, is probably one of the reasons for its success.

The posterior approach does have some disadvantages, however, and these may be avoided with an anterior approach, as first described by Mollard[2] (Lyons, France), and subsequently adopted and modified by Davies and Cywes[3] (South Africa) and Yazbeck[4] (Canada), among others: muscles are not divided, the urorectal fistula (which is most often present) is identified first without the need to split the posterior rectal wall, the puborectalis sling is more easily identified and preserved, and a more physiologic anorectal angle can be created.

F.I. Luks, M.D.

References

1. DeVries PA, Peña A: Posterior sagittal anorectoplasty. *J Pediatr Surg* 17:638–643, 1982.
2. Mollard P, Marechal JM, Jaubert de Beaujeu MJ: Surgical treatment of high imperforate anus with definition of the puborectalis sling by an anterior perineal approach. *J Pediatr Surg* 13:499–504, 1978.
3. Davies MRQ, Cywes S. The use of a lateral skin-flap perineoplasty in congenital anorectal malformations. *J Pediatr Surg* 19:577–580, 1984.
4. Yazbeck S, Luks F, St-Vil D: Anterior perineal approach and three-flap anoplasty for imperforate anus: Optimal reconstruction with minimal destruction. *J Pediatr Surg* 27:190–195, 1992.

Appendicitis in Children and Young Adults: Doppler Sonographic–Pathologic Correlation

Patriquin HB, Garcier J-M, Lafortune M, et al (Hôpital Sainte-Justine, Montreal)

AJR Am J Roentgenol 166:629–633, 1996 10–37

Background.—The use of high-frequency compression sonography has enabled better diagnosis and treatment in children with acute abdominal pain. When the appendix is difficult to locate, color Doppler sonography appears to be a useful adjunct to gray-scale sonography. It was determined whether the normal appendix yields arterial Doppler signals, whether an acutely inflamed appendix contains more signals than a normal appendix, whether necrosis affects the Doppler pattern, and whether a specific Doppler flow pattern is seen in recurrent and chronic appendicitis.

Methods.—Patients aged 1 to 25 years with 1 or more episodes of acute right-sided abdominal pain and a clinical suspicion of appendicitis were assessed prospectively. Twenty-five healthy subjects were also examined. Sonography was done with 3-5 or 5 MHz transducers for the abdominal examination and 7 MHz linear for the compression assessment. Low-flow settings, with the highest color Doppler gain possible, were used.

Findings.—The appendix was found in 10 of the healthy subjects. Signals were difficult to find, with 1 or 2 tiny color pixels identified in 4 patients and no signals in the appendix in 6. Thirteen of 30 patients undergoing surgery had pathologically proved uncomplicated appendicitis. More than 4 color Doppler signals were found easily in the appendix throughout the greater part of its length in all of these patients. The mean resistive index in spectral analysis was 0.54. An increased number of signals was observed when intestinal loops in the right lower quadrant were compressed gently and assessed with color Doppler. In 11 patients with acute appendicitis with focal necrosis, the appendix was abnormally thick on gray-scale images. No Doppler signals were detected in 1 of these patients, and few signals were found in 5. The mean resistive index was 0.54. The tip of the appendix showed no signals in 8 children, and in 2, the surrounding tissue showed more than 4 signals with high diagnostic flow. Of 3 patients with recent exacerbations of chronic appendicitis, 1 had a single Doppler signal at the tip of the appendix, and another had a thickened appendix with few color Doppler signals. In the third patient, an ill-defined right lower quadrant mass and the thickened bladder wall adjacent to it yielded abundant color Doppler signals. Another 3 patients with right lower quadrant pain had numerous color Doppler signals and high diastolic flow arising from structures in the right iliac fossa. In these patients, the appendix could not be found. Two had Crohn's disease.

Conclusion.—The vascularity of the appendix as visualized by Doppler sonography was well correlated with the inflammatory site as seen pathologically. Most of the appendix is hypervascular in patients with acute appendicitis. The vascularity and number of Doppler signals are reduced with necrosis and perforation, especially at the tip.

▶ From a center where ultrasound has been used for many years as an adjunct to the diagnosis of appendicitis comes this testimony to how sophisticated this modality has become. There is now more to positive ultrasound result than a simple "noncompressible enlarged tubular structure in the right lower quadrant." As one would expect, early appendicits is associated with hyperemia, which, thanks to Doppler, makes the appendix easier to find. Ultrasound may, thus, become more sensitive in precisely those cases that may be difficult to diagnose clinically. The progression to focal hypovascularity, ischemia, and necrosis is logical and correlated with the pathophysiology of perforated appendicitis.

F.I. Luks, M.D.

Is a Histologically Normal Appendix Following Emergency Appendicectomy Always Normal?

Wang Y, Reen DJ, Puri P (Our Lady's Hosp for Sick Children, Dublin)

Lancet 347:1076–1079, 1996 10–38

Background.—Often, a surgically removed appendix is subsequently found to be histologically normal. However, focal appendicitis has been found in some of these appendixes. Altered cytokine expression, indicating an inflammatory response, has been noted in several gastrointestinal conditions. Therefore, cytokine expression was investigated in histologically normal and abnormal appendix specimens.

Methods.—The expression of tumor necrosis factor-α (TNF-α) and interleukin-2 (IL-2) was measured, using in situ hybridization, in 31 histologically normal appendixes from patients with a clinical diagnosis of acute appendicitis, 10 appendixes with histologic evidence of acute appendicitis, and 12 normal appendixes from patients who underwent elective abdominal surgery.

Results.—In the appendixes with histologic evidence of inflammation, there was intense expression of TNF-α mRNA in germinal centers with moderate expression in the submucosa and in the lamina propria. There was also intense expression of IL-2 mRNA in the lamina propria with moderate expression in germinal centers. Both were expressed in the muscular layer and serosa. In contrast, there was almost no expression of either TNF-α or IL-2 mRNA in the normal appendixes. In 7 of the 31 histologically normal appendixes from patients with clinically diagnosed appendicitis, the patterns of TNF-α and IL-2 mRNA expression were similar to those in the inflamed appendixes, though expression was less intense and did not extend into the muscle layers and serosa.

Conclusions.—A subgroup of histologically normal appendixes in patients with a clinical diagnosis of appendicitis demonstrate altered cytokine expression, indicating an inflammatory response.

► To every surgeon who has ever performed an appendectomy for "very early" appendicitis and was told by the pathologist that the appendix was normal, take heart and ask: "Yes, but did you check for TNF-α?" This study is interesting because of the relationship between clinically suspected (but histologically refuted) inflammation and elevated expression of mRNA for TNF-α and IL-2. Although this knowledge may offer solace to the surgeon, it does not necessarily justify an appendectomy; the progression from TNF-overexpression to clinical appendicitis and rupture would by no means be evident, even if the demonstration of cytokine activitation were to be found in *all* false positive appendixes (rather than in 7 of just 31 cases).

F.I. Luks, M.D.

Randomized, Single-blinded Trial of Laparoscopic Versus Open Appendectomy in Children: Effects on Postoperative Analgesia

Lejus C, Delile L, Plattner V, et al (Bloc Opératoire de Chirurgie Pédiatrique, Nantes, France)

Anesthesiology 84:801–806, 1996 10–39

Introduction.—The most common reason for laparoscopy in children is appendectomy. Laparoscopic cholecystectomy has known benefits in adults, but the results of laparoscopic appendectomy are less clear. The postoperative period after appendectomy was compared in children undergoing a laparoscopic vs. an open procedure.

Methods.—The prospective, randomized trial included 63 children, aged 8 to 15 years, who were scheduled for appendectomy. Those weighing less than 20 kg were excluded. They were randomly assigned in the operating room to open or laparoscopic surgery. The children, parents, and nurses were unaware of which procedure the child had. During laparoscopic appendectomy, intra-abdominal pressure was maintained at less than 12 cm H_2O. The procedure was done through 2 incisions in the right and left lower quadrants. The appendix was removed using a 3.5 endoloop ligature. The open procedures were done through a standard McBurney's incision. Postoperative analgesia was provided with self-administered (PCA) IV boluses of nalbuphine, 25 $\mu g \cdot kg^{-1}$. The children made pain ratings every 3 hours when awake, on a 10-cm visual analogue scale

(VAS). The children, parents, and nurses all rated the overall quality of analgesia over the first 3 postoperative days.

Results.—The 2 groups were comparable in terms of demographic characteristics, preoperative dose of opioid analgesia, and delay between the last dose of dextromoramide and the loading dose of nalbuphine. The macroscopic appearance of the appendix also was similar in the 2 groups. Patients undergoing laparoscopy had significantly longer operative and anesthesia times. During the first day, the median patient-controlled analgesia nalbuphine dose was similar: 414 μg/per kilogram in the open surgery group and 562 μg/per kilogram in the laparoscopy group. Neither was there any significant difference on the second day. There were no significant differences in visual analogue scale pain scores during the 3 days after surgery. Shoulder pain occurred in 35% of children in the laparoscopy group vs. 10% in the open surgery group. No significant differences were found in the children's, parents', and nurses' ratings of analgesia. There were no differences in delays of regular feeding, sedation, nausea, vomiting, or urinary retention.

Conclusions.—Laparoscopic appendectomy in children offers no significant advantages over traditional open appendectomy. There are no differences in pain scores, analgesic usage, or delays in eating or walking. Unlike previous studies—which were neither randomized nor blinded—this trial finds no improvement in the postoperative period with laparoscopic vs. open appendectomy.

▶ The basis for this elegant study (patients were truly blinded, and wore 3 plastic strip bandages even if they only had 1 incision!) is a question many colleagues have been grappling with: What are the true benefits of laparoscopy in pediatric surgery? Rapid recovery is the rule in children after any operation, open or endoscopic; early return to work is not exactly relevant; and pain after laparoscopy is not really less than that experienced after laparotomy, only short-lived (not an easy concept for young children).

In the final analysis, the size of the incision is probably the most important factor, particularly for young children whose scar may grow as they do. Therefore, laparoscopy in children should not try to compete with "mini-laparotomies," such as appendectomy and pyloromyotomy. Laparoscopic appendectomy is certainly feasible but not really better (and, one could argue, more expensive) than its open counterpart. This is essentially the authors' conclusion. The team from Nantes is very well versed in laparoscopy and has creatively applied this modality to a great number of pediatric surgical conditions, and this only adds credence to their article.

F.I. Luks, M.D.

11 Oncology

Introduction

The last several years have seen a major movement toward the molecular basis for the pathogenesis of malignant disease. As a consequence, more and more manuscripts are emphasizing the importance of genetics and molecular events in the pathogenesis, early diagnosis, and treatment of cancer. However, important information can still be learned from large, randomized prospective trials, as well as from large institutional series that have extensive experience in the treatment of patients with cancer. This overview will attempt to emphasize some of these new developments.

Since the discovery of the *BRCA-1* and *BRCA-2* genes, important information is being obtained regarding the prevalence of these genetic mutations in various populations. For example, a search for *BRCA-1* mutations will be most productive in young Jewish women with a family history of breast cancer. We are beginning to see a better definition of the pathobiology, prognosis, and genetic linkage studies for both *BRCA-1* and *BRCA-2*. However, genetic studies are not limited to breast and ovarian cancer. Similar relationships have been defined for the molecular genetics and management of hereditary nonpolyposis colorectal cancer (HNPCC) and for the development of colorectal cancer in general. Studies on genetic mutations are also being expanded into less common gastrointestinal malignancies such as hepatocellular carcinoma and pancreatic cancer. With the use of polymerase chain reaction (PCR), one is able to identify K-*ras* mutations in pancreatic adenocarcinoma from routine cytologic smears.

Once again, percutaneous techniques are being used in the molecular diagnosis of exocrine pancreatic cancer. Similarly, new markers are being used as clinical aid to the management of other common malignancies. An example that immediately comes to mind is lymphatic blood vessel invasion in breast cancer. Similar studies are being performed in human colorectal carcinoma with factors such as angiogenetic factor and thymidine phosphorylase.

New diagnostic aids, however, are not limited to molecular analyses. New tests such as positron emission tomographic scanning in abdominal malignancy and spiral CT angiography for preoperative planning in patients with epigastric tumors are being used. The use of laparoscopy in the staging of abdominal malignancies is becoming increasingly important, especially in concert with more standard techniques such as US and CT.

Not only is the staging process more accurate with these new techniques, but it is also often possible to avoid unnecessary larger procedures and thereby reduce costs.

Clinical trials, especially of the randomized prospective format, remain an important means of answering clinical questions and therefore of influencing future clinical decision making. This past year has seen important trials on adjuvant chemotherapy for gastric cancer, utilization of lymphadenectomy in melanoma, perioperative chemotherapy in breast cancer, and preoperative radiation therapy in resectable rectal cancer. Not all important observations, however, result from randomized prospective trial. Many are made from carefully designed prospective analyses of large patient series, usually from single institutions. Examples are regional vs. systemic chemotherapy in the treatment of colorectal carcinoma metastatic to the liver or resection of nonresectable metastatic disease after neoadjuvant chemotherapy.

In this era of increasing managed care and careful cost analysis, more studies are being designed to analyze an individual surgeon's performance with regard to cost. These studies attempt to reduce the length of stay and the resultant costs by, for example, using early postoperative feeding after open colon resection. As more studies like these are performed, it becomes clear that a need exists to define and measure outcome results so that the most cost-effective and efficient patient care will be delivered in the future.

Finally, influence on clinical practice has come about through maturation of studies addressing such issues as the sequencing of chemotherapy and radiation therapy after conservative surgery for early-stage breast cancer, as well as straight and colonic J-pouch anastomoses after low anterior resection of the rectum.

In summary, I have attempted to select manuscripts that will influence and potentially improve the practicing surgeon's care of patients with malignancy. To this end, I have selected some relatively technical and basic science publications to introduce the practicing surgeon to the vocabulary and parameters for the molecular and genetic events associated with the development of common malignancies. Outside pressures will continue to influence the practicing surgeon toward efficient, more cost-effective care with improved patient satisfaction. This year's selections will, I hope, help accomplish these goals.

Timothy J. Eberlein, M.D.

New Diagnostics

Dynamic Contrast-Enhanced Magnetic Resonance Imaging of the Breast Combined With Pharmacokinetic Analysis of Gadolinium-DTPA Uptake in the Diagnosis of Local Recurrence of Early Stage Breast Carcinoma

Mussurakis S, Buckley DL, Bowsley SJ, et al (Univ of Hull, England; Kingston Gen Hosp, England)

Invest Radiol 30:650–662, 1995 11–1

Objective.—The value of dynamic contrast-enhanced MR imaging of the breast for detecting local recurrences of early stage breast cancer was studied in a prospective series of 50 women who underwent breast-conserving surgery and received radiotherapy.

Methods.—Thirty-four percent of the patients were examined as a routine follow-up measure, whereas the rest had clinical and/or mammographic reasons for the procedure. The breast was imaged using a 1.5-Tesla MR system (Signa: General Electric, Milwaukee, Wis) and a breast coil. Dynamic studies were performed by acquiring 25 sequential images at each of 4 preselected sections, covering any suspect lesion by using a radiofrequency-spoiled fast-GRASS sequence. Images were acquired before, during, and after the injection of dimeglumine gadopentetate. They were interpreted without knowledge of the clinical or imaging data. Contrast uptake was estimated by using a pharmacokinetic model based on the wash-in and wash-out rates and the amplitude of uptake.

Results.—Ten patients had local recurrences diagnosed histologically. They were scanned an average of 6 years after initial conservation surgery. The 40 patients without recurrent disease were examined an average of 2 years after surgery. Most of the MR features exhibited at least some overlap between benign and malignant lesions. Only benign lesions had a well-defined contour, and only malignant masses had a poorly defined (but not spiculated) contour. Lesions that were hypointense after contrast injection were always benign. Malignant lesions enhanced to a greater degree and more rapidly than did benign masses. There were indeterminate mammographic findings with 5 of the 9 patients who had locally recurrent invasive cancer. Two of 40 patients without recurrence had falsely positive MR findings.

Conclusions.—Dynamic MR imaging is required to reliably detect locally recurrent breast cancer in women undergoing conservation surgery. Pharmacokinetic analysis of gadolinium uptake may be performed to obtain parametric images that retain good spatial resolution and provide added information on the vascularity and permeability of the region.

▶ Local recurrence after breast conservation treatment, especially in patients who receive radiation therapy, can be extremely difficult to diagnose. This often leads to unnecessary biopsy, which generates only further scar tissue and/or disfigurement of the breast. Core-needle biopsy has been proposed as a potential alternative. This paper proposes an expensive, yet noninvasive, technique for diagnosing potential recurrence using dynamic contrast-enhanced MRI of the breast. In addition to pharmacokinetic analysis of gadolinium (Gd)-DTPA uptake, it can also be of aid in the diagnosis of local recurrence of early stage breast carcinoma.

Pharmacokinetic analysis of Gd-DPTA can provide additional information with regard to vascularity and other aspects that may distinguish benign from malignant lesions. There are, however, several caveats with this technique. First, it requires a fair investment of time to familiarize the user with it. Second, virtually all of the tumors in this study were invasive carcinomas, so using this technique for recurrence with DCIS is yet to be determined. Also, the minimal size of recurrence has also not been determined by this study. Finally, this technique may be more widely implemented only after technical advances that allow rapid scanning of the entire breast are found. Currently, these techniques are limited to a few experimental centers.

T.J. Eberlein, M.D.

PET Scans of Abdominal Malignancy

Blahd WH, Brown CV, Khonsary SA, et al (West Los Angeles Veterans Affairs Med Ctr; Univ of California, Los Angeles)

World J Surg 20:245–247, 1996 11–2

Introduction.—The introduction of positron emission tomography (PET) has enabled evaluation of the chemical and metabolic changes caused by a number of disease processes. This diagnostic modality has promise in the evaluation of functional changes associated with cancer.

PET Technique.—The PET scanner is used to measure the radiation emitted by radioactive tracer molecules as they are taken up by specific organ cells; these data are translated into an image by tomographic computer reconstruction. Cancer cells have been shown to exhibit accelerated glucose membrane transport. Therefore, administration of radiolabeled 2-fluoro-2-deoxy-D-glucose (FDG), which is metabolized intracellularly and remains trapped within the cell, demonstrates cancer cell glycolytic activity in essentially all human cancers. Accuracies of 80% or more have been demonstrated with PET-FDG. It can detect abnormalities before structural changes and has been shown to correlate with the rate of tumor growth.

Applications.—PET-FDG has been shown to have greater accuracy than CT in the preoperative staging and detection of residual tumor or recurrence after treatment of colorectal cancer (Fig 1). It has demonstrated changes in FDG uptake in colorectal lesions after radiotherapy and can thus be useful in evaluating the effects of palliative therapy. Metastatic liver lesions and lymphoma can also be detected by PET-FDG.

Conclusions.—Whole-body PET-FDG imaging enables the functional evaluation of tumor activity and growth, which has utility in the detection

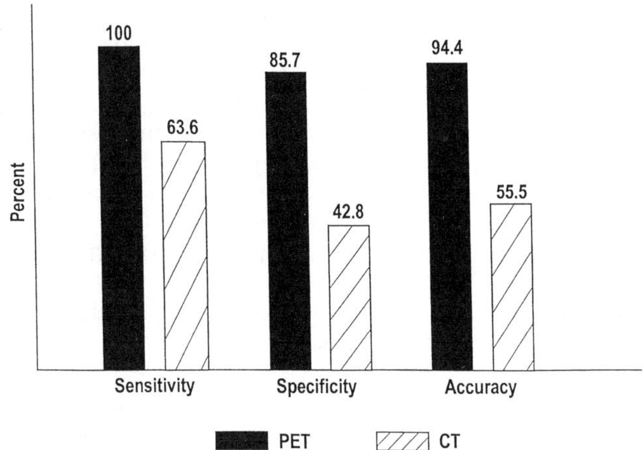

FIGURE 1.—Comparative efficacy of positron emission tomography (*PET*) and CT for detecting residual recurrent colorectal tumor (n = 18). (Courtesy of Blahd WH, Brown CV, Khonsary SA, et al: PET scans of abdominal malignancy. *World J Surg* 20:245–247, copyright 1996 by Springer-Verlag.)

of primary tumors and tumor recurrence and in the evaluation of the efficacy of therapy.

► Positron emission tomography, now with FDG, is much more effective than CT for detecting residual recurrent colorectal tumor. This ability to detect cancer is related to the fact that malignant tissue has a high rate of aerobic and anaerobic glycolysis, as well as accelerated glucose membrane transport. Previous studies have shown that essentially all human cancers accumulate FDG. Thus PET-FDG scans will be particularly important, especially when used in the whole-body imaging mode. PET-FDG imaging can detect cancers suspected from other clinical tests, determine occult spread and thereby influence therapy, and may be most effective in distinguishing scar from recurrent malignancy.

T.J. Eberlein, M.D.

Prospective Comparison of Laparoscopy, Ultrasonography and Computed Tomography in the Staging of Gastric Cancer

Stell DA, Carter CR, Stewart I, et al (Royal Infirmary, Glasgow, Scotland)

Br J Surg 83:1260–1262, 1996 11–3

Background.—Gastric cancer continues to be a common malignancy. Preoperative staging is routinely done using ultrasonography (US) and CT, though both modalities have limitations for this purpose. The accuracies of US, CT, and laparoscopy in the staging of gastric adenocarcinoma were compared.

Methods and Findings.—One hundred three patients were included in the study. Histologic assessment showed metastases to the liver in 27 patients, to lymph nodes in 49, and directly to the peritoneum in 13. For each type of metastasis, all 3 modalities had a specificity of 92% to 100%. However, laparoscopy was more sensitive in detecting hepatic, nodal, and peritoneal metastases. The relative efficacy of laparoscopy was best in demonstrating hepatic metastases. Nodal and peritoneal metastases detection with US and CT was very poor. No significant morbidity and no mortality were associated with laparoscopy.

Conclusion.—Laparoscopy is a safe, sensitive, and specific modality for staging gastric carcinoma. Accurate staging is becoming increasingly important in planning management by nonoperative palliative methods.

► This paper reports on 103 consecutive patients. I have chosen it because I believe that laparoscopy is finding an ever-important role in the staging evaluation of patients with abdominal malignancy. According to Table 2 of the article, laparoscopy performed significantly better than either US or CT. In fact, only 1 patient had liver metastases missed by laparoscopy, and these same lesions were missed by US and CT. With respect to nodal metastases, laparoscopy was much less sensitive; however, it was significantly better than either US or CT. With respect to peritoneal metastases, laparoscopy sensitivity was improved and was significantly better than US or CT.

Detection of peritoneal seeding was somewhat limited in this study in that a single viewing port was used without the aid of dissecting or manipulating instruments. Certainly, if a more thorough laparoscopic evaluation were performed, it would seem reasonable that a higher sensitivity would be seen with respect to peritoneal metastases. Authors of some studies have believed that laparoscopy has not been sensitive enough in the staging of gastric cancer; however, in this series, 37% of the patients did not undergo surgery, largely because of laparoscopy staging information. Thus, laparoscopy will reduce costs and length of stay if the philosophy is not to perform extended resection in the face of regional or metastatic disease. Obviously, if results of laparoscopy are negative, conversion to an open procedure and attempted curative resection could be undertaken at the same time.

T.J. Eberlein, M.D.

Spiral CT Angiography for Preoperative Planning in Patients With Epigastric Tumors: Comparison With Arteriography

Freund M, Wesner F, Reibe F, et al (Univ of Kiel, Germany)

J Comput Assist Tomogr 20:786–791, 1996 11–4

Background.—Spiral CT can obtain large amounts of data in a short time, permitting examination during the arterial phase of IV contrast injection. This CT angiographic (CTA) technique has been evaluated for use in many parts of the body, including the abdomen. In patients with epigastric tumors, the relationship of the disease to the adjacent blood vessels is crucial in determining the surgical approach. The use of CTA for preoperative assessment in patients with epigastric tumors was investigated.

TABLE 4.—Results of Computed Tomography Angiography and Arteriography for Portal Vein

	CTA	Arteriography
Anatomy	22/22	22/22
Variations	0/22	0/22
Thrombosis	1/22	1/22
Displacement	7/22	5/22
Compression	5/22	3/22
Encasement	2/22	1/22

(Courtesy of Freund M, Wesner F, Reibe F, et al: Spiral CT angiography for preoperative planning in patients with epigastric tumors: Comparison with arteriography. *J Comput Assist Tomogr* 20:786–791, 1996.)

Methods.—Twenty-two patients with epigastric disease underwent CTA and plain film arteriography. For CTA, the patients received 150 mL of contrast material at a flow rate of 4 mL/sec. After 30 seconds, spiral CT scanning of the epigastrium was performed, with axial images reconstructed at 2-mm increments. Standard arteriography was performed with the use of a transfemoral catheter placed into the epigastric arteries. The 2 techniques were compared for their ability to depict the arteries and portal vein and to depict blood vessel involvement by disease.

Results.—Both techniques successfully visualized the blood vessels in all patients. Furthermore, both techniques visualized an anatomical variation, i.e., a right hepatic artery arising from the superior mesenteric artery. Blood vessel involvement with disease was demonstrated in 22 cases with CTA vs. 15 with angiography. Conventional angiography missed 2 cases of compression of the celiac trunk and 2 cases of displacement, 2 cases of compression, and 1 case of encasement of the portal vein (Table 4).

Conclusions.—Spiral CT angiography is useful for preoperative evaluation of patients with epigastric tumor. Although the smaller arterial branches are better appreciated with conventional arteriography, the portal vein and its intrahepatic branches are better appreciated on CTA. Both techniques show good correlation in terms of disease involvement, particularly when axial slices are used additionally. Because of its minimal invasiveness, CTA may replace conventional angiography for some patients.

▶ I have included this manuscript because spiral CT angiography is rapidly replacing plain film arteriography. It obviously would be associated with less morbidity because the injection for spiral CT is made intravenously. Obviously, the risk of anaphylaxis or a paravenous injection is still present. However, spiral CT angiography is routinely performed on an outpatient basis. Although plain film conventional arteriography is also performed as an outpatient procedure at our institution, costs for the spiral CT angiography are less.

Because most patients with intra-abdominal malignancy obtain CT scans, the potential for cost savings is also present if they were to undergo spiral

CT angiography. With respect to portal vein demonstration, spiral CT angiography seems to be superior to conventional arteriography because the latter technique indirectly causes opacity in the portal vein. Another advantage of spiral CT angiography is the possibility of post-processing and reprojecting images from any angle because of the 3-dimensional nature of the acquired data.

T.J. Eberlein, M.D.

Gastric

Prognostic Factors in Resectable Gastric Cancer: Results of EORTC Study No. 40813 on FAM Adjuvant Chemotherapy

Lise M, Nitti D, Marchet A, et al (Università di Padova, Padua, Italy; EORTC Data Ctr, Brussels, Belgium; Ospedale Civile di Padova, Padua, Italy; et al)

Ann Surg Oncol 2:495–501, 1995 11–5

Introduction.—There is no consensus on what is considered to be adequate surgical treatment of gastric carcinoma. The effect of prognostic factors on survival and time of recurrence were evaluated in a randomized clinical trial on adjuvant FAM2 chemotherapy. Adequate surgery was also investigated as an independent prognostic factor.

Methods.—A total of 314 patients from 28 European institutions were randomized to receive chemotherapy with either the FAM2 regimen or control arm. The extent of surgery and lymphadenectomy was noted. The prognostic factors included the following: patient age, sex, and performance status; preoperative laboratory data; tumor stage and category; and treatment approach. The influence of these factors on time of recurrence and survival were evaluated.

Results.—The median follow-up was 80 months. The overall 5-year survival rate was 43%. The median survival was 3.7 years. For stage II and stage III patients, respectively, the 5-year survival rate was 72% and 32%. There were no significant differences between survival times. Treated patients had a significant advantage over untreated patients in time of recurrence. The surgical complication rate was not significantly different according to the extent of lymphadenectomy performed. Significant differences in survival were noted for T and N category, hemoglobin (Hb) level, and stage of disease (Table 2). Survival was significantly better for patients with subtotal vs. total gastrectomy, no splenectomy vs. splenectomy, and patients with "adequate" vs. "doubtful" or "inadequate" surgery (Table 2 and Figure 3).

Conclusion.—Prognostic factors for duration of survival of patients with resectable gastric cancer were T and N category, adequacy of surgery, and Hb level. Adjuvant chemotherapy was of borderline significance. For time of recurrence, prognostic factors were T and N category, adequacy of surgery, and adjuvant chemotherapy.

▶ This is a very significant multi-institutional European trial. Although, there is no overall improvement in survival with adjuvant FAM chemotherapy, this

TABLE 2.—Prognostic Factors With a Statistically Significant Effect on Survival and Disease-Free Interval at Univariate Analysis

Variable	Pts (N)	Log rank p (duration of survival)	Log rank p (time to progression)
Hb			
WHO 0	242	0.011	0.109
WHO 1–2	54		
T category			
T1	12	<0.001	<0.001*
T2	126		
T3	144		
T4	29		
N category			
NO	81	<0.001	<0.001*
N1	115		
N2	86		
N3	27		
Stage			
II	81	<0.001	<0.001
III	228		
Surgical procedure			
Gastric resection	184	0.002	0.011
Total gastrectomy	119		
Splenectomy			
No	198	0.004	0.111
Yes	95		
Adequacy of surgery			
Adequate	102	<0.001	<0.001*
Doubtful	131		
Inadequate	76		
Adequacy of surgery (stage II patients)			
Adequate	66	0.007	<0.001
Doubtful	13		
Adequacy of surgery (stage III patients)			
Adequate	36	0.022*	0.093*
Doubtful	118		
Adequate	71		
Adjuvant chemotherapy			
Yes	155	0.308	0.021
No	159		

In some cases the total number of patients is not 314 because some data are not available.
*Test for linear trend.
Abbreviation: WHO, World Health Organization (performance status scale).
(Courtesy of Lise M, Nitti D, Marchet A, et al: Prognostic factors in resectable gastric cancer: Results of EORTC study no. 40813 on FAM adjuvant chemotherapy. *Ann Surg Oncol* 2:495–501, 1995.)

study emphasizes the tumor and nodal stage in addition to adequacy of surgery as important criteria for survival. After surgical and pathologic data were compared, lymphadenectomy was classified as "adequate" when the extent of lymph node dissection was wider than the lymph node metastatic diffusion, "partially adequate" or "doubtful" when these coincided, and "inadequate" when the dissection did not encompass metastatic diffusion. When using these criteria, as demonstrated in Figure 3, adequacy of surgery is very important in determining overall survival. Stage of presentation as well as tumor and nodal metastases are also extremely important. None of this information is new, especially when reviewing the large Pacific Basin

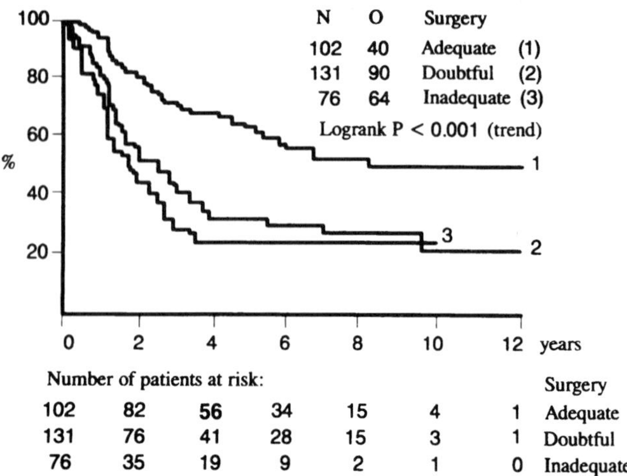

FIGURE 3.—Regional node involvement according to extent of lymphadenectomy. (Courtesy of Lise M, Nitti D, Marchet A, et al: Prognostic factors in resectable gastric cancer: Results of EORTC study no. 40813 on FAM adjuvant chemotherapy. *Ann Surg Oncol* 2:495–501, 1995.)

trials, but this extensive study underscores the importance of accurate staging as well as thorough and "adequate" surgery.

T.J. Eberlein, M.D.

Laparoscopic Staging for Gastric Cancer

Lowy AM, Mansfield PF, Leach SD, et al (Univ of Texas, Houston)
Surgery 119:611–614, 1996 11–6

Background.—Computed tomography scanning has traditionally been used to stage intraabdominal disease. However, it has not always been adequately sensitive in detecting small-volume metastatic disease in the liver and peritoneal cavity. Recent improvements in CT technology may improve its sensitivity in these settings. Laparoscopy has been used to stage gastric cancer, but its value is controversial. The usefulness of laparoscopy for staging gastric adenocarcinoma was evaluated in patients who also underwent CT scanning with the advanced technologies.

Methods.—Staging laparoscopy was performed on 71 patients with gastric adenocarcinoma with CT indications of resectable disease. The laparoscopy findings were compared with pathologic findings, particularly in patients with negative or equivocal CT findings.

Results.—Laparoscopy was completed in 69 of the 71 patients, including 41 patients who underwent laparotomy with curative intent and 38 patients who underwent resection of all gross tumors (Fig 1). There was pathologic evidence of hepatic metastases in 3 patients with a negative CT scan of the liver; these metastases were detected by laparoscopy in 1 of the patients. Laparoscopy detected disease in 16 of the 17 patients with peritoneal metastases. This allowed laparotomy to be avoided in 12 (17%)

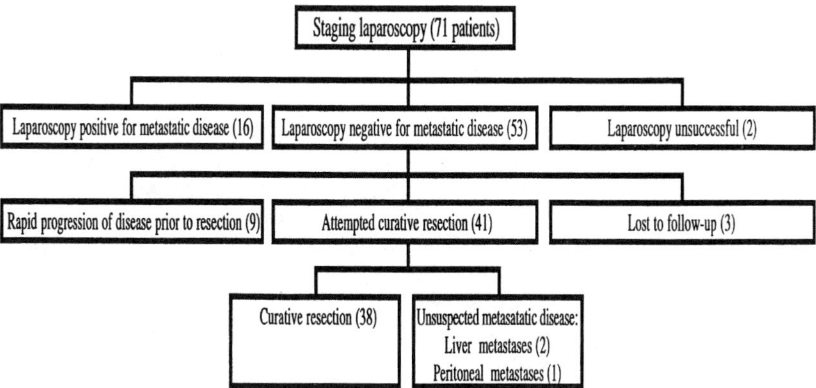

FIGURE 1.—Staging laparoscopy in 71 patients with potentially resectable gastric cancer. (Courtesy of Lowy AM, Mansfield PF, Leach SD, et al: Laparoscopic staging for gastric cancer. *Surgery* 119:611–614, 1996.)

patients. Laparotomy was performed in 3 patients with occult peritoneal diseases only in the context of a clinical trial.

Conclusion.—Combined CT and laparoscopic staging allowed a resectability rate of 93% for patients with gastric adenocarcinoma who under-

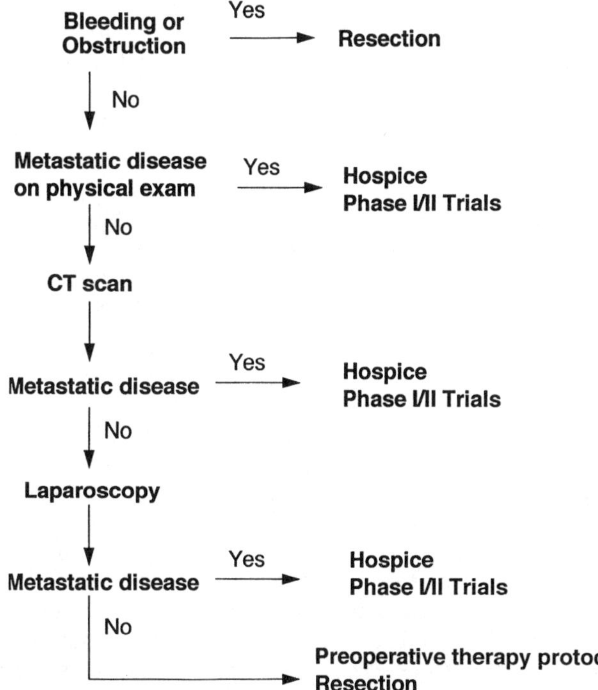

FIGURE 2.—Work-up of biopsy proven gastric cancer. (Courtesy of Lowy AM, Mansfield PF, Leach SD, et al: Laparoscopic staging for gastric cancer. *Surgery* 119:611–614, 1996.)

went a potentially curative resection. Therefore, laparoscopic staging should be included in the algorithm for the management of gastric cancer (Fig 2). Although laparoscopy has an increased cost, cost savings will ultimately be realized because of the decreased morbidity and decreased hospitalization for patients who avoid unnecessary laparotomy.

▶ Staging laparoscopy has become more popular, both because it is very effective and because it is a cost-effective method to detect metastatic disease and, therefore, makes it possible to avoid costly surgery laparotomy. In this article, 71 patients with biopsy-proven gastric cancer underwent staging laparoscopy. Not all patients who have a biopsy proven cancer, however, undergo laparoscopy, as can be seen in Figure 2. A very elegant algorithm is used. Unless the patient has bleeding or an obstruction, metastatic disease is sought by physical examination or CT scan. If none is found, then laparoscopy is performed. In the patients who had negative laparoscopies, 41 underwent attempted curative resection and 38 of those patients were successfully treated with surgery.

Laparoscopy has found an important role in the diagnosis and staging of pancreatic cancer, islet call tumors, and hepatocellular carcinoma. In these patients, if metastatic disease is documented, celiotomy is avoided as well as attempt at resection in the face of metastatic disease. As has been documented previously, laparoscopy is associated not only with shorter hospitalization, but also with diminished postoperative pain and a more rapid return to normal activities. In the case of patients with pancreatic or gastric cancer, this would also presumably avoid delays in initiation of experimental treatment trials.

T.J. Eberlein, M.D.

Brain

Distribution of Epidermal Growth Factor Receptor Gene Amplification in Brain Tumours and Correlation to Prognosis

Diedrich U, Lucius J, Baron E, et al (Neurologische Universitätsklinik, Göttingen, Germany; Institut für Humangenetik der Universität, Göttingen, Germany)

J Neurol 242:683–688, 1995 11–7

Introduction.—Epidermal growth factor receptor (EGFR) gene amplification in human brain tumors is most common in gliomas. Meningiomas lack this kind of mutation, even in malignant tumors for which the EGFR is strongly expressed. The distribution of gene amplification at the EGFR, epidermal growth factor (EGF), and transforming growth factor-alpha (TGF-α) loci in gliomas and meningiomas were analyzed.

Methods.—Seventy-five gliomas and 31 meningiomas underwent EGFR gene amplification. The EGF and TGF-α loci lacked amplification and rearrangement of DNA sequences in these two tumor types. Histological diagnosis, malignancy grade, age, sex, and clinical course were reviewed.

Results.—Twenty-three of 75 gliomas showed EGFR gene mutations. No EGFR gene mutations were found in 31 meningiomas. The EGFR gene

TABLE 3.—Median Survival Times and Median Patient Age in Relation to EGFR Gene Mutations and Malignancy Grade of Gliomas

Grade (WHO)	EGFR gene mutation	*n*	Median age (years)	Median survival time without progression of tumour (month)	Median survival time (month)
I - IV	+	23	59.4	5*	6†
	−	52	44.7	11	12
I/II	+	2	59.5	3	5
	−	17	27.8	> 36	> 38
III	+	8	53.6	5.5‡	9
	−	16	39.9	11	14
IV	+	13	63.4	4	7
	−	19	62.7	5	6

P values of significant differences (log-rank test): *0.0024, †0.0046, ‡0.0380.

Abbreviations: EFGR, epidermal growth factor receptor; *WHO,* World Health Organization.

(Courtesy of Diedrich U, Lucius J, Baron E, et al: Distribution of epidermal growth factor receptor gene amplification in brain tumours and correlation to prognosis. *J Neurol* 242:683–688, copyright 1995 by Springer-Verlag.)

mutations were not restricted to any histological entity within the gliomas. There was a significant increase from 0% to 41% in the frequency of gene mutations of gliomas, with an overall frequency of 31%. The average age of patients whose gliomas carried an EGFR gene amplification was 59.4 years, compared with an average age of 44.7 years for those whose gliomas lacked an EGFR gene mutation. The median survival time ranged from 5–9 months for patients with grade I–III gliomas with EGFR gene mutation (Table 3). The occurrence of EGFR gene mutation was not associated with a worse prognosis for patients with glioblastomas. Although other investigations have reported that EGFR gene amplification precedes loss of chromosome 10 in primary glioblastomas, this was not so in this cohort. Glioblastomas in patients older than 64 years of age lacked loss of chromosome 10 in the presence of EGFR gene mutations.

Conclusion.—Most patients whose gliomas carried an EGFR gene mutation, even when the tumor was graded as benign, had a poor prognosis compared to patients with glioblastomas. Findings were not in agreement with other reports stating that EGFR gene amplification requires loss of chromosome 10 in primary glioblastomas. Chromosome 10 was not found in any patients with glioblastoma who were older than 64 years of age.

► This is a relatively small series of patients. It is interesting that EGFR gene amplification correlated with prognosis and, most importantly, with a shorter period until progression of the tumor. The EGFR ligand may be important in other diseases, such as medullary carcinoma of the thyroid. Therefore, genetic mutations such as these may have implications for more aggressive multimodality treatment. Although this aggressive behavior of tumors was seen in young patients anecdotally, 1 limitation of this study is that it is not age-corrected. Furthermore, it has always been assumed that EGFR gene amplification has been associated with chromosome 10 loss.

This may be true in younger patients, but in older patients, loss of chromosome 10 is not a precondition for such amplification.

T.J. Eberlein, M.D.

Melanoma

The Role of Selective Lymphadenectomy in the Management of Patients With Malignant Melanoma

Glass LF, Fenske NA, Messina JL, et al (Univ of South Florida College of Medicine, Tampa)

Dermatol Surg 21:979–983, 1995 11–8

Background.—There is evidence to suggest that long-term survival for patients with intermediate thickness malignant melanoma (MM) and regional lymph node metastasis have a significantly reduced long-term survival rate in comparison with those who have no nodal involvement. Studies on the utility of regional lymph node dissection in these patients, however, have been inconclusive. A clinical experience with selective lymphadenectomy involving lymph node mapping and sentinel node biopsy in patients with intermediate thickness MM was reported.

Methods.—Preoperative and intraoperative lymph node mapping using lymphoscintigraphy to locate the sentinel node was performed in 132 patients with MM and a tumor thickness greater than 0.76 mm. There were 78 men and 54 women with a mean age of 53 years. The mean Breslow thickness of the tumor was 2.2 mm. The sentinel node was defined as the first node in the node basin most likely to harbor micrometastasis. Complete lymph node dissection was performed only if the sentinel node was found to harbor micrometastatic disease.

Results.—Thirty-one of the 132 patients (23%) had positive sentinel node biopsies and underwent complete lymph node dissection under general anesthesia. The sentinel node was found to be the only node involved in 23 of the 31 patients. Forty-one of 47 (87%) sentinel nodes identified in these 31 patients contained micrometastasis, compared with only 44 of the 531 (8%) excised nonsentinel nodes.

Conclusions.—Selective lymphadenectomy based on the results of lymphatic mapping is an effective method for staging patients with intermediate thickness cutaneous MM. Both the preoperative and intraoperative mapping procedures should be performed after the initial biopsy but before performing wide local excision.

▶ This is a very interesting paper by the group at the University of South Florida College of Medicine. The authors extend their earlier work and that of Morton's group at the John Wayne Cancer Center. Several points with this technique need emphasis. In melanoma patients, unlike breast cancer patients, sentinel lymph nodes can be defined with relative certainty, especially in patients with melanoma in the extremities. Removal of the sentinel node can be performed easily under local anesthesia, and this provides the opportunity not only for standard histologic review but also immunocytochemistry and/or molecular biological studies. A negative sentinel node biopsy can potentially spare the patient a regional lymph node dissection. In this series, only 1 patient had subsequent metastasis developed when the sentinel node biopsy was negative. Although specialized equipment is necessary, the technique itself is quite simple to learn and fairly easy to perform. A randomized multicenter trial is currently evaluating this selective approach to lymphadenectomy. We are anxiously awaiting the results.

T.J. Eberlein, M.D.

Efficacy of an Elective Regional Lymph Node Dissection of 1 to 4 mm Thick Melanomas for Patients 60 Years of Age and Younger

Balch CM, Soong S-J, Bartolucci AA, et al (Univ of Texas, Houston; Univ of Alabama at Birmingham; Univ of Kansas, Kansas City; et al)

Ann Surg 224:255–266, 1996 11–9

Background.—The value of immediate, elective regional lymph node dissection continues to be debated. A prospective, multicenter, randomized trial was performed to determine whether elective lymph node dissection (ELND) improves survival rates among patients with intermediate-thickness melanoma.

Methods and Findings.—Seven hundred forty patients with stage I or II melanoma were stratified by tumor thickness, anatomical site, and ulceration and randomly assigned to ELND or nodal observation. They were followed for a median of 7.4 years. Tumor ulceration, trunk site, tumor thickness, and patient age independently influenced survival. Although overall 5-year survival was comparable in the ELND and observation groups, it was significantly better in patients aged 60 years or younger undergoing ELND. Among these patients, the 5-year survival rate was better with ELND in patients with tumors 1 to 2 mm thick, those without tumor ulceration, or those in both categories. Survival was lower in patients older than 60 years undergoing ELND compared with observation. When crossover patients were included in the analysis, ELND was associated with a significantly improved 5-year survival rate in patients with tumors 1 to 2 mm thick, those without tumor ulceration, and those 60 years of age or younger with 1 to 2 mm thick tumors or no ulceration (Figs 3 and 6).

Conclusion.—Surgical treatment is beneficial in selected patients with clinically occult regional metastases. Because distant disease is still developing in some of these patients, however, this analysis should be considered to be interim.

► This is a prospective, multi-institutional trial of over 700 patients conducted by the Intergroup Melanoma Surgical Program. Overall 5-year survival was not significantly different for patients who received ELND. In looking at subcategories of these patients, however, there appeared to be small statistically significant improvement in survival for patients under the

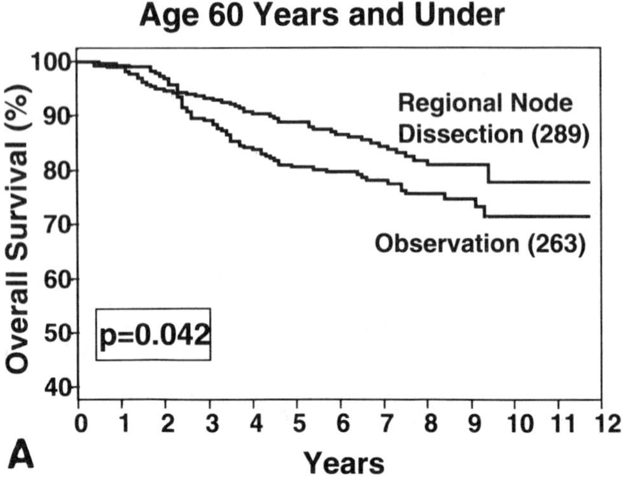

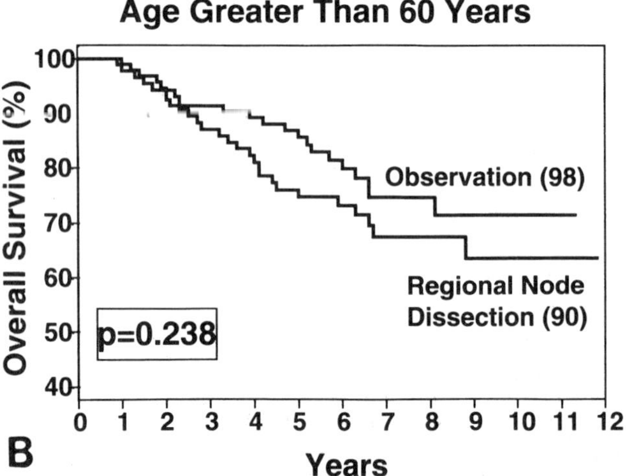

FIGURE 3.—Survival rates by age group based on randomized intent. (Courtesy of Balch CM, Soong S-J, Bartolucci AA, et al: Efficacy of an elective regional lymph node dissection of 1 to 4 mm thick melanomas for patients 60 years of age and younger. *Ann Surg* 224:255–266, 1996.)

age of 60 years (Fig 3), patients with tumor thickness of 1–2 mm (Fig 6, A), and patients without tumor ulceration (Fig 6, B). In this article, no mention is made of the morbidity of ELND. Morton, Reintgen, and others[1,2] have shown quite conclusively that for extremity melanoma, lymphatic mapping for early-stage disease appears to be preferable to ELND. In these studies (a randomized trial is pending), a negative sentinel node biopsy correlates extremely well with a negative lymph node dissection. Thus, a negative sen-

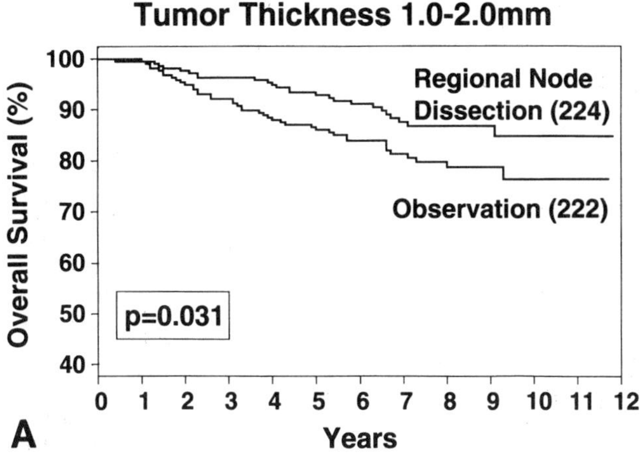

Without Tumor Ulceration

Overall Survival (%)

100
90
80
70
60
50
40

Regional Node Dissection (280)

Observation (262)

p=0.018

0 1 2 3 4 5 6 7 8 9 10 11 12

Years

B

FIGURE 6.—Survival rates by subgroups based on actual treatment received according to tumors 1 to 2 mm thick (**A**) or without ulceration (**B**). This includes patients in all age groups. (Courtesy of Balch CM, Soong S-J, Bartolucci AA, et al: Efficacy of an elective regional lymph node dissection of 1 to 4 mm thick melanomas for patients 60 years of age and younger. *Ann Surg* 224:255–266, 1996.)

tinel node biopsy would, in theory, spare the patient the morbidity of a full lymph node dissection.

T.J. Eberlein, M.D.

References

1. Morton DL, Wen DR, Wong JM, et al: Technical details of intraoperative lymphatic mapping for early stage melanoma. *Arch Surg* 127:392–399, 1992.
2. Reintgen D, Cruse CW, Wells K, et al: The orderly progression of melanoma nodal metastases. *Ann Surg* 220: 759–767, 1994.

Thirty-Five Years of Isolated Limb Perfusion for Melanoma: Indications and Results

Vrouenraets BC, Nieweg OE, Kroon BBR (Netherlands Cancer Inst, Amsterdam)

Br J Surg 83:1319–1328, 1996 11–10

Objective.—Isolated limb perfusion (ILP) is a controversial treatment for melanoma. In ILP, high-dose cytostatic chemotherapy is given locoregionally to a limb that is isolated from the rest of the body by vascular ligation and artificial circulation. This permits very high doses of the chemotherapy drug—usually melphalan—to the limb, while minimizing systemic exposure. Although ILP has been used for many years, its true value remains unknown because of shortcomings in the available research. The literature on ILP as a treatment for melanoma was reviewed.

Findings.—All reports of ILP that included a control group of nonperfused patients and/or included objective response rates were reviewed. Many retrospective studies of ILP have appeared; however, they are inadequate to determine the value of this form of adjuvant therapy. Preliminary data from 1 large trial—the European Organization for Research and Treatment of Cancer–World Health Organization–North American Perfusion Group trial—suggest that ILP may aid locoregional control in patients with melanomas of 1.5–3.0 mm in thickness who do not have elective lymph node dissection. However, there is no definite survival advantage. Therefore, ILP does not seem to be indicated as a treatment for "high-risk" patients with primary melanoma.

Similarly, there are no data to prove that ILP can prevent locoregional recurrence after resection of recurrent limb melanoma. One small study found that ILP could prevent limb recurrence for a while, but results do not justify routine use of the technique. Any survival advantage in this situation will have to be established by a large international trial comparing ILP with simple excision or laser ablation.

Isolated limb perfusion does appear to be the therapeutic procedure of choice in patients with locally inoperable limb melanoma. In this group of patients, ILP provides a good chance of eliminating all macroscopic disease. This can improve the symptoms and avoid the need for amputation, with mild limb and systemic toxicity. However, the limb recurrence rate is high and the duration of response is brief. Prospective studies are needed to compare ILP with other treatments in patients with locally inoperable limb melanoma.

Summary.—The evidence does not support the use of ILP for primary melanoma or recurrent limb melanoma. However, it is the treatment of choice for recurrent limb melanoma that is not suitable for local treatment. Further research is needed into this and other potential indications for ILP in melanoma.

▶ I have included this very nicely written review of ILP simply because of the relative confusion regarding the utilization and results of ILP. The references are up to date and the review is nicely categorized according to prophylactic and therapeutic trials.

British isolated limb perfusion may have the potential of playing a larger role in the management of melanoma, if it is used as a prophylactic treatment. However, prospective randomized trials are not available. From the 1 trial that is being performed by the World Health Organization, a possible reduction in local/regional recurrence is being seen for intermediate thickness melanoma. However, a survival advantage has not been demonstrated.

In patients with recurrent limb melanoma, ILP may delay the occurrence of local/regional metastases, but again survival advantage is not identified. This would seem somewhat logical because ILP is a local/regional treatment. The only way it would have a major impact on survival is to eradicate disease confined to the extremity. This obviously is a very small number of patients because most patients with recurrence would either already have metastatic disease, or would have no evidence of the need for further treatment. There is a small number of patients, however, who have a local/regional recurrence and no evidence of metastatic disease. Although these patients may not benefit in terms of overall survival, ILP offers a very important potential treatment for diminishing an often difficult local problem.

T.J. Eberlein, M.D.

Gallbladder

Is Radical Surgery in Locally Advanced Gallbladder Carcinoma Justified?

Bloechle C, Izbicki JR, Passlick B, et al (Univ Hosp Eppendorf, Germany; Univ of Hamburg, Germany)

Am J Gastroenterol 90:2195–2200, 1995 11–11

Introduction.—Although patients with early gallbladder carcinoma have 5-year survival rates after surgical treatment of 90% to 100%, locally advanced gallbladder carcinoma is regarded to have a dismal prognosis. However, advances in diagnosis, perioperative care, and understanding of the natural history of gallbladder carcinoma has led to a trend toward more aggressive treatment of advanced disease. The effectiveness of radical surgery for the management of locally advanced gallbladder carcinoma was studied retrospectively.

Methods.—Review of the records of patients treated surgically for malignant gallbladder tumors over a 9-year period identified 66 patients with carcinoma that was staged pT2 or more advanced. Of the 66 patients, 25 underwent primarily palliative surgical procedures, including palliative cholecystectomy, hepaticojejunostomy, and segment III bypass procedures. The remaining 41 patients underwent procedures with curative intent, including cholecystectomy and regional lymphadenectomy, en bloc resection of the gallbladder with liver segment and regional lymphadenectomy, and extended right hepatectomy and regional lymphadenectomy. Complete tumor resection (R0) was achieved in 29 patients, and 9 patients had

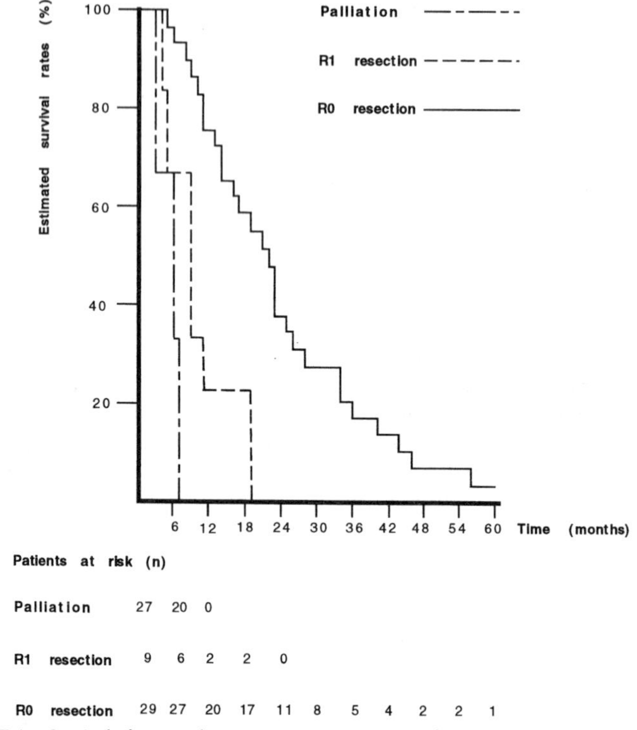

FIGURE 1.—Survival after complete resection (R0, n = 29) and incomplete resection (R1, n = 9; R2, n = 27) of locally advanced gallbladder carcinoma (pT2–pT4), $P < 0.01$ (log-rank test). (Courtesy of Bloechle C, Izbicki JR, Passlick B, et al: Is radical surgery in locally advanced gallbladder carcinoma justified? *Am J Gastroenterol* 90(12):2195–2200, 1995.)

microscopic residual tumor (R1). Survival was calculated and compared among treatment groups and according to surgical outcome.

Results.—Postoperative morbidity and mortality rates were 20% and 1.5%, respectively. The mean survival was 4.5 months in patients who underwent palliative procedures, 25.1 months in patients who underwent R0 resection, and 8.1 months in patients who underwent R1 resection (Fig 1). The particular type of procedure did not significantly affect survival. In patients with R0 resection and no distant metastases, survival was not affected by local tumor progression or tumor invasion into the regional lymph nodes.

Conclusions.—Radical surgical procedures resulting in complete surgical excision of locally advanced gallbladder carcinoma significantly improve survival rates, with a 20% morbidity rate and a 1.5% mortality rate. Future study should evaluate the impact of adjuvant treatment modalities.

► Carcinoma of the gallbladder is a silent cancer that is often diagnosed at advanced stage. This is a retrospective study with the objective of evaluating the effectiveness of radical surgery in locally advanced gallbladder carcinoma. These authors showed that local tumor progression and even invasion into regional lymph nodes did not seem to have an impact on survival in a negative fashion as long as there was no evidence of distant metastases and complete tumor resection was achieved. This has an important caveat that needs emphasis. The importance of the skill of the operating surgeon and familiarity with the anatomy and potential sources of spread of tumor are extremely important. Even in the experienced hands of the reporting surgeons, the morbidity and mortality rates were 20% and 1.5%.

Although an improvement in diagnostic techniques as well as perioperative care would support a more aggressive approach, surgery remains the primary treatment of choice. Better results will be obtained only with better adjuvant therapies.

T.J. Eberlein, M.D.

Pancreas

Polymerase Chain Reaction-based K-*ras* Mutation Detection of Pancreatic Adenocarcinoma in Routine Cytology Smears

Apple SK, Hecht JR, Novak JM, et al (Univ of California, Los Angeles; Johns Hopkins Hosp, Baltimore, Md)
Am J Clin Pathol 105:321–326, 1996 11–12

Purpose.—It can be very difficult to make the cytologic diagnosis of pancreatic carcinoma, especially the distinction between benign atypia and well-differentiated adenocarcinoma. Many pancreatic cancers are associated with mutation of codon 12 in the K-*ras* oncogene. In difficult cases, the diagnosis of pancreatic cancer might be improved through detection by polymerase chain reaction (PCR) followed by restriction endonuclease digestion. A PCR-based detection method for the diagnosis of pancreatic carcinoma in routine cytologic smears was investigated.

Methods.—The study included pancreatic cytology specimens from 60 patients: 46 with adenocarcinoma of the pancreas, 2 with islet cell tumors, and 12 with benign lesions. The DNA was extracted from the slides, and a fragment that represented K-*ras* exon 1 and spanning codon 12 was amplified by PCR. The amplification process used a single base mismatch incorporated at the 31st nucleotide of the 5'-primer and a wild-type 3'-primer. This produced a Bst-N1 recognition site with the wild-type codon 12, but not the mutant allele. The results, which were available in 24 to 48 hours, were compared with those of clinical follow-up.

Results.—Five of the 46 cases of adenocarcinoma were false-negative on cytomorphologic analysis. The new PCR-based technique detected K-*ras* codon 12 mutations in 44 of these 46 cases, including cancers of all grades and histologic types. No such mutations were identified in the benign cases or islet cell tumors. The K-*ras* mutation was also detected in 12 cases of metastatic pancreatic carcinoma. The mutation was detected in samples that contained as few as 5 cells with a ratio of 1:1,000 tumor to nontumor cells. All 5 cases that had been false-negative on cytomorphologic analysis were positive by K-*ras* mutation analysis.

Conclusion.—A PCR-based technique for detection of K-*ras* mutations in pancreatic adenocarcinoma uses routine cytology slides and produces results in 1 or 2 days. It may help to make the diagnosis of pancreatic cancer more sensitive in ambiguous cases and reduce the risks, discomfort, and costs associated with surgical exploration for definitive diagnosis.

Molecular Diagnosis of Exocrine Pancreatic Cancer Using a Percutaneous Technique

Evans DB, Frazier ML, Charnsangavej C, et al (Univ of Texas, Houston)
Ann Surg Oncol 3:241–246, 1996 11–13

Background.—The diagnosis of pancreatic adenocarcinoma is commonly established by the cytologic findings of CT-guided percutaneous fine-needle aspiration (FNA) of the pancreas. However, false-negative FNA results are common. Most patients with exocrine pancreatic cancer have the K-*ras* oncogene, characterized by point mutations at codon 12. The feasibility of detecting the K-*ras* mutation by extracting DNA from the FNA material discarded during cytologic slide preparation was investigated.

Methods.—Twenty-five patients with a pancreatic mass who underwent CT-guided FNA and in whom pancreatic adenocarcinoma was cytologically or histologically diagnosed were studied. The FNA sample was centrifuged, and the DNA was extracted from the supernatant. The DNA was amplified with 15 cycles of polymerase chain reaction (PCR) using primers K-*ras* 5^1 and K-*ras* 3^1, then digested with BstNI (to remove the wild-type K-*ras* codon 12, which has a BstNI restriction site not found on mutant K-*ras* codon 12). The PCR and digestion steps were repeated, then subjected to gel electrophoresis (Fig 1).

Results.—Each specimen yielded a median of 3.33 μg of DNA. Mutant K-*ras* DNA was detected in 21 of the 25 samples, including the samples from 6 of 8 patients with potentially resectable disease and from 15 of 17 patients with locally advanced or metastatic disease. All of these patients had positive cytology results.

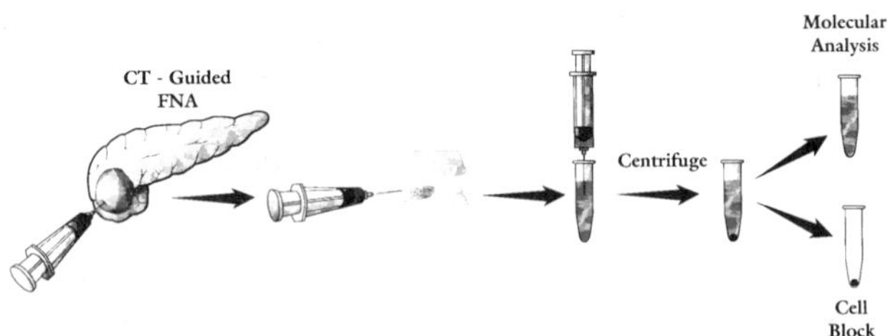

FIGURE 1.—Illustration of the steps involved in processing a fine-needle aspiration specimen in the dedicated radiology-cytology diagnostic suite. The material submitted for molecular analysis would ordinarily be discarded. (Courtesy of Evans DB, Frazier MI, Charnsangavej C, et al: Molecular diagnosis of exocrine pancreatic cancer using a percutaneous technique. *Ann Surg Oncol* 3:241–246, 1996.)

Conclusion.—The extraction of DNA for PCR analysis from the material usually discarded from FNA samples is feasible and does not interfere with FNA preparation for cytologic analysis. This technique provides objective data that can be used as an adjunct to cytologic analyses of FNA specimens. Molecular analysis may be useful at institutions without cytopathologists experienced in the interpretation of pancreatic FNA specimens.

▶ These 2 articles deal with a similar technique: PCR-based amplification of DNA extracted from slides with mismatched primers that introduce a BstN1 restriction endonuclease cleavage site at codon 12 of the wild-type, but not mutant, K-*ras*.

In the article by Apple and colleagues (Abstract 11–12), 44 of 46 cases of pancreatic cancer and none in the 12 benign or 2 islet cell tumor cases showed K-*ras* codon 12 mutations. In the article by Evans and colleagues, 21 of 25 specimens demonstrated mutated K-*ras* DNA.

Figure 1 in the Evans article demonstrates the methodology that is quite simple and can easily be performed even retrospectively on cytology smears. This technique requires no special handling, is cost effective, and may augment the ability to diagnose pancreatic carcinoma.

T.J. Eberlein, M.D.

Pancreaticoduodenectomy: Does It Have a Role in the Palliation of Pancreatic Cancer?

Lillemoe KD, Cameron JL, Yeo CJ, et al (Johns Hopkins Med Insts, Baltimore, Md)

Ann Surg 223:718–728, 1996 11–14

Objective.—Recent data indicate that patients with pancreatic carcinoma have improved survival after pancreaticoduodenectomy even with

TABLE 5.—Perioperative Complications

	Palliative Pancreatico-duodenectomy (N = 64)	Palliative Bypass (N = 62)	Significance
Hospital mortality (%)	1.6	1.6	NS
Complications (%)			
Delayed gastric emptying	27	16	NS
Pancreatic fitsula	11	2	NS
Cholangitis	2	10	NS
Biliary anastomotic leak	2	3	NS
Cardiac	2	2	NS
Pneumonia	2	2	NS
None	58	68	NS
Length of postoperative stay	18.4 days	15.0 days	$p < 0.03$

NS=not significant.

(Courtesy of Lillemoe KD, Cameron JL, Yeo CJ, et al: Pancreaticoduodenectomy: Does it have a role in the palliation of pancreatic cancer? *Ann Surg* 223:718–728, 1996.)

TABLE 6.—Survival and Quality of Life

	Palliative Pancreatico-duodenectomy	Palliative Bypass
Median survival (mos)	12.0	9.0
Mean survival (mos)	15.3	11.4
Actual survival (%)		
1 year	62.5	38.7
2 years	15.6	8.1
3 years	6.3	0
5 years	1.6	0
Hospital readmissions (patients)	7	12
Reoperations (patients)	0	3

(Courtesy of Lillemoe KD, Cameron JL, Yeo CJ, et al: Pancreaticoduodenectomy: Does it have a role in the palliation of pancreatic cancer? *Ann Surg* 233:718–728, 1996.)

lymph node involvement and positive margins. Unresectable pancreatic carcinoma usually is treated palliatively with biliary and gastric bypass. Perioperative complications and overall survival in patients undergoing pancreaticoduodenectomy were compared with those in patients undergoing standard surgical palliation.

Methods.—Prospective data were collected on 64 patients aged 37–85 years who underwent palliative pancreaticoduodenectomy and had positive margins between 1986 and 1994, and 62 patients aged 41–82 years who underwent standard surgical palliation, mostly biliary and gastric bypass, because of local invasion with no evidence of metastatic disease between 1986 and 1991. Survival was analyzed statistically.

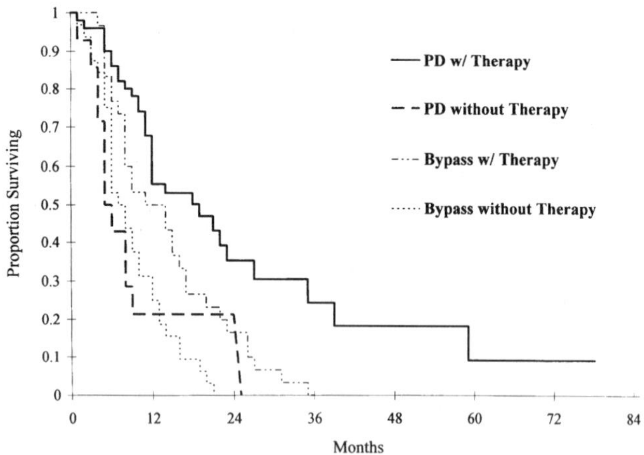

FIGURE 2.—The actuarial survival curves for patients undergoing palliative pancreaticoduodenectomy (*PD*) with (*W/*, n = 50) and without (*n* = 14) postoperative chemotherapy and radiation therapy and palliative bypass with (*W/*, *n* = 30) and without (n = 32) therapy. (Courtesy of Lillemoe KD, Cameron JL, Yeo CJ, et al: Pancreaticoduodenectomy: Does it have a role in the palliation of pancreatic cancer? *Ann Surg* 223:718–728, 1996.)

Results.—Hospital mortality and complications were similar in the 2 groups, but the pancreaticoduodenectomy group had a significantly longer hospital stay (Table 5). Postoperative chemotherapy and radiation therapy were administered to 48% of the unresected group and 78% of the pancreaticoduodenectomy group. Overall survival was significantly improved for the pancreaticoduodenectomy group (Table 6). Postoperative adjuvant therapy improved survival significantly (Fig 2).

Conclusion.—For patients with pancreatic cancer, pancreaticoduodenectomy improves survival significantly over standard palliative surgery without increasing perioperative morbidity and mortality.

▶ These authors compared, retrospectively, a group of consecutive patients undergoing pancreaticoduodenectomy for pancreatic cancer who had gross or microscopic evidence of adenocarcinoma at the surgical resection margin with a group of consecutively identified patients who had unresectable disease because of local invasion but had no evidence of metastatic disease. The vast majority of this latter group underwent biliary and gastric bypass. As expected, median survival was less for the palliative bypass group. It should be noted that the very acceptable operative mortality is attributable to the experience of the authors at this institution. Similarly, the nonsignificant risk of complication is also the result of the experience of these authors. Thus, trying to perform these types of operations in patients with marginally resectable disease may result in significantly different complications in a community setting. Palliative pancreaticoduodenectomy resulted in a marginally significant increased hospital stay. However, re-admission and re-operation were more frequent in the palliative bypass group (Table 6).

As is seen in Figure 2 of this paper, there is a suggestion that palliative pancreaticoduodenectomy with postoperative chemotherapy and radiation therapy may confer a significant survival advantage to patients treated with palliative surgery but without these adjuvant treatments. Obviously this implies having minimal morbidity and mortality from the surgery but also significant experience in radiation therapy techniques to minimize the morbidity of this very intensive treatment for these patients. Treatment of this disease, however, will benefit significantly from the introduction of newer adjuvant therapies and/or diagnosis at an earlier time. However, in specialized centers, palliative surgery, especially in combination with postoperative adjuvant multimodality therapy, may have significant benefit in a small number of patients.

T.J. Eberlein, M.D.

bcl-2 and p53 Expression in Resectable Pancreatic Adenocarcinomas: Association With Clinical Outcome

Sinicrope FA, Evans DB, Leach SD, et al (Univ of Texas, Houston)
Clin Cancer Res 2:2015–2022, 1996 11–15

Introduction.—The fifth most common cause of cancer-related death in the United States is pancreatic carcinoma, and the prognosis continues to be poor. The selection of patients for anticancer treatment may be improved by correlation of patient outcome with genetic markers. The process of apoptosis, or programmed cell death, seems to be regulated by the *bcl-2* proto-oncogene and the *p53* gene. The expression and regulation of the p53 and bcl-2 proteins and their prognostic significance in resectable pancreatic adenocarcinoma were examined.

Methods.—In 35 archival pancreatic and 6 ampullary adenocarcinomas, bcl-2 and p53 expression was analyzed, along with their relationship to overall survival. Fifteen patients were treated with 5-fluorouracil and irradiation after surgery, and 21 patients were treated with 5-fluorouracil and irradiation before surgery; 5 had only surgery.

Results.—In 22 of 40 tumors (55%), cytoplasmic bcl-2 was detected and in 20 of 37 (54%) tumors, nuclear p53 proteins were detected with specific monoclonal antibodies. There was no relationship between bcl-2 and p53 expression. Preoperative chemoradiation resulted in no histologic response

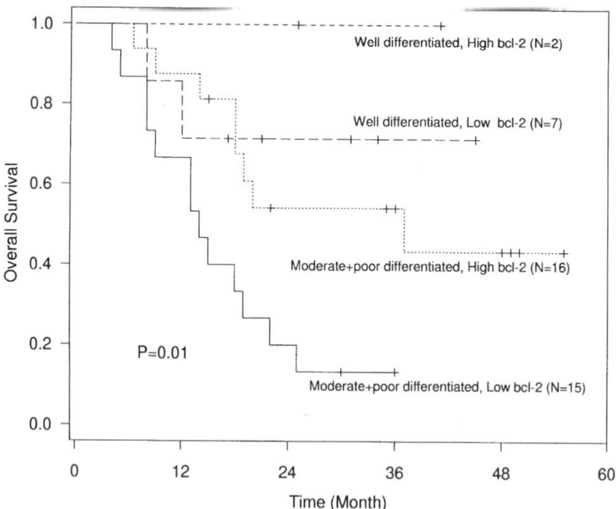

FIGURE 3.—Multivariate analysis of overall survival stratified by the combined variable of bcl-2 protein expression and histologic grade. High bcl-2 refers to > 25% bcl-2–positive tumor cells with medium-to-strong intensity; low bcl-2 refers to ≥ 25% bcl-2–positive tumor cells with weak intensity. Overall survival differences among the 4 categories were significant ($P = 0.010$). Statistical significance was preserved when the first 3 categories were combined and compared with tumors with moderate and poor differentiation and low bcl-2 ($P = 0.002$). (Courtesy of Sinicrope FA, Evans DB, Leach SD, et al: bcl-2 and p53 expression in resectable pancreatic adenocarcinomas: Association with clinical outcome. *Clin Cancer Res* 2:2015–2022, 1996.)

with bcl-2 or p53. Twenty-one of 41 cases had lymph node involvement, and poor overall survival was predicted by lymph node involvement. In well-differentiated tumors and in those with increased bcl-2 expression, there was a trend toward improved survival (Fig 3). Clinical outcome was not related to p53 expression. At a median follow-up of 34.7 months, 24 patients had died, 15 were alive without evidence of disease, and 2 had recurrent disease. The median survival was 19 months.

Conclusion.—In pancreatic carcinomas, bcl-2 and p53 proteins were widely expressed. The single most important predictor of overall survival was nodal status, according to the multivariate analysis. The only stronger prognostic variable than nodal status alone was the combined variable of bcl-2 expression and histologic grade. Preoperative biopsy specimens can be used to evaluate these features, which cannot be said for nodal status.

▶ *bcl-2* is a proto-oncogene that encodes an integral membrane protein that protects cells from apoptosis and, in fact, has been thought to play a role in resistance to apoptotic stimuli, including multiple anticancer drugs and irradiation. It is not surprising, therefore, that in resectable pancreatic adenocarcinoma, a trend toward improved survival is seen in well-differentiated tumors and in those with increased bcl-2 expression.

This group from M.D. Anderson Cancer Center has constructed a model that predicts for survival by showing that moderately and poorly differentiated tumors with low bcl-2 expression have an extremely poor survival. While nodal status has been associated with predicting poor overall survival, by using histologic grade and bcl-2 expression, one would be able to evaluate and predict survival in preoperative biopsy specimens. This might also help in selecting patients who might benefit from neoadjuvant or adjuvant therapies, in spite of successful surgical excisions.

T.J. Eberlein, M.D.

Outcomes

Comparison of Individual Surgeon's Performance: Risk-adjusted Analysis With POSSUM Scoring System

Sagar PM, Hartley MN, MacFie J, et al (Royal Liverpool Univ, England; Scarborough Hosp, England; Warrington Hosp, England)

Dis Colon Rectum 39:654–658, 1996 11–16

Introduction.—There is growing public interest in rating the performance of individual hospitals and surgeons. Such comparisons are misleading, however, if no form of risk-adjusted analysis is performed. In comparing the outcomes of colorectal resection among different surgeons, an allowance must be made for differences in case mix and patient fitness. A simple and well-validated scoring system was used for risk-adjusted comparison of the performance of 5 different surgeons.

Methods.—The Physiological and Operative Severity Score for Enumeration of Morbidity and Mortality (POSSUM) (Table 1) was used to determine the morbidity and mortality risk of 438 patients who underwent

TABLE 1.—Physiologic Score

	Score			
	1	2	4	8
Age	<60	61–70	>71	JVP
Cardiac signs	No failure	Cardiac medications	Edema	
Respiratory	No dyspnea	SOBOE	Limiting dyspnea	SOB at rest
Blood Pressure				
Systolic	110–130	131–170	>170	
Diastolic		100–109	90–99	<90
Pulse	50–80	81–100	101–120	>120
		40–49		<40
Glasgow Coma Score	15	12–14	9–11	<9
Hemoglobin	13–16	11.5–12.9	10.0–11.4	<10.0
		16.1–17.0	17.1–18.0	>18.0
White cell count	4–10	10.1–20.0	>20	
		3.0–4.0	<3.0	
Urea	<7.5	7.6–10.0	10.1–15.0	>15.0
Sodium	>135	131–135	126–130	<126
Potassium	3.5–5.0	3.2–3.4	2.9–3.1	<2.8
		5.1–5.3	5.4–5.9	>5.9
Echocardiogram	Normal		Atrial fibrillation	Any other abnormal rhythm

Operative Severity Score

	Score			
	1	2	4	8
Operative severity	Minor	Moderate	Major	Major†
No. of procedures	1		2	>2
Total blood loss (ml)	<100	101–500	501–999	>999
Peritoneal soiling	None	Minor (serous fluid)	Local pus	Free feces blood or pus
Presence of malignancy	None	Primary only	Positive nodes	Distant metastases
Mode of surgery	Elective		Emergency resus of >2 hours possible	Distant metastases Immediate

Abbreviations: JVP, jugular venous pulse; *SOBOE,* shortness of breath on exertion.

(Courtesy of Sagar PM, Hartley MN, MacFie J, et al: Comparison of individual surgeon's performance: Risk-adjusted analysis with POSSUM scoring system. *Dis Colon Rectum* 39(6):654–658, 1996.)

colorectal resection. Each patient was operated on by 1 of 5 study surgeons. The predicted morbidity and mortality rates were compared with the observed crude rates for each of the 5 surgeons.

Results.—The crude incidence of morbidity varied substantially by operating surgeon, from 14% to 31%. Thirty-day mortality rates varied as well, from 4.5% to 6.9%. There were no significant differences, however, on the risk-adjusted analysis. The overall observed:expected ratio for the entire study sample was 0.87 for mortality and 0.97 for morbidity.

Conclusions.—Comparing surgeons on the basis of their crude operative mortality and postoperative morbidity rates can produce misleading results. Risk-adjusted analysis, with use of the POSSUM system, shows that most of the variation in outcome is related to the surgeons' case mix and the patients' physiologic status. Such risk-adjusted analyses allow meaningful comparisons of surgical performance.

▶ As we enter an era of much tighter scrutiny by HMOs and institutions that measure quality as well as productivity, a simple means of comparison among surgeons has traditionally been incidence of morbidity and mortality. I've included this article because it demonstrates that the incidence of morbidity may vary sharply among surgeons; when risk-adjusted analysis is applied, however, a more meaningful comparison is obtained.

A simple scoring system, POSSUM, has been developed for use in general surgery. The system has been utilized fairly extensively. Obtaining a POSSUM score is relatively quick and is usually obtained from the case history. This technique also has value when comparing outcome among multiple institutions.

As seen in Table 4 of the original article, surgeon A had a higher rate of morbidity, yet the risk-adjusted morbidity rate (Table 5) showed this surgeon's morbidity to be no different than the other 4 surgeons studied.

As further scrutiny of individual surgical practice is undertaken, development of better standardized systems for comparison of information will be necessary. This article will stimulate discussion in this regard.

T.J. Eberlein, M.D.

Safe and Effective Early Postoperative Feeding and Hospital Discharge After Open Colon Resection

Choi J, O'Connell TX (Kaiser Permanente Med Ctr, Los Angeles)

Am Surg 62:853–856, 1996 11–17

Objective.—The safety of early feeding after open colon resection was investigated.

Background.—Postoperative feeding is normally begun after colon resection when postoperative ileus has resolved. It is believed that this delay prevents nausea and vomiting and allows the anastomosis to heal, but delayed feeding can prolong the time IV fluid is needed and delay hospital discharge. It has been reported that patients can be fed before signs of return to bowel function after laparoscopic and laparoscopic-assisted colon resection. It is unclear whether early feeding and hospital discharge are possible after open colon resection.

Methods.—An early postoperative feeding protocol was used in 41 patients (group A) who had open colon resection. There was no routine use of postoperative nasogastric tube, a clear liquid diet was started on postoperative day 2, and a regular diet was started on day 3 as tolerated. Patients were discharged after the regular diet was tolerated. A control group (group B) consisted of an additional 41 patients who had open colon resection and followed a traditional feeding protocol. The surgical procedures were similar for both groups and were performed by one surgeon.

Results.—In group A, a clear liquid diet was begun earlier than in group B. Tolerance of the clear liquid diet was similar in both groups. A nasogastric tube was needed in 4 patients from group B, but no patient in group A required such a tube. The mean hospital stay was 4.2 days for group A

TABLE 3.—Results

	Group A	Group B
Tolerate feeding	37/41 (90%)	35/41 (85%)
Start clear liquid diet (days)	2	4.9 (range 4–7)
Hospital discharge (days)	4.2 (range 3–8)	6.7 (5–34)
Discharge by POD 4 (patients)	27/41 (66%)	0/41

Abbreviation: POD, postoperative day.
(Courtesy of Choi J, O'Connell TX: Safe and effective early postoperative feeding and hospital discharge after open colon resection. *Am Surg* 62:853–856, 1996.)

and 6.7 days for group B. By day 4, 67% of patients in group A had been discharged, compared to none in group B (Table 3). There were no readmissions within 2 weeks for nausea or vomiting. Morbidity and mortality were similar for both groups.

Conclusions.—In these patients after open colon resection, early postoperative feeding and early hospital discharge were safe. It is unnecessary to delay feeding until signs of ileus resolution. The feeding and discharge results of this protocol after open colon resection are similar to results reported after laparoscopic colon resection.

► I have selected this paper because it raises an issue that we in the northeast are facing: trying to minimize length of stay after bowel surgery. This article is not a randomized prospective trial but rather a study of consecutive patients. However, in reviewing the article, the demographics are remarkably similar for the 2 groups of patients. As can be seen in Table 3, starting a clear liquid diet early results in early hospital discharge, reducing by 33% the length of stay. A concern among surgeons in delaying the onset of oral intake has been the risk of nausea, vomiting, and abdominal distention, or possibly anastomotic leak. This study showed that even the patients who received early feeding had no greater risk of emesis or abdominal distention. Early feeding has been used in laparoscopic surgical procedures and yet the anastomoses are virtually identical. Increased risk of leak is not identified and this conclusion has also been verified by the current study. The use of nonopiate analgesics during the postoperative period may also further improve results. Nonopiates were not used in the present study.

T.J. Eberlein, M.D.

Sarcoma

Analysis of Prognostic Factors in 1,041 Patients With Localized Soft Tissue Sarcomas of the Extremities

Pisters PWT, Leung DHY, Woodruff J, et al (Mem Sloan-Kettering Cancer Ctr, New York)

J Clin Oncol 14:1679–1689, 1996 11–18

Introduction.—Several attempts have been made to identify prognostic factors for local recurrence, distant metastasis, and tumor-related mortality in extremity soft-tissue sarcoma, but the results have been inconsistent. Specific independent adverse clinicopathologic factors for event-free survival were identified in a cohort of consecutively treated patients with extremity soft-tissue sarcomas.

Methods.—Data were collected prospectively from 1,041 adult patients with localized extremity sarcomas (stage IA to IIIB) over an 8-year period. Almost all patients were treated with surgical resection by limb-sparing surgery or amputation. Some patients received adjuvant chemotherapy or radiation therapy. Univariate and multivariate analyses were used to analyze patient, tumor, and pathologic factors for independent prognostic factors for the end points of local recurrence, distant recurrence, disease-specific survival, and postmetastasis survival.

Results.—Most patients (80%) had localized primary sarcomas at the initial visit. The lesions were 5 cm or larger in 53% of patients and smaller than 5 cm in 41% of patients. Lesion size was not determined in 6% of patients who had undergone resection of their sarcomas at another institution. The proximal lower extremity was the most common anatomical site and most lesions were located beneath the investing fascia. The 5-year survival rate was 76% for local recurrence and 75% for distant recurrence. The median follow-up was 3.95 years. For local recurrence, the significant independent adverse prognostic factors were age greater than 50 years, recurrent disease at initial visit, microscopically positive surgical margins, and the histologic subtypes fibrosarcoma and malignant peripheral-nerve tumor (Table 3). The significant independent adverse prognostic factors for distant recurrence were intermediate tumor size, large tumor size, high histologic grade, deep location, recurrent disease at initial visit, and the histologic subtypes leiomyosarcoma and nonliposarcoma (Table 4). Large tumor size, high grade, deep location, recurrent disease at initial visit, the histologic subtypes leiomyosarcoma and malignant peripheral-nerve tumor, microscopically positive surgical margins, and lower extremity site were adverse factors for disease-specific survival. Tumor larger than 10 cm was the only adverse prognostic factor for postmetastasis survival. The relative hazards for the development of distant metastasis from high- and low-grade tumors changed over time; the hazard rate for high-grade tumors was most acute in the first 30 months after surgery (Fig 1). After 30 months, the hazard rate for metastases decreased, but did not plateau.

TABLE 3.—Analyses of Local Recurrences

Variable	5-Year LR-Free Rate (%)	Univariate *P*	Selection Into Cox Model (Score *P*)	Model Coefficient	SE	RR	95% CI
Age, years							
≤ 50	79.9						
> 50	70.7	.016	.0011	0.45	0.16	1.6	1.1–2.1
Sex							
Female	74.9						
Male	76.0	.69					
Presentation							
Primary	79.2						
Recurrence	60.3	.0001	.0001	0.68	0.17	2.0	1.4–2.7
Size (cm)							
< 5	80.2						
5–10	72.6						
> 10	72.8	.025*					
Site							
Upper extremity-proximal	70.8						
Upper extremity-distal	72.1						
Lower extremity-proximal	78.6						
Lower extremity-distal	75.1	.31*					
Location							
Proximal	76.9						
Distal	73.6	.53					
Depth							
Superficial	79.4						
Deep	74.1	.26					
Grade							
Low	73.6						
High	76.2	.55					
Symptoms							
No pain	75.6						
Painful	75.8	.91					
Bone or neurovascular invasion							
Absent	76.8						
Present	55.0	.015					
Histology							
Liposarcoma	73.9						
Malignant fibrous histocytoma	76.2						
Synovial sarcoma	87.6						
Fibrosarcoma	60.1		.0058	0.59	0.21	2.5	1.4–4.4
Leiomyosarcoma	82.8						
Malignant peripheral-nerve tumor	68.7		.0010	0.89	0.30	1.8	1.2–2.7
Other tumors	76.3	.0006*					
Microscopic surgical margins							
Negative	80.0						
Positive	59.9	.0001	.0001	0.57	0.17	1.8	1.3–2.5

*Log-rank tests of no differences among categories vs. any differences among categories.

Abbreviation: LR, local recurrence.

(Courtesy of Pisters PWT, Leung DHY, Woodruff J, et al: Analysis of prognostic factors in 1,041 patients with localized soft tissue sarcomas of the extremities. *J Clin Oncol* 14:1679–1689, 1996.)

TABLE 4.—Analyses of Distant Recurrences

Variable	5-Year DR-Free Rate (%)	Univariate *P*	Selection Into Cox Model (Score *P*)	Model Coefficient	SE	RR	95% CI
Age, years							
≤ 50	75.0						
> 50	71.8	.10					
Sex							
Female	75.0						
Male	71.7	.21					
Presentation							
Primary	73.6						
Recurrence	71.9	.87	.015	0.42	0.17	1.5	1.0–2.1
Size (cm)							
< 5	83.5						
5–10	66.8		.0001	0.65	0.18	1.9	1.3–2.8
> 10	59.6	.0001*	.028	0.41	0.16	1.5	1.0–2.0
Site							
Upper extremity-proximal	79.5						
Upper extremity-distal	76.7						
Lower extremity-proximal	70.3						
Lower extremity-distal	73.0	.049*					
Location							
Proximal	72.4						
Distal	74.7	.72					
Depth							
Superficial	90.2						
Deep	67.5	.0001	.0007	0.91	0.25	2.5	1.5–4.1
Grade							
Low	93.0						
High	63.3	.0001	.0001	1.5	0.24	4.3	2.6–6.9
Symptoms							
No pain	74.6						
Painful	66.9	.041					
Bone or neurovascular invasion							
Absent	74.0						
Present	63.5	.061					
Histology							
Liposarcoma	79.4		.0031	−0.44	0.17	0.64	0.46–0.90
Malignant fibrous histocytoma	75.9						
Synovial sarcoma	63.5						
Fibrosarcoma	93.8						
Leiomyosarcoma	67.4		.024	0.52	0.23	1.7	1.0–2.6
Malignant peripheral-nerve tumor	67.4						
Other tumors	55.9	.0001*					
Microscopic surgical margins							
Negative	74.1						
Positive	70.3	.13					

*Log-rank tests of no differences among categories vs. any differences among categories.

Abbreviation: DR, distant recurrence.

(Courtesy of Pisters PWT, Leung DHY, Woodruff J, et al: Analysis of prognostic factors in 1,041 patients with localized soft tissue sarcomas of the extremities. *J Clin Oncol* 14:1679–1689, 1996.)

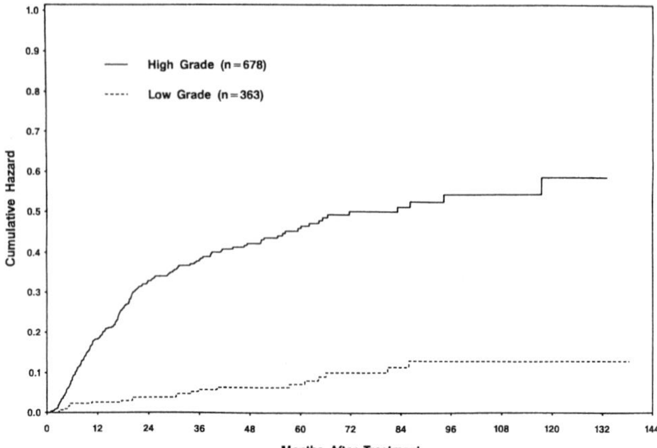

FIGURE 1.—Cumulative hazard of developing distant metastasis by histologic grade as a function of time from initial treatment at Memorial Sloan-Kettering Cancer Center. (Courtesy of Pisters PWT, Leung DHY, Woodruff J, et al: Analysis of prognostic factors in 1,041 patients with localized soft tissue sarcomas of the extremities. *J Clin Oncol* 14:1679–1689, 1996.)

Within the 30-month period, metastasis developed in 177 patients. Of these, only 10 patients had low grade-tumors.

Conclusion.—Specific adverse prognostic factors were identified for local recurrence, distant recurrence, tumor-related mortality, and postmetastasis survival. These data may be considered reliable for re-evaluation of the current staging systems for soft-tissue sarcoma, design of clinical trials, and identification of individual patients at high risk for disease recurrence and death.

▶ This is an extremely large, prospectively collected database from Memorial Sloan-Kettering Cancer Center. The major finding of this analysis is that different prognostic factors influence local recurrence, especially recurrent disease at presentation and microscopically positive surgical margins (see Table 3). In contrast, the more traditional prognostic markers of tumor size, histologic grade, and deep location were important for predicting distant recurrence (see Table 4). As seen in Figure 1, tumor grade is important in the development of distant metastasis, but this effect is most marked in the early post-treatment period. Because the development of distant metastasis is associated with tumor-related mortality, it was not surprising that the prognostic factors observed to result in an increased risk for distant metastasis were similar to those for tumor-related mortality. In summary, the adverse prognostic factors for local recurrence in extremity soft-tissue sarcomas are different from those for distant metastasis and disease-specific survival. These authors also emphasize the fact that an increased risk is associated with presentation with locally recurrent disease or microscopically positive surgical margins. Patients who have these features that result in local recurrence are at increased risk for subsequent local recurrence, distant recurrence, and tumor-related mortality.

T.J. Eberlein, M.D.

Breast

The Prognostic Value of Lymphatic and Blood Vessel Invasion in Operable Breast Cancer

Lauria R, Perrone F, Carlomagno C, et al (Università degli Studi di Napoli "Federico II," Napoli, Italy; Seconda Università di Napoli, Italy; CNR-ACRO, Napoli, Italy)

Cancer 76:1772–1778, 1995 11–19

Introduction.—In addition to axillary node metastasis and the size of the primary tumor, both lymphatic vessel invasion (LVI) and blood vessel invasion (BVI) by tumor emboli have been assumed to have potential prognostic value. This remains to be proved, however, in part because of varying methods of pathologic assessment and a lack of multivariate analysis in many studies.

Objective.—To document the prognostic value of LVI and BVI, both univariate and multivariate survival analyses were carried out in a retrospective sample of 1,408 consecutive patients with operable breast cancer. Fourteen percent of patients were primarily treated by quadrantectomy followed by radiotherapy rather than radical (12%) or modified radical (74%) mastectomy.

Findings.—Lymphatic vessel invasion was detected in 34% of cases and BVI in 4% of cases. The 2 findings correlated with one another, and both correlated closely with the presence and number of axillary metastases. Mortality was 23.5% after a median follow-up of 7 years. Both LVI and BVI were associated with shortened survival on univariate analysis (Fig 3). On multivariate analysis, LVI (but not BVI) significantly and indepen-

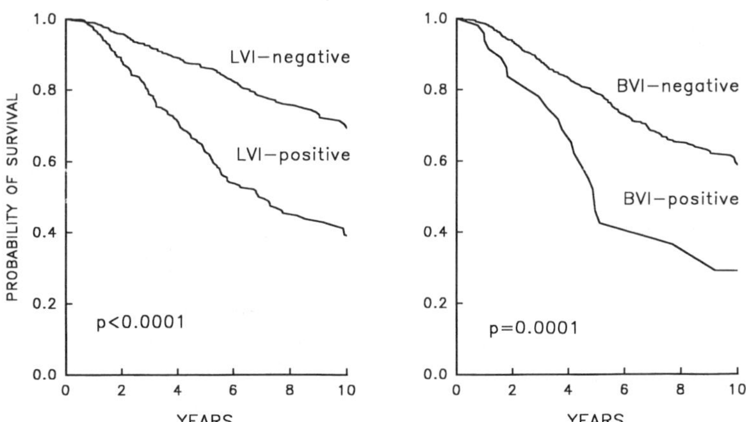

FIGURE 3.—Survival according to LVI and BVI Status. *Abbreviations: LVI*, lymph vessel invasion; *BVI*, blood vessel invasion. (Courtesy of Lauria R, Perrone F, Carlomagno C, et al: The prognostic value of lymphatic and blood vessel invasion in operable breast cancer. *Cancer* 76:1772–1778, Copyright © 1995 American Cancer Society. Reprinted by permission of Wiley-Liss, Inc., a subsidiary of John Wiley & Sons, Inc.)

TABLE 4.—Multivariate Analysis: Relative Risk of Death (95% CI) on the Node-Negative Sample

	All tumor types (516 cases, 67 events)	Ductal carcinomas (377 cases, 55 events)
Postmenopausal vs. premenopausal	1.06 (0.65–1.75)	1.12 (0.63–1.99)
LVI+ vs. LVI–	2.44 (1.41–4.24)	2.26 (1.26–4.03)
T2 vs. T1	0.84 (0.50–1.39)	0.91 (0.52–1.60)
T3 vs. T1	3.66 (1.59–8.43)	4.99 (1.92–12.9)
G3 vs. G1–G2	—	1.63 (0.93–2.86)
Adjuvant vs. no adjuvant	0.89 (0.52–1.54)	1.05 (0.58–1.90)

Abbreviations: CI, confidence interval; *LVI,* lymph vessel invasion; *T,* tumor; *G,* grade.

(Courtesy of Lauria R, Perrone F, Carlomagno C, et al: The prognostic value of lymphatic and blood vessel invasion in operable breast cancer. *Cancer* 76:1772–1778, Copyright © 1995 American Cancer Society. Reprinted by permission of Wiley-Liss, Inc., a subsidiary of John Wiley & Sons, Inc.)

dently influenced survival (Table 4). The prognostic value of LVI was independent of tumor size and the number of involved nodes.

Conclusions.—The presence of LVI is prognostically significant in women with operable breast cancer. It identifies a high-risk group of node-negative patients who would be expected to benefit from adjuvant measures.

▶ This article documents that LVI is a poor prognostic indicator for patients with node-negative breast cancer. All of us are striving to identify factors, which taken alone or in combination, will identify patients who will benefit from adjuvant therapy. I think most investigators agree that patients with positive lymph nodes will benefit from adjuvant systemic therapy. This article clearly suggests (but with inadequate numbers) that BVI is also a poor prognostic feature. In our clinic, LVI is treated as a positive node. Estrogen-receptor negative status, extensive intraductal component–positive, and a poorly differentiated histology are other features that are associated with a higher risk of recurrence. This suggests a possible benefit from systemic adjuvant therapies. We will anxiously await other molecular and genetic markers as they are identified.

T.J. Eberlein, M.D.

Pyruvate Utilization, Phosphocholine and Adenosine Triphosphate (ATP) Are Markers of Human Breast Tumor Progression: A ^{31}P- and ^{13}C-Nuclear Magnetic Resonance (NMR) Spectroscopy Study

Singer S, Souza K, Thilly WG (Brigham and Women's Hosp, Boston; Harvard Med School, Boston; Massachusetts Inst of Technology, Cambridge)

Cancer Res 55:5140–5145, 1995 11–20

Background.—Too little is known about the biochemical changes that accompany tumor development in the human breast. A better understanding of the biochemical phenotype of normal breast tissue, compared to that of cancer cells, might help clarify the biochemical events and lead to useful

TABLE 2.—Phosphate Metabolite Concentrations (Mole Percentage ± SD) in Perchloric Acid Extracts Prepared From Six 75% Confluent T-flasks of Normal Breast Epithelial Cell Strain (76N) Compared to Primary Breast Cancer Cell Lines (21PT and 21NT) and Metastatic Breast Cancer Cells (21MT-2)

	Mole percentage of metabolite ± SD			
Metabolite	76N cells* (n = 3)	21PT cells† (n = 4)	21NT cells‡ (n = 3)	21MT-2 cells§ (n = 4)
PE	6.7 ± 1.9	7.5 ± 1.0	12.8 ± 0.4‖	11.4 ± 3.8
PC	0.4 ± 0.2	7.1 ± 0.5¶	5.8 ± 0.6‖	10.0 ± 1.1**
GPE	2.2 ± 0.9	3.1 ± 0.8	3.0 ± 0.7	2.5 ± 1.9
GPC	2.1 ± 0.4	6.0 ± 0.6¶	6.8 ± 0.2	3.1 ± 1.4**
PCr	2.8 ± 0.5	0.5 ± 0.1¶	0.4 ± 0.02	0.7 ± 0.4
β-ATP	15.8 ± 1.4	11.3 ± 1.4¶	9.3 ± 0.4‖	9.5 ± 2.2
β-ADP	3.1 ± 1.6	3.0 ± 0.8	4.5 ± 1.0	2.9 ± 0.8
UDPG	4.0 ± 0.8	2.9 ± 1.3	1.5 ± 0.2	2.8 ± 2.5
NAD^+ + NADH	8.9 ± 1.6	15.2 ± 3.4¶	16.9 ± 1.9	14.0 ± 2.2

*Normal breast.
†Primary breast cancer derived, nontumorigenic.
‡Primary breast cancer derived, tumorigenic.
§Metastatic.
‖Level significantly different ($P < 0.05$) when compared to 21PT cells.
¶Level significantly different ($P < 0.05$) when compared to 76N cells.
**Level significantly different ($P < 0.05$) when compared to 21NT cells.
(Courtesy of Singer S, Souza K, Thilly WG: Pyruvate utilization, phosphocholine and adenosine triphosphate (ATP) are markers of human breast tumor progression: A ^{31}P- and ^{13}C-Nuclear magnetic resonance (NMR) spectroscopy study. *Cancer Res* 55:5140–5145, 1995.)

markers of progression. Studies to date have focused on breast cancer cell lines derived from metastases.

Objective and Methods.—Metabolite levels and fluxes were studied by ^{31}P- and ^{13}C-nuclear MR spectroscopy in normal human breast epithelial cells (76N), 2 primary breast tumor cell lines (21PT, 21NT), and a metastatic cell line (21MT-2).

Findings.—The phosphocholine (PC) content of the primary breast cancer cell lines was increased 16- to 19-fold compared to the normal breast epithelial cell line, and PC was increased 27-fold in metastatic cells (Table 2). The tumor cells exhibited a 30% decrease in adenosine triphosphate compared to normal breast epithelium, an 83% decrease in phosphocreatine and a 2-fold increase in the level of NAD^+ + NADH. The flux of pyruvate used to generate mitochondrial energy, compared to that used to replenish tricarboxylic acid cycle intermediates, was reduced 50% in primary breast cancer cells and 89% in metastatic cells.

Conclusion.—The major reactions involved in phosphatidylcholine metabolism are outlined in Fig 2. Progression from normal breast epithelium to primary and metastatic cancer may be accompanied by a progressive decline in mitochondrial energy production.

▶ This study uses nuclear MR spectroscopy to measure key metabolite levels and fluxes in normal and malignant breast cells. The study offers great hope because this technique is able to detect very subtle but predictive changes in the evolution of benign to malignant and malignant to metastatic breast cancers. Although the technology does not currently exist to convert

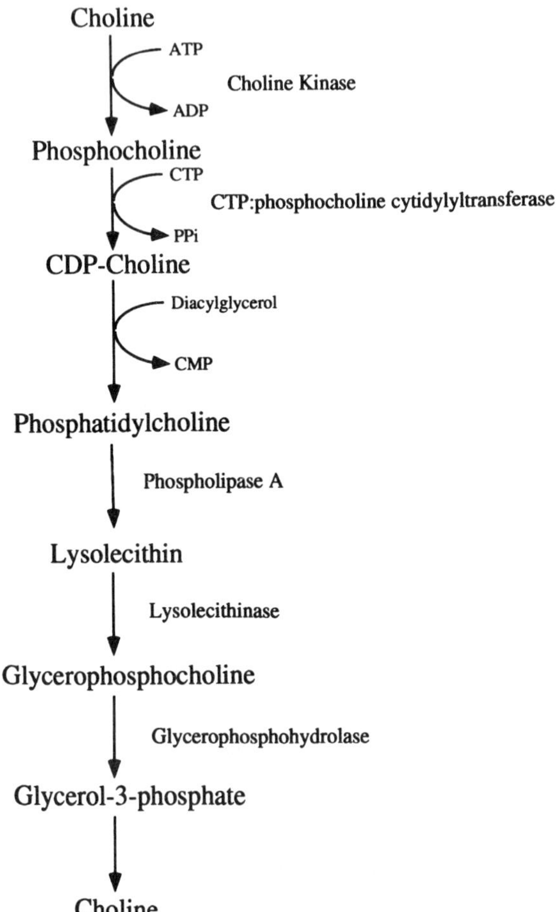

FIGURE 2.—Major Reactions in Synthesis and Breakdown of Phosphatidylcholine. (Courtesy of Singer S, Souza K, Thilly WG: Pyruvate utilization, phosphocholine and adenosine triphosphate (ATP) are markers of human breast tumor progression: $A^{31}P$- and ^{13}C-nuclear magnetic resonance (NMR) spectroscopy study. *Cancer Res* 55:5140–5145, 1995.)

this new-found knowledge to nuclear MR imaging, it does offer the hope of choosing patients that will potentially benefit from more aggressive treatment regimens. For example, sensitivities to various chemotherapy agents should be able to be determined using these techniques. These authors have previously shown that they can predict cell death much earlier than standard trypan blue exclusion, when Rhodamine (a mitochondrial poison) is used to treat malignant cells.

Although this study utilizes cultured tumor lines, in theory the same type of result can be obtained with fresh tumor specimens. This might make a much more predictable and objective analysis of human tumors and their potential response to various cytotoxic agents.

T.J. Eberlein, M.D.

Randomized Cooperative Study of Perioperative Chemotherapy in Breast Cancer

Sertoli MR, Bruzzi P, Pronzato P, et al (Genova Univ, Italy; Istituto Nazionale per la Ricerca sul Cancro, Genova, Italy; Sampierdarena Hosp, Genova, Italy; et al)

J Clin Oncol 13:2712–2721, 1995 11–21

Introduction.—Experimental evidence and the prevailing theoretical model underlying therapeutic planning for patients with malignancies suggests that longer delays in initiating therapy allow a greater increase in resistant cells in both the primary tumor and in the micrometastases. It was hypothesized, therefore, that reducing the interval between surgery and chemotherapy would increase treatment efficacy. To test this hypothesis, the effects of perioperative chemotherapy on survival and relapse-free survival (RFS) in patients with early breast cancer were studied.

Methods.—A total of 600 patients with clinical stages T1–3A, N0–1, M0 breast cancer were randomly assigned to receive either 1 cycle of combination chemotherapy 48–72 hours after surgery or no perioperative chemotherapy. The perioperative cycle (PC) cyclophosphamide, 600 mg/m^2; epidoxorubicin, 600 mg/m^2; and fluorouracil, 600 mg/m^2 (CEF). Further treatment was determined by nodal status, with node-negative patients receiving no further treatment and node-positive patients receiving 11 further cycles of CEF alternated with 6 cycles of cyclophosphamide, 600 mg/m^2; methotrexate, 40 mg/m^2; and fluorouracil, 600 mg/m^2 (CMF)

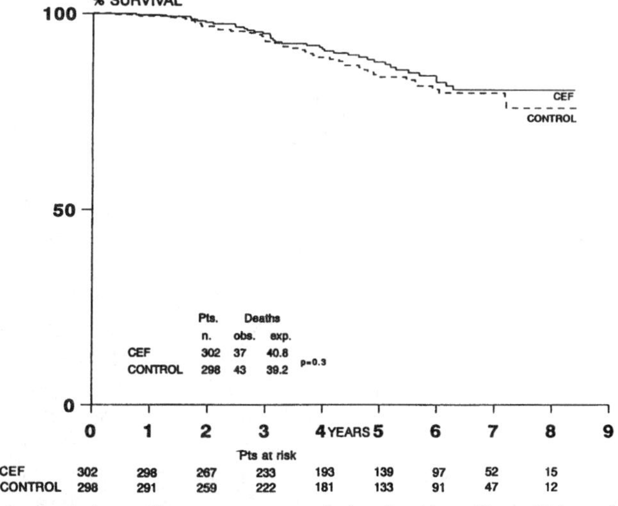

FIGURE 1.—Survival according to treatment: cyclophosphamide, epidoxorubicin, and fluorouracil (*CEF*) in a perioperative cycle (PC) or no PC (*CONTROL*). Both groups received the same long-term chemohormonal treatment. The number of patients at risk is shown for each yearly interval. Median follow-up was 5 years, 7 months. Patients are indicated by *Pts.; obs.* indicates observed; *exp.* indicates expected. (Courtesy of Sertoli MR, Bruzzi P, Pronzato P, et al: Randomized cooperative study of perioperative chemotherapy in breast cancer. *J Clin Oncol* 13:2712–2721, 1995.)

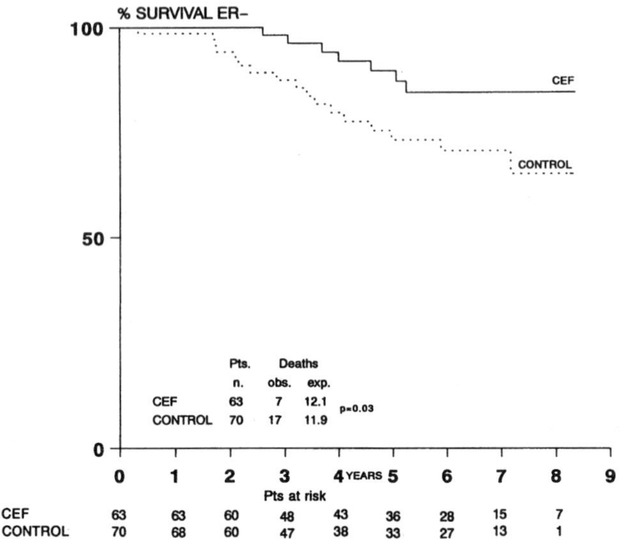

FIGURE 2.—Survival according to treatment analyzed in estrogen receptor–negative (*ER*−) patients. Number of patients at risk is shown for each yearly interval. *CEF* indicates cyclophosphamide, epidoxorubicin, and fluorouracil; *Pts.*, patients; *exp.*, expected. (Courtesy of Sertoli MR., Bruzzi P, Pronzato P, et al: Randomized cooperative study of perioperative chemotherapy in breast cancer. *J Clin Oncol* 13:2712–2721, 1995.)

if they had previously received PC. Node-positive patients who had not received PC were given 6 cycles of CEF alternated with 6 cycles of CMF, begun within 30 days of surgery. Overall survival and relapse-free survival (RFS) were compared in those receiving and not receiving PC, and the toxicity of PC was assessed.

Results.—The 5-year overall survival rates were 88% in the PC group and 84% in the control group (Fig 1). Analysis of survival by tumor size, nodal status, menopausal status, and estrogen receptor (ER) status indicated a significant survival advantage associated with PC only in patients with ER negativity (Fig 2). The 5-year RFS rates were 76% in the PC group and 70% in the control group. Perioperative cycle treatment had a significant RFS benefit in postmenopausal, but not premenopausal, women; in node-negative, but not node-positive, women; and in ER−, but not ER+, patients. Treatment by PC with CEF had mainly gastrointestinal toxicity. It did not affect surgical wound healing. In the long term, toxic side effects were similar in both treatment groups.

Conclusion.—There was no overall survival benefit but there was a borderline significant benefit in RFS associated with perioperative chemotherapy. Estrogen receptor status is the most important predictor of perioperative chemotherapy's effectiveness. Further study is needed to examine the impact of different perioperative chemotherapy regimens.

▶ This manuscript describes one of a number of perioperative or neoadjuvant-type chemotherapies for early stage breast cancer. In this particular study, perioperative chemotherapy consisted of a multidrug regimen of CEF. This was given immediately after the surgical procedure. In general, these patients were relatively aggressively treated with adjuvant therapy. The overall survival rate was unchanged between groups; however, as seen in Figure 2, in the subcategory of ER-negative tumor patients, perioperative chemotherapy seemed to confer survival advantage.

In addition to examining survival, it would be helpful to identify other tumor parameters that might predict response to this aggressive regimen of adjuvant therapies. As important as the positive results in ER-negative tumor patients were, should we take from this study the idea that ER-positive patients do not require perioperative chemotherapy? Certainly, ER-negative tumor status, together with extensive intraductal tumor and lymphatic or blood vessel invasion, appears to be associated with a higher risk of recurrence and diminished survival. However, only through large randomized trials will we be able to look at other parameters, such as angiogenesis and HER2/neu expression, in an effort to help the patients who will optimally benefit from this aggressive treatment.

T.J. Eberlein, M.D.

Self-Reported Breast Implants and Connective-Tissue Diseases in Female Health Professionals: A Retrospective Cohort Study

Hennekens CH, Lee I-M, Cook NR, et al (Harvard Med School, Boston; Harvard School of Public Health, Boston)

JAMA 275:616–621, 1996 11–22

Background.—Basic research, case reports, and case series have raised concern about an increased risk of connective-tissue diseases among women with silicone breast implants. Though such descriptive studies are useful for formulating hypotheses, they are not adequate for testing them. Recent analytic studies, including case-control and cohort studies, have shown that the hazard of connective-tissue disease among such women is apparently not significant. However, small increases in risk could not be excluded. The relationship between breast implants and connective-tissue disease was investigated.

Background.—Data were obtained on a cohort of 395,543 female health care professionals who completed questionnaires for the Women's Health Study. Between 1962 and 1991, 10,830 women had breast implants, and 11,805 were diagnosed as having connective-tissue diseases.

Findings.—Women with breast implants had a relative risk of 1.24 of any connective tissue disease. The findings for other connective-tissue diseases, including mixed, were significant. Findings for rheumatoid arthritis, Sjögren's syndrome, dermatomyositis or polymyositis, and scleroderma were of borderline significance. The findings for systemic lupus erythematosus were nonsignificant. No clear trends were noted in the relative risks associated with increasing duration of breast implants.

Conclusions.—Consistent with previously published findings, these results suggest a small increased risk of connective-tissue diseases among women with breast implants. Also consistent with previous data, the current findings exclude the existence of a great risk.

▶ This is a retrospective cohort study of the Women's Health Study. It reports a very small increase of connective-tissue disease among women who have breast implants. It does exclude a large risk of connective-tissue disorders in this patient population. The study confirms the results from two other very important studies from the Mayo Clinic[1] and the Nurses' Health Study.[2] These other studies also failed to show any great increased risk of connective tissue disorders in women with breast implants. While the design of this study is self-reporting, it is also limited somewhat by the fact that the authors were unable to correlate the results with either the type of breast implant (silicone, gel-filled, saline-filled, etc.), nor were they able to correlate with documented complications such as rupture, etc. Nonetheless, the very large number of patients enrolled in the study makes a major contribution in that it excludes great risks of connective-tissue disease following breast implants.

T.J. Eberlein, M.D.

References

1. Gabriel SE, O'Fallon WM, Kurland LT, et al: Risk of connective-tissue disease and other disorders after breast implantation. *N Engl J Med* 330:1697–1702, 1994.
2. Sanchez-Guerrero J, Colditz GA, Karlson EW, et al: Silcone breast implants and the risk of connective-tissue diseases and symptoms. *N Engl J Med* 332:1666–1670, 1994.

Long-term Follow-up of Elderly Patients With Operable Breast Cancer Treated With Surgery Without Axillary Dissection Plus Adjuvant Tamoxifen

Martelli G, DePalo G, Rossi N, et al (Istituto Nazionale Tumori, Milan, Italy)
Br J Cancer 72:1251–1255, 1995 11–23

Rationale.—Nearly one third of new breast tumors are found in women older than 70 years of age. The best approach to these patients remains uncertain, in part because other diseases and impaired function preclude formal clinical trials. Nonrandomized studies have suggested that tamoxifen is a useful first-line treatment for selected elderly women with breast cancer.

Study Population.—This study evaluated limited surgery—without axillary dissection—combined with tamoxifen therapy in older patients with no clinically evident lymph node involvement. The study group included 321 patients 70 years of age and older who were diagnosed with operable primary breast cancer and clinically negative axillary nodes between 1982

TABLE 2.—Patient Distribution by Pathologic Tumor Size, ER, PgR, and Site of Recurrence

	Pathological stage																
Events	*pT1*		*pT2*		*pT3*	*pT4b*		*Total*		ER^+	ER^-	*Not performed*	*Total*	PgR^+	PgR^-	*Not performed*	*Total*
Local relapse	12/219	5.4%	3/77	3.9%	0/1	2/24	8.3%	17/321	5.3%	8	7	2	17	6	9	2	17
Axillary node involvement	9/219	4.1%	2/77	2.5%	0/1	3/24	12.5%	14/321	4.3%	13	—	1	14	9	4	1	14
Distant metastasis	8/219	3.6%	13/77	16.9%	0/1	2/24	8.3%	23/321	7.2%	18	2	3	23	13	7	3	23
Total	29/219	13.2%	18/77	23.3%	0/1	7/24	29.1%	54/321	16.8%	39/239	9/28	6/54	54/321	28/190	20/77	6/54	54/321

Abbreviations: pT, pathologic tumor size; *ER,* estrogen receptor; PgR, progesterone receptor.

(Courtesy of Martelli G, DePalo G, Rossi N, et al: Long-term follow-up of elderly patients with operable breast cancer treated with surgery without axillary dissection plus adjuvant tamifoxen. *Br J Cancer* 72:1251–1255, 1995.)

and 1990 (Table 2). The median age at the time of diagnosis was 77 years. More than two thirds of primary tumors were less than 2 cm.

Treatment.—The primary tumor was removed with at least 2 cm of normal tissue. All patients had negative surgical margins. Nearly two thirds of tumors were infiltrating ductal carcinomas. Patients received 20 mg of tamoxifen daily, starting at the time of surgery, and were followed at 4 month intervals for 3 years and then every 6 months. Mammography was done annually.

Results.—The median follow-up was 5 years, and 172 patients were followed longer than 5 years. Seventeen patients relapsed locally a median of 33 months after tumor excision. Cumulative rates of local relapse at 5 and 10 years were 5.4% and 8.7%, respectively. Fourteen patients had axillary node disease develop ipsilaterally; the cumulative incidence rates were 4.3% at 5 years, and 5.9% at 10 years. Disseminated disease developed in 6.2% of patients at 5 years and 13.4% at 10 years. Five patients had new primary tumors develop ipsilaterally, and 5 had tumors in the contralateral breast. Six years after treatment, the overall relapse-free survival rate was 76%.

Implications.—Breast conservation surgery, when combined with tamoxifen therapy, may be just as effective as more radical surgery in preventing locoregional relapse in older women with breast cancer. It may be best to limit axillary node dissection to those patients whose lymph nodes are clinically involved.

► This is a retrospective analysis of 321 elderly patients. Excluding the patients with large tumor size, there was a very acceptably low probability of developing either local or axillary recurrence, despite the fact that patients were treated without axillary lymph node dissection (see Table 2). Thus, it may seem reasonable not to treat elderly woman with small breast cancers with radiation therapy or with axillary lymph node dissection, but with adjuvant tamoxifen. Multi-focal disease, positive margins, and extensive intraductal components may be contraindications. The best way to resolve this question, however, will be through a randomized prospective trial. In the meantime, careful selection and adherence to some of the principles indicated in this article will be of help.

T.J. Eberlein, M.D.

Conservative Treatment Versus Mastectomy in Early Breast Cancer: Patterns of Failure With 15 Years of Follow-up Data

Arriagada R, for the Institut Gustave-Roussy Breast Cancer Group (Institut Gustave-Roussy, Villejuif, France)

J Clin Oncol 14:1558–1564, 1996 11–24

Purpose.—Of 6 randomized trials that compared limited surgery and radiotherapy with mastectomy for women with early breast cancer, all but 1 have found no differences in overall or relapse-free survival. The authors

TABLE 2.—Relative Risks of Death Associated With 4 Prognostic Factors in a Multivariate Cox Model Including 179 Patients

Characteristic	No. of Patients	Beta Coefficient	SE	RR	*P*
Age, years					
< 35	7	0.9195	0.5618	2.5	.003
36–50	78	0	—	1*	
51–65	81	−0.2307	0.3259	0.8	
66+	13	1.2255	0.4269	3.4	
Clinical size of tumor (mm)					
≤ 10	79	0	—	1*	.001
11+	100	1.0197	0.3024	2.8	
Histologic grading					
I	56	0	—	1*	.01
II	80	1.0015	0.3743	2.7	
III	43	1.0059	0.4020	3.1	
No. of positive axillary nodes					
0	121	0	—	1*	.003
1–3	39	0.0126	0.3460	1.0	
4+	19	1.2829	0.3945	3.6	
Prognostic score†					
< 1.000	64	0	—	1*	10^{-4}
1.001–2.000	60	0.5742	0.3870	1.8	
2.001+	55	1.4997	0.3557	4.5	

*Reference category.

†Sum of corresponding beta coefficients for each patient. For example, a patient who is 67 years of age with a tumor of 15 mm, grade 1, and 2 involved axillary nodes will have a prognostic score of 2.2578 (1.2255 + 1.0197 + 0 + 0.0126.

(Courtesy of Arriagada R, for the Institut Gustave-Roussy Breast Cancer Group: Conservative treatment versus mastectomy in early breast cancer: Patterns of failure with 15 years of follow-up data. *J Clin Oncol* 14:1558–1564, 1996.)

have previously reported the 5- and 10-year results of 1 of these trials. The long-term results, including an analysis of the patterns of failure with each treatment, were analyzed in this study.

Methods.—One hundred seventy-nine patients with early-stage breast cancer were randomized to undergo conservative treatment or mastectomy. All patients had tumors no larger than 20 mm at macroscopic examination. Axillary dissection with frozen-section examination was performed in all patients. Those who had positive lymph nodes were further randomized to receive either lymph node irradiation or no further treatment. Follow-up was at least 14 years. The analysis of patterns of failure used a competing risk approach, which does not assume that the analyzed events are independent of each other. Multivariate analysis was performed to assess prognostic factors associated with survival and treatment failure (Table 2).

Results.—Patients who underwent conservative treatment and mastectomy had similar outcomes in terms of overall survival, distant metastasis, contralateral breast cancer, new primary malignancy, and locoregional recurrence rate (Fig 1). There were no significant differences in outcome for node-positive patients who received irradiation or no irradiation. Local recurrences and distant metastases were most likely to occur within the first 10 years of follow-up. A prognostic score comprising patient age,

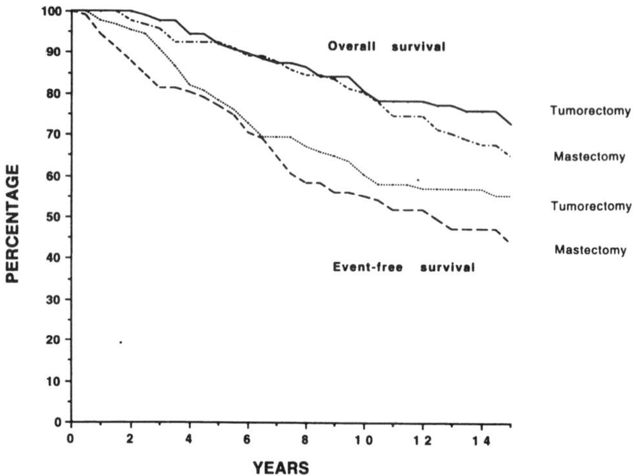

FIGURE 1.—Overall survival (P = .19, log-rank test) and event-free survival (P = .23, log-rank test) according to treatment group. (Courtesy of Arriagada R, for the Institut Gustave-Roussy Breast Cancer Group: Conservative treatment versus mastectomy in early breast cancer: Patterns of failure with 15 years of follow-up data. *J Clin Oncol* 14:1558–1564, 1996.)

tumor size, histologic grade, and number of positive axillary lymph nodes permitted the identification of 3 distinct prognostic groups.

Conclusions.—Long-term follow-up supports the conclusions of previous reports that limited surgery followed by systematic breast irradiation is a safe treatment option for women with early breast cancer. The prognostic score described in this study is easily calculated from available clinical and histologic data and is very accurate in the prediction of overall and event-free survival.

▶ This is a follow-up study from the Institut Gustave-Roussy in France of a randomized trial that compared tumorectomy and breast irradiation with modified radical mastectomy. There are 15 years of follow-up data. As seen in Figure 1, overall survival and event-free survival is virtually indistinguishable between tumorectomy and mastectomy. These authors were able to separate their patients into prognostic groups through the utilization of F4 prognostic factors in a multivariant Cox model for the factors associated with prognosis for age, tumor size, histologic grading, and number of positive axillary nodes.

This study further verifies the results of other randomized trials, and demonstrates that conservative treatment with breast irradiation is not only safe, but also has similar effectiveness to mastectomy with respect to long-term local control and overall survival.

T.J. Eberlein, M.D.

The Sequencing of Chemotherapy and Radiation Therapy After Conservative Surgery for Early-stage Breast Cancer

Recht A, Come SE, Henderson IC, et al (Beth Israel Hosp, Boston; Harvard Med School, Boston; Dana-Farber Cancer Inst, Boston; et al)

N Engl J Med 334:1356–1361, 1996 11–25

Introduction.—More and more patients with early-stage breast cancer who are considered at increased risk of systemic metastases are receiving breast-conserving treatment plus adjuvant chemotherapy. Although the order of chemotherapy and radiation therapy for patients with early-stage invasive breast cancer can affect the clinical results, there have been no randomized trials of this issue. The effects of treatment sequence—that is, giving chemotherapy or radiotherapy first—on the clinical outcomes of patients undergoing conservative surgery for early-stage breast cancer were assessed.

Methods.—The randomized trial included 244 patients with clinical stage I or II breast carcinoma who were deemed to be at substantial risk of distant metastases. This determination included axillary lymph node status, estrogen receptor status, or both. After breast-conserving surgery, the patients were assigned to receive either a 12-week course of chemotherapy followed by radiation therapy, or the same treatments in the opposite order. Surviving patients were followed up for a median of 58 months.

Results.—The 5-year actuarial rate of recurrent cancer at any site was 38% in the patients receiving radiotherapy first and 36% in those receiving chemotherapy first. The distant metastasis rates in these groups were 31% vs. 25%. The overall survival was 73% for the radiotherapy-first group and 81% for the chemotherapy-first group. The crude 5-year local recurrence rate was 5% in the radiotherapy-first group vs. 14% in the chemotherapy-first group. For distant regional recurrence or both, the crude 5-year rates were 32% for the radiotherapy-first group vs. 20% for the chemotherapy-first group. The differences in recurrent rates were borderline significant.

Conclusions.—In patients undergoing conservative surgery for early-stage breast cancer who are at increased risk of metastases, giving postoperative chemotherapy before radiotherapy produces a lower systemic recurrence rate and thus better overall results. The risk of local recurrence is lower when radiotherapy is given first, however. Although the results suggest that chemotherapy should be given before radiation, the subgroup analyses are of low statistical power, and the results cannot necessarily be applied to other treatment regimens.

► An increasing number of women are undergoing breast conservation. For women with tumors larger than 1 cm as well as pathologic features such as a lymphatic vessel invasion or estrogen-negative status, sequencing of chemotherapy and radiation therapy is not clear. This study, from the Joint Center for Radiation Therapy at Harvard, presented a randomly designed trial in which chemotherapy was given either before or after radiation therapy.

Although the overall survival for both treatments was equivalent in this study, the patients who were treated with radiation therapy first had a reduced risk of local recurrence but a higher risk of systemic disease than in the patients who received chemotherapy first. The increased risk of local recurrence in patients receiving chemotherapy first may be minimized by careful attention to the type of surgery performed and the resection margins, as well as the details of radiotherapy technique.

There are, however, a few cautionary notes with this study. The first is that the duration of chemotherapy was 12 weeks, and therefore extrapolation to longer or more intense regimens may be misleading. As stated earlier, careful attention to the type of surgery and the margin of resection may actually minimize the risk of local recurrence in patients treated with chemotherapy first. Certainly, patients with a large risk of systemic disease (4 or more positive nodes) would benefit from systemic treatment and wide negative margins.

T.J. Eberlein, M.D.

Five Versus More Than Five Years of Tamoxifen Therapy for Breast Cancer Patients With Negative Lymph Nodes and Estrogen Receptor-Positive Tumors

Fisher B, Dignam J, Bryant J, et al (Natl Surgical Adjuvant Breast and Bowel Project)

J Natl Cancer Inst 88:1529–1542, 1996 11–26

Introduction.—Women with advanced breast cancer and those with primary operable breast cancer and positive axillary lymph nodes have been known to receive benefit from tamoxifen therapy. To assess the effectiveness of adjuvant tamoxifen therapy in women with histologically negative lymph nodes and estrogen receptor–positive tumors, the National Surgical Adjuvant Breast and Bowel Project began a randomized clinical trail (B-14) in 1982 with 2,800 women. Questions persisted on how long the benefits would be expected to persist, the duration of tamoxifen administration necessary, and the adverse effects from prolonged therapy with tamoxifen. Findings were described after 10 years of follow-up of this study.

Methods.—In the original trial, women received either tamoxifen at 20 mg/day or placebo. Those women who were treated with tamoxifen who remained disease free after 5 years received either another 5 years of therapy or 5 years of placebo. The study evaluated the data to compare 5 years of tamoxifen therapy with more than 5 years of tamoxifen therapy.

Results.—A significant advantage was seen in women who received tamoxifen for the first 5 years. Their disease-free survival (69% vs. 58%), distant disease-free survival (76% vs. 67%), and survival (80% vs. 76%) were significantly better than those of women who did not initially receive tamoxifen therapy. In the incidence of contralateral breast cancer, tamoxifen therapy was associated with a 37% reduction. For those who then discontinued tamoxifen therapy after the initial 5 years of therapy, there was more of an advantage in disease-free survival (92% vs. 86%) and distant disease-free survival (96% vs. 90%). For those who stopped using tamoxifen, survival was 96% compared with 94% for those who continued treatment. In the women treated with tamoxifen for more than 5 years, there was a higher incidence of thromboembolic events. The incidence of second cancers was not increased with tamoxifen therapy, except for endometrial cancer.

Conclusion.—After 10 years of follow-up, the benefit from 5 years of tamoxifen therapy persisted. However, no additional benefit was obtained from continuing therapy with tamoxifen for more than 5 years.

▶ This article shows that 5 years of tamoxifen therapy in node-negative patients with breast cancer has persistent benefit through 10 years of follow-up. An additional 5 years of treatment did not improve overall survival. There was a higher risk of thromboembolic events in the group that received tamoxifen. Although many different types of tumors were identified in the tamoxifen-treated group, endometrial cancer was the only malignancy associated with a higher incidence in the tamoxifen-treated group. This paper probably provides the strongest objective data to support cessation of tamoxifen therapy after 5 years of treatment. I, therefore, recommend it to surgeons who deal with patients with breast cancer.

T.J. Eberlein, M.D.

Genetics

Allelic Loss on Chromosomes 4q and 16q in Hepatocellular Carcinoma: Association With Elevated α-Fetoprotein Production

Yeh S-H, Chen P-J, Lai M-Y, et al (Natl Taiwan Univ, Taipei)
Gastroenterology 110:184–192, 1996 11–27

Background.—Evaluation of human hepatocellular carcinomas (HCC) by restriction fragment length polymorphism analysis has frequently demonstrated allelic loss on chromosomes 4q and 16q.

Objective and Methods.—The method of microsatellite polymorphism analysis was used to better define the chromosomal regions involved in an attempt to positionally clone the putative tumor-suppressor genes. DNA samples were derived from 42 pairs of hepatocellular cancers (larger than 5 cm) and corresponding nonneoplastic liver tissue. Loss of heterozygosity at chromosomes 4q and 16q was studied using 13 and 12 sets of microsatellite polymorphic markers, respectively.

Findings.—Allelic loss on chromosome 16q was identified in 70% of cases; the common region was mapped to 16q22-23. Allelic loss at 4q occurred in 77% of cases, with the common region mapped to 4q12-23. Allelic loss of 4q correlated significantly to cancers characterized by increased serum α-fetoprotein (AFP) but not to those associated with normal AFP levels.

Discussion.—Allelic loss on chromosomes 4q and 16q is very frequent in HCC. Hopefully, it will soon be possible to precisely clone the tumor-suppressor genes presumably present at these sites. Further studies of the gene on chromosome 4q might clarify how AFP is expressed in HCC.

▶ As with tumors such as breast cancer and colon cancer, an oncogene has not been described in HCC. This article examined more extensively the loss of heterozygosity (LOH) analysis on chromosomes 4q and 16q. They showed allelic loss on chromosome 16q was 70%, with an even higher frequency of 77% found on chromosome 4q. More importantly, the allelic loss of chromosome 4q was significantly associated with hepatocellular carcinoma that had an elevated serum α-AFP. This frequent LOH in hepatocellular carcinoma is used for the presence of a putitive tumor-suppressor gene in this region, deletion of which would inactivate its function, and thus lead to tumor growth. The correlation of LOH at this region with AFP elevation in HCC suggests that loss of such a putitive tumor suppressor gene can also remove the repression of AFP gene expression. Thus, this potential tumor-suppressor gene could not only be important in down-regulating the activities of genes promoting hepatocyte growth but could also be involved in postnatal repression of AFP expression. Further positional cloning of these putitive tumor suppresser genes in the loci described in this paper will hopefully be accomplished in the near future.

T.J. Eberlein, M.D.

Gene Modification of Primary Tumor Cells for Active Immunotherapy of Human Breast and Ovarian Cancer

Philip R, Clary B, Brunette E, et al (Applied Immune Sciences, Inc, Santa Clara, Calif; Duke Univ, Durham, NC)

Clin Cancer Res 2:59–68, 1996 11–28

Background.—Attempts to use genetically modified tumor cells to induce protective immunity have led to encouraging results in animals. There is interest in using a vaccine made from cytokine gene-modified tumor tissue to treat human breast and ovarian cancers, but an efficient method of gene transfer is needed. Retroviral vectors are hampered by efficiency and safety concerns. An alternative is to use cationic liposomes to facilitate the transfection of primary and cultured cells by adeno-associated virus (AAV) plasmids.

Objective.—An AAV-based expresssion plasmid, pMP6IL2, was used in conjunction with cationic liposomes to deliver genes into freshly isolated, uncultured cells from human breast and ovarian tumors (Fig 3). The goal was to produce tumor cells that would secrete interleukin 2 (IL-2).

Results.—Significant amounts of IL-2 were detected in primary breast and ovarian tumor cells, as well as in tumor-cell lines. Transfection with a non-AAV plasmid containing the same expression cassette induced expression of IL-2 in the tumor-cell line, but not in primary tumor cells. The

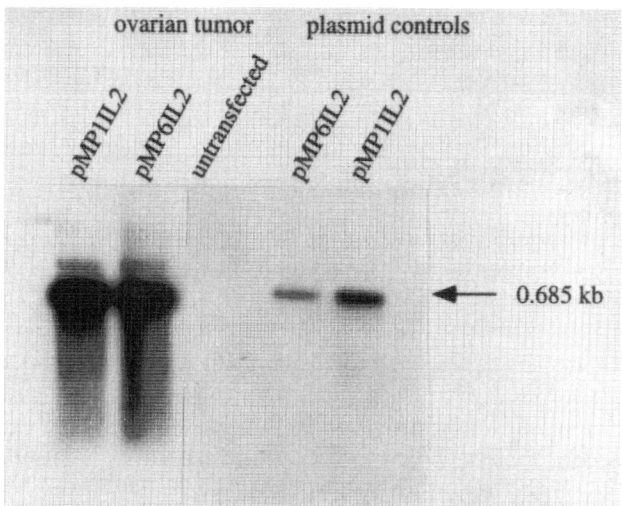

FIGURE 3.—Southern blot analysis of primary ovarian tumor cells transfected with pMP1IL-2 or pMP6IL-2 complexed to DDAB:DOPE. Transfected cells were harvested 7 days after transfection, and genomic DNA was prepared. Genomic DNA was digested with *Pvu*II/*Hinc*II. As a control, plasmids were cut with loaded lug/lane enzymes. One μg DNA was loaded per lane. The blots were probed with a ^{32}P-labeled IL-2 fragment. (Courtesy of Philip R, Clary B, Brunette E, et al: Gene modification of primary tumor cells for active immunotherapy of human breast and ovarian cancer. *Spine* 2:59–68, 1996.)

particular liposome composition used for transfection was not a critical factor. Transfected breast cancer cells continued to express IL-2 for up to 28 days after being lethally irradiated. From 20% to 50% of the tumor-cell line and primary tumor cells were transfected. Immunostaining for IL-2 demonstrated the transgene in at least 40% of primary tumor cell preparations, despite the fact that the preparations consisted of mixed cell populations.

Conclusions.—It is possible to efficiently express biologically active cytokines in primary tumor cells using a liposome-based system of AAV plasmid DNA. This may make it easier to develop efficient gene-based immunotherapy for cancer.

▶ This article describes an alternative method for facilitating transfection of primary ovarian and breast cancers by using cationic liposomes. Transfecting a gene into a tumor normally requires the tumor to be actively growing, and this method avoids that problem. Using the AAV plasmid tranfections, the authors obtain efficient expression of the cytokine gene (Fig 3) and offer a mechanism for avoiding the necessity of actively dividing tumor cells. They are able to demonstrate this technology in several tumors which clearly implies the ability to use this technology on a wide range of primary tumors.

T.J. Eberlein, M.D.

▶ The next 2 articles concern *BRCA1* mutations. Although neither is a definitive study, they are both very important in the examination of this genetic mutation and its effect on various populations with breast cancer.

T.J. Eberlein, M.D.

BRCA1 **Mutations in a Population-Based Sample of Young Women with Breast Cancer**

Langston AA, Malone KE, Thompson JD, et al (Fred Hutchinson Cancer Research Ctr, Seattle; Univ of Washington, Seattle)
N Engl J Med 334:137–142, 1996 11–29

Background.—It is accepted that inherited mutations in the *BRCA1* gene correlate with a high risk of breast and ovarian cancers in some families. It remains uncertain, however, whether and to what extent these mutations contribute to breast cancer in the general population.

Objective.—The frequency and types of *BRCA1* mutations were examined in 80 women who received a diagnosis of breast cancer before 35 years of age, and who were not selected on the basis of family history. The participants were from a large population-based study of early-onset breast cancer.

Methods.—Genomic DNA was analyzed for *BRCA1* mutations by analyzing single-strand conformation polymorphisms and by screening with allele-specific oligonucleotides. Alterations were defined by DNA sequencing.

Findings.—Six of the 80 women studied were found to have germ-line mutations of *BRCA1*. In addition, 4 rare sequence variations of uncertain functional significance were identified. Two mutations and 3 sequence variations were found among 39 women who reported no family history of breast or ovarian cancers. Of 73 unrelated subjects forming a reference population, none had a *BRCA1* mutation and only 1 had one of the sequence variants.

Implication.—Mutation of *BRCA1* may be present in 10% or more of younger women with breast cancer, and is not limited to those with a positive family history.

▶ It is now accepted that *BRCA1* and *BRCA2* mutations are associated with a high risk of breast and/or ovarian cancer in some families. The purpose of this paper was to illuminate the contribution of *BRCA1* mutations to breast cancer in the general population. These authors studied 80 women who had been diagnosed with breast cancer before 35 years of age but were not selected on the basis of family history. Approximately 10% of this cohort of patients had alterations in *BRCA*. Five of the 6 mutations have been identified previously in high risk families and include 3 of the most common mutations identified to date. Therefore, large population-based screening studies will be necessary to establish the frequency, penetrance, and relative importance of each of the variations in the sequence of the *BRCA1* in patients with a history of breast cancer, as well as those women unaffected by this disease. It is clear that mutations in *BRCA1* not associated with a familial history may still be important in the development of sporadic breast cancer.

T.J. Eberlein, M.D.

Germ-Line *BRCA1* Mutations in Jewish and Non-Jewish Women With Early-Onset Breast Cancer

FitzGerald MG, MacDonald DJ, Krainer M, et al (Massachusetts Gen Hosp, Charlestown; Harvard School of Public Health, Boston; Dana-Farber Cancer Inst, Boston)

N Engl J Med 334:143–149, 1996 11–30

Background.—Familial breast cancers are assoicated with mutations in a germ-line allele of the *BRCA1* gene, but the frequency of mutations in non-familial cases remains uncertain.

Objective and Methods.—Mutations of *BRCA1* were sought in 418 women given a diagnosis of breast cancer at 40 years of age or earlier. In 30 women who developed breast cancer at or before 30 years of age, a complete mutational analysis was performed by automated nucleotide sequencing and a protein-truncation assay. In addition, in 39 of the women 40 years of age or younger who were Ashkenazi Jews, an allele-specific polymerase chain reaction assay was used to identify a *BRCA1* mutation that is prevalent in this population, 185delAG.

Findings.—Four of the women who had breast cancer develop before 30 years of age (13%) had definite chain-terminating mutations of *BRCA1*, and one had a missense mutation. Two of the 4 Jewish women in this group had the 185delAG mutation. Of 39 Jewish women who had breast cancer at or before 40 years of age, 8 (21%) had the 185delAG mutation (Table 3).

Implications.—A search for *BRAC1* mutations will be most productive in young Jewish women with breast cancer. An increased risk of early-onset cancer in women who carry the 185delAG mutation indicates that intensified screening should begin at an early age, but screening of the general Ashkenazi Jewish population is not yet warranted.

▶ The patients in this study have a specific *BRCA1* mutation, 185delAG, that is prevalent in the Ashkenazi Jewish population. In this study of young breast cancer patients, 21% of the Jewish women under 40 years of age had this mutation. Some caution is warranted, however, in interpreting the risk of breast cancer associated with this mutation in women who do not have a family history of breast cancer. This is because the penetrance of this allele is unknown in women in the general population who do not have a history of breast cancer. Once penetrance of this allele is identified in the general population, identification of this mutation, especially in young Jewish women, will require formulation of guidelines for genetic counseling and prevention at an early age.

T.J. Eberlein, M.D.

TABLE 3.—Incidence of the *BRCA1* Mutation 185delAG Among Jewish Women With the Onset of Breast Cancer at or Before the Age of 40*

185delAG Present	No. of Women (%)	Mean Age at Onset	Bilateral Breast Cancer	Family History of Breast Cancer: Definite‡	Family History of Breast Cancer: 1st-Degree Relative	Family History of Breast Cancer: 1st- or 2nd-Degree Relative	Relatives With Breast Cancer†
		yr		*no. of women (%)*			*no./no. at risk (%)*
Yes	8 (21)	36	2 (25)	0	4 (50)	7 (88)	10/43 (23)
No	31 (79)	36	1 (3)	3 (10)	11 (35)	13 (42)§	20/168 (12)¶
Total	39 (100)	36	3 (8)	3 (8)	15 (38)	20 (51)	30/211 (14)

*The 185delAG mutation was identified by allele-specific PCR amplification in 39 Jewish women with breast cancer diagnosed at or before the age of 40. The number of cases of breast cancer among the first- and second-degree female relatives of known 185delAG carriers was obtained from the family history.

†Values shown are the numbers of female relatives with breast cancer as a fraction of all female first- and second-degree relatives.

‡A definite family history was defined as the presence of breast cancer in three or more paternal or maternal relatives in two or more generations.

§$P=0.02$ for the comparison with women with the 185delAG mutation.

¶$P=0.06$ for the comparison with women with the 185delAG mutation.

(Reprinted by permission of *The New England Journal of Medicine* from FitzGerald MG, MacDonald DJ, Krainer M, et al: Germ-line *BRCA1* mutations in Jewish and non-Jewish women with early-onset breast cancer. *N Engl J Med* 334:143–149,)

Molecular Genetic Basis of Colorectal Cancer Susceptibility
Cunningham C, Dunlop MG (Univ of Edinburgh, Scotland)
Br J Surg 83:321–329, 1996 11–31

Background.—A better understanding of the mechanisms underlying colorectal carcinogenesis will facilitate the development of new treatments and preventive strategies. The identification of persons at high risk is an important goal. The molecular genetic basis of colorectal cancer susceptibility was discussed.

Discussion.—Two syndromes are responsible for most known genetic susceptibility to colorectal cancer: familial adenomatous polyposis (FAP), and hereditary nonpolyposis colorectal cancer (HNPCC). With prophylaxis, patients with FAP now account for less than 0.2% of colorectal cancers. However, HNPCC accounts for up to 5% of colorectal cancer cases.

Germline mutations in the adenomatous polyposis coli (*APC*) gene cause FAP. Through genetic linkage analysis, *APC* has been localized to the long arm of chromosome 5. Somatic *APC* gene mutations have been found in early adenomas and dysplastic aberrant crypt foci, believed to be precursors of adenomas. Thus, the initiation of adenoma formation in FAP apparently requires inactivation of both *APC* copies. These findings demonstrate the pivotal role of *APC* mutations in the genesis of colorectal cancer. Accurate predictive testing for FAP is now possible using genetic linkage analysis or mutation analysis.

Four different genes have been implicated in the etiology of HNPCC. These are human homologues of yeast and bacterial DNA repair genes, known as *h*MSH2 on chromosome 2p, *h*MLH1 on chromosome 3p, *h*PMS1 on chromosome 2q, and *h*PMS2 on chromosome 7q. Penetrance is likely to be only 70% to 80%. In addition, there are no clinical pathognomonic features of HNPCC, except for early onset cancer with a familial aggregation. Thus, HNPCC is a more difficult problem than FAP for researchers and clinicians. Cancers that occur in the HNPCC syndrome tend to arise in the proximal colon. Colorectal cancer is the only malignancy in some families, whereas others have a segregation of uterine, ovarian, gastric, upper urinary tract, pancreatic, small bowel, and skin cancers.

Conclusions.—The identification of mutations in the *APC* gene in affected persons can be used to minimize the requirement for clinical screening in relatives at risk. Testing to identify persons for early diagnosis and treatment will soon become routine in other more common, less defined heritable forms of colorectal cancer.

▶ This is a very nice review article that is quite understandable. It does not discuss all aspects of molecular genetics, but deals primarily with the *APC* gene and the recently discovered DNA mismatch repair genes in colorectal cancer. These are extremely important in the onset of colorectal tumor. The central role that *APC* and the mutator genes play in colorectal cancer is now more clear. It is even possible that changes in other cancer genes may be induced by defects in the mismatch repair genes. As the molecular basis of HNPCC is unraveled, it will have considerable influence on colorectal cancer screening; this may lead to a rational approach to population screening in predisposition syndromes. Familiarity with this work will help the general surgeon understand the patients who should be screened and what alternative interventions may be offered. This will take on a similar importance and urgency as with the *BRCA1* inherited malignancies.

T.J. Eberlein, M.D.

Hereditary Breast Cancer: Pathobiology, Prognosis, and BRCA1 and BRCA2 Gene Linkage

Marcus JN, Watson P, Page DL, et al (Creighton Univ, Omaha, Neb; Vanderbilt Univ, Nashville, Tenn; McGill Univ, Montreal; et al)
Cancer 77:697–709, 1996 11–32

Background.—*BRCA1* is a breast cancer susceptibility gene that is present in approximately half of the families with hereditary breast cancer (HBC) and ovarian cancer, but it is rare in families with male breast cancer. *BRCA2* is another major breast cancer susceptibility gene that only moderately increases the risk of ovarian cancer and is present in most families with male HBC. However, these genes may also occur in patients with sporadic cancer. Identifying the genes involved could be facilitated by determining the special characteristics of the corresponding tumors. Therefore, the distinctive histopathologic, DNA cytometric, and prognostic features were investigated in patients with HBC and sporadic cancer.

Methods.—A total of 272 women in 52 families with HBC were identified. Tumor blocks and/or slides were available for 182 carcinomas in 156 of these women for study and comparison with 187 specimens from 181 women with breast cancer without a family history. The patients with HBC were classified in 2 groups: those with detected *BRCA1* gene linkage

TABLE 7.—Status of the Study Patients at the End of Follow-up

	Hereditary Breast Cancer		
	BRCA1 Related	Other	Comparison Series
Dead of breast cancer	14 (19.4)	20 (30.3)	32 (24.6)
Alive with recurrent breast cancer	1 (1.4)	9 (13.6)	3 (2.3)
Dead, disease free*	1 (1.4)	4 (6.1)	37 (28.5)
New primary cancers*	20 (27.8)	13 (19.7)	10 (7.7)
Living, disease free*	36 (50)	20 (30.3)	48 (36.9)
Median follow-up	3.6 yr	5.0 yr	8.3 yr

Note: Values are numbers of study patients with percentages in parentheses.
*These were censored categories in the breast cancer–specific survival analysis.
(Courtesy of Marcus JN, Watson P, Page DL, et al: Hereditary breast cancer: Pathobiology, prognosis, and BRCA1 and BRCA2 linkage. *Cancer* 77:697–709, Copyright © 1996 American Cancer Society. Reprinted by permission of Wiley-Liss, Inc., a subsidiary of John Wiley & Sons, Inc.)

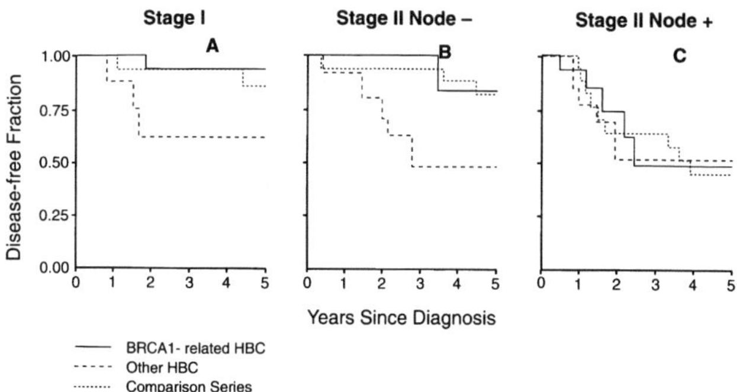

FIGURE 2.—Disease-free survival in "no special type" carcinomas for *BRCA1*-related hereditary breast cancer (*HBC, solid lines*) and other HBC (*heavy dashed lines*). Differences in disease-free fractions between these HBC groups were significant for stage I patients (**A**, $P = 0.011$) and stage II node-negative patients (**B**, $P = 0.033$) but not for stage II node-positive cases (**C**, $P = 0.84$). The comparison series was not used in statistical analysis of the recurrence rates. (Courtesy of Marcus JN, Watson P, Page DL, et al: Hereditary breast cancer: Pathobiology, prognosis, and BRCA1 and BRCA2 linkage. *Cancer* 77:697–709, Copyright © 1996 American Cancer Society. Reprinted by permission of Wiley-Liss, Inc., a subsidiary of John Wiley & Sons, Inc.)

or with presumed *BRCA1* gene linkage (because of a family history of ovarian cancer but no male breast cancer) and those classified as other HBC cases (Table 7). Clinical information was derived from patient records. The specimens were analyzed for histopathologic classification and grading and with quantitative DNA flow cytometry.

Results.—When compared with the comparison group, the 2 HBC groups had a significantly younger age and more early-stage disease at diagnosis. No significant differences were noted in the incidence of any histologic type, but patients in the other HBC category had significantly more of the combined tubular-lobular group (TLG) diagnoses than did the comparison group and the *BRCA1*-linked group. *BRCA1*-related HBCs had significantly fewer diploid tumors than did cancers in the other HBC and comparison groups. The mean S-phase fraction was similar in diploid cancers in the 3 groups but was significantly higher in the aneuploid tumors of the *BRCA1*-related HBC group than in the other 2 groups. Survival rates did not differ significantly among the 3 groups. The *BRCA1*-related HBC group had a lower stage-adjusted recurrence rate (Fig 2).

Conclusions.—Breast cancer associated with mutations of the *BRCA1* gene have a distinctive pathobiology characterized by a high incidence of aneuploid tumors, a lower aneuploid DNA index, and greater tumor cell proliferation. Therefore, it is proposed that the *BRCA1* mutation mediated accelerated cell proliferation. However, the prognosis in these patients was better than that in the other HBC group and comparable to that of the comparison group.

▶ This is a very interesting paper that looks at *BRCA1*-related HBC cases and compares them with 187 predominantly non-HBC cases. In spite of being more frequently aneuploid and having strikingly higher proliferation rates, *BRCA1*-related HBC appears to be associated with lower recurrence rates than other types of HBC.

The significance of earlier-stage disease in the *BRCA1*-related group still is unclear. Is this a biological difference or perhaps due to a greater awareness on the part of the patient and therefore much greater surveillance? Although this study focused on histopathology and DNA cytometry, it would be interesting to make similar correlates with other markers such as hormone receptors, angiogenesis, and oncogene expression.

T.J. Eberlein, M.D.

Overview of Natural History, Pathology, Molecular Genetics and Management of HNPCC (Lynch Syndrome)

Lynch HT, Smyrk T, Lynch JF (Creighton Univ, Omaha, Neb)
Int J Cancer 69:38–43, 1996 11–33

Background.—Molecular genetic research has discovered the genetic factors underlying a number of hereditary cancers (Table 1). A substantial proportion of the cases of colorectal carcinoma are hereditary, although

TABLE 1.—Genes Implicated in Hereditary Cancers.

Cancer/cancer syndrome	Gene	Chromosomal location
Breast, ovary	*BRCA1*	17q21
Breast	*BRCA2*	13q12–13
SBLA/Li-Fraumeni	*p53*	17p13
Breast	*AT*	11q22–23
Retinoblastoma	*RB1*	13q14
Lynch syndrome/HNPCC	*MSH2*	2p
	MLH1	3p21.3–23
	PMS1	2q31–33
	PMS2	7p22
Turcot's syndrome		
predominance of glioblastoma multiforme	*PMS2*	7p22
	MLH1	3p21.3–23
predominance of cerebellar medulloblastoma	*APC*	5q21
Familial adenomatous polyposis	*APC*	distal to 5'
Hereditary flat adenoma syndrome	*APC*	proximal to 5'
Melanoma	*MLM* (p16/MTS-1)	9p21
Neurofibromatosis	*NF1*	17q11.2
Von Hippel-Lindau	*VHLS*	3p25
Medullary thyroid	*RET*	10q11.2
Wilms' tumor	*WT1*	11p13

(Courtesy of Lynch HT, Smyrk T, Lynch JF: Overview of natural history, pathology, molecular genetics, and management of HNPCC (Lynch syndrome). *Int J Cancer* 69:38–43, 1996. Reprinted by permission of Wiley-Liss, Inc., a subsidiary of John Wiley & Sons, Inc.)

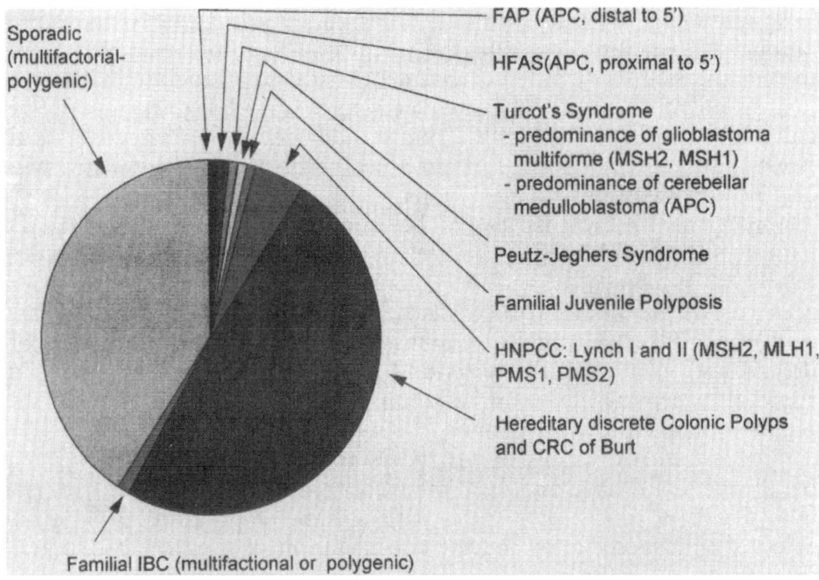

FIGURE 1.—Extant heterogeneity in hereditary colorectal cancer. *Abbreviations: FAP,* familial adenomatous polyposis; *HFAS,* hereditary flat adenoma syndrome; *HNPCC,* hereditary nonpolyposis colorectal cancer; and *CRC,* colorectal carcinoma. (Courtesy of Lynch HT, Smyrk T, Lynch JF: Overview of natural history, pathology, molecular genetics, and management of HNPCC (Lynch syndrome). *Int J Cancer* 69:38–43, 1996. Reprinted by permission of Wiley-Liss, Inc., a subsidiary of John Wiley & Sons, Inc.)

the underlying genetic factors appear to be heterogeneous (Fig 1). The clinical, pathologic, and genetic features of hereditary nonpolyposis colorectal cancer (HNPCC) were discussed, together with its differential diagnosis and management.

Features of HNPCC.—Hereditary nonpolyposis colorectal cancer confers a high risk of colorectal carcinoma in affected families. Colorectal carcinomas typically arise proximal to the splenic flexure and tend to form multiple carcinomas if the patient is not treated with a subtotal colectomy. Particular extracolonic malignancies are common and include carcinomas of the endometrium, ovary, small intestine, biliary tract, ureter, renal pelvis, stomach, and pancreas, whereas the risk of lung cancer is decreased. Compared with sporadic colon cancer, poorly differentiated carcinomas and cancers producing extracellular mucin are more common with HNPCC. It has been hypothesized that adenomas are more likely to progress to carcinoma and progress more quickly in association with HNPCC. However, it has also been suggested that colorectal cancer has a better prognosis if it is associated with HNPCC than if it is sporadic. Hereditary nonpolyposis colorectal cancer has been associated with genes on chromosome 2p and chromosome 3p, genes that regulate DNA mismatch repair. Defects in these short repeat sequences produce microsatellite instability and allow replication errors.

Differential Diagnosis.—Several other colorectal cancers demonstrate familial aggregations, including the hamartomatous polyposis syndromes, the hereditary discrete polyp-carcinoma phenomenon, and familial adenomatous polyposis (FAP). The attenuated form of FAP is particularly difficult to differentiate from HNPCC, but should be suspected in patients with fewer than 100 adenomas, with proximal predominance, combined with upper gastrointestinal manifestations.

Management.—Patients should be carefully counseled regarding the natural history of HNPCC, the limitations of DNA testing, and the potential for psychological and social consequences of testing before undergoing DNA predictive testing. Those who are found to have genetic evidence of HNPCC should be counseled regarding surveillance for colorectal and extracolonic cancers and prophylactic treatment, including subtotal colectomy and total abdominal hysterectomy and bilateral salpingo-oophorectomy in women.

Conclusion.—Advances in the understanding of the molecular genetic basis of HNPCC have improved the identification of patients at high risk for colorectal cancer. For these patients, the importance of frequent colonoscopic surveillance and the consideration of prophylactic surgical treatment are emphasized.

▶ Hereditary nonpolyposis colorectal cancer now has provided a model for studying the molecular genetics leading to colorectal carcinoma. Patients with HNPCC are at high risk for the development of colorectal carcinoma. Table 1 nicely summarized the genes that are implicated in hereditary cancer, in particular, those associated with Lynch syndrome (HNPCC). Although knowledge of these chromosomal locations may not be necessary for the general surgeon, certainly familiarity with these genetic markers and their locations on chromosomes will be extremely helpful as general surgeons obviously will be involved in identifying patients, referring them for genetic counseling, and eventually intervening surgically in this patient population.

Hereditary nonpolyposis colorectal cancer is not a polyposis syndrome. However, individuals who have this syndrome do form adenomas, and there is at least strong circumstantial evidence that adenomas are precursor lesions to malignancy in this syndrome. When the adenomas do occur, they are more likely to progress to carcinoma than are adenomas in the general population. Thus, the syndrome forms an excellent model for the study of the genetic changes that occur in the transition from normal epithelia to frank malignancy.

This paper will be particularly useful for general surgeons because obtaining appropriate genetic counseling for patients will not only be mandatory but will be necessary to provide a full understanding of the natural history, limitations, and eventual recommendations regarding patents with this diagnosis.

T.J. Eberlein, M.D.

Colorectal

Management of Early Invasive Colorectal Cancer: Risk of Recurrence and Clinical Guidelines

Kikuchi R, Takano M, Takagi K, et al (Takano Hosp, Kumamoto, Japan; Fujiyoshi Clinic, Kumamoto, Japan; Oita Med Univ, Japan)

Dis Colon Rectum 38:1286–1295, 1995 11–34

Purpose.—Early invasive cancer (EIC) of the large bowel can be treated with bowel resection, local resection, or endoscopic polypectomy. Because endoscopic polypectomy is increasingly used in clinical practice, more cases of EIC are reported. However, guidelines for the treatment of EIC that incorporate the new technology have not yet been defined. The development of new clinical guidelines for the treatment of EIC was studied.

Methods.—Between 1982 and 1989, 182 patients with a mean age of 61.3 years were diagnosed with colorectal EIC and underwent resection. Follow-up was for at least 5 years or until death. Only patients with EIC in which malignant cells extended through the muscularis mucosa into the submucosa but did not deeply invade the muscularis propria were included in the study. Patients were divided into 3 groups based on the level of invasion. Of the 182 patients, 64 had slight submucosal invasion (sm1), 82 had intermediate submucosal invasion (sm2), and 36 had tumor invasion that extended to the inner surface of the muscularis propria (sm3).

Results.—All tumors were adenocarcinomas. Thirty-nine patients with sm1 (60.9%) and 35 patients with sm2 (42.7%) underwent endoscopic polypectomy or local resection, and all 36 patients with sm3 underwent colectomy. Thirteen patients (7.1%) had lymph node metastasis, 4 of whom had sm2 and 9 had sm3. Four patients with sm2 had local recurrence. Statistical analysis revealed that level of invasion, configuration, and location were significant risk factors for the development of lymph node metastasis or local recurrence, whereas lymphovascular invasion, histologic grade, and diameter were not.

Conclusions.—Preoperative assessment of the level of submucosa invasion in patients with EIC may decrease the rate of unnecessary surgery in patients with sessile polyps. Appropriate new guidelines for the treatment of EIC of the large bowel should group patients according to submucosal invasion level.

► The depth of invasion of colon cancer has been known to be associated with risk of recurrence. This has been particularly important in the management of polyps with microscopic invasive cancer. This article assesses the level of invasion using a sub-classification. The authors divide depth of invasion into three levels: level 1, slight invasion of muscularis mucosa; level 2, with intermediate invasion; and, level 3, with carcinoma invasion extending to the inner surface of the muscularis propria. Briefly, these authors conclude that early invasive carcinoma with slight invasion (level 1) can be cured with local resection or endoscopic polypectomy. Intermediate lesions with microscopic negative margins can be followed. However, if carcinoma is detected near the resection margin, either additional bowel resection or very careful follow-up would be desirable. Level 3 invasion would require bowel resection and risk of distant metastases, especially, if lymphovascular invasion or rectal location is suspected. In summary, the level of invasion, the configuration of the tumor, and its location are significant factors in the prediction of lymph node metastases and local recurrence.

T.J. Eberlein, M.D.

Rectal Cancer: The Influence of Tumor Proliferation on Response to Preoperative Irradiation

Willett CG, Warland G, Coen J, et al (Harvard Med School, Boston)

Int J Radiat Oncol Biol Phys 32:57–61, 1995 11–35

Purpose.—Preoperative irradiation in patients with advanced rectal cancer may bring about marked tumor regression or downstaging. Several physical features of rectal tumors associated with a higher likelihood of tumor regression or downstaging after irradiation have been identified, including small lesion size, mobility, and exophytic morphology. The relationship between a rectal tumor's pretreatment proliferative state and its pathologic response to irradiation was studied.

Methods.—Between 1975 and 1994, 39 women and 83 men (with a mean age of 66 years) with locally advanced rectal cancer underwent preoperative irradiation followed by tumor resection or laparotomy. All patients had undergone tumor biopsy before the start of radiation therapy. The pretreatment tumor biopsies were scored for proliferative dependent antigen (Ki-67) immunostaining, proliferating cell nuclear antigen (PCNA) immunostaining, and the number of mitoses per 10 high-powered fields (hpf). All surgical specimens were examined for residual disease.

Results.—Patients whose rectal tumors were mobile, smaller, or proliferative as determined by Ki-67, PCNA, and mitotic activity scores had higher tumor regression rates than patients who did not have these features (Table 1). All 3 proliferative markers were assessed in 95 patients. For these patients, overall proliferative activity was graded on a 3-point scale, where 0 indicated that none of the 3 markers showed increased proliferation, and 3 indicated that all 3 markers showed increased proliferation. When the 3-point scoring system was used to grade proliferative activity, the incidence of marked pathologic regression after irradiation was strongly correlated with the pretreatment proliferative activity of these tumors (Table 2). In addition to tumor proliferative activity, lesion size was also associated with the likelihood of marked pathologic regression after preoperative irradiation. Further stratification revealed that marked tumor regression occurred most frequently in smaller tumors with high proliferative activity scores.

TABLE 1.—Incidence of Marked Pathological Regression by Pretreatment Variables

Variable	No. pts.	Incidence of regression
A. Clinical Stage		
Mobile tumor	18	11 (61%) p=0.005
Locally advanced tumor	104	27 (26%)
B. Tumor size		
Less than 5 cm	41	21 (51%) p=0.002
5 cm or greater	74	16 (22%)
(7 Pts unevaluable)		
C. Tumor grade		
Well/moderately well differentiated	105	33 (31%) p= NS
Poorly differentiated	15	4 (27%)
(2 Pts unevaluable)		
D. Ki-67 Staining		
Minimal	9	2 (22%)
Moderate	39	9 (23%) p= NS*
Extensive	66	24 (36%)
(8 Pts unevaluable)		
E. PCNA staining		
Minimal	20	2 (10%)
Moderate	43	16 (37%) p=0.02†
Extensive	41	17 (41%)
(18 Pts unevaluable)		
F. Mitoses/10 hpf		
Less than 22	77	18 (23%) p=0.002
22 or greater	41	19 (46%)
(4 Pts unevaluable)		

*Difference between minimal and moderate vs. extensive Ki-67 staining was not statistically significant (P = 0.20).

†Difference between minimal vs. moderate and extensive PCNA staining was statistically significant (P = 0.02).

(Reprinted by permission of the publisher from Willett CG, Warland G, Coen J, et al: Rectal cancer: The influence of tumor proliferation on response to preoperative irradiation. *Int J Radiat Oncol Biol Phys* 32:57–61, Copyright 1995 by Elsevier Science Inc.)

TABLE 2.—Incidence of Marked Pathological Regression by Proliferative Score

Proliferative score	Incidence of regression
0	0/8 (0%)
1	7/27 (26%)
2	11/37 (30%)
3	14/23 (61%)
Total	32/95 (34%)

Difference between scores were statistically significant (P = 0.006).

(Reprinted by permission of the publisher from Willett CG, Warland G, Coen J, et al: Rectal cancer: The influence of tumor proliferation on response to preoperative irradiation. *Int J Radiat Oncol Biol Phys* 32:57–61, Copyright 1995 by Elsevier Science Inc.)

Conclusions.—Ki-67, PCNA, and mitotic activity are markers of a rectal tumor's proliferative status. The response of the tumor to preoperative irradiation is closely associated with its pretreatment proliferative activity score.

► It is now widely accepted that regression of rectal carcinoma and downstaging of tumors is possible after preoperative radiation. Some randomized prospective trials examine whether this impacts favorably on survival. The article addresses an extremely important question: how to identify patients that might benefit from preoperative radiation. As seen in Table 1, locally advanced tumors and large tumors tend not to respond as well to preoperative radiation therapy; somewhat in contrast to conventional wisdom. However, proliferative activity as demonstrated by Ki-67 staining and PCNA staining, as well as the high mitotic index, predict for regression following preoperative radiation therapy. This may help to predict which tumors may regress after irradiation (as well as those unlikely to regress), and therefore, may help to identify patients that would be candidates for eventual local excision or coloanal anastamosis as an alternative to abdominoperineal resection.

T.J. Eberlein, M.D.

Local Recurrence Rate in a Randomised Multicentre Trial of Preoperative Radiotherapy Compared With Operation Alone in Resectable Rectal Carcinoma

Påhlman L, for the Swedish Rectal Cancer Trial (Univ of Upsala, Sweden)
Eur J Surg 162:397–402, 1996 11–36

Background.—Previous studies have reported reduced local recurrence rates in patients with resectable rectal carcinoma who receive preoperative irradiation. The effect of short-term high-dose preoperative radiotherapy on local recurrence and postoperative mortality was evaluated in a prospective randomized trial.

Methods.—Over a 3-year period, 1,168 patients with resectable rectal carcinoma were randomly assigned to treatment with surgery alone or radiotherapy at 25 Gy in 5 fractions in 1 week and surgery within the next week. Operations that yielded tumor specimens with tumor-free margins were considered curative. The tumors were staged. Local recurrence rates after a minimum of 2 years follow-up were determined.

Results.—The overall local recurrence rates were 9% in the irradiated group and 24% in the surgery alone group. Significantly lower local recurrence rates were also seen in the irradiated group than in the surgery alone group among patients with curative operations and among patients with all stages of disease (Table 2), regardless of the type of surgical procedure (Table 3). Distant metastases developed within 2 years in 17% of the irradiated group and 20% of the surgery alone group among those with curative operations.

TABLE 2.—Local Recurrence Rates by Dukes' Stage for All Resected Tumors

	Irradiated group Local Dukes' stage				Surgery alone group Local Dukes' stage			
	A	B	C	Total	A	B	C	Total
Distant metastases	0/5	0/11	2/26 (8)	2/42 (5)	0/4	0/12	5/25 (20)	5/41 (12)
Locally not cured	0	2/6 (33)	1/8 (13)	3/14 (21)	0	2/8 (25)	6/11 (55)	8/19 (42)
Uncertain local cure	0/2	5/13 (39)	8/28 (27)	13/43 (17)	1/3 (33)	5/8 (63)	19/32 (59)	25/43 (58)
Curative surgery	6/174 (3)	7/165 (4)	20/115 (17)	33/454 (7)	13/147 (9)	24/145 (17)	56/162 (35)	93/454 (20)
Total	6/181 (3)	14/195 (7)	31/177 (18)	51/553 (9)	14/154 (9)	31/173 (18)	86/230 (37)	131/557 (24)

Note: Figures are numbers (%) of patients.

(Courtesy of Påhlman L, for the Swedish Rectal Cancer Trial: Local recurrence rate in a randomised multicentre trial of preoperative radiotherapy compared with operation alone in resectable rectal carcinoma. *Eur J Surg* 162:397–402, 1996.)

TABLE 3.—Local Recurrence Rates by Operation

Operation	Irradiated group			Surgery alone group		
	Not curative	Curative	Total	Not curative	Curative	Total
Anterior resection	3/37 (8)	15/206 (7)	18/243 (7)	8/33 (24)	33/194 (17)	41/227 (18)
Abdominoperineal resection	14/61 (23)	17/243 (7)	31/304 (10)	28/66 (42)	59/256 (23)	87/322 (27)
Other procedures	1/1 (100)	1/5 (20)	2/6 (33)	2/4 (50)	1/4 (25)	3/8 (38)

Note: Figures are numbers (%) of patients.

(Courtesy of Påhlman L, for the Swedish Rectal Cancer Trial: Local recurrence rate in a randomised multicentre trial of preoperative radiotherapy compared with operation alone in resectable rectal carcinoma. *Eur J Surg* 162:397–402, 1996.)

Conclusions.—Short-term high-dose preoperative radiotherapy reduces the local recurrence rate by approximately 65% in patients with resectable rectal carcinoma. Longer follow-up is needed to determine the effect of preoperative radiotherapy on overall survival.

▶ This is a randomized prospective trial of almost 1,200 patients allocated to receive preoperative radiation followed by operation within a week or surgery alone. As has been seen in other randomized trials in the United States and abroad, this trial shows a substantial decrease in local recurrence rate compared to Dukes' stage (Table 2) or operation performed (Table 3).

This is a superbly done trial and these investigators have approximately 15 years of experience with this regimen. This is actually a high-dose, short-term radiotherapy regimen. Therefore, it is possibly more cost-effective. However, no trial has yet compared this regimen with more conventional preoperative radiation therapy regimens. There is concern among some radiation therapists that because of the high fraction doses, there may be possible late toxicities. In other Swedish series that utilized this same regimen, however, this has not been substantiated.

In the surgery-alone treatment group, there is approximately a 24% local recurrence rate. Some surgeons may consider this high. However, as emphasized in the article, the surgeons who participated in this trial were not subspecialists and, therefore, the authors felt this reflected a better representation of general surgeons who perform this type of surgery.

Another concern was the possible overtreatment of patients with Dukes' A and possibly Dukes' B lesions. These authors have not made any comment about survival, and we will anxiously await the further evaluation after a 5-year median follow-up has been achieved. However, there already seems to be at least a numerical advantage to patients who receive this regimen of preoperative radiation therapy.

T.J. Eberlein, M.D.

Male and Female Sexual and Urinary Function After Total Mesorectal Excision With Autonomic Nerve Preservation for Carcinoma of the Rectum

Havenga K, Enker WE, McDermott K, et al (Mem Sloan-Kettering Cancer Ctr, New York)

J Am Coll Surg 182:495–502, 1996 11–37

Background.—Conventional surgery for rectal carcinoma can result in sexual dysfunction. Most studies of this complication focus on sexual function in men younger than 60 or 65 years of age. The current study included men and women of all ages who underwent total mesorectal excision with automatic nerve preservation by abdominoperineal resection or low anterior resection for rectal carcinoma.

Methods.—Eighty-two men and 54 women responded to a survey on postoperative sexual and urinary function. These 136 patients represented 78% of the patients eligible for the study.

Findings.—Eighty-six percent of the patients younger than 60 years of age and 67% of the patients 60 years of age and older were still able to have intercourse. Eighty-five percent of the women still experienced arousal with vaginal lubrication. Ninety-one percent were able to achieve orgasm. Eighty-seven percent of the men were still able to have an orgasm. Male sexual dysfunction was significantly associated with abdominoperineal resection (compared with low anterior resection) and an age of 60 years or more. Most patients reported few or no problems with urinary function. None had serious urinary dysfunction, such as neurogenic bladder.

Conclusions.—Autonomic nerve preservation with total mesorectal excision minimizes sexual and urinary dysfunction in patients who undergo surgery for rectal carcinoma. Sexual function can be preserved in most men and women, especially those younger than 60 years of age and after low anterior resection.

▶ This is a retrospective postoperative study of sexual and urinary function in 136 patients who submitted to standardized questionnaires. Abdominoperineal resection at 60 years of age or greater was associated with an increase in male sexual dysfunction. The majority of the patients had very few complaints related to urinary dysfunction. Obviously, the success of these types of procedures rest on the surgeon's ability to identify the nerves. Autonomic nerve preservation consists of identification and preservation of the pelvic hypogastric (sympathetic) as well as splanchnic (parasympathetic) nerve trunks together with a pelvic autonomic nerve plexus. These nerves are often difficult to identify and are usually totally ignored by most surgeons who perform low anterior resection and/or abdominoperineal resection. A corollary technical point is that these authors rarely mobilize the autonomic nerves and plexuses. Additionally, internal iliac lymph nodes are also rarely dissected. In these patients, local control is 8.3% and 5-year survival rate (in patients with Dukes' B or C tumors) is

74.2%. As surgery for rectal tumors becomes more refined, these techniques may increasingly improve the lifestyles of postoperative patients.

T.J. Eberlein, M.D.

Randomized Comparison of Straight and Colonic J Pouch Anastomosis After Low Anterior Resection

Hallböök O, Påhlman L, Krog M, et al (Univ Hosp, Linköping, Sweden; Academic Hosp, Uppsala, Sweden; Central Hosp, Gävle, Sweden; et al)

Ann Surg 224:58–65, 1996 11–38

Objective.—Most patients with rectal cancer are now offered resection with sphincter preservation. The surgery involves a low anastomosis that can lead to poor bowel function as a result of the loss of the rectal reservoir. Although use of a colonic J-shaped pouch is associated with better functional outcome, the safety and efficacy of the procedure has not been tested in clinical trials. Reconstructions with traditional straight anastomosis and the colonic J-pouch anastomosis were compared in a randomized study.

Methods.—Patients from 4 centers were randomly allocated to receive either a straight (n = 52) or a colonic J pouch (n = 45) anastomosis (Fig 1). Bowel function was evaluated in 93 patients after 2 months and in 89 after 1 year. Questionnaires were used to determine frequency of bowel function, degree of urgency, grade and frequency of incontinence, differentiation between gas and stool, ability to evacuate in less than 15 minutes, sensation of incomplete evacuation, effect on well-being, and any required medication. Results were analyzed statistically.

Results.—Significantly more patients with straight anastomosis rather than J-pouch anastomosis had leakage (8 vs. 1) and anastomotic stricture

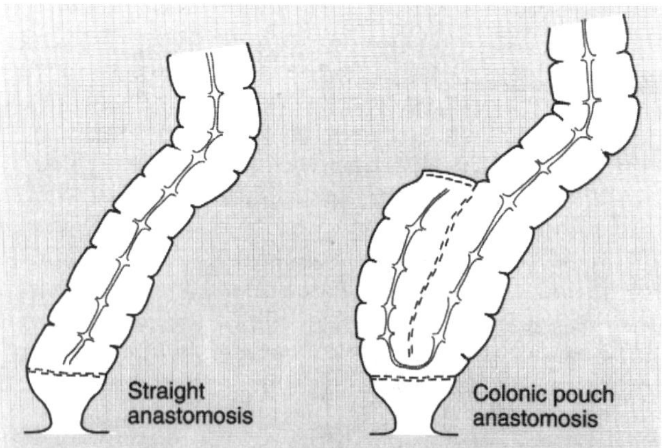

FIGURE 1.—The patients were randomly allocated to reconstruction with either a straight or a colonic J-pouch anastomosis. (Courtesy of Hallböök O, Påhlman L, Krog M, et al: Randomized comparison of straight and colonic J pouch anastomosis after low anterior resection *Ann Surg* 224:58–65, 1996.)

TABLE 6.—Postoperative Functional Outcome

	Two Months			One Year		
	Straight (n = 50)	Pouch (n = 43)	p	Straight (n = 47)	Pouch (n = 42)	p
Frequency of bowel movements 24 hr [median (interquartile range)]	6.4 (4.5–8.1)	2 (1.5–2.5)	<0.001*	3.5 (2.4–4.5)	2 (1.3–2.3)	<0.001*
Nocturnal bowel movements	31 (62%)	13 (30%)	0.0019†	11 (24%)	3 (7%)	0.042†
Ability to defer defecation > 30 min (%)			<0.001*			<0.001*
Always	8	44		15	49	
Often	22	35		40	44	
Sometimes	36	21		30	5	
Never	34	0		15	2	
Composite score of incontinence, 0–18 [median (interquartile range)]	7 (2.8–13)	1.5 (0–5)	<0.001*	5 (2–9)	2 (0–5.3)	0.0018*
Unable to differentiate gas from stool	22 (44%)	5 (12%)	<0.001†	8 (17%)	4 (10%)	0.36†
Regular use of retarding medication	21 (42%)	3 (7%)	<0.001†	19 (40%)	1 (2%)	<0.001†
Regular use of bulking medication	10 (20%)	18 (42%)	0.026†	10 (21%)	21 (50%)	0.071†

*Wilcoxon rank sum test.

†Fisher's exact test.

(Courtesy of Hallböök O, Påhlman L, Krog M, et al: Randomized comparison of straight and colonic J pouch anastomosis after low anterior resection. *Ann Surg* 224:58–65, 1996.)

TABLE 7.—Postoperative Functional Outcome With Regard to Evacuation

	Two Months			One Year		
	Straight (n = 50)	Pouch (n = 43)	p	Straight (n = 47)	Pouch (n = 42)	p
Ability to evacuate the bowel < 15 min (%)			0.54*			0.073*
Always	50	56		55	34	
Often	28	23		26	39	
Sometimes	14	21		15	20	
Never	8	0		4	7	
Sensation of incomplete evacuation (%)			0.033*			0.10*
Never	13	32		9	22	
Sometimes	29	39		52	50	
Often	40	21		32	23	
Always	18	8		7	5	
Regular use of enema or suppository to evacuate the bowel [no. (%)]	0	3 (7)	0.095†	0	4 (10)	0.046†

*Wilcoxon rank sum test.
†Fisher's exact test.
(Courtesy of Hallböök O, Påhlman L, Krog M, et al: Randomized comparison of straight and colonic J pouch anastomosis after low anterior resection. *Ann Surg* 224:58–65, 1996.)

(7 vs. 3). The J-pouch group had significantly improved bowel function (Table 6). The J-pouch group rated overall bowel function higher at 1 year than the straight anastomosis group (Table 7). At 1 year there were no local recurrences, but 5 patients in each group had indications of distant metastases.

Conclusion.—Use of the colonic J pouch after low anterior resection for rectal cancer gave improved bowel function at 2 months and 1 year when compared with the straight anastomosis.

► This is a randomized, prospective series of 100 patients who were treated with either straight or colonic J-pouch anastomosis for sphincter-saving procedures for rectal cancer. This work builds on the results not only from ileoanal pull-through procedures but also from coloanal anastomoses where J- pouch reconstruction is often associated with better functional outcome. In this study, frequency of bowel movements and nocturnal bowel movement as well as incontinence were much less in patients with pouch reconstruction. This was particularly true in the early postoperative phase (Table 6, 2 months) but was also significant at 1 year. It is of interest that patients with J-pouch reconstruction had, especially in the long term, a slightly increased need for utilization of enemas or suppositories to evacuate their bowel. Although one would intuitively feel that J-pouch reconstruction may be associated with higher complications, and this was technically true in this series, there were actually more symptomatic anastomotic leaks in the straight reconstruction group compared with the J-pouch reconstruction group. These excellent results may well be attributable to the technical abilities of the surgeons involved. However, it seems that once the technical aspects of J-pouch reconstruction are mastered, a better functional outcome results for the patient, using this type of reconstruction.

T.J. Eberlein, M.D.

Clinical Utility of External Immunoscintigraphy With the IMMU-4 Technetium-99m Fab′ Antibody Fragment in Patients Undergoing Surgery for Carcinoma of the Colon and Rectum: Results of a Pivotal, Phase III Trial

Moffat FL Jr, for the Immunomedics Study Group (Univ of Miami, Fla)

J Clin Oncol 14:2295–2305, 1996 11–39

Background.—Radioimmunodetection (RAID), in which scintigraphic imaging is performed after administration of radiolabeled monoclonal antibodies against various tumor antigens, appears to offer important information beyond that provided by conventional diagnostic modalities (CDM). IMMU-4, which is a murine monoclonal antibody specific for anti–carcinoembryonic antigen (CEA), has given promising results in RAID. Previous open-label studies have examined the use of IMMU-4 ^{99m}Tc-Fab' RAID (CEA-Scan) in patients who had colorectal cancer. This method was evaluated to determine whether it provided diagnostic information and influenced decisions regarding treatment in patients who had colorectal carcinoma.

Methods.—Two hundred ten patients who were awaiting surgery for advanced recurrent or metastatic colorectal carcinoma were included. Each patient underwent external scintigraphy 2–5 hours and 18–24 hours after receiving CEA-Scan by IV injection. The patients also underwent imaging with CDM. The results of the imaging studies were compared with the surgical and histologic findings.

Results.—The anti–carcinoembryonic antigen scan was more sensitive than CDM in the extrahepatic abdomen (55% vs. 32%) and in the pelvis (69% vs. 48%). In the liver, the findings of CEA-Scan were complementary to those of CDM. Analysis of 122 patients who had known disease showed a positive predictive value of 98% when both imaging studies were positive, compared with a value of 68% to 70% with either study alone. Accuracy was also higher when the 2 studies were used together. For the 88 patients who had occult disease, accuracy increased from 33% to 61% when CEA-Scan was combined with CDM. Overall, CEA-Scan was deemed of potential clinical benefit in 42% of patients. Two patients showed human antimouse antibodies after a single injection of CEA-Scan. None of 19 patients had antibodies after 2 injections of CEA-Scan.

Conclusions.—This imaging technique is safe and valuable for the detection and localization of colorectal cancer. It is inexpensive and readily available and provides high-quality images, thereby yielding clinically significant information that is not obtained by CDM. Antibody reactions are rare. When the results of both CEA-Scan and CDM are positive, the positive predictive value may be high enough to obviate the need for histologic confirmation.

▶ Radioimmunodetection has been investigated during the past several decades. This article deals with 2 phase III prospective protocols. The authors used a CEA-Scan in more than 200 patients. The protocols included patients with recurrent or metastatic colorectal cancer who had 1 or more tumor deposits visualized by conventional modalities. The second protocol included patients suspected of having tumor-recurrence but there was no definitive abnormality on conventional modality scanning. The specificity of the CEA-Scan was relatively low (see Table 2 of original article). Its sensitivity was greater, however, than that of conventional modalities.

When used alone, CEA-Scan did not offer significant improvement over conventional modalities. When combined with conventional modalities, however, the positive predictive value approached 100% (98%). This finding implies that the utility of CEA-Scan, when combined with conventional radiographic tests, may have the potential for avoiding laparotomies in both patients without recurrence and patients in whom the extent of tumor is beyond the technical ability of surgical removal.

Another unique feature to this study is that the CEA-Scan RAID conjugate used murine monoclonal antibody fragments from which the Fc portion had been removed. This almost completely eliminated the development of human antimouse antibody reactivity. As the technology improves, high-quality and rapid imaging without the risk of development of mouse anti human antibody will be possible. This group is also analyzing the influence of CEA-Scan in surgical decision making.

T.J. Eberlein, M.D.

Detection of K-*ras* Mutations in Stools of Patients With Colorectal Cancer by Mutant-enriched PCR

Nollau P, Moser C, Weinland G, et al (Universitätskrankenhaus Eppendorf, Germany; Israelitisches Krankenhaus, Hamburg, Germany)

Int J Cancer 66:332–336, 1996 11–40

Background.—Because early diagnosis of colorectal cancer significantly improves survival, the development of new sensitive and specific diagnostic tests is important. Assays of the discovered mutations of oncogenes and tumor-suppressor genes may become important diagnostic tools. The mutant-enriched polymerase chain reaction (PCR) is a new, rapid, nonradioactive technique, based on 2 consecutive PCRs with intermediate restriction digest to eliminate wild-type alleles, which can be used to detect K-*ras* mutated tumor cells in the stool. The assay accuracy was evaluated by comparing the results of mutant-enriched PCR of stool DNA and of PCR-mediated restriction fragment length polymorphism (RFLP) analysis of tumors from patients with colorectal cancer.

Methods.—Polymerase chain reaction–mediated RFLP analysis was done to detect mutations at codons 12 and 13 of K-*ras* genes in 50 sporadic colorectal tumors. Stool samples were collected before surgery. Mutant-enriched PCR, using semi-nested pairs of primers, was done on stool samples from 11 healthy donors, to determine the optimal number of cycles for each PCR to detect mutations. For detection of codon 12 mutation, 20 cycles were done in the first PCR and 38 in the second PCR. For detection of codom 13 mutation, 16 cycles were done in the first PCR and 38 in the second. These procedures were followed for the mutant-enriched PCR analysis of stool samples from the 16 patients with previously detected K-*ras* tumor mutations, stool samples from 7 other randomly selected patients with no detected K-*ras* tumor mutations, and a stool sample from 1 patient with non-Hodgkin's lymphoma. The nucleotide exchanges in both tumors and stools were analyzed with sequencing.

Results.—Mutations were detected with mutant-enriched PCR in the stool samples of 12 of the 16 patients with detected tumor mutations (including 9 of 12 with codon 12 mutations and 3 of 4 with codon 13 mutations) and in 1 of the 12 patients without detected tumor mutations at the 2 tested codons. These results were reproducible in 3 to 5 experiments with each sample. The DNA sequencing revealed identical nucleotide exchanges in the stool samples and tumors of all of these patients. Re-analysis of the tumor DNA from the 1 patient with mutations discovered in the stool but not the tumor was done with mutant-enriched PCR and revealed a mutant tumor fragment with the nucleotide exchange corresponding to that found in the stool sample.

Conclusions.—K-*ras* mutated tumor cells can be detected in the stools of patients with colorectal cancer with good sensitivity, specificity, and reproducibility, using mutant-enriched PCR, which suggests that this may be an applicable routine diagnosis technique. However, it can only be done to analyze mutations with known localization. Therefore, further research is needed to localize other mutations and to develop similar techniques in order to adequately screen for colorectal cancer.

▶ This article demonstrates the power of detecting K-*ras* mutations using PCR-mediated RFLP analysis. Detection of these mutations was not 100%. In fact, only 13 of 16 stool samples in which K-*ras* mutations had been identified from tumors were detected in stool samples.

A technical limitation of this type of study is that a more sensitive detection of point-mutated genes appears to be the error frequency of the polymerases used for amplification of *ras* genes from stool samples. This study used only single stool samples and, therefore, the diagnostic sensitivity may be improved by increasing the number of samples tested per patient.

Although this analysis is relatively quick, and will be easily adjusted to automation, it is limited to analysis of mutations with known localization. Although K-*ras* mutations occur in 30% to 40% of colorectal tumors, analysis of other frequently mutated genes (p53, APC) also may improve results.

T.J. Eberlein, M.D.

Clinicopathologic and Prognostic Significance of an Angiogenic Factor, Thymidine Phosphorylase, in Human Colorectal Carcinoma

Takebayashi Y, Akiyama S-I, Akiba S, et al (Kagoshima Univ, Japan; Taiho Pharmaceutical Co Ltd, Saitama, Japan)

J Natl Cancer Inst 88:1110–1117, 1996 11–41

Objective.—Tumor growth and metastasis depend on the development of new blood vessels, which is promoted by platelet-derived endothelial cell growth factor (PD-ECGF). A previous study revealed that thymidine phosphorylase (dThdPase) is the same protein as PD-ECGF. A series of primary colorectal carcinomas was reviewed to determine their expression of dThdPase, the relationship of this enzyme to angiogenesis and clinicopathologic findings, and its prognostic value.

Methods.—One hundred sixty-three surgical specimens of colorectal carcinoma were included. Immunostaining of endothelial cells for factor VIII was performed to enable counting of microvessels. In the same sections, dThdPase expression was studied with use of the purified monoclonal antibody against dThdPase. Both assessments were performed without knowledge of the clinicopathologic findings. Survival analysis was performed to determine the prognostic significance of dThdPase.

Results.—The mean number of microvessels counted in a 400 × field was 17.5 in dThdPase-positive specimens vs. 9.3 in dThdPase-negative specimens. Thymidine phosphorylase status was significant associated with tumor size, extent of invasion, lymph node metastases, and lymphatic and venous invasion (Fig 4). On Cox regression analysis, with adjustment

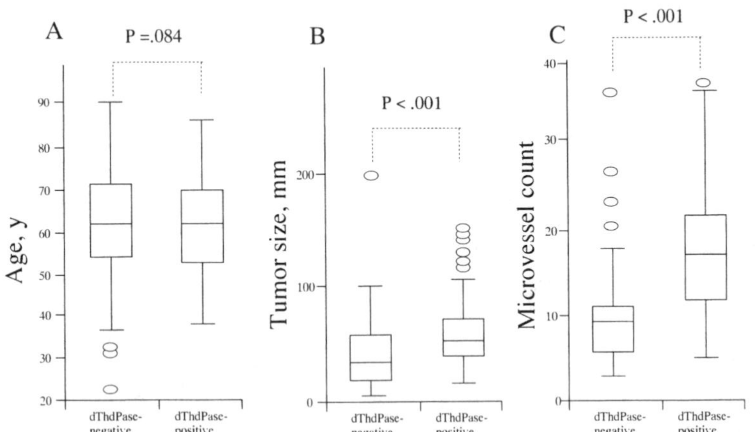

FIGURE 4.—Distribution of age, tumor size, and microvessel count as a function of dThdPase. In each panel, the *box* corresponds to the interquartile ranges, with the *lower boundary* of the *box* representing the 25th percentile and the *upper boundary* representing the 75th percentile. The *line* inside the *box* represents the mean value. The *vertical line* represents the 5th and 9th percentiles, and the *open ovals* represent the outliers. *P* values were calculated by Student's *t* test (2-sided). (Courtesy of Takebayashi Y, Akiyama S-I, Akiba S, et al: Clinicopathologic and prognostic significance of an angiogenic factor, thymidine phosphorylase, in human colorectal carcinoma. *J Natl Cancer Inst* 88:1110–1117, 1996.)

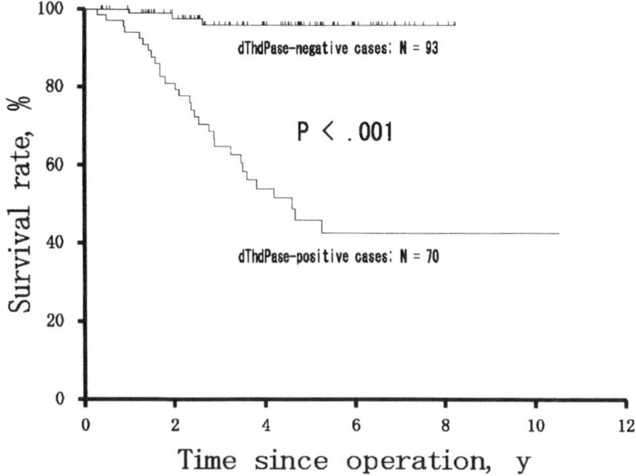

FIGURE 5.—Kaplan-Meier survival curves of patients with colorectal carcinoma. Comparison of survival curves for patients whose tumors stained positive for dThdPase with those patients whose tumors were classified as negative for dThdPase expression. *Curves* present the results for all patients. The 95% confidence intervals (*CIs*) on the curves for dThdPase-negative cases at 1, 3, and 4 years were 0.97–1.00, 0.91–1.00, and 0.91–1.00, respectively. The 95% CIs on the curves for dThdPase-positive cases at 1, 3, and 4 years were 0.88–0.99, 0.56–0.79, and 0.41–0.67, respectively. *Tick marks* represent observations. (Courtesy of Takebayashi Y, Akiyama S-I, Akiba S, et al: Clinicopathologic and prognostic significance of an angiogenic factor, thymidine phosphorylase, in Human colorectal carcinoma. *J Natl Cancer Inst* 88:1110–1117, 1996.)

for Dukes' stage and microvessel count, dThdPase expression was a significant prognostic factor for poor disease outcome (Fig 5).

Conclusions.—A high level of dThdPase expression in colorectal carcinoma is linked to more extensive development of new blood vessels, poor clinical and laboratory findings, and a poor clinical outcome. The way in which dThdPase mediates angiogenesis, tumor invasiveness, and metastatic ability remains to be determined. However, dThdPase inhibitors may be a useful part of therapy for colorectal carcinoma.

► These investigators have shown that dThdPase and PD-ECGF are the same protein. This study looked at 163 patients who had colorectal carcinoma. The authors showed that dThdPase tumors had higher microvessel counts and were large and more extensive (Fig 4). In addition, they showed that these tumors were associated with a much poorer prognosis (Fig 5). These are very similar findings to those by Folkman and colleagues[1, 2] in breast cancer.

The exact mechanism of dThdPase in angiogenesis and tumor growth is still unknown; however, involvement of this enzyme in angiogenesis and especially in the development of invasive tumors and metastatic tumors would suggest a possible mechanism to help inhibit tumors. There are already phase I trials in progress in breast cancer that use a similar strategy. These investigators have already begun to develop strategies in which inhibitors of this enzyme are used in the therapy of patients who have colorectal carcinomas.

T.J. Eberlein, M.D.

References

1. Folkman J, Klagsburn M: Angiogenic factors. *Science* 235:442–447, 1987.
2. Folkman J: What is the evidence that tumors are angiogenesis dependent? *J Natl Cancer Inst* 82:4–6, 1990.

Curative Reoperations for Locally Recurrent Rectal Cancer

Suzuki K, Dozois RR, Devine RM, et al (Mayo Clinic and Mayo Found, Rochester, Minn)

Dis Colon Rectum 39:730–736, 1996 11–42

Background.—Evidence suggests that the outcome of reoperation for locally recurrent rectal cancer may not be as bad as is generally assumed. Morbidity, survival and related factors, and patterns of failure among patients undergoing further surgery in an attempt to cure locally recurrent rectal cancer were reported.

Methods.—Two hundred twenty-four patients with a preoperative diagnosis of recurrent rectal cancer underwent reoperation between 1981 and 1988 at 1 center. Sixty-five of these patients had additional surgery with the goal of achieving no gross or microscopic residual disease at tumor margins postoperatively.

Findings.—No deaths occurred within 30 days of the repeat surgery. Fourteen patients had a total of 17 complications necessitating hospitalization and/or surgical intervention. Extended procedures, involving partial or complete removal of surrounding organs or structures, were asso-

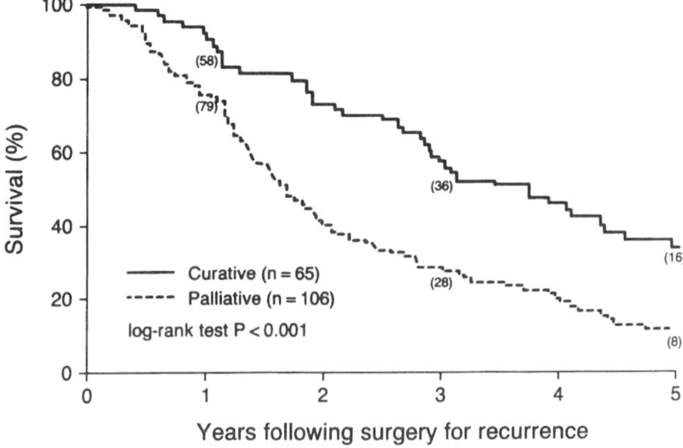

FIGURE 2.—Survival after surgery for recurrence in patients with curative resection vs. microscopic residual disease or gross residual disease. (Courtesy of Suzuki K, Dozois RR, Devine RM, et al: Curative reoperations for locally recurrent rectal cancer. *Dis Colon Rectum* 39(7):730–736, 1996.)

ciated with a longer operating time, a longer hospital stay, and more transfusions than were more limited procedures. Survival was 57% at 3 years and 34% at 5 years. The median survival was 44.7 months. Survival was better after curative resection than after palliative procedures (Fig 2). Women and patients without pain tended to have better survivals. The cumulative probability of local failure was 24% at 1 year, 41% at 3 years, and 47% at 5 years. The cumulative risk of distant metastasis was 30% at 1 year, 51% at 3 years, and 62% at 5 years.

Conclusion.—Complete excision of locally recurrent rectal cancer is safe and beneficial in a significant number of patients with locally recurrent cancer. The encouraging 3- and 5-year survival rates in this study suggest that an aggressive approach in selected patients is reasonable.

► Sixty-five patients who underwent extensive surgery with an intention of cure for recurrent rectal cancer are reported. The overall point of the article is that long-term survival (see Fig 2) is possible even in patients with recurrent pelvic tumor.

However, these patients were relatively highly selected. In fact, they were from a subset of 176 patients, 106 of whom also underwent operation but had either gross or microscopic tumor after reoperation. Thus, in a rough sense, reoperation with intent to cure is possible in approximately one quarter to one third of patients (48 other patients had evidence of extrapelvic tumor at the time of evaluation). No specific factors were identified as being associated with survival, although the presence of pain was marginally significant in reducing survival.

Obviously, this type of surgery does come at a cost, as over 30% of the patients had some sort of complication, oftentimes requiring rehospitalization or another surgical procedure. The bottom line is that this group of surgeons have extensive experience in evaluating these types of patients. Only a minority of patients, in fact, will be resectable for cure, and then at a relatively high cost. Especially in patients who have had radiation and chemotherapy in the treatment of their primary tumor, reoperation can be technically difficult and associated with high morbidity. Nonetheless, in patients with recurrence confined to the pelvis, long-term survival is possible.

T.J. Eberlein, M.D.

Resection of Nonresectable Liver Metastases From Colorectal Cancer After Neoadjuvant Chemotherapy

Bismuth H, Adam R, Lévi F, et al (Hôpital Paul Brousse, Villejuif, France; Univ of Paris-Sud)

Ann Surg 224:509–522, 1996 11–43

Purpose.—Liver metastases from colorectal cancer are best treated by resection; however, this is possible in only 10% of patients. The rest do not live long, even if they have a partial response to chemotherapy. Chemo-

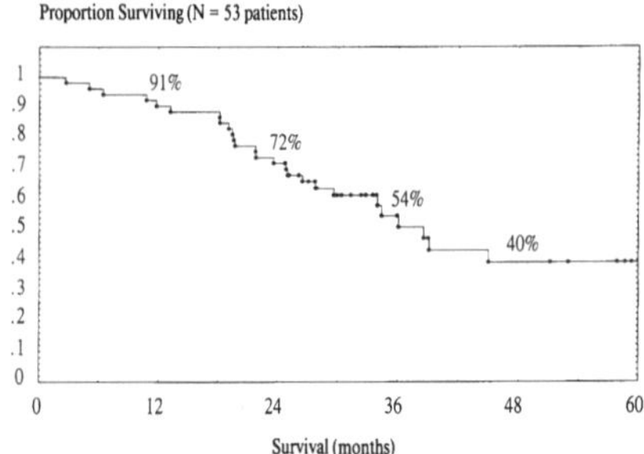

FIGURE 6.—Cumulative survival after liver resection, after systemic chronomodulated chemotherapy for all unresectable liver metastases. (Courtesy of Bismuth H, Adam R, Lévi F, et al: Resection of nonresectable liver metastases from colorectal cancer after neoadjuvant chemotherapy. *Ann Surg* 224:509–522, 1996.)

therapy, however, could be effective enough to permit secondary resection of the liver metastases. The results of curative hepatectomy in patients with liver metastases that were downstaged by chemotherapy were reviewed.

Methods.—The experience included 53 patients with colorectal cancer and metastases to the liver. In each case, the liver metastases were considered unresectable because of multinodular lesions (45% of patients), extrahepatic disease (25%), or ill-located or large lesions (15% each). All

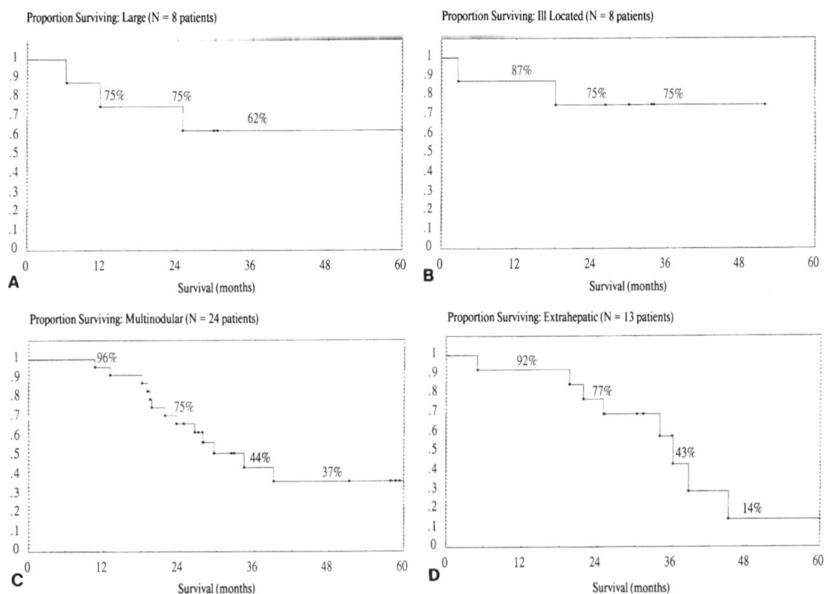

FIGURE 7.—Survival after resection of colorectal liver metastases, according to the cause of primary unresectability. **A,** previously unresectable because of the large size of the tumor; **B,** previously unresectable because of ill-located tumors; **C,** previously unresectable because of multinodular tumors; **D,** previously unresectable because of associated extrahepatic disease. (Courtesy of Bismuth H, Adam R, Lévi F, et al: Resection of nonresectable liver metastases from colorectal cancer after neoadjuvant chemotherapy. *Ann Surg* 224:509–522, 1996.)

patients had their metastases downstaged by means of chronomodulated systemic chemotherapy, consisting of 5-fluorouracil, folic acid, and oxaliplatin. The decision to perform secondary hepatectomy was made after a mean 8 months of chemotherapy. Thirty-seven patients had a major hepatectomy, i.e., more than 3 segments, and 16 had less extensive surgery. Twenty-five patients had associated surgical procedures as well, including 2-stage hepatectomy in 5 patients and pulmonary resection in 3.

Results.—None of the patients died during or within the first 2 months after surgery. Twenty-six percent of patients had complications, most involving the hepatectomy site. Survival was 54% at 3 years and 40% at 5 years (Fig 6). Survival varied according to the reason for initial unresectability; survival was better for patients with large or ill-located tumors than in those with multinodular tumors or extrahepatic disease (Fig 7). Of 34 patients with hepatic recurrences, 15 were managed by repeat surgery.

Conclusions.—In some patients with liver metastases from colorectal cancer, neoadjuvant chemotherapy may downstage tumors sufficiently for hepatic resection. In terms of survival, the results are comparable to those achieved in patients undergoing primary hepatectomy. With an aggressive surgical approach—including repeat hepatectomy and extrahepatic surgery—these patients may have a reasonable chance of long-term survival.

► Patients who have metastatic colorectal tumor confined to the liver have the potential for long-term survival if surgical resection is possible. Unfortunately, in the patients who are not able to undergo resection, survival is extremely poor, even if they have partial response to adjuvant chemotherapy. This study reports on a very aggressive regimen of neoadjuvant chemotherapy to downstage the liver with possible inclusion of extra liver metastases excision, as well as the willingness to perform repeat hepatectomy. By using this very aggressive approach, survival is comparable to that obtained with a primary liver resection (40%—see Fig 6). In addition to this very aggressive approach, reproducing these excellent results also requires excellent judgment and excellent technical skill. Another point to be underscored, is that this is a highly selected series of patients; yet, they would be anticipated to have the poorest survival. The regimen of chemotherapy is reasonably toxic, yet complications in these patients were at a very acceptable rate. There were no operative deaths.

In studying Figure 7, it is interesting to note that the patients that seemed to do the best were patients with either large tumors or ill-located tumors that then responded to the neoadjuvant chemotherapy. As might be anticipated, patients with multinodular tumors, or extrahepatic extension still had a very poor survival. Others have shown[1] in hepatocellular carcinoma that an aggressive neoadjuvant chemotherapy regimen and an aggressive surgical approach may improve the long-term survival of a population of patients expected to have uniformly poor prognoses.

T.J. Eberlein, M.D.

Reference

1. Meta-Analysis Group in Cancer: Reappraisal of hepatic arterial infusion in the treatment of nonresectable liver metastases from colorectal cancer. *J Natl Cancer Inst* 88:252–258, 1996.

Randomized Study on Preoperative Radiotherapy in Rectal Carcinoma

Cedermark B, for the Stockholm Colorectal Cancer Study Group (Karolinska Hosp, Stockholm)

Ann Surg Oncol 3:423–430, 1996 11–44

Introduction.—In the mid-1980s, a Swedish study found that preoperative radiotherapy in patients with operable rectal cancer reduces the pelvic recurrence rate, but at the cost of an increase in postoperative mortality. Another study performed about the same time—using a 3-portal technique to a relatively small target volume instead of an anteroposterior opposed portal technique to a larger volume—found no increase in postoperative mortality. Outcomes in a new study of preoperative radiotherapy, using a high dose of radiation given over a short time, in patients with operable rectal cancer were assessed.

Methods.—The study included 557 patients with histologically proved, clinically resectable adenocarcinoma of the rectum. All were less than 80 years old, and those who were scheduled for local excision or who had received previous pelvic irradiation were excluded. The patients were assigned to preoperative irradiation followed by surgery or to surgery only. Patients in the radiotherapy group received 25 Gy of radiation to the rectum and pararectal tissues over a period of 5–7 days. The target was the intersection of the central axes of 4 beams and included the anal canal, rectum, mesorectum, presacral nodes, and lymph nodes of the iliac artery, lumbar spine, and obturator foramens. Follow-up was complete up to a median of 50 months. Eighty-six patients underwent potentially curative surgery.

TABLE 3.—Postoperative Complications in Irradiated and Nonirradiated Patients

Postoperative complication	Radiotherapy (%) (N = 272)	Surgery (%) (N = 285)
Wound sepsis	41 (15)	16 (6)
Septicemia	3 (1)	3 (1)
Anastomotic leak	12 (4)	8 (3)
Wound dehiscence	6 (2)	5 (2)
Bowel obstruction	13 (5)	16 (6)
Others	51 (19)	40 (14)
None	161 (59)	206 (72)

(Courtesy of Cedermark B, for the Stockholm Colorectal Cancer Study Group: Randomized study on preoperative radiotherapy in rectal carcinoma. *Ann Surg Oncol* 4:423–430, 1996.)

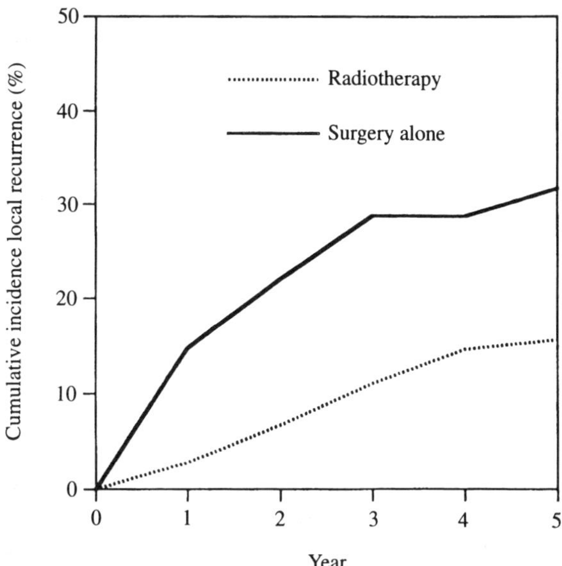

FIGURE 1.—Cumulative incidence of pelvic recurrence after curative surgery. (Courtesy of Cedermark B, for the Stockholm Colorectal Cancer Study Group: Randomized study on preoperative radiotherapy in rectal carcinoma. *Ann Surg Oncol* 4:423–430, 1996.)

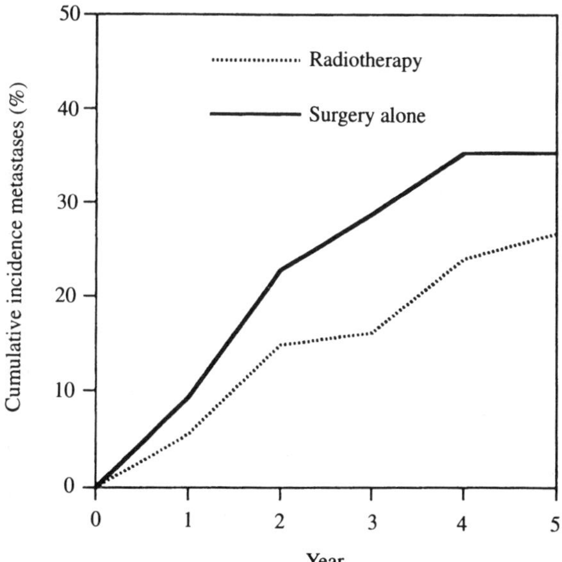

FIGURE 2.—Cumulative incidence of distant metastases after curative surgery. (Courtesy of Cedermark B, for the Stockholm Colorectal Cancer Study Group: Randomized study on preoperative radiotherapy in rectal carcinoma. *Ann Surg Oncol* 4:423–430, 1996.)

TABLE 7.—Incidence of Pelvic Recurrence in Curatively Operated Patients in Relation to Tumor Stage

Tumor stage	No. pts.	Events (%)	RH	Log-rank p	
Dukes' A	Rt+	98	5 (5)	0.5	0.246
	Rt−	78	7 (9)	1.0	
Dukes' B	Rt+	69	9 (13)	0.4	0.020
	Rt−	79	24 (30)	1.0	
Dukes' C	Rt+	63	12 (19)	0.5	0.031
	Rt−	92	31 (34)	1.0	

Abbreviation: RH, relative hazards.
(Courtesy of Cedermark B, for the Stockholm Colorectal Cancer Study Group: Randomized study on preoperative radiotherapy in rectal carcinoma. *Ann Surg Oncol* 4:423–430, 1996.)

Results.—Postoperative complications, especially wound sepsis, were more frequent in the radiotherapy group (Table 3). Postoperative mortality was 2% in the radiotherapy group and 1% in the surgery-only group. The locoregional recurrence rate was 10% in the radiotherapy group vs. 21% in the surgery-only group (Fig 1). For patients undergoing curative surgery, the distant metastasis rate was 19% in the radiotherapy group vs. 26% in the surgery-only group (Fig 2). The pelvic recurrence rate was significantly lower in patients with Dukes' stage B and C tumors (Table 7). Survival was similar overall, but it was better for patients undergoing curative surgery after radiotherapy (Fig 4).

Conclusions.—The short-term, high-dose preoperative radiotherapy regimen used in this study can improve the results of curative surgery for

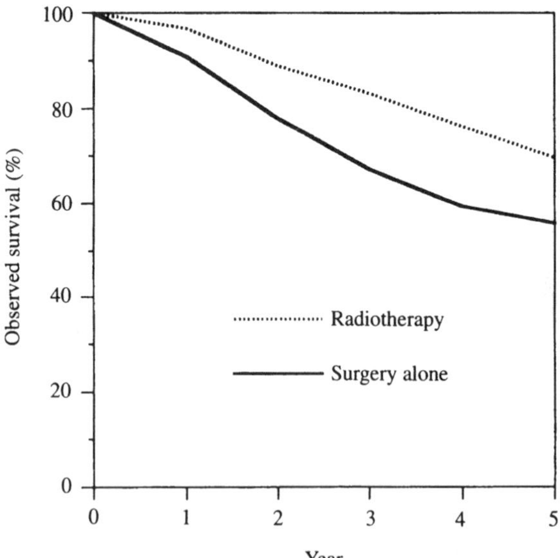

FIGURE 4.—Overall survival in the 49 patients after curative surgery. (Courtesy of Cedermark B, for the Stockholm Colorectal Cancer Study Group: Randomized study on preoperative radiotherapy in rectal carcinoma. *Ann Surg Oncol* 4:423–430, 1996.)

rectal cancer. Preoperative radiotherapy reduces the risk of local and distant recurrence and increases survival. The risk of postoperative mortality may still be increased for certain patient subgroups.

▶ This study is a randomized prospective trial comparing preoperative radiotherapy, followed by surgery or surgery alone. As was seen in earlier trials by this group, reduction in pelvic recurrence was identified in the irradiated group. What is particularly intriguing with this current study is that there was also a reduction in distant metastases in the radiation group, resulting in an overall improved survival (see Figs 2 and 4). As has been documented in other preoperative radiation therapy trials, the postoperative complication rate was increased in patients receiving radiation therapy (see Table 3). However, the serious complications appeared to be no greater in the group receiving radiation therapy than in the group with surgery alone.

As identified in Table 7 of this article, the radiation therapy group had fewer patients with Dukes' B and Dukes' C cancer. This likely is because of a downstaging in the radiation therapy group. It was not seen in the previous trials by this group, but has been reported in other trials of preoperative radiation therapy. This may have important implications in the increase in overall survival in the radiation therapy group because there was a decrease in the rate of metastases in the patients receiving preoperative radiation therapy. This perhaps, as the authors speculated, was related to a reduction in local recurrence, contributing to a reduction in distant metastases. Another notation is that in this trial, a 4-field approach was used for delivery of the radiation therapy, in contrast to a 2-field approach in the earlier trials. This may well have also contributed to the observation of reduced pelvic recurrence and to the reduction of lymph node metastases downstaging and, therefore, improved overall survival.

T.J. Eberlein, M.D.

Results of Local Excision for Rectal Carcinoma

Obrand DI, Gordon PH (McGill Univ, Montreal)
Can J Surg 39:463–468, 1996 11–45

Introduction.—For patients with low-lying invasive rectal carcinoma, abdominoperineal resection remains the standard treatment. Some patients, however, would benefit from local excision. Criteria for selecting patients for local excision are mobile lesions that are located in the distal one third of the rectum, are polypoid, occupy less than one third of the rectum, and have no lymph node involvement. Local excision of rectal carcinomas as the primary treatment was described.

Methods.—Nineteen patients had local excision of rectal carcinomas as their primary treatment for cure. The median age of the patients was 73 years; they were all followed for gross morphology, depth of invasion and size of carcinoma, rate of survival, complication of operation, rates of recurrence, and adequacy of the margins of excision. The patients underwent endorectal ultrasonography and abdominal ultrasonography or computed tomography. The technique involves using a Parks or Pratt retractor for exposure. The excision includes 1 cm of normal rectal wall, and the defect is closed transversely.

Results.—No intraoperative complications were seen. Urinary retention and bleeding were each found in 1 patient after the operation. Local recurrences occured in 5 patients (26%). In 3 patients (60%), salvage operations were performed and were successful in 2. There was a survival rate of 82% for 5 years. In patients with inadequate margins of excision and ulcerative lesions, the recurrence rate was higher. No matter which method of resection was used, ulcerative lesions had a higher recurrence rate. Recurrence was not correlated with the size or grade of the carcinoma.

Conclusion.—In selected patients, local excision of rectal carcinoma can be performed successfully. Because up to 60% of local recurrences can be treated successfully, diligent follow-up is necessary.

► I have selected this paper, although it describes a retrospective series, to show that it is possible to offer alternative therapy for patients with rectal carcinoma. The key, however, is that these patients require careful selection. The surgery itself can be done with relatively little morbidity. This series, as well as previous ones, show that salvage is possible in patients who have rerecurrence of tumor. The size of the lesion did not seem to predict recurrence in this series. A technical note is that excision is, in fact, full thickness. In addition to full thickness excision, margin evaluation is extremely important. It is noteworthy that in this series, 3 of the 5 patients who had recurrence had either minimal margins of normal tissue or unassessable margins.

Another important issue is that the patient must be reasonably compliant and reliable because close follow-up is extremely important, especially if the salvage procedure is expected to be successful. Although adjuvant therapy was not utilized in this series, both adjuvant therapy with radiation alone and radiation combined with chemotherapy have been shown to diminish the risk of local recurrence. Utilization of these adjuvant therapies will certainly expand the possibilities of this option for the management of rectal carcinoma.

T.J. Eberlein, M.D.

Regional Versus Systemic Chemotherapy in the Treatment of Colorectal Carcinoma Metastatic to the Liver: Is There a Survival Difference? Meta-Analysis of the Published Literature

Harmantas A, Rotstein LE, Langer B (Univ of Toronto)

Cancer 78:1639–1645, 1996 11–46

Introduction.—In North America, colorectal carcinoma is one of the leading causes of death; 18% of patients at initial diagnosis have metastases, with half of these having metastatic disease isolated to the liver. Therapies include resection, conventional IV chemotherapy, or chemotherapy with 5-fluorouracil or floxuridine, which is a derivative of 5-fluorouracil. An analysis of the literature was conducted to determine whether regional infusion chemotherapy with 5-fluorouracil or floxuridine results in better survival than systemic chemotherapy.

Methods.—This analysis of the literature included 149 articles or abstracts, and of these, 6 clinical trials were used for this study. For each treatment modality, 1- and 2-year survival rates were retrieved after conducting a test for the homogeneity of the treatment, using a test statistic.

Results.—Data from all 6 clinical trials showed that those who received regional infusion chemotherapy had a 12.9% increase in survival at 1 year when compared with those who received systemic chemotherapy. The 2-year rate of survival was 7.5%. One of the clinical trials, however, seemed biased, and when that trial was eliminated, summary survival rates calculated with the 5 remaining trials showed that at 1 year, regional infusion chemotherapy with floxuridine produced a 10% increase in survival and a 6% increase in survival at 2 years when compared with conventional therapy.

Conclusion.—There is a modest survival benefit with hepatic artery infusion chemotherapy when compared with systemic chemotherapy. However, the quality of survival must also be taken into consideration. Future studies should consider other modalities of therapy and the quality of life after therapy.

▶ This meta-analysis of the literature compares regional infusion chemotherapy with either 5-fluorouracil or floxuridine. A review of the literature showed that at 1 and, to a lesser extent, 2 years, there is a survival advantage for patients treated with regional infusion chemotherapy.

It should be noted that only 1 of the individual trials showed a statistically significant survival advantage with regional chemotherapy. Thus the conclusions of this manuscript are clearly the result of the type of analysis and statistical methodology. However, many of the trials, although statistically not significant, showed a trend toward improved survival. One of the complicating issues surrounding evaluation of this type of trial is allowing cross-over in patients receiving systemic treatment and having documented progression. An exclusion of these cross-over patients in the meta-analysis was reflected in improved survival at 1 and 2 years.

Another issue regarding regional infusion chemotherapy is the toxicity. Most proponents of this type of chemotherapy believe that the toxicity is, if anything, reduced. However, complications from hepatic arterial cannulation, as well as hepatic toxicities, in fact minimize the potential advantage of regional chemotherapy. Although survival is identified in these individual trials, quality of life is not thoroughly evaluated. Until better chemotherapeutic and other systemic agents are identified, treatment of metastatic colorectal disease in the liver will remain difficult at best.

T.J. Eberlein, M.D.

Tumor Immunology/Vaccine

Vaccine Therapy for Cancer

Linehan DC, Goedegebuure PS, Eberlein TJ (Harvard Med School, Boston)
Ann Surg Oncol 3:219–228, 1996 11–47

Background.—Research has demonstrated a cell-mediated immune response to cancer. It is now possible to isolate tumor-specific cytotoxic T-lymphocytes (CTLs) from solid tumors, draining lymph nodes, metastatic effusions, and peripheral blood. However, attempts to use cancer vaccines in active specific immunotherapy have not been successful in clinical trials. The immunobiology of the cell-mediated immune response to cancer was reviewed, with a focus on what is known about the major histocompatibility complex (MHC)-restricted interaction between tumor cells and CD8+ or CD4+ T cells (Fig 1). Recent advances in the identification of tumor-associated antigens (TAAs) recognized by tumor-specific CTLs in melanoma and other cancers were also reviewed.

Vaccine Therapy for Cancer.—Despite major advances in the study of TAAs and the CTL response to certain cancers, no clinically effective cancer vaccine has been developed. The immune repertoire of patients with cancer includes T cells that recognize and lyse tumor cells. Thus, the task is to find the best tumor antigens and manipulate the immune system to elicit an effective antitumor response in vivo. The goal of current strategies that employ genetically modified tumor cell vaccines transfected with

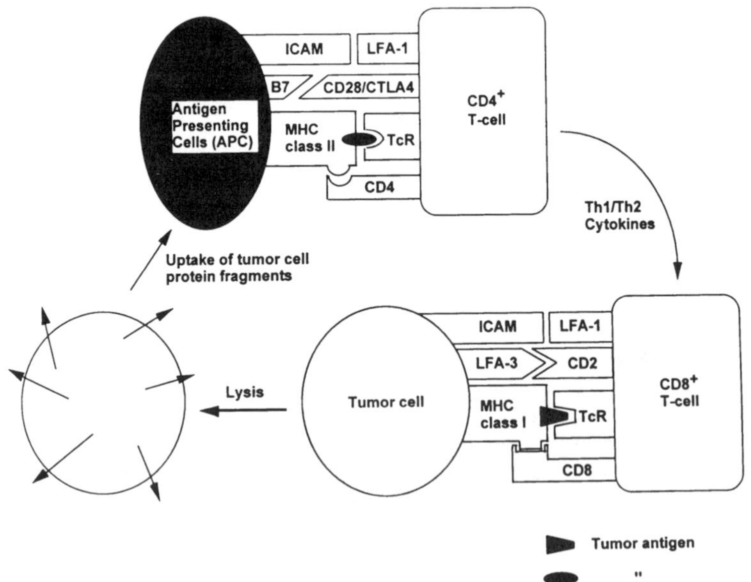

FIGURE 1.—Schematic representation of the cell-mediated immune response to cancer cells. (Courtesy of Linehan DC, Goedegebuure PS, Eberlein TJ: Vaccine therapy for cancer. *Ann Surg Oncol* 3:219–228, 1996.)

genes expressing cytokines and co-stimulatory molecules is to increase the adequacy of tumor-specific T-cell help. As more antigenic peptide epitopes recognized by tumor-specific CTLs are identified, more peptide-based vaccines for active specific immunotherapy trials will be developed, not only in melanoma, but in several other types of cancer. The ideal candidate for an effective peptide antigen is unique to tumor cells and able to bind to the particular MHC allele that presents antigen on the cell surface. However, such an antigen has not yet been discovered. Currently, researchers are focusing on tissue-specific, not tumor-specific, antigens. Though much effort has been devoted to identifying a solitary tumor-specific antigen consistently expressed by all tumors, none has been found. A polyvalent vaccine is widely believed to be the only therapeutic strategy that will be effective against antigenically heterogeneous targets such as cancer.

Conclusions.—Several TAAs and antigenic peptide epitopes have recently been identified in melanoma and other cancers, which has enabled immunotherapy researchers to focus on the development of anticancer vaccines. Immunotherapists are cautiously optimistic about their search for effective cancer vaccines.

▶ This is a fairly comprehensive review of possible vaccine therapies. It deals not only with the CD8 cytotoxic side of the immune response, but also the CD4 positive MHC Class II identification of antigen (see Fig 1). As more and more antigens are identified, as well as better strategies for the use of the identified antigen to stimulate an endogenous immune response, we will see more and more of these types of protocols. Because their ultimate efficacy may be in an adjuvant setting, it would be of use to general surgeons who treat large numbers of patients where these strategies may play a role after primary resection of their malignancy.

T.J. Eberlein, M.D.

12 Plastic, Reconstructive, and Head and Neck Surgery

Introduction

As time has gone on and this author has had an opportunity to garner more experience in this job, some conceptual questions have come to mind as the selection process unfolds. The principal question is what does the reader want from my section of the YEAR BOOK? Perhaps we need a series of focus groups convened between the readers and myself in desirable locations such Oahu, Madrid, Buenos Aires, and others, but I sincerely doubt the publisher will spring for the project. So, in the absence of other data (which may exist but of which I am blissfully ignorant), intuitive reasoning will have to suffice. Different readers probably have different reasons, and probably several groups exist. Our offering in this section this year is an effort (hopefully) to meet these different needs. Please remember, though, that the recommendations are but one man's opinion, and what I considered a knockout paper and discussion you may find either inane or incredibly esoteric. Nevertheless, considerable effort and thought has been poured into the selection, and I am certain that this observation is equally true of the remainder of the YEAR BOOK. Please use the menu below to pick and choose those dishes that may stimulate your palate.

Three fourths of the selections are in the arena of head and neck neoplasms. In that group of selections are the subcategories of diagnosis, technology or nonconventional therapy, adjuvant therapy, quality of life (QOL), and the biggest subcategory, appropriately, surgical treatment. In addition, several articles were included primarily because of their excellent review attributes in the discussion section of the papers.

This year I included but one diagnostic imaging paper, namely, the use of MRI in the management of parapharyngeal space tumors. Check out the MRI images in the original paper. In technology and/or nonconventional therapy were several interesting and almost conjectural papers. The manuscript on guided navigation in tumor surgery is another glimpse into the future. The paper on radiosurgery for recurrent cranial base tumor may also have some futuristic overtones, and that paper as well as the description of the use of brachytherapy with simultaneous vascularized flap coverage for salvage bring the reader up to the cutting edge of treatment of persistent and/or recurrent disease. Both are excellent. Included in this subsection is also a report of 1-year results with the use of photodynamic therapy.

Several papers are included to comply with this author's opinion that surgeons must stay abreast of the adjuvant therapy developments in oncology. Two papers on the N0 neck, each from a somewhat different perspective, are included to provide the reader with some information for decisions about the use of radiotherapy in the postoperative period. Also included is an extremely provocative paper from France on the use of chemotherapy *alone* as primary therapy with complete clinical response and 5-year results. Read this paper carefully if you wish; some significant design problems exist.

Papers written from a surgical point of view include decisions about radiotherapy vs. resection for carcinoma in situ of the larynx, patient selection in near-total laryngectomy, the adverse effect of homologous blood in patients with laryngeal cancer, and an article on posterolateral neck dissection. Also included is a paper that effectively dispels the myth of "emergency laryngectomy" being a procedure that would increase the risk of tracheostomal recurrence after laryngectomy. The final paper in this section would receive my unqualified recommendation for a read of the original manuscript, "Carotid Artery Resection for Head and Neck Cancer." I didn't agree with the conclusions, but the discussion of the workup of patients for potential carotid artery resection will give the reader the contemporary diagnostic approach.

Three papers in a miscellaneous surgical therapy category include a cadaver study of the anatomy of the mandible with respect to decisions about marginal mandibulectomy, a surgical salvage paper on use of the pectoralis major flap for management of carotid artery exposure, and finally and most provocatively, a paper on fine-needle aspiration and thyroid surgery in the community hospital. This last paper reached some conclusions that are extremely troubling. We'll simply plant that seed alone and hope the reader will be sufficiently curious to pursue.

Again this year we have included 2 papers on QOL measurement in head and neck cancer patients. One was included for the excellent review of the current status (evaluation of QOL assessment in head and neck cancer) and the other not for the conclusions but for the effort, namely, a longitudinal assessment of QOL in laryngectomy patients.

In the skin cancer group are 3 papers, 2 on the management of metastases from cutaneous squamous cell carcinoma of the skin and the other on the prognostic outcome in melanoma patients with the technique of biopsy of the primary.

The last section is miscellaneous but includes several papers picked just because of their excellent review of that topic within the body of the discussion. These items include head and neck cancer in HIV patients and mycobacterial nodal disease in the neck. Related articles on the head and neck but not of the neoplastic theme included a paper on the efficacy of bedside tracheostomy in the ICU and an article on the use of color Doppler in penetrating injuries of the neck.

Outside of the head and neck, again in an effort to satisfy various tastes, another trauma-related subject was the use of emergency free flap coverage for complex injuries of the lower extremities from Austria. The results are impressive.

Two breast papers are available for perusal, and both have an economic tenor to the subject. The first, from England, was an effort to answer the question about rationing of breast reduction surgery. The premise was curious and perhaps somewhat humorous, but the conclusions were neither. The second paper attempted to compare free or microvascular transfer vs. pedicle transverse rectus abdominis myocutaneous flap reconstruction of the breast, an important paper that compared cost (I won't give away the ending).

A truncal reconstruction paper was included on the use of rectus turnover flaps for reconstruction of large midline abdominal wall defects—a difficult problem, but I am not certain the technique advocated is the solution, yet an excellent review of the problem. The final paper is another chapter in the culture epithelial keratinocyte saga just to keep the reader up to date on the subject of the development of "artificial" skin.

Edward A. Luce, M.D.

Head and Neck

Magnetic Resonance Imaging and the Management of Parapharyngeal Space Tumors

Miller FR, Wanamaker JR, Lavertu P, et al (Cleveland Clinic Found, Ohio)
Head Neck 18:67–77, 1996 12–1

Background.—The parapharyngeal space (PPS), described by many authors, extends from the skull base to the hyoid bone; it is bound medially by the fascia surrounding the pharyngeal constrictors and laterally by the ramus of the mandible and the medial pterygoid muscle. It has an anterior and posterior compartment—prestyloid and poststyloid, respectively—separated by the styloid process. Differentiating a prestyloid from a poststyloid mass is critical in diagnosis and treatment. Most neoplasms in the PPS consist of minor salivary gland tumors or ectopic salivary gland tumors, tumors of the deep lobe of the parotid, and tumors of neurogenic origin. Most are benign. Magnetic resonance imaging is currently considered the best imaging modality for assessing PPS tumors. One experience with the assessment and management of PPS tumors was reviewed.

Methods and Findings.—The records of 51 patients who had undergone surgical excision of a PPS tumor at one center between 1980 and 1992 were reviewed. Computed tomographic and MRI findings were compared.

Only 18% of the tumors in the series were malignant. The symptom most commonly associated with a benign PPS mass was an otherwise asymptomatic pharyngeal or neck mass. On physical assessment, most patients with benign PPS lesions had a pharnygeal mass with displacement of the tonsil and/or soft palate. Cranial nerve deficits were more likely to occur with schwannomas or paragangliomas. Symptomatic pain, trismus, otalgia, and cranial nerve deficits were more likely to occur in patients with malignant than with benign tumors. In 6 patients, CT could not distinguish a PPS mass from a tumor of the deep lobe of the parotid. On MRI, tumors of the PPS were clearly identified in relation to the carotid sheath structures. The relationship of the mass to the deep lobe of the parotid gland was also clear in 20 of 21 patients. Sixty-one percent of the tumors were removed through a transcervical approach. Twenty-eight percent were removed by a transparotid approach. Four patients underwent a combined transparotid-mandibulotomy approach. A combined lateral skull base and transcervical approach was used in 2 patients with lesions of the PPS extending into the jugular foramen and skull base. Sixty-four percent of the 14 patients treated by a transparotid approach had a significant facial nerve palsy. Five of the 31 patients undergoing transcervical removal of a PPS tumor had mild marginal mandibular nerve weakness.

Conclusion.—Magnetic resonance imaging enables superior soft-tissue resolution and visualization in multiple planes and, thus, is the imaging modality of choice for diagnosing tumors in the PPS. Because most PPS tumors are benign, MRI permits the selection of the operative technique with the least morbidity.

▶ This is a clean, concise discussion of the use of imaging to better differentiate PPS tumors and, perhaps most importantly, avoid angiography in most cases. The illustrations that accompany this article are excellent cross-sectional depictions of the PPS and its contents.

E.A. Luce, M.D.

Virtual Image Guided Navigation in Tumor Surgery: Technical Innovation

Wagner A, Ploder O, Enislidis G, et al (Univ-Clinic for Maxillofacial Surgery, Vienna; Artma Biomedical, Inc, Vienna)

J Craniomaxillofac Surg 23:271–273, 1995 12–2

Objective.—Current virtual reality systems permit the user to interact with the computer-generated "virtual world" by means of a data glove and an immersive head-mounted display. However, to be used in medicine, the virtual reality system must realistically simulate the way tissues act during surgery. Recent years have seen the development of head-up displays, suggesting that interventional video tomography (IVT) could become a useful surgical visualization technique. An IVT system for use in image-guided surgical navigation was described.

The IVT System.—The underlying principle of IVT is the fusion of stereophotometric analysis with 6-degree-of-freedom, electronic, three-dimensional (3-D) sensor data. Structures visualized on planar cephalograms or CT and MRI scans are projected in their correct spatial position on the IVT image. The system uses 3-D sensors attached to a head-mounted camera worn by the surgeon, to the patient's head, and to the stereotactic surgical instruments. Three-dimensional reconstructions of anatomic structures are created by stereophotometric analysis from planar cephalograms, with orientation provided by digitized radiopaque markers on the patient.

The surgeon uses the video input provided by the head-mounted camera to confirm the position of structures located on conventional images. Before the operation, the system can simulate a pathway for the surgical instruments and display it in its spatial relationships to anatomic structures (Fig 1). During the operation, the virtual images are overlaid on the live

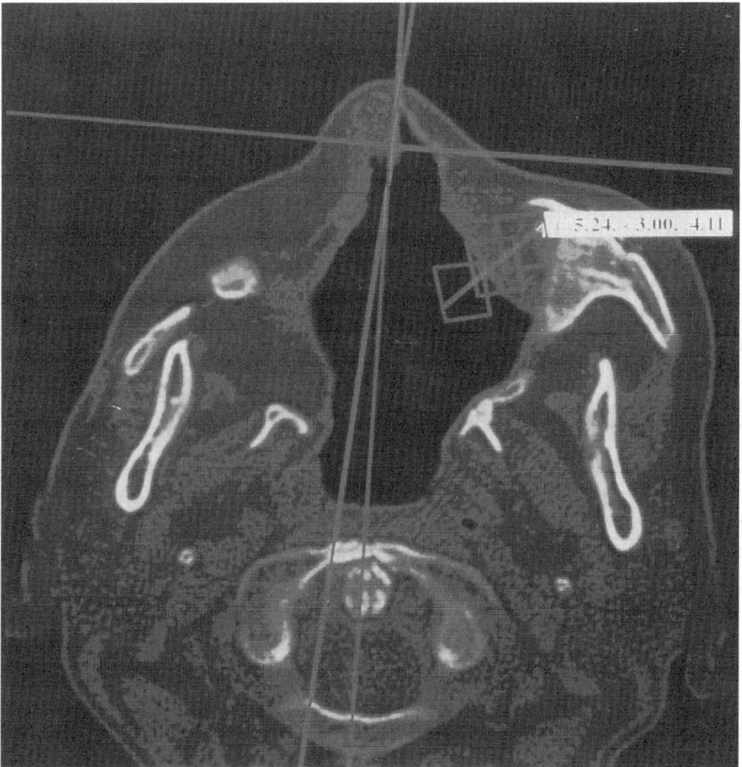

FIGURE 1.—Virtual coordinates and access path to region suspected of being a tumor recurrence. (Courtesy of Wanger A, Ploder O, Enislidis G, et al: Virtual image guided navigation in tumor surgery: Technical innovation. *J Craniomaxillofac Surg* 23:271–273, 1995.)

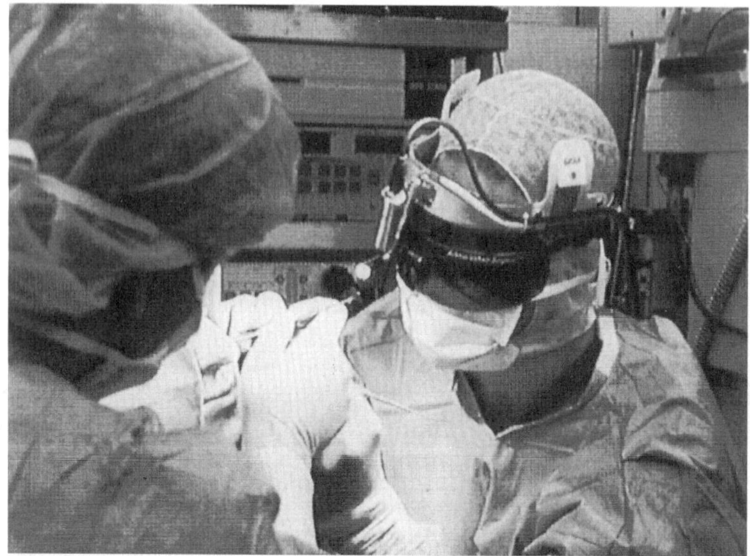

FIGURE 4.—Surgeon with head-up display, head-mounted camera, and a miniature head lamp. (Courtesy of Wanger A, Ploder O, Enislidis G, et al: Virtual image guided navigation in tumor surgery: Technical innovation. *J Craniomaxillofac Surg* 23:271–273, 1995.)

image from the head-mounted video camera, appearing on the surgeon's head-up display (Fig 4).

Discussion.—The IVT system described provides a practical, head-up virtual reality display to help in guiding surgical instruments to marked anatomic structures. It permits fusion of live images with real-time visualization of digitially processed medical images. It also provides for preoperative simulations of the operative approach, which can be transparently transferred to the surgical environment. In addition, the IVT system defines a virtual halo in stereotactic space, providing an alternative to Mayfield frame registration.

▶ This is a fascinating element of high technology that might be worthy of the reader's perusal of the original article. My impression of the approach is that the learning curve is probably quite significant, yet it could hold great promise for the diagnosis of possible radiotherapy-recurrent disease in the larynx or pharynx. Actually this guided navigation system is the mechanical and hardware analogue of the experienced surgeon, who will mentally "register" the CT data for recall during surgery (although CT scans always should be available in the operating room at the time of the diagnostic procedure).

E.A. Luce, M.D.

Radiosurgery for Recurrent Cranial Base Cancer Arising From the Head and Neck

Firlik KS, Kondziolka D, Lunsford LD, et al (Univ of Pittsburgh, Pa)

Head Neck 18:160–166, 1996 12–3

Background.—Head and neck tumors that invade the cranial base can pose a difficult treatment challenge. Although therapeutic modalities such as conventional surgery, fractionated radiotherapy, and chemotherapy are available, residual tumor frequently remains after such treatment. This can eventually lead to local recurrences, for which treatment options are limited. An additional boost of fractionated radiation can be delivered to adjacent fields in some instances; however, dose delivery is generally hampered by previous irradiation regimens. Stereotactic radiosurgery, which delivers a single high dose of radiation to a well-defined tumor volume, with a steep fall-off in the radiation dose into the surrounding structures, may provide a treatment alternative. This procedure is not contraindicated by proximity to the brain stem, cranial nerves, and major vessels, or by previous delivery of fractionated radiotherapy. Experience with radiosurgery for cranial base residual or recurrent tumors from head and neck cancers is described.

Patients and Methods.—Twelve patients undergoing radiosurgery for recurrent or residual head and neck cancer involving the cranial base were studied. The primary tumor had been resected in all 12 patients. Initial treatment included fractionated radiotherapy in 11 and chemotherapy in 4 patients. Selection criteria for radiosurgery included a tumor size of less than 2.5 cm in mean diameter, a well-identified tumor on imaging, and patients who were free of systemic disease or who had actively managed systemic disease. Contraindications included tumor extent below the foramen magnum, tumors that were attached to a mobile structure, poor Karnofsky performance status, and large tumor volume. Contrast-enhanced MRI was used to define irregular tumor borders, and target selection and dose planning were done by the neurologic surgeon, radiation oncologist, and radiation physicist. In all but 1 patient, the 50% isodose line was used to encapsulate the tumor margin. A 201-source Cobalt 60 gamma unit was used for radiosurgery. During the procedure, the patient's head was held with the stereotactic frame and was rigidly suspended within the gamma knife collimator helmet so that precise radiation delivery was accomplished. Follow-up imaging was done for 8 of the 12 tumors at 4 to 17 months after radiosurgery.

Results.—After radiosurgery, 2 of the 8 tumors with postoperative imaging were unchanged, 3 had decreased in size, and 2 were no longer apparent. No complications or worsening of symptoms were noted. Four of the 12 patients died before follow-up imaging could be performed, but death was not attributable to local progression of the radiosurgically treated lesion. Mean survival after radiosurgery was 10.5 months. Seven patients (58%) are still living.

Conclusion.—Radiosurgery is a fairy noninvasive method that can safely and effectively provide local control for recurrent cranial base cancers stemming from the extracranial head and neck. This technique also offers a considerable benefit over other methods in terms of preserving quality of life. Patients with failed fractionated radiation or surgical resection, as well as those who are poor medical candidates, should be considered for radiosurgery. Although results thus far appear to be promising, longer follow-up and more clinical experience are needed to clarify further the overall role of radiosurgery in patients with head and neck cancer.

▶ Of course, these results are not breathtaking—2 of 12 patients had disappearance of their tumor, and 3 others were "decreased" in size. Yet, few other options remain for these patients. Because of the prior use of fractionated radiotherapy, the structures are not amenable to further external radiotherapy. Intracavitary brachytherapy would be a nightmare to undertake. The most exciting aspect of the paper, as the editorial comment from the University of Florida attached to the main paper states, is the possible extrapolation of these results to extracranial sites and, in particular, in selected head and neck tumors as *primary* treatment. My guess is, as our imaging becomes more accurate and refined with the use of MRI, "pinpoint registration" of the tumor will be possible for delivering an accurate dose with the gamma knife. This can be followed by (speculation is running wildly at this point) further external beam therapy of the peripheral fields.

E.A. Luce, M.D.

Salvage Treatment for Inoperable Neck Nodes in Head and Neck Cancer Using Combined Iridium-192 Brachytherapy and Surgical Reconstruction

Cornes PGS, Cox HJ, Rhys-Evans PR, et al (Royal Marsden Hosp, London)
Br J Surg 83:1620–1622, 1996 12–4

Introduction.—In advanced instances of head and neck cancer, dissection or radical radiotherapy can often achieve a cure. Options for salvage treatment by surgery or radiotherapy are limited if the disease is inoperable and fixed and the neck has been irradiated to a radical dose. Brachytherapy—the surgical implantaion of radioactive sources within and around the tumor—allows a high dose to be delivered to the tumor. However, necrosis and tissue fibrosis have been known to occur with brachytherapy, which can result in ulceration and contracture similar to that in uncontrolled cancer. Brachytherapy re-irradiation for patients with isolated neck relapses of head and neck cancer were described.

Methods.—Radical-dose radiotherapy to the neck had been performed on 39 patients, 25% of whom also had neck dissection. The patients were divided into 2 groups. Thirteen had the neck disease approached through the previously irradiated skin, which was elevated to debulk the underly-

TABLE 2.—Grades of Severe Late Radiation Toxicity in the 2 Treatment Groups

Grade	Group 1 (n = 13)	Group 2 (n = 26)	Total (n = 39)
5	0	0	0
4	4	0	4
3	2	3	5
Total	6	3	9

Note: Toxicity used the grading system of the European Organization for Research and Treatment of Cancer and the Radiotherapy and Oncology Group of the USA

(Courtesy of Cornes PGS, Cox HJ, Rhys-Evans PR, et al: Salvage treatment for inoperable neck nodes in head and neck cancer using combined iridium-192 brachytherapy and surgical reconstruction. *Br J Surg* 83:1620–1622, 1996, Blackwell Science Ltd.)

ing tumor. As soon as early wound healing had occurred, cannulas to the skin were loaded with radioactive iridium-192 wire. Twenty-six patients had their previously irradiated skin excised over the planned treatment area. After as much of the tumor as possible was excised and hollow cannulas were placed, the site was resurfaced with pedicled cutaneous or myocutaneous flaps, including 17 deltopectoral, 7 pectoralis major, and 2 latissimus dorsi flaps. Side effects from radiotherapy were recorded.

Results.—At 1 year from the time of the procedure, the overall actuarial probability of local contol in the neck was 63%. There was a 38% probability of survival to 24 months. There were 4 minor surgical complications, in the group of 13, and there were 2 major surgical complications, together with 7 minor surgical complications, in the group of 26. A comparison of radiation toxicity revealed that 6 of the 13 had severe late radiation toxicity and 3 of the 26 had radiation toxicity (Table 2).

Conclusion.—The unmodified operative technique resulted in an unacceptable (6 of the group of 13 patients) rate of serious morbidity with symptoms caused by chronic nonhealing ulceration or severe contractile cutaneous and subcutaneous fibrosis. In fact, the symptoms were as severe as the progressive cancer that the treatment was supposed to avoid. Serious toxicity was reduced by resurfacing with unirradiated skin.

▶ Brachytherapy (application of high-dose local radiotherapy by means of radium-loaded catheters) is one method—probably the only method—for addressing "inoperable" postradiation recurrence in the neck. The most common example, in our experience, has been the patient who has a postradiation, postneck dissection recurrence with involvement of the carotid. Resection leaves microscopic disease on the carotid. The use of brachytherapy and catheters in combination with a muscle flap markedly diminishes the incidence of early and late complications, in our experience.

The authors viewed their results differently, namely, that the benefit obtained was from excision of irradiated skin and provision of vascularized skin by means of either a deltopectoral cutaneous or a pectoralis major myocutaneous flap. This reviewer reasons that the major benefit comes from the provision of vascularized tissue (pectoralis major muscle alone) rather than excision of the irradiated skin. The point is not a minor one because a deltopectoral flap has a much higher incidence of complications than the rotation of a pectoralis major muscle alone. Probably the best compromise is to raise an island of skin situated on the pectoralis major muscle (because the arc of rotation is relatively short to the neck) and either use or not use it, depending on the assessment of the native neck skin after completion of the procedure.

E.A. Luce, M.D.

Treatment of Head and Neck Cancer With Photodynamic Therapy: Results After One Year

Dilkes MG, DeJode ML, Gardiner Q, et al (Royal London Hosp)

J Laryngol Otol 109:1072–1076, 1995 12–5

Background.—Current surgery and radiotherapy for head and neck tumors are often accompanied by significant morbidity, disfigurement, and disabling side effects. One year's experience using photodynamic therapy (PDT), a new treatment method that uses specific wavelengths of light to activate photosensitizing chemicals preferentially absorbed by tumor cells, in the treatment of head and neck tumors was described.

Methods.—Over 1 year, 17 treatments with PDT were administered to patients for whom standard therapy was inappropriate or for whom adjunctive therapy seemed potentially helpful. For 15 treatments, a second-generation photosensitizing agent, *meta*-tetrahydroxyphenylchlorin (*m*-THPC), was administered intravenously. After a wait of 96 hours, a copper vapor laser, pumping a rhodamine dye laser, irradiated the tumor at a wavelength of 652 nm for a total light dose of 20 J/cm^2. One treatment was with Photofrin 2, an early agent, and one was with δ-aminolevulinic acid, a topical agent. Different waiting times and light intensities were required for these agents.

Results.—In all cases, erythema at the irradiated site was followed by tumor sloughing that continued for up to 4 weeks. Significant pain associated with 3 tumors was reduced after treatment. All patients receiving *m*-THPC had pain at the injection site, and all patients experienced pain at the tumor site for up to 3 weeks. Some were unable to eat solid food for up to 1 week, but all remained able to swallow liquids.

Conclusion.—Although the duration and size of this study were too limited to allow evaluation of efficacy, it appears that PDT, especially with *m*-THPC, may have a role in the treatment of head and neck tumors.

► Both primary and adjunctive therapy seem to be encouraging areas for the use of PDT. The problem still is delivery to more ischemic and less well-vascularized tumor areas, analogous to that of radiotherapy in large primaries. The difficulty is in achievement of a wider margin between tumoricidal effect and sparing of normal tissues. Photodynamic therapy, though, holds considerable promise, so keep an eye out for future reports.

E.A. Luce, M.D.

Nodal Failures in Patients With N0 N+ Oral Squamous Cell Carcinoma Without Capsular Rupture

Brugère JM, Mosseri VF, Mamelle G, et al (Institut Curie, Paris; Institut Gustave Roussy, Villejuif, France; Centre Claudius Regaud, Toulouse, France; et al)

Head Neck 18:133–137, 1996 12–6

Objective.—A multicenter retrospective analysis sought to determine whether postoperative irradiation of the neck after lymph node dissection prevents cervical node recurrence (NR) in patients with squamous cell carcinoma of the oral cavity without palpable lymph nodes (N0). Analysis was limited to patients who were histologically N+ without capsular rupture (N+ CR−) and to those with histologically negative nodes (N−).

Methods.—Patients included in the analysis were 680 men with a mean age of 56 years and 99 women with a mean age of 58 years. Most tumors were on the mobile part of the tongue (58%) or the floor of the mouth (35%). Tumors were classified as T1 in 291 cases, T2 in 407 cases, and T3 in 81 cases. All 7 centers at which patients were treated followed a policy of neck dissection for N0 patients. Postoperative irradiation of the neck was delivered, in most cases, at a mean dose of 55 to 60 Gy over 6 weeks.

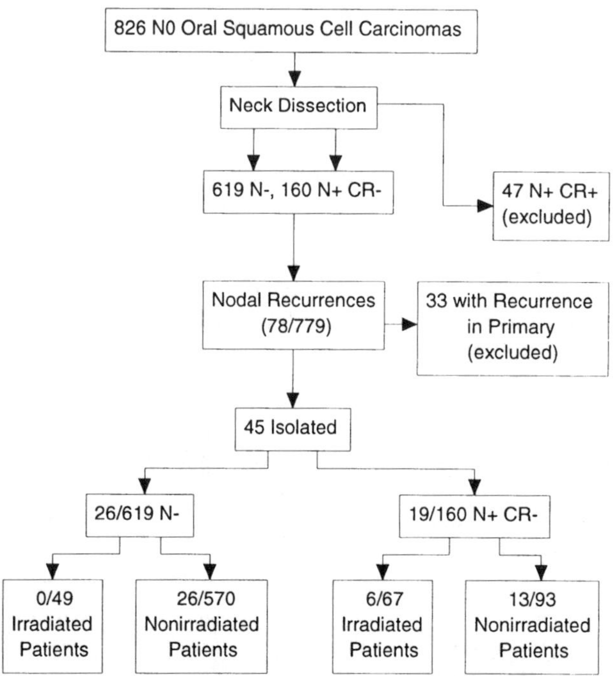

FIGURE 1.—Distribution of 826 N0 oral squamous cell carcinomas. *Abbreviation: CR,* capsular rupture. (Courtesy of Brugère JM, Mosseri VF, Mamelle G, et al. Nodal failures in patients with N0 N+ oral squamous cell carcinoma without capsular rupture. *Head Neck* 18:133–137, 1996. Reprinted by permission of John Wiley & Sons, Inc.)

Thirteen local complications and 4 postoperative deaths were reported. Patients were followed for at least 3 years and for an average of more than 6 years.

Results.—Positive nodes were identified in 20% of patients, with the highest rate in those with carcinoma of the mobile tongue. Postoperative cervical irradiation was administered to 67 of 160 N+ CR− patients and to 49 of 619 patients with histologically negative nodes (N−). Nodal recurrences developed in 78 patients; they constituted local recurrence in 33 patients and isolated recurrence in 45. The isolated cases occurred in 4% of the N− patients and in 12% of the N+ CR− patients. None of the N− patients with isolated nodal recurrence had received postoperative irradiation. The rate of NR in N+ CR− patients, however, did not differ between irradiated and nonirradiated patients (Fig 1). Nodal recurrence rates did not differ according to the level of the positive nodes or to number of lymph nodes invaded. The site of 14 of 45 isolated NRs was a nondissected suprahyoid region. One third of the 779 patients were subsequently given a diagnosis of a second primary cancer. Cancer was the cause of death in 141 of 494 deceased patients; 40 deaths were attributed to isolated cervical failure.

Conclusion.—Because isolated neck recurrences are uncommon in patients with N0 oral squamous cell carcinoma, postoperative irradiation can be limited to N+ CR+ patients and to those with more than 3N+ CR−. Following this management policy allows radiotherapy to be reserved for second primary cancers, which are common in these patients.

▶ This paper is a worthwhile addition to our body of knowledge of the behavior of oral cavity squamous cell carcinoma in that the results have a direct clinical application. If the recurrence rate in the neck in patients with clinically negative but pathologically positive lymph node disease is as low as this series would indicate, then postoperative radiation therapy is not sufficiently efficacious to warrant the loss of that modality for possible future new primaries or metachronous disease. Two caveats are evident: the absence of extracapsular rupture and fewer than 3 positive nodes. Please note that this is a retrospective study, hamstrung by a number of limitations.

E.A. Luce, M.D.

Extracapsular Spread in the Clinically Negative Neck (N0): Implications and Outcome

Alvi A, Johnson JT (Univ of Pittsburgh, Pa)
Otolaryngol Head Neck Surg 114:65–70, 1996 12–7

Background.—Extracapsular spread (ECS) of tumors of the head and neck from metastasized cervical nodes is an indication of poor prognosis. Whether this holds true for ECS in nodes from patients with clinically negative necks (N0) at the time of diagnosis was studied.

Methods.—A review was made of the medical records of all patients over a 4-year period who had squamous cell carcinoma of the head and neck and who were N0 at the time of manifestation but subsequently underwent neck dissection. The site and stage of disease, the treatment, outcome, and recurrence of disease, and the presence of ECS were noted.

Results.—Of 109 patients whose charts were reviewed, 37 (34%) had occult nodal metastasis, of whom 18 (49%) also had ECS. After at least 2 years' follow-up, patients with positive nodes were significantly less likely to be disease free (40%) than those with no positive nodes (82%). Patients with nodal disease and ECS were less likely to be still free of disease after 2 years than were those with positive nodes but no ECS. The sample size was too small to prove a significant difference. The presence of ECS did not affect the results of postoperative radiation or the rate of recurrence of tumor.

Conclusion.—Although ECS is a poor prognostic finding for patients with N0 clinical staging, N0 stage is difficult to diagnose clinically. Radiation therapy does not improve the outcome for those patients with ECS.

▶ Actually the incidence may be even higher because this study excluded all those cases in which nodes greater than 1 cm were seen on imaging techniques. The authors also did not enumerate which patients received preoperative radiotherapy, also likely to affect the results. Finally, the numbers are much too small to begin to draw conclusions about the efficacy of radiotherapy in clinically negative but pathologically positive nodes with ECS. Yet the authors have sufficiently emphasized the point of prognostic value in neck dissection in both staging of disease and provision of information for treatment planning.

E.A. Luce, M.D.

Cisplatin-Fluorouracil Exclusive Chemotherapy for T1-T3N0 Glottic Squamous Cell Carcinoma Complete Clinical Responders: Five-Year Results

Laccourreye O, Brasnu D, Bassot V, et al (Univ Paris V; Univ Paris VI)
J Clin Oncol 14:2331–2336, 1996 12–8

Introduction.—The usual approaches to laryngeal preservation in patients with stage T1–T3N0 glottic squamous cell carcinoma are vertical partial laryngectomy and radiation therapy. However, the local recurrence rate is high. Induction chemotherapy with cisplatin and fluorouracil has been used in an attempt to increase the local control rate, with the intention of carrying out standard therapy in clinical complete responders (CCRs). However, many of these patients have declined standard therapy and gone on to experience excellent long-term control and survival. The results of cisplatin-fluorouracil exclusive chemotherapy (EC) in T1–T3N0 CCRs were reviewed.

Patients.—From 1985 to 1992, 178 consecutive patients with T1–T2 glottic squamous cell carcinoma were treated with cisplatin-fluorouracil induction chemotherapy. Fifty-eight of these patients (31%) were CCRs, all suitable for radiation therapy or partial laryngeal therapy. In nonrandomized fashion, 21 of these patients underwent EC with cisplatin and fluorouracil (EC-CCR). The rest had partial laryngectomy or radiation therapy (IC-CCR). Forty-six patients were followed for at least 5 years.

Outcomes.—Five-year actuarial survival was 95% in the EC-CCR group and 86% in the IC-CCR group. Five-year local control rate was 71% and 97%, respectively, with local recurrence being significantly more likely in the EC-CCR group. Six patients in the EC-CCR group received salvage surgery or radiation therapy. Five-year actuarial second primary tumor rate was about 14% in each group. Chemotherapeutic toxicity was similar in the 2 groups.

Conclusions.—Some patients with T1–T3N0 glottic squamous cell carcinoma have "chemocurable" tumors, this study suggests. In these patients, EC with cisplatin and fluorouracil can preserve the laryngeal structure and permit long-term survival. The use of chemotherapy could avoid the need for radiation and surgery, which would then be options in case of local recurrence and/or second primary tumor. The results of this retrospective study await confirmation.

▶ This is an intriguing and provocative study. Readers should keep in mind, though, a couple of observations: first, the group of investigators are experienced chemotherapists with the capability to keep complication rates to a minimum. They used up to 6 treatment courses, although offering the opinion that "complete response should be evident by the third course or cycle." The second observation is that a statistically significant higher incidence of local regional recurrence was present in those 21 patients who did not elect either radiation therapy or partial laryngectomy after a complete response to chemotherapy. This statistically increased local regional recurrence did not affect survival, but this is a *small* group of patients, and might well do so in larger numbers. The intriguing aspect, of course, is the identification of a potentially chemocurable group of patients. The authors speculate, on the basis of the 21 noncompliant patients who refused chemotherapy or radiation therapy as well as the proportion of the patients who had no histologically identifiable disease in the partial laryngectomy group (60%), that perhaps as many as two thirds of those patients who have complete response to chemotherapy are "chemocurable." More questions than answers in this study, but it's worth reading.

E.A. Luce, M.D.

Carcinoma in Situ of the Glottic Larynx: Excision or Irradiation?

Nguyen C, Naghibzadeh B, Black MJ, et al (Sir Mortimer B Davis-Jewish Gen Hosp, Montréal; McGill Univ, Montréal)

Head Neck 18:225–228, 1996 12–9

Background.—Carcinoma in situ (CIS) of the glottic larynx is generally treated by vocal cord stripping, which can include cordectomy, surgical diathermy, electrocoagulation, cryonecrosis, or laser therapy. Yet, although vocal cord stripping is considered the standard treatment in many facilities, other centers favor radiotherapy (RT). A retrospective evaluation of the effects of vocal cord stripping and RT on the outcome of patients with laryngeal CIS was undertaken at McGill University.

Patients and Methods.—Thirty-four patients (median age, 67 years) with histologically proven CIS of the glottis were included in the study. Patients had been treated between 1974 and 1994 and had been followed up for at least 24 months (median follow-up, 96 months). Vocal cord stripping was performed in 21 patients who were considered appropriate candidates by the head and neck surgeon. The remaining 13 patients, with only biopsy for diagnosis, underwent RT using cobalt to 6 MV photon external beam, with parallel opposed portals covering the larynx only. Study end points included local recurrence, occurrence of an invasive tumor, and overall survival.

Results.—No patients were lost to follow-up. Of the 21 patients who underwent vocal cord stripping as initial therapy, 11 experienced recurrent CIS. Six of these 11 were salvaged using another cord stripping, and 5 underwent RT using a dose of 5,000 cGy in 20 fractions. All were free of disease after subsequent treatment, making the salvage rate 100% for patients in the cord stripping group with recurrent CIS. Of the 13 patients initially treated with RT, an invasive subglottic tumor developed in 1 individual at 36 months after initial therapy. This patient later died of his tumor. At 15 years, the overall actuarial survival for both treatment groups was 95%; corresponding rates for the cord stripping and the RT groups were 100% and 87%, respectively. Subsequent nonlaryngeal primary tumors did not occur in any of the patients in the cord stripping group. In contrast, 2 patients from the RT group did experience a second head and neck primary, including a palate CIS, treated by local excision, in 1 patient, and an early tonsil carcinoma, treated surgically, in the second patient.

Conclusion.—Treatment of laryngeal CIS remains controversial. Both RT and vocal cord stripping provide excellent local control, although 48% of the patients in the cord stripping group required additional treatment because of recurrence. In terms of convenience, however, stripping has the advantage of therapy completion in a short period, compared with a minimum of 4 to 5 weeks required to complete RT. At present, the authors perform vocal cord stripping in patients with newly diagnosed glottic CIS, reserving RT for patients with recurrent lesions, and for those with medical contraindications to general anesthesia or unreliable follow-up.

▶ This is a good study because the duration of follow-up is sufficient for recurrence rates to become evident. In fact, the recurrence rate for vocal cord stripping is about 50%, with half that group treated either with restripping or RT. I do have some concerns about the reexcision group, because the follow-up for the entire study may not have been sufficient to ascertain the ultimate outcome of this much smaller subset of patients. Regardless, the pertinent point is close follow-up. If one suspects compliance as a problem, certainly RT is indicated, because the natural history of untreated CIS is not good. A significant number of those patients will end with loss of the larynx, because they will likely have invasive carcinoma develop, and will probably present late.

E.A. Luce, M.D.

Near-Total Laryngectomy: Patient Selection and Technical Considerations

Suits GW, Cohen JI, Everts EC (Oregon Health Sciences Univ, Portland)
Arch Otolaryngol Head Neck Surg 122:473–475, 1996 12–10

Introduction.—Numerous methods have been developed to restore or preserve speech in patients treated for laryngeal cancer. The near-total laryngectomy, described by Pearson et al. in 1980, has successfully preserved speech when performed at the center that developed the procedure. A review of 39 patients who underwent near-total laryngectomy sought to identify perioperative factors associated with success.

Methods.—The patients underwent the procedure according to the method of Pearson et al. Charts were analyzed for various factors, such as site of the primary lesion, use of radiation therapy, incidence of aspiration, speech results, and disease-specific survival. The patient group included 30 men and 9 women with a mean age of 62 years; mean follow-up was 36 months.

Results.—Site of the primary lesion was pyriform sinus in 15 patients, glottic in 13, and supraglottic in 11. Four lesions were stage II, 20 were stage III, and 15 were stage IV. Distant metastasis occurred in 8 patients (21%) during follow-up and local recurrence in 4 (11%). Five patients died of disease and 30 were alive with no evidence of disease. Voice quality was judged good in 29 patients and poor in 5; 4 patients failed to develop speech through their fistula. Aspiration was absent or minimal in 76% of patients and severe in 21%. Patients with a postoperative pharyngocutaneous fistula were more likely to have severe aspiration and poor voice outcome.

Discussion.—Overall, the results with near-total laryngectomy in this series of patients are comparable to those of previous reports. Careful selection of patients and attention to surgical technique are required to create a functional myomucosal speaking shunt after near-total laryngectomy. Patients at high risk for pharyngocutaneous fistula and irreversible aspiration through the shunt are candidates for total laryngectomy with tracheoesophageal puncture.

► This operation has not always worked as well for others as for Pearson. This series is worthy for 2 points: First, a confirmation in selected patients that near total laryngectomy is a worthwhile option, and second, that some patients are quite poor candidates. This latter group includes irradiated patients and those with advanced medical disease. Total laryngectomy and immediate tracheoesophageal puncture is a good alternative, yet some patients may not be particularly good candidates for that procedure either, and would benefit from an anatomic muscular shunt for speech

E.A. Luce, M.D.

Blood Transfusions in Laryngeal Cancer: Effect on Prognosis

León X, Quer M, Maestre L, et al (Universitat Autònoma, Barcelona)

Head Neck 18:218–224, 1996 12–11

Background.—Blood transfusions have an immunosuppressive effect, which could potentially lead to a worse prognosis for patients with cancer. Previous studies of this possibility, in cancers of different locations, have yielded conflicting results. Several different transfusion-related immune effects have been proposed to explain the effects of transfusion on cancer prognosis. The question is whether transfusion has a direct negative influence on prognosis or whether patients with a worse prognosis are more likely to receive transfusions. The prognostic impact of blood transfusion in patients with laryngeal and hypopharyngeal carcinoma was analyzed.

Methods.—The retrospective study included 269 patients with laryngeal and hypopharyngeal carcinoma who were undergoing major surgical procedures. All were studied for at least 3 years. Twenty variables—including clinical, treatment, and pathologic variables—were analyzed per patient. Any blood component administered within 1 week before to 2 weeks after the surgery was considered a perioperative transfusion.

Results.—Perioperative transfusions were given in 32% of patients, all of whom received packed red blood cells. There was no difference in global actuarial 5-year control between groups: 63% for patients receiving transfusion vs. 67% for those without transfusion. The only independent prognostic factors on multivariate analysis were, in order, regional disease stage, resection margin status, and presence of extracapsular spread.

Conclusions.—Perioperative homologous blood transfusion does not appear to affect prognosis in patients with laryngeal and hypopharyngeal cancer, multivariate analyses suggest. Autologous transfusion can avoid the small risks posed by homologous blood exposure. Furthermore, because mild to moderate anemia does not affect wound healing, reducing the number of transfusions done could be an effective means of reducing both the risks and costs of transfusion.

▶ This article outlines as concisely as possible the current controversy about the use of homologous blood transfusions in patients with cancer, in this instance head and neck cancer. The authors found no difference in survival in a group of 269 patients, of whom one third received transfusions. This reviewer has to confess that his grasp of the details of "multivariate analysis used in Cox multiple regression method" is not sufficient to accept the conclusions reached, of course, except on faith alone. Perhaps the message here should be that we avail ourselves more of the use of autologous transfusion, which realistically could be accomplished in most cases. More than three fourths of the patients receive 2 or less units of blood, which, to follow the authors' numbers, would reduce the overall number of patients who would require homologous blood to about 8% of the total.

E.A. Luce, M.D.

The Posterolateral Neck Dissection

Diaz EM Jr, Austin JR, Burke LI, et al (Univ of Texas, Houston)

Arch Otolaryngol Head Neck Surg 122:477–480, 1996 12–12

Introduction.—The postauricular or suboccipital lymph node drainage groups, important for managing metastatic disease, are not addressed in the classic radical neck dissection. The posterolateral neck dissection was described as effective in controlling regional metastases from cutaneous malignancies of the posterior region of the scalp. As part of a multidisciplinary treatment approach, the effectiveness of the posterolateral neck dissection was evaluated for its ability to provide regional control of metastatic disease to the posterior triangle from head and neck primary tumors.

Methods.—A review of 55 patients (46 male and 9 female) treated with a posterolateral neck dissection during a 10-year period was conducted. A total of 58 operations were performed, as 3 patients had bilateral dissections. In this group, 35 had melanomas, 10 had squamous cell carcinoma, and 10 had various other histologic types. Patients were followed up for a minimum of 3 years. They were evaluated for histologic type and site of primary tumors, extent of surgery performed, pathologic findings, other therapies provided, and clinical outcome. They were reviewed for recurrence at either the primary site or the regional site, surgical morbidity, and development of distant metastases.

Results.—In 89% of patients, disease was controlled at the site of the primary tumor. This was true for 94% of patients with melanoma. In 93% of patients, regional disease was controlled, and this was true for 89% of patients with melanoma. In 16 patients, the trapezius muscle was sacrificed. In 1 patient, the internal jugular vein was removed, and in 14 patients, the spinal accessory nerve was intentionally sacrificed to achieve adequate margins of resection. Postoperative complications were rare, with 16 patients having complications, which included wound dehiscence, infection, and seroma formation. There were no deaths. There were 2 iatrogenic spinal accessory nerve injuries.

Conclusion.—Control of regional metastatic disease to the posterior neck from head and neck primary tumors is provided by the functional posterolateral neck dissection, considered to be an effective surgical therapy. The spinal accessory nerve or the internal jugular does not need to be removed routinely.

▶ This approach to the posterior neck is much more sensible than the radical procedure described 35 years ago. In my experience, only a minor lateral release of the trapezius at the occiput is necessary to resect the suboccipital nodes, and preservation of the spinal accessory nerve is almost uniformly possible. By retracting the trapezius posteriorly and the sternocleidomastoid muscle anteriorly, a comprehensive clean-out of the posterior triangle can be accomplished. Of course, inferiorly an arbitrary division line has to be established for nodal resections because the nodes will then continue onward through the supraclavicular fossa into the mediastinum. All these statements (and the paper as well) hinge on the assumption that only the posterior compartment is the area of interest, *and* that nearly one half of the patients received some type of adjuvant therapy, usually radiotherapy.

E.A. Luce, M.D.

Risk Factors of Tracheostomal Recurrence After Laryngectomy for Laryngeal Carcinoma

Yuen APW, Wei WI, Ho WK, et al (Univ of Hong Kong)

Am J Surg 172:263–266, 1996 12–13

Background.—Patients with tracheostomal recurrence after total laryngectomy for laryngeal cancer have a poor prognosis. Such recurrences are more likely for patients with preoperative tracheostomy, subglottic involvement, advanced tumors, and lymph node metastases; these factors may be interrelated. Independent risk factors for tracheostomal recurrence were assessed by multivariate analysis.

Methods.—The study included 322 patients undergoing total laryngectomy for laryngeal carcinoma. The patients were 285 men and 37 women, mean age 62 years. If the patient had an existing tracheostomy, the tracheostomy tract and overlying skin were removed at the time of laryngectomy. Postoperative external radiotherapy was given as indicated. The potential risk factors for tracheostomal recurrence analyzed were sex, age, tumor stage, sites of involvement, preoperative airway obstruction, preoperative tracheostomy, extent of surgery, radiotherapy, and resection margin. The patients were followed for a mean of 44 months.

Results.—The rate of tracheostomal recurrence was 5%. The recurrence rate was 17% in patients with carcinoma in the resection margins, 5% in those with clear margins, and 0% in those with dysplasia or carcinoma in situ. Two of 2 patients with a pathologic tracheal resection margin involving tumor had tracheostomal recurrences. Significant risk factors on univariate analysis included subglottic involvement, postcricoid extension, and preoperative airway obstruction. On multivariate analysis, postcricoid extension and subglottic involvement remained significant, although preoperative airway obstruction did not. The tracheostomal recurrence rate was 2% in patients with neither of these risk factors vs. 10% in those with one or both risk factors. All patients with tracheostomal recurrence died of their tumor in a mean of 4 months.

Conclusions.—The independent risk factors for tracheostomal recurrence after laryngectomy for laryngeal carcinoma are subglottic and postcricoid involvement. Preoperative tracheostomy per se does not increase the risk of such recurrence. When the independent risk factors are present, performing emergency laryngectomy to avoid tracheostomy will not prevent tracheostomal recurrence. High-risk patients with subglottic and postcricoid involvement should be targeted for preventive measures, such as thyroidectomy or radiation covering the tracheostomal and superior mediastinal region.

▶ This type of information simply has not been available in the past, and effectively dispels the myth that a preoperative tracheostomy will increase the incidence of tracheostomal recurrence. If the primary presentation of a patient with laryngeal carcinoma has been airway obstruction, many of those patients have had a tracheostomy followed by emergency laryngectomy because of the assumption that such patients would be more at risk for tracheostomal recurrence, if any hiatus existed between the tracheostomy and the definitive procedure. This paper provides evidence that emergency laryngectomy is of no value (at least from that aspect) and the tracheostomy can be performed and the patient assessed with some element of leisure.

The only problem with this hypothesis is that patients who have sufficiently neglected disease as to have airway obstruction may be more likely to be noncompliant with a treatment program. Once the airway obstruction has been relieved, some of these patients are at risk for refusing further therapy at that juncture and "signing out AMA."

E.A. Luce, M.D.

Carotid Artery Resection for Head and Neck Cancer

Okamoto Y, Inugami A, Matsuzaki Z, et al (Akita Univ, Japan; Research Inst of Brain and Blood Vessels, Akita, Japan)

Surgery 120:54–59, 1996 12–14

Introduction.—For patients with head and neck cancer involving the carotid artery, carotid artery resection may offer the only hope of cure or palliation. There is currently no way to identify which patients are at risk for neurologic injury after such resection. Interposition grafting may reduce the risk but can be technically difficult. An experience with carotid artery resection in patients with head and neck cancer was described, including a positron emission tomography (PET) test to determine the adequacy of hemispheric collateral blood flow.

Methods.—Twenty-four patients with head and neck cancer involving the carotid artery were studied. Ten patients who had tumor adherent to the carotid artery underwent en bloc resection to the tumor with the internal and common carotid arteries. The arteries were then replaced by autogenous saphenous vein grafts. The graft was covered by a muscle flap in all patients. The other 14 patients had suspected tumor involvement near the skull base, too close for interposition grafting. Twelve patients had no clinical deficit on internal carotid artery balloon test occlusion. These patients underwent preresection [^{15}O] H_2O PET cerebral blood flow studies, with and without balloon test occlusion.

Results.—One patient who underwent interposition grafting had a wound infection, which led to carotid rupture and death. There were no other cases of skin necrosis, mucocutaneous fistula, carotid rupture, or wound infection. Ten of 14 patients undergoing balloon test occlusion had either no change or less than a 10 mL/100 mL/min reduction in cerebral blood flow. In all 10, cerebral blood flow stayed above 35 mL/100 mL/min. These patients underwent en bloc tumor resection. In 4 of the 10, the tumor was separated from the carotid artery, which was salvaged. The 4 patients who had inadequate collateral blood flow did not have en bloc resection and died within 8 months.

Conclusions.—In patients undergoing carotid artery resection for head and neck cancer, the artery should be reconstructed, if possible, with interposition grafts and covered with nonirradiated, well-vascularized tissue. If no reconstruction is planned, an internal balloon occlusion test should be done. If there is no clinical deficit, PET can provide a quick quantitative determination of cerebral blood flow. This test may help to reduce the risk of cerebral infarction because of inadequate collateral flow.

▶ Such an article appears in head-and-neck literature every couple of years and usually is one of advocacy for resection for advanced cancer of the neck. This article, though, is the most sophisticated that this reviewer has read from the standpoint of a preoperative workup and is worth reading for that reason alone.

One must quibble, however, with their results: actually the 12-month survival in patients with *squamous cell* carcinoma (excluding the thyroid cancers) was 1 of 6 in the resected without reconstruction group and 1 of 6 in the reconstructed group. Informed consent, then, requires a patient to be aware that the ultimate survival after 1 year is in the neighborhood of 10% to 15%.

This article may well set the standard of care for workup of patients with carotid artery resection, namely, a balloon occlusion preliminary test with neurologic monitoring, followed by a PET scan to assess the adequacy of the ipsilateral hemispheric collateral blood flow. This article does *not* answer the question of whether carotid artery resection with reconstruction vs. resection alone yields the best results for this group of patients.

Of course, the other approach, as outlined in the included article by Okamoto, is that of carotid artery resection, plus or minus reconstruction.

E.A. Luce, M.D.

The Dentate Adult Human Mandible: An Anatomic Basis for Surgical Decision Making

Haribhakti VV (Jaslok Hosp and Research Centre, Bombay, India)

Plast Reconstr Surg 97:536–541, 1996 12–15

Background.—The critical aesthetic and functional significance of the mandible influences the current surgical approach to it. When a tumor approaches but does not invade the bone, rim resection to preserve cortical continuity is favored. Segmental resection is generally preferred when tumor invades the bone. However, there is little agreement on the precise definition and design of each procedure. The internal anatomy of the mandible was reviewed in detail to evolve a rational surgical approach to the management of malignant invasion.

Methods.—Thirty-six adult dentate mandibles from formalin-fixed cadavers were examined. Six sections from each bone were prepared. The location of the mandibular and mental foramina, the precise location of the inferior alveolar canal in relation to the external cortical rim, and the lingual and buccal cortices on either side were studied.

Findings.—The height of the mandibular foramen ranged from 31% to 40% of the maximum height of bone in 44% of the specimens and from 41% to 50% in half the specimens. This measurement was more than 50% in 6% of the specimens. The canal was almost flush with the lingual cortex all along the ramus, running closer to the lingual cortex in the body.

Conclusion.—Most specimens studied had a conspicuous medullary core with a thin cortical rim 2 to 4 mm thick. The inferior alveolar nerve coursed consistently within the anterior segment of the ramus and dipped significantly in the body. Thus, rim resections cannot include the entire medullary core and nerve. Segmental resections can spare the posterior segment of the ramus in selected patients (Fig 5).

▶ This study was well performed but perhaps misses the point somewhat. The point is not whether we can resect the nerve with a rim resection. The point in a marginal mandibulectomy (perhaps a better term than rim) is resection of the soft-tissue tumor, the periosteum, and the adjacent *cortex* of the mandible. As proven in the classic study by Marchetta decades ago, if a tumor-free margin can be clinically ascertained between the primary and the adjacent mandible, the periosteum will not be involved. The marginal mandibulectomy is a useful procedure when the tumor abuts, but does not

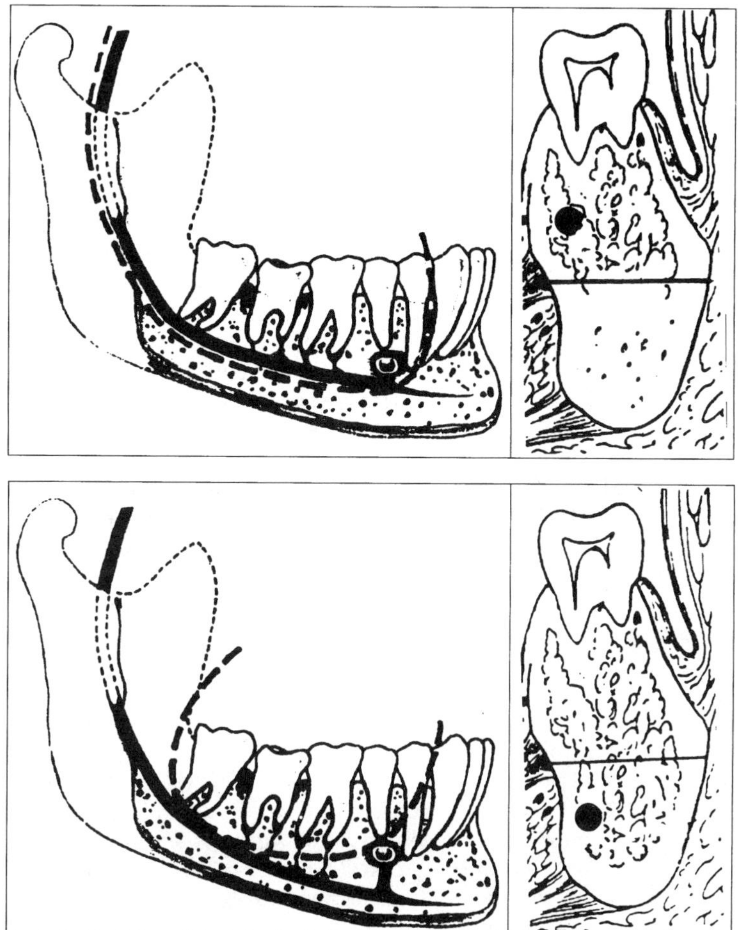

FIGURE 5.—Top, rim resection: line of section, in theory. **Bottom,** rim resection: line of section, in practice. (Courtesy of Haribhakti VV: The dentate adult human mandible: An anatomic basis for surgical decision making. *Plast Reconstr Surg* 97:536–541, 1996.)

invade, the mandible, as it provides a more secure margin than the sacrifice of the periosteum alone. One must agree with the authors that once the tumor invades the medullary portion of the mandible, all bets are off.

E.A. Luce, M.D.

Management of Carotid Artery Exposure With Pectoralis Major Myofascial Flap Transfer and Split-thickness Skin Coverage

Leemans CR, Balm AJM, Gregor RT, et al (The Netherlands Cancer Inst, Amsterdam)

J Laryngol Otol 109:1176–1180, 1995 12–16

Background.—Exposure of the major cervical blood vessels, a life-threatening sequela of radical oncological surgery, occurs most often after salvage surgery following radiotherapy. The preferred method of reconstruction in cases of carotid artery exposure is the pectoralis major flap transfer. The 8 patients reported here were successfully treated through use of the myofascial variant instead of a myocutaneous flap.

Patients and Methods.—The 8 cases represent 3% of patients who underwent neck dissection procedures from 1989 to 1994. The 6 men and 2 women who developed carotid exposure ranged from 44 to 78 years of age. Five had undergone previous radiotherapy (54Gy to 70Gy) and 2 were malnourished. The interval between surgery and the identification of carotid artery exposure ranged from 7 to 60 days. For protection of the carotid artery, patients underwent pectoralis major myofascial flap transfer with split-thickness graft coverage.

Results.—The reconstructive procedures were successful in all 8 patients with observed or imminent carotid artery exposure. Devitalized tissue was removed in the course of reconstruction for protection of the artery. Wound healing occurred in 2 to 4 weeks, and cosmesis was acceptable. Patients were able to be discharged on a normal diet within 4 weeks.

Conclusion.—Rapid intervention is needed when skin flap necrosis leads to postoperative exposure of the carotid artery. This infrequent complication occurs most often in the presence of preoperative radiation therapy, salivary contamination of the neck, malnutrition, and cachexia. The myofascial modification used in these cases is preferred to the bulkier myocutaneous flap because the former does not have to be twisted and distortion of the donor area does not occur.

▶ This is a brief, concise discussion of one of the most feared complications in head and neck surgery: carotid artery exposure in the presence of salivary fistula and radiated tissues. It emphasizes all the important points in management and describes a useful modification. My only caveat would be to carefully examine for compression of the pedicle after transfer of the flap. This modification probably twists the flap less than other approaches that turn the deep side of the pec major muscle into the depths of the neck, yet may also compress the pedicle at the clavicle.

E.A. Luce, M.D.

Fine-Needle Aspiration Cytology and Thyroid Surgery in the Community Hospital

Maxwell JG, Scallion RR, White WC, et al (Univ of North Carolina at Chapel Hill; New Hanover Regional Med Ctr, NC; Coastal Area Health Education Ctr, Wilmington, NC)

Am J Surg 172:529–535, 1996 12–17

Introduction.—Many centers consider fine-needle aspiration biopsy (FNAB) to be the initial diagnostic test of choice in patients with thyroid nodules. This procedure is widely preferred over radionuclide scanning or US. The use and value of FNAB of the thyroid were reviewed.

Methods.—All patients undergoing FNAB of the thyroid during 1993 were reviewed. In addition, a review of all patients undergoing thyroid surgery during the same year was done to see whether they had had FNAB beforehand. Finally, all thyroid surgery cases from 1987 to 1994 were reviewed to determine the yearly percentage of malignancy.

Results.—In 1993, 53 patients underwent 55 FNABs. Although the results of FNAB provided an indication for thyroid surgery in 21 patients, only 12 (57%) actually had surgery. Preoperative FNAB was done in just 20 (48%) of 42 patients undergoing surgery for a thyroid nodule. Three of these 20 patients had cancer. The FNAB correctly predicted 2 of the

TABLE 5.—Clinical Practice Guideline for Thyroid Masses

Step	Clinical Presentation	Appropriate Action
1	Patient presents with thyroid mass	History and physical examination
2	Is patient euthyroid?	History, physical examination, free T4 and TSH
3	Is mass solitary?	Physical examination, ? ultrasound
4	If mass is solitary, or if uncertain	FNAB with or without guidance by ultrasound
5	FNAB Class 1	Repeat FNAB
6	FNAB Class 2, 3, 4, or 5	Depending on age > 20 < 60 years, female gender, size < 2 cm, no history of irradiation Observe patient at intervals of 3 to 6 months Repeat FNAB if course inconsistent with presumed diagnosis
7	FNAB Class 6, 7, or 8	Surgical biopsy especially if patient < age 20, > age 60 and/or male gender (Lobectomy or hemi-thyroidectomy as a minimum procedure for biopsy)

cancers; it was correct in 18 of the 20 patients. In the 8-year review of thyroid surgery cases, the malignancy rate ranged from 11% to 29% per year and was unrelated to the increasing number of patients having FNAB each year.

Conclusions.—Fine-needle aspiration biopsy did not play a central role in the diagnosis of thyroid nodules at this institution. Although it is a highly accurate diagnostic test, FNAB plays a minor role in surgical decision making at this institution. Surgeons may miss essential details of the pathologic report and the pathologist may lack important patient information. Different clinicians use different FNAB techniques and may not repeat the biopsy when the specimen is inadequate. Physicians performing FNAB may lack up-to-date information on the skill of pathologists at their institution. They also may be unaware that the diagnostic confidence level of FNAB differs for papillary thyroid carcinoma vs. follicular thyroid neoplasm. There is a clinical practice guideline for the use of FNAB in patients with possible thyroid malignancy (Table 5).

▶ These numbers are, well, shocking, for lack of a better word. Only half of the patients in whom a FNAB indicated surgical excision was appropriate actually received an operation. One of 6 patients who either had a benign or an inadequate FNAB had a thyroidectomy done. One fourth of the FNABs were inadequate (a relatively high number), yet only 2 patients had a repeated FNAB. The authors are to be congratulated for the candid publication of these results from a community institution, and perhaps a similar type of "quality assurance" should be done at every major medical center that does thyroid surgery.

E.A. Luce, M.D.

Evolution of Quality of Life Assessment in Head and Neck Cancer

Morton RP (Green Lane Hosp, Auckland, New Zealand)

J Laryngol Otol 109:1029–1035, 1995 12–18

Introduction.—Quality of life has multiple dimensions and reflects occupational, family, and economic experiences, in addition to physical, psychological, and social well-being. The impact of a disease depends on chronicity, the degree to which it is perceived as a threat, and the disability that the disease and treatment create. Head and neck cancer can seriously affect speaking, swallowing, and breathing and can result in considerable disfigurement. The quality of life of patients who have head and neck cancer is very important because of the tremendous personal psychological investment in the head and neck. The historical development of evaluating quality of life in patients who had head and neck cancer was reviewed, and key developments and their application in clinical practice were discussed.

Traditional Approach.—The focus of medical care was traditionally on treatment and control of disease, with only secondary interest in the concerns of the patient. Quality of life has only recently become an

TABLE 2.—Domains of Inquiry That Should Be Considered When Planning a Questionnaire to Investigate Quality of Life in Head and Neck Cancer

(1) Physical functioning (day-to-day activity).
(2) Symptoms (disease- and treatment-specific).
(3) Emotional functioning (anxiety/depression, etc.).
(4) Role functioning (family/occupation, etc, roles).
(5) Social functioning (interaction at home, with friends).
(6) Coping ability.
(7) Financial impact.
(8) Health status.
(9) Sexuality.
(10) Global index (single item, patient-generated).

(Courtesy of Morton RP: Evolution of quality of life assessment in head and neck cancer. *J Laryngol Otol* 109:1029–1035, 1995.)

important consideration, even when cancer has had a profound effect on the patient. Although blatant disregard for the patient's psychological welfare was not uncommon into the 1960s, quantitative assessment of quality of life in patients who had cancer began in the 1940s.

Quality of Life in Head and Neck Cancer: 1950 to 1985.—Early studies came from clinicians and generally focused on one disease, one operation, and one life domain, such as physical or psychological status. Later studies became quantitative and correlated quality of life outcomes with specific variables, such as treatment modality and preoperative counseling. The first longitudinal study was in 1982, but follow-up was only 6 months. Since then, only two other studies have had longer follow-up.

Quality of Life in Head and Neck Cancer: 1985 to 1994.—There has been increased attention to quality of life in research. One prospective, randomized study used quality of life indices to evaluate toxicity in patients who had head and neck cancer and were receiving radiation therapy; more studies like this are needed.

Discussion.—Techniques for evaluating quality of life are evolving with help from social scientists. Quality of life has become an outcome measure in cancer treatment. When survival outcomes are comparable, quality of life outcomes may determine the preferred treatment. Clinicians should acquaint themselves with the methodology of this rapidly growing area of medicine (Table 2).

▶ In the current struggle to assess the appropriate role and importance of the different treatment modalities of surgery, radiation therapy, chemotherapy and the place of reconstruction, 3 outcomes need to be measured: survival, function, and quality of life. We and our patients need the data from all 3 to make the appropriate decisions.

E.A. Luce, M.D.

Longitudinal Assessment of Quality of Life in Laryngeal Cancer Patients

List MA, Ritter-Sterr CA, Baker TM, et al (Univ of Chicago; Northwestern Univ, Chicago; Loyola Univ, Maywood, Ill)

Head Neck 18:1–10, 1996 12–19

Background.—Quality of life and performance outcome in patients with head and neck cancer are key considerations in evaluating treatment alternatives, providing patient care, and developing rehabilitative services. Although patients with head and neck cancer can experience substantial dysfunction and psychosocial problems, quality of life measures have rarely been included in cancer treatment protocols. Instruments that measure quality of life specifically in patients with head and neck cancer have recently been developed. Most prospective studies of these patients have focused on a narrow range of quality of life components, such as functional speech, voice quality, and ability to swallow. Quality of life and performance outcome over time were evaluated in patients with laryngeal cancer.

Methods.—Evaluations of 21 patients with laryngeal cancer were conducted at various times within 6 months of treatment. Group 1 had total laryngectomy, group 2 had hemilaryngectomy, and group 3 had radiotherapy only. The Performance Status Scale for Head and Neck Cancer Patients, the Functional Assessment of Cancer Therapy–Head and Neck Version, and the Karnofsky Performance Status Rating Scale were used.

Results.—As expected, performance recovery varied among groups. Group 1 recovered the most slowly and did not return to normal functioning by 6 months. Most patients in group 2 achieved normal functioning by 3 months. Little overall dysfunction was seen in group 3. Overall quality of life was similar for all groups. There was a significant correlation between performance status and the Functional Assessment of Cancer Therapy—Head and Neck Version and a slight correlation between performance status and the physical subscale of this instrument. There was no association between ability to eat or speak and overall quality of life or specific quality of life dimensions, such as emotional well-being.

Conclusion.—Evaluation of patients with head and neck cancer must not only include physiologic data but also assessment of quality of life and multiple dimensions of life experience. The use of the Performance Status Scale for Head and Neck Cancer Patients and the Functional Assessment of Cancer Therapy–Head and Neck Version in such patients is supported.

▶ This study, from the aspect of conclusions only, is not worth much despite the authors' efforts. Two crippling, and perhaps fatal, flaws were present in the design: the absence of any pretreatment data (as admitted to by the authors) and the inability to stratify patients for stage. The paper should not be read for the conclusions but rather as an excellent model for both instruments and methods that can be successfully applied to larger studies. The authors examined one site—larynx—and made a concerted effort to do prospective observations, a big step in the right direction.

E.A. Luce, M.D.

Metastatic Cutaneous Squamous Cell Carcinoma of the Head and Neck Region

Tavin E, Persky M (New York Univ)

Laryngoscope 106:156–158, 1996 12–20

Background.—The numerous risk factors associated with squamous cell carcinoma of the head and neck region—as well as the many specialties involved with its treatment—have caused confusion in the literature concerning this particular disease. The authors of the present report sought to clarify some of the issues surrounding metastatic cutaneous squamous cell carcinoma, using 31 years of treatment experience with lesions in the head and neck region.

Patients and Methods.—A retrospective review of patients with squamous cell carcinoma of the skin in the head and neck region who had been recorded in the tumor registry of New York University Medical Center between 1961 and 1992 was undertaken. Excluded from the analysis were patients with squamous cell carcinoma originating on the lips, the external auditory canal, or any mucosal surfaces, as well as those with Bowen's disease or carcinoma in situ. Thirty-seven patients, including 29 men and 8 women, met the study criteria, and the hospital records of the admission during which the metastases in these patients were treated were reviewed. Patients' ages ranged from 47 to 87 years, with an average age of 70 years.

Results.—The most common primary site, noted in 9 patients (24%), was the cheek or preauricular region, and the most common metastatic site, found in 23 patients (62%), was the level I neck lymph nodes. Seven patients (19%) had metastases at the initial presentation, 19 patients (51%) had recurrence at the primary site before metastases developed (average time from treatment of the primary tumor to tumor recurrence was 21 months), and 11 (30%) developed metastasis, even though the primary tumor had been controlled. The average time from treatment of the primary tumor to the occurrence of metastases was 19 months among the 30 patients who did not have metastatic disease at initial presentation. Curative treatment, consisting of surgery or radiation therapy or a combination thereof, was attempted in 31 patients, whereas the remaining 6 patients were treated with palliative methods. Information was available for 23 patients at 2 years posttreatment, with 10 of these patients remaining free of disease, for a 43% 2-year, disease-free survival. At 5 years after treatment, this rate had decreased to 36%. Eleven of the 31 patients receiving curative treatment died of their disease during the mean 49-month follow-up period.

Conclusion.—In this study, metastatic disease was noted in 9.9% of patients with cutaneous squamous cell carcinoma of the head and neck, usually presenting as nodal lesions in the upper neck and parotid gland. The risk of metastasis was found to increase when recurrence of the primary tumor had transpired. Large, multicenter, prospective, randomized studies are needed before a consensus concerning preferred treatment strategies can be reached.

▶ Because squamous cell carcinoma of the skin metastasizes so infrequently, no one clinician will have the opportunity to see a gamut of such patients (fortunately). The points made by the authors are important, i.e., that the majority of the patients will have a recurrence in the primary site as a herald of regional metastasis. Recurrence of squamous cell carcinoma, in contrast to basal cell carcinoma, should be viewed with trepidation and treated aggressively. The mortality rate in this series and others is quite significant. Only about one third of the patients were free of disease at 5 years.

What is also impressive about the results was the disproportionate number of cases drawn from the scalp, forehead, and temple; perhaps lesions in this area are more virulent and aggressive. Regardless, the operation of choice is parotidectomy in addition to neck dissection. What we need are better prognostic and predictive factors in the analysis of the primary lesion in both squamous and basal cell carcinomas.

E.A. Luce, M.D.

Parotid and Neck Metastases From Cutaneous Squamous Cell Carcinoma of the Head and Neck

Khurana VG, Mentis DH, O'Brien CJ, et al (Royal Prince Alfred Hosp, Sydney, Australia; Univ of Sydney, Australia)

Am J Surg 170:446–450, 1995 12–21

Purpose.—About 20% of cutaneous malignancies are squamous cell carcinomas (SCC). Regional lymph node metastases, often to the nodes associated with the parotid gland, occur in approximately 5% of cases of cutaneous SCC. There is little information on the clinical outcomes of parotid gland and neck metastases in patients with cutaneous SCC or on the proper extent of parotidectomy. An experience with the management of parotid gland and neck metastases from cutaneous SCC is presented, with an emphasis on patterns of recurrence and survival and an analysis of prognostic factors.

Methods.—The combined retrospective/prospective study included 75 patients with parotid gland and neck metastases from cutaneous SCC of the head and neck treated during an 11-year period. Thirty-nine percent of patients had neck metastases alone, 44% had parotid gland metastases alone, and 17% had both neck and parotid metastases. Nine percent of patients had abnormal facial nerve function when first seen at the study hospital, and 21% had immunodeficiency states. Recurrence and survival analyses were performed in subgroups, 1 including only the 70 patients

TABLE 1.—Surgical Treatment in 68 Patients With Metastatic Cutaneous Squamous Cell Carcinoma of the Head and Neck

Surgery	No. Operations
Parotidectomy	43
Superficial	34
Near total conservative	3
Total conservative	2
Total radical	4
Neck dissection	59
Selective	14
Modified radical	14
Radical	31
Total	102

(Reprinted by permission of the publisher from Parotid and neck metastases from cutaneous squamous cell carcinoma of the head and neck, Khurana VG, Mentis DH, O'Brien CJ, et al, *Am J Surg,* 170:446–450, copyright 1995 by Excerpta Medica Inc.)

with unilateral disease and another including only the 59 surgically treated patients with unilateral disease who did not receive preoperative radiotherapy. Parotidectomy was superficial and neck dissection radical in most cases (Table 1). Prognostic factors analyzed included the presenting metastatic site, the tumor pathology, and the use of postoperative radiotherapy.

Results.—Of 68 surgically treated patients, 71% had histologic extranodal spread and 18% had perineural invasion. The lesions were poorly differentiated in 47% of patients, and 60% had clear surgical margins. Postoperative radiotherapy was used in 74% of patients. Of 61 patients followed up for at least 1 year, 43% had recurrent SCC. There were 12 recurrences in the parotid gland, 7 in the neck, and 7 in both the neck and parotid gland. Two-year cumulative local disease control was 60%. There was no difference in local control between patients undergoing surgery alone or surgery with postoperative radiotherapy, although the latter were in a higher-risk group. The only significant prognostic factor for local recurrence was histologic involvement of the surgical margins.

Metastases developed in 18% of patients followed up until recurrence or for at least 1 year. The 5-year cumulative disease-specific survival was 61%.

Conclusions.—Cutaneous SCC with metastases to the parotid gland and/or neck appears to be an aggressive tumor, tending toward infiltrative growth and multiple recurrences. There is continuing controversy about the extent of parotidectomy in such cases. The high rate of involved surgical margins in this study questions the use of a conservative, facial, nerve-sparing surgical approach. Postoperative radiation does not necessarily improve control of metastases, although this could be related to the selection of patients for irradiation. Distant metastases are more of a danger for patients with neck involvement than for those with parotid disease alone.

▶ This is a sizable series from a very busy unit in an area with one of the highest incidences of skin cancers in the world—Australia.

One of the principal therapeutic questions is, "Do we spare the facial nerve or not?" Please note that the authors had a 40% incidence of positive margins. Our experience with clinically evident disease in the parotid (metastatic from skin cancer) is that the metastatic deposit frequently extends to the plane of cranial nerve VII. As such, parotidectomy, either superficial or total with sparing of the nerve, often has a very thin margin about the deep plane of the tumor. The 2 choices are sparing of the nerve with postoperative radiation therapy vs. total parotidectomy with sacrifice of the nerve and immediate nerve graft with postoperative radiotherapy. If, clinically, the mass is larger than 2 cm, the likelihood is that one will violate the tumor with any effort at a total parotid with preservation of the nerve.

E.A. Luce, M.D.

Influence of Biopsy on the Prognosis of Cutaneous Melanoma of the Head and Neck

Austin JR, Byers RM, Brown WD, et al (Univ of Texas, Houston)

Head Neck 18:107–117, 1996 12–22

Background.—The diagnosis of melanoma relies on the histologic assessment of a biopsy specimen. However, the appropriate extent of the biopsy is controversial. To date, no study has concentrated on the outcomes of biopsy of cutaneous melanoma of the head and neck.

Methods.—One hundred fifty-nine patients with head and neck melanoma treated between 1983 and 1991 were studied. Median follow-up was 38 months. Patient age, sex, treatment type, biopsy mode, presence of residual melanoma in re-excision, lesion location, presence of ulceration, Clark's level, Breslow thickness, and histologic type were included in the analysis.

Findings.—Seventy-nine patients had excisional biopsies; 48, incisional biopsies; and 32, other procedures, such as shave, needle biopsy, cauterization, and cryotherapy. The location of the lesion before treatment differed significantly between patients who underwent excisional biopsies and those who underwent other biopsy types. Type of biopsy was significantly associated with survival rate. Mortality was 31.3% among patients who underwent incisional biopsy, 25% among those who underwent other types of biopsy, and 8.9% among patients who underwent excisional biopsy. Distant metastases developed in 31.3%, 28.1%, and 10.1%, respectively. Local and regional recurrence rates did not differ significantly among the 3 groups, nor did any of the other variables studied. In a multivariate analysis, presence of tumor in the reexcision specimen, biopsy type, and nodal disease were independent prognostic factors.

Conclusion.—Type of biopsy may influence the clinical outcome of cutaneous melanoma of the head and neck. A biopsy that cuts through the tumor appears to worsen outcome. Also, the development of distant metastasis is significantly associated with a biopsy that removes less than the whole tumor.

► I have 2 problems with this article. The first is conceptual—if excisional biopsies are excisional, and re-excision is performed to insure minimal local recurrence, then why should excisional biopsy have a better survival rate than incisional? The second has to do with the retrospective nature of the study and a possible selection factor of patients who had incisional rather than excisional biopsy, namely, substantially larger surface area tumor (a factor that the authors admitted to). Nevertheless, the operative gut instinct is that an excisional biopsy, if possible, should put the patient at less risk than a cut through a gross tumor as a biopsy maneuver.

E.A. Luce, M.D.

Human Immunodeficiency Virus-Associated Squamous Cell Carcinomas of the Head and Neck Presenting as Oral and Primary Intraosseous Squamous Cell Carcinomas

Langford A, Langer R, Lobeck H, et al (Rudolf Virchow Univ, Berlin; Humboldt Univ, Berlin; Univ Clinic, Essen, Germany)

Quintessence Int 26:635–654, 1995 12–23

Background.—Patients with HIV appear to be at greater risk for certain neoplasms, which frequently originate in the area of the head and neck or the oral cavity. At present, the clinical, radiologic, and histologic characteristics of HIV-related head and neck carcinomas have not been well described, and primary intraosseous squamous cell carcinoma in patients infected with HIV have never been reported. Clinical features, histologic traits, treatment, and clinical follow-up of 6 patients with HIV-associated squamous cell carcinoma of the head and neck are described in detail in the present report.

Observations.—Clinical presentation in these 6 patients included a painful necrotizing ulcer in the floor of the oral cavity; a defect of the alveolar process, measuring approximately 3.6 cm × 7.0 mm, in the left mandible; a slightly painful ulceration in the area of the right mandible extending to the floor of the oral cavity; pain irradiating into the mandible, odynophagia, deviation of the tongue to the left, and an indurated mucosal area; a painful, massive tumor with central ulceration involving the entire right side of the tongue; and homogeneous leukoplakia on the left cheek, accompanied by leukoplakia with a nonhomogeneous surface and erythroplakia localized on the lingual side of the left mandible, extending from the canine to the second premolar. Biopsy specimens were obtained in all patients. Histologic evaluation showed features of well-differentiated carcinoma in 2 patients, including islands of keratinizing stratified epithelium with multiple keratin pearls, and hyperchromatic atypical cells. The tumor also was found to be encapsulated by infiltrating lymphocytes, eosinophils, and mast cells. In another patient, carcinoma in situ with focal infiltration of the tumor in the underlying stroma was found. A moderately differentiated solid tumor was noted in another patient, and well-differentiated carcinomas were diagnosed in the remaining 2 patients. Immunohistochemical studies revealed the presence of cytokeratins 19. These were typically expressed in the suprabasal cellular layers and found in scattered foci within the tumors of all 6 patients. In 3 patients, tumor cells in organized formation or in scattered arrangements were found to express differentiation-related keratins, including cytokeratin 4, 5, or 13. As an indication of keratinization, focally arranged tumor cells in these 3 patients expressed cytokeratin 10/11. Single cells positive for the proliferation marker Ki 67 were noted within the tumors. Immune histologic evaluations of viral antigens were negative. The serologic parameters of all 6 patients showed a reduction in cellular immunity.

Treatment consisted of surgery plus irradiation or radiotherapy alone, the latter of which provided a good local response of reduced tumor size but also was accompanied by severe local side effects, including heavy persistent oral ulcers, mucositis, xerostomia, and skin epitheliolysis. Four patients subsequently died at 5, 7, 12, and 12 months, respectively, after the onset of their initial symptoms. Two patients were without recurrence at 3 and 6 months posttreatment, respectively, and both have remained free of AIDS-associated symptoms to date.

Conclusions.—Neoplastic diseases are a leading cause of morbidity and mortality in patient with AIDS, reportedly affecting more than 40% of such patients. Prognosis was poor in the patients described herein, and response to therapy was relatively unfavorable. Follow-up studies of previously reported cases and reports of new cases that provide thorough descriptions of the initial lesion, applied treatment strategies, and the clinical outcome of emerging lesions are of utmost importance, as such data will permit evaluation of different therapeutic schemes, leading to the development of helpful management guidelines.

▶ This is the best review and description of head and neck cancer in patients with AIDS that I have had the opportunity to read. This article pulls together information from disparate sources and is a concise discussion.

Clearly, the prognosis in these patients is not good, not only because of their young age, but obviously because of their immunosystem depression. Yet, in a very small number of patients, (5 of the 6 were treated definitively), surgery followed by radiation therapy appeared to be preferable to radiation therapy alone. Two of the 6 cases were of primary intraosseous carcinoma of the mandible, a distinctly rare variant, and these patients presented with nerve pain and loosening of teeth, rather than the classic presentation of ulcer in the mouth. This atypical presentation delays diagnosis in these patients, and this diagnosis should be considered in patients with such a clinical picture.

These patients do not handle radiotherapy particularly well; they develop mucositis more frequently and with lower doses than the standard population. The prophylactic and therapeutic measures suggested by the authors should be instituted in all such patients.

Most importantly, therapy should not be withheld.

E.A. Luce, M.D.

Mycobacterial Disease of the Head and Neck: Current Perspective

Cleary KR, Batsakis JG (Univ of Texas, Houston)

Ann Otol Rhinol Laryngol 104:830–833, 1995 12–24

Background.—Mycobacterial disease has shown a rise in incidence in most of the industrialized world, including the United States. Factors that contribute to this increase include HIV, immigration from areas where tuberculosis is common, disease transmission in congregate settings, and deterioration of the health care infrastructure. The growth in case rates for tuberculosis and nontuberculous mycobacterial disease, and the impact of these changes on the practice of the head and neck surgeon are reviewed.

Tuberculosis.—From 1985 to 1992, tuberculosis case rates increased primarily in men (92%) from 25 to 44 years of age (>80%). This age group also accounted for two-thirds of extrapulmonary cases. Racial-ethnic minorities and the foreign-born were overrepresented in tuberculosis cases.

Nontuberculous Mycobacterial Disease.—Species of nontuberculous mycobacteria (NTM), recognized as human pathogens in only the past 40 years, number more than 50. Although rare before 1980, NTM infections are now a common cause of opportunistic infections in patients with AIDS, and are not limited to males or to members of racial-ethnic minorities. The most commonly reported NTM is the *Mycobacterium avium-intracellulare* complex (MAC), once rare outside of rural areas. Whereas only 37 cases of disseminated MAC disease were reported in the literature before the AIDS epidemic, as many as 25% of patients with AIDS have widespread disease from MAC.

Clues that suggest NTM infection include overlying skin inflammation in cervical lymphadenopathy, abscess formation, and unilateral cervical lymphadenopathy. Chest x-rays are often normal; fever, malaise, or weight loss are absent, as is a history of exposure to adults with pulmonary tuberculosis. Most cases of mycobacterial cervical lymphadenitis in children are caused by mycobacteria other than *M. tuberculosis.* Bilateral cervical lymph node involvement is very unusual in NTM infection. Acid-fast staining in histologic sections is not reliable as the sole diagnostic measure for NTM. Because of the subjectivity of histopathologic interpretation, diagnosis must be based on objective identification of the NTM species using molecular strategies. Excisional biopsy is the preferred method for both diagnosis and treatment of NTM lymphadenitis.

▶ Written by a pathologist, this article is a brief and concise summary of the emerging problem of mycobacterial disease of the cervical lymph nodes in head and neck medicine and surgery. With the AIDS epidemic and other immunocompromised states, mycobacterial nodal disease of tubercular origin has become more prevalent in adults. Myobacterial nodal disease of children, which is much more commonly nontubercular, may also be more prevalent now than in the past.

E.A. Luce, M.D.

Bedside Tracheostomy in the Intensive Care Unit

Wease GL, Frikker M, Villalba M, et al (William Beaumont Hosp, Royal Oak, Mich)

Arch Surg 131:552–555, 1996 12–25

Background.—Tracheostomy has recently taken on an important role in the care of chronically ventilator-dependent patients in the ICU. One experience with bedside tracheostomy was reviewed.

Methods.—The medical records of all 204 adults who underwent elective bedside tracheostomy in the ICU between 1983 and 1988 were reviewed. The group included 107 men and 97 women (mean age, 63.6 years). Tracheostomy was indicated by chronic ventilator dependence in 87% of patients, airway protection in 6%, and pulmonary toilet in 5%.

Findings.—Major complications occurred in 2.9%. One patient died of tube obstruction. In addition, there were 2 episodes of bleeding that necessitated reoperation, 1 tube entrapment that necessitated operative removal, 1 nonfatal respiratory arrest, and 1 bilateral pneumothorax. Minor complications occurred in 3.4% of patients. There were 5 episodes of minor bleeding, 1 tube dislodgement in a tracheostomy with a well-developed tract, and 1 episode of mucus plugging. The 1 late complication was tracheal stenosis.

Conclusions.—In the ICU, tracheostomy can be performed at the bedside. The mortality and morbidity rates are comparable to those associated with operative tracheostomy. This procedure is also significantly cost-efficient.

► Actually, bedside tracheostomy was the usual site and protocol for those of us of a certain older generation. The procedure was performed in a ward bed, illumination was provided by a gooseneck lamp, and there was no suction or cautery. Publication of series in the late 1960s and early 1970s of the difference in complication rates between ward and operating room tracheostomies (lower morbidity and mortality) was an impetus to perform the procedure in the operating room if possible. The full cycle back to the bedside in the ICU has been possible because of much better illumination (good headlights) and portable cautery. There are some criticisms, however, regarding the design of this study. First, no controls are available for this retrospective chart review, and the reader's appreciation has been enhanced by a more sophisticated cost analysis. No longer can we simply compare the cost of a single event, such as average cost of the tracheostomy in the operating room vs. the charge for bedside tracheostomy. What we need is a comparison of the cost of the complications in group A vs. group B, length of stay, and the cost of long-term complications. Regardless, a 3% incidence of major complications for the series is perfectly admirable.

E.A. Luce, M.D.

Color Doppler Sonography in Penetrating Injuries of the Neck

Montalvo BM, LeBlang SD, Nuñez DB Jr, et al (Univ of Miami, Fla)

AJNR Am J Neuroradiol 17:943–951, 1996 12–26

Background.—Different methods have been advocated for the diagnostic workup of arterial injuries in stable patients who have penetrating neck trauma. Most investigators recommend an integrated clinical and radiographic workup in these patients. However, screening angiography, a costly procedure, is negative in as many as 83% of patients. The value of color Doppler sonography in the screening of patients with penetrating traumatic neck injuries was investigated prospectively.

Methods and Findings.—Fifty-two patients who had gunshot wounds or lacerations were included. The findings of color Doppler sonography were compared with those of angiography in 44 patients, with surgical findings in 4, and with clinical status in 4. Color Doppler sonography correctly detected all 6 serious injuries of the carotid arteries and all 4 injuries of the vertebral arteries, which were diagnosed with angiography. Reversible narrowing of the internal and external carotid arteries in 1 patient was missed on sonography. In addition, sonography failed to show 2 normal vertebral arteries.

Conclusions.—In clinically stable patients who have zone II or III injuries and no evidence of active bleeding, color Doppler sonographic screening is as accurate as angiography. Such patients in whom sonographic findings are complete and normal may need no further imaging studies or neck explorations. Angiography may be beneficial in patients who have incomplete or technically suboptimal sonographic findings. Further information may be obtained from CT of the neck in patients who have gunshot wounds. In patients who have a serious injury detected on sonography and are candidates for surgery or intervention, angiography should be done for procedure planning and branch vessel examination.

▶ This paper, published in the nonsurgical (radiology) literature, addresses the use of angiography and the nonoperative workup of penetrating wounds of the neck. The results, as the authors caution, must be regarded as preliminary and need corroboration by other studies. Yet, the preliminary data would indicate that color Doppler sonography can screen those patients who do not have a vascular injury, thereby reserving angiography for a demonstrable lesion on Doppler exam. From the perspective of this reviewer, that application might be appropriate at this juncture in zones II and III; angiography should continue to be used for assessment of zone I injuries.

The questions that arise with respect to design are those of patient selection, because of the 106 patients, 22 went to surgery and only half the remainder were included in the study. Of course, color Doppler sonography will not, in all likelihood, diagnose significant venous injuries either.

E.A. Luce, M.D.

Breast and Miscellaneous

Emergency Free Flap Cover in Complex Injuries of the Lower Extremities

Ninković M, Schoeller T, Benedetto K-P, et al (Univ Clinic of Plastic and Reconstructive Surgery, Innsbruck, Austria; Univ of Innsbruck, Austria)
Scand J Plast Reconstr Hand Surg 30:37–47, 1996 12–27

Background.—The advent of microsurgical techniques, such as free-tissue transfer, has revolutionized the manner in which complex injuries of the lower extremities are currently managed, having made possible the reconstruction or salvaging of injured or amputated limbs. The indications, operative techniques, and potential for emergency flap transfers (performed either at the completion of primary debridement or within 24 hours after injury) and salvage free-tissue transfer in patients with complex injuries to the lower leg were reviewed.

Patients and Methods.—Nineteen patients (mean age, 32 years) underwent immediate reconstructive procedures for high energy trauma-related injuries to the lower extremities, associated with serious soft-tissue damage. Radical débridement and primary repair of injured structures, including nerves, tendons, vessels, and muscles, were performed, as was initial bone stabilization, using external fixators, in the 13 patients with associated tibial fractures, including 3 Gustilo type IIIB and 10 Gustilo type IIIC. In these 13 patients, a second operation was done 8 to 12 weeks later to remove the fixator and fix the fractures internally using AO plates. All bone defects measured less than 5 cm. After these initial procedures, emergency free-flap reconstruction was undertaken. All procedures were completed within 24 hours of the initial injury. Latissimus dorsi and scapular muscle flaps were used in 14 and 2 patients, respectively, and a free groin flap was used in 1 patient. A salvage free-flap transfer was done in 2 patients with complete below-knee amputations associated with avulsion of soft tissue, in an effort to preserve length of stump and knee joint function. Median follow-up was 3.5 years (range, 4 months to 8 years).

Results.—In all 19 patients, the emergency free flaps survived without evidence of deep infection or osteomyelitis. There was very little morbidity associated with the procedures, and the need for secondary operations was minimal. Three patients experienced thrombosis of the flap anastomosis, necessitating revision with an interposition vein graft, and 1 patient had partial necrosis of the flap distally, requiring excision and direct closure. Two hematomas, both at the donor site, also occurred and were managed by incision and drainage. One fracture required revision fixation and revision bone grafting; all other fractures healed without complications.

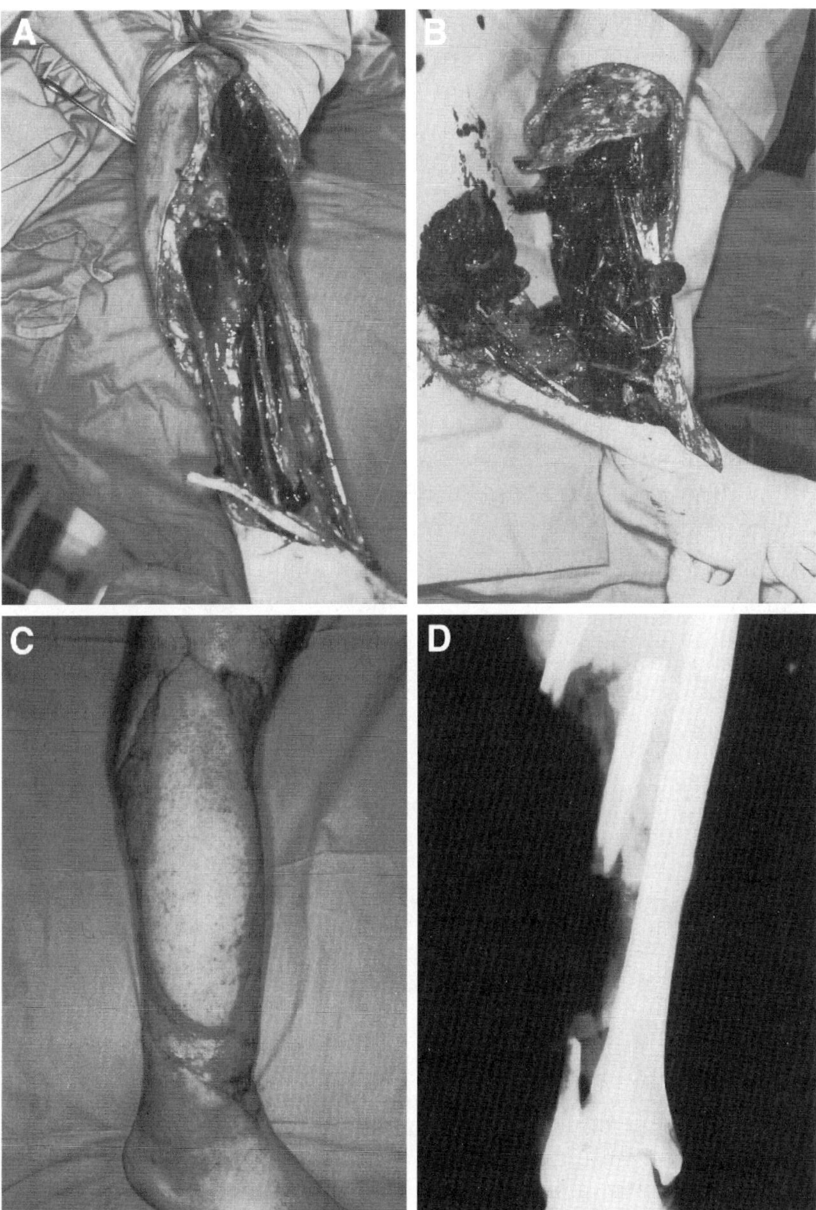

FIGURE 3.—*Case 1.* (**a**) Operative view after radical débridement and exposure of neurovascular bundles, bone, and tendons. (**b**) Harvested latissimus dorsi flap. (**c**) Postoperative view. (**d**) Result 11 months later. (Courtesy of Nonković M, Schoeller T, Benedetto K-P, et al: Emergency free flap cover in complex injuries of the lower extremities. *Scand J Plast Reconstr Hand Surg* 30:37–47, 1996.)

Median time to full weight-bearing was 4.5 months, and all patients had good functional results. Hospital stay also was reduced, with a median stay of 23 days (range, 17 to 43 days).

Conclusion.—Emergency free-flap cover of soft-tissue defects in complex injuries of the lower limb is associated with many advantages, including reductions in morbidity, flap failure, deep bony or soft tissue infections, and hospital stay, as well as improved functional and cosmetic outcomes. Emergency and salvage flaps are time-consuming procedures, however, and should be performed by a surgical team experienced in microsurgical reconstruction and management, after first thoroughly assessing the patient's suitability for such procedures. In patients undergoing such procedures, the timing of wound closure is a critical concern. The most important aspect of early wound care is radical débridement, done under tourniquet control. Surgically clean wounds can then be closed within 12 hours of injury, whereas complex untidy wounds should be converted to surgically clean wounds to permit primary closure. In patients with complex contaminated wounds, coverage with muscle flaps after proper débridement is recommended. The authors prefer to use pure muscle flaps with split thickness skin grafts, which provide better protection against reulceration, particularly in weight-bearing areas. In patients with large primary defects who will require several secondary operations during the reconstruction process, musculocutaneous flaps are useful. Skin islands may be used to enhance blood supply of the distal aspect of a large musculocutaneous flap, and to facilitate contouring of the extremity (Fig 3).

▶ The authors make their points well, but I suggest the following caveats for the reader. First, the injuries must have been moderate in this series, insofar as no bone defect was larger than 5 cm. Second, the reoperation rate of 16% is considerably greater than optimal. Third, and perhaps most importantly, is that these were isolated injuries of the lower extremity alone without trauma elsewhere. Still, there is no quibbling with the results. The absence of osteomyelitis, satisfactory length of stay, and assumption of weight-bearing by the patients are all impressive results.

E.A. Luce, M.D.

Should Breast Reduction Surgery Be Rationed? A Comparison of the Health Status of Patients Before and After Treatment: Postal Questionnaire Survey

Klassen A, Fitzpatrick R, Jenkinson C, et al (Univ of Oxford, England; Radcliffe Infirmary, Oxford, England)

BMJ 313:454–457, 1996 12–28

Purpose.—Hospitals in the state-funded British National Health Service still offer breast reduction surgery. However, there are questions about whether this and other cosmetic procedures are justified in such a system. Such operations are likely to be excluded from future service contracts

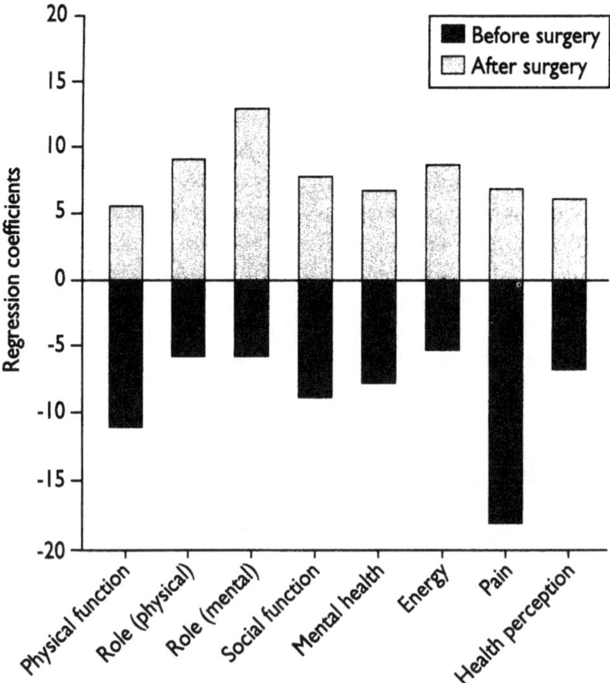

FIGURE 1.—Differences in age-adjusted mean SF-36 scores of patients undergoing breast reduction and those in the general female population. (Courtesy of Klassen A, Fitzpatrick R, Jenkinson C, et al: Should breast reduction surgery be rationed? A comparison of the health status of patients before and after treatment: Postal questionnaire survey. *BMJ* 313:454–457, 1996.)

unless there is evidence to show that they should be included. The benefits of breast reduction surgery were evaluated by before-and-after health status assessments.

Methods.—The study included 166 women referred for breast reduction surgery. A questionnaire was sent to each patient before the operation. The questionnaires included several well-validated health status measurement tools, including the "short form 36" (SF-36) health questionnaire, the general health questionnaire, and Rosenberg's self-esteem scale. Follow-up questionnaires were sent to as many women as possible 6 months after the operation. The SF-36 data were compared with those of a previously studied, random sample of women. The patients' scores before and after surgery were compared with those of the general population of women.

Results.—The patients waited an average of 100 days for an outpatient appointment after the date of referral. Eighty-five patients had breast reduction surgery after spending an average of 146 days on the waiting list. Most breast reductions were done for physical indications. Postoperative questionnaires were sent to 74 patients, and 58 (68%) responded. The greatest difference in any score between the patients and the general female population was in the pain dimension of the SF-36. The patients differed from the general population on all 8 dimensions of this study instrument, suggesting that they were in poorer health than the general population (Fig 1). After breast reduction surgery, the patients reported themselves to be in significantly better health than the general population. There was great improvement in Rosenberg's self-esteem scale and moderate improvement in general well-being on the general health questionnaire. The proportion of patients rated as having possible psychiatric disturbance decreased from 41% before to 11% after surgery.

Conclusions.—Women undergoing breast reduction surgery show significant improvement in health status after their operations. The benefits may be compared with those produced by other interventions, such as treatment for peptic ulcer or rheumatoid arthritis. This information should be considered in making resource allocation decisions regarding breast reduction and possibly other cosmetic procedures.

▶ Although some significant design problems, at least from this reader's perspective, exist in this study, the paper represents the essence of what we need to examine for a large number of surgical procedures. Breast reduction perhaps is a more obvious case, but the world of surgery abounds with such examples. The authors used curious language by stating that their purpose was to examine "cosmetic" operations, then proceeded to establish that physical function and health and well-being were substantially enhanced after breast reduction surgery. They reached the conclusion that breast reduction surgery should not be excluded from service contracts. Questions that remain to be answered include exactly how big were the breasts, and some others, but the study represents a good start.

Incidentally, the average wait for a patient to obtain an appointment in the National Health Service for breast reduction, after referral by a general practitioner, was 3 months, and another 6 months before surgery was accomplished. Would patients in the United States tolerate such a hiatus?

E.A. Luce, M.D.

Comparison of Resource Costs of Free and Conventional TRAM Flap Breast Reconstruction

Kroll SS, Evans GRD, Reece GP, et al (Univ of Texas, Houston)
Plast Reconstr Surg 98:74–77, 1996 12–29

Background.—Because the free transverse rectus abdominis myocutaneous (TRAM) flap is associated with less donor-site morbidity and a better blood supply and has a success rate similar to that achieved with the conventional TRAM flap, it is being used increasingly. There have been concerns, however, regarding the cost of the free TRAM flap. The resource costs of performing breast reconstruction with the free TRAM flap or the conventional TRAM flap were compared. In addition, the costs of performing bilateral mastectomy and reconstruction were compared with those of unilateral mastectomy and reconstruction.

TABLE 1.—Cost Components, in 1993 Dollars

Cost Component	Dollar Value
Operating room (1 hour)	548.00
Hospital day, initial reconstruction, free TRAM	1,218.00
Hospital day, initial reconstruction, conventional TRAM	1,113.00
Hospital day, revision	670.00
Surgicenter day	530.00
Staff surgeon (1 hour)	156.00
Surgical assistant (1 hour)	43.00
Anesthesia personnel cost (1 hour)	119.00

Abbreviation: TRAM, transverse rectus abdominis myocutaneous.
(Courtesy of Kroll SS, Evans GRD, Reece GP, et al: Comparison of resource costs of free and conventional TRAM flap breast reconstruction. *Plast Reconstr Surg* 98:74–77, 1996.)

Methods.—The resource costs, defined as the costs required of the hospital, were reviewed for all patients who underwent mastectomy and immediate breast reconstruction between 1986 and 1994. These costs included hourly personnel costs, costs for each day of the hospital stay, laboratory work, and recovery room costs for the initial reconstruction and any subsequent revisions (Table 1).

Results.—Of the 154 patients who had completed breast reconstruction with TRAM flaps, 95 had free TRAM flaps and 59 had conventional TRAM flaps. There was only a 4.1% difference in the total resource costs for the initial procedure in these 2 groups, with conventional TRAM flaps costing nonsignificantly less than free TRAM flaps. The revision costs were slightly higher in the conventional TRAM flap group, however, because of longer hospital stays. The mean resource cost of unilateral mastectomy with reconstruction was $17,840, compared with $18,729 for bilateral mastectomy with reconstruction, a 5% difference.

Conclusions.—The conventional TRAM flap has a slight cost advantage over the free TRAM flap for the initial procedure. The difference, however, is not statistically significant. Similarly, the costs of performing bilateral mastectomy with immediate reconstruction are not significantly higher than those of performing unilateral mastectomy with immediate reconstruction.

▶ The growing body of evidence would indicate that immediate breast reconstruction is preferable to delayed reconstruction and that free (microvascular) TRAM flap is preferable over pedicle reconstruction from the standpoint of esthetics, ultimate results, etc. This paper tells us that those better results do not cost more.

The only caveat is this study was performed at one of the most experienced microvascular surgery centers in the country. To obtain an equivalent cost without a pedicled flap, free flaps have to be performed with a very low complication rate.

E.A. Luce, M.D.

Rectus Turnover Flaps for the Reconstruction of Large Midline Abdominal Wall Defects

DeFranzo AJ, Kingman GJ, Sterchi JM, et al (Bowman Gray School of Medicine/Baptist Hosp, Winston-Salem, NC)
Ann Plast Surg 37:18–23, 1996 12–30

Background.—Synthetic materials may be needed for reconstruction of large midline defects of the abdominal wall. However, these reconstructions commonly fail. The synthetic material may pull away from the perimeter of the defect, or the mesh may erode into the viscera. Bilateral rectus turnover flaps were used to reconstruct large midline defects of the abdominal wall.

Technique.—The reconstructive technique used the rectus abdominis muscle, which is innervated in segments by the seventh through twelfth intercostal nerves. Below the arcuate line, the posterior rectus sheath is composed solely of the transversalis fascia, which is usually extremely thin. Thus, a hernia would be likely to develop below the arcuate line if the entire muscle and anterior rectus sheath were simply turned over (Fig 2). The reconstruction started with incision of the anterior rectus sheath from above the costal margin to the level of the arcuate line for upper and middle abdominal hernias and to the pubis for hernias involving the upper, middle, and lower abdomen. About 1 cm of sheath was then freed from the underlying rectus muscle, and blunt dissection was done around the lateral border and posterior to the muscle. With the segmental arteries and nerves and the muscular attachments divided as necessary, the muscle was turned over. This made the anterior sheath into a posterior sheath layer below the muscle. After the peritoneum and sheath were closed, the muscle was closed as a third layer. Prolene (polypropylene) mesh, when used,

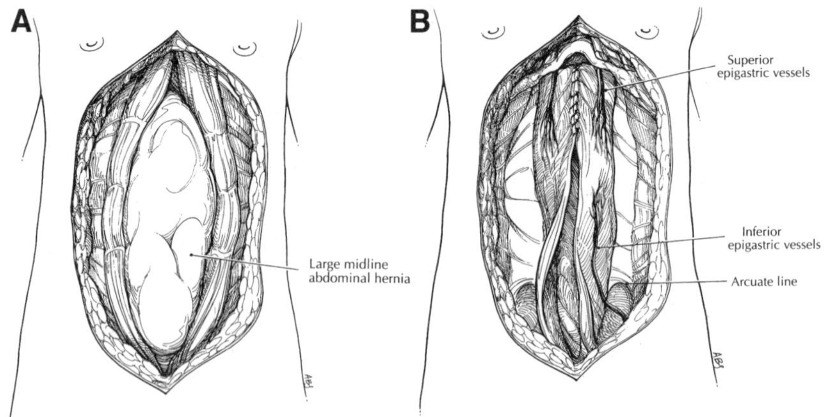

(*Continued*)

FIGURE 2 (cont.)

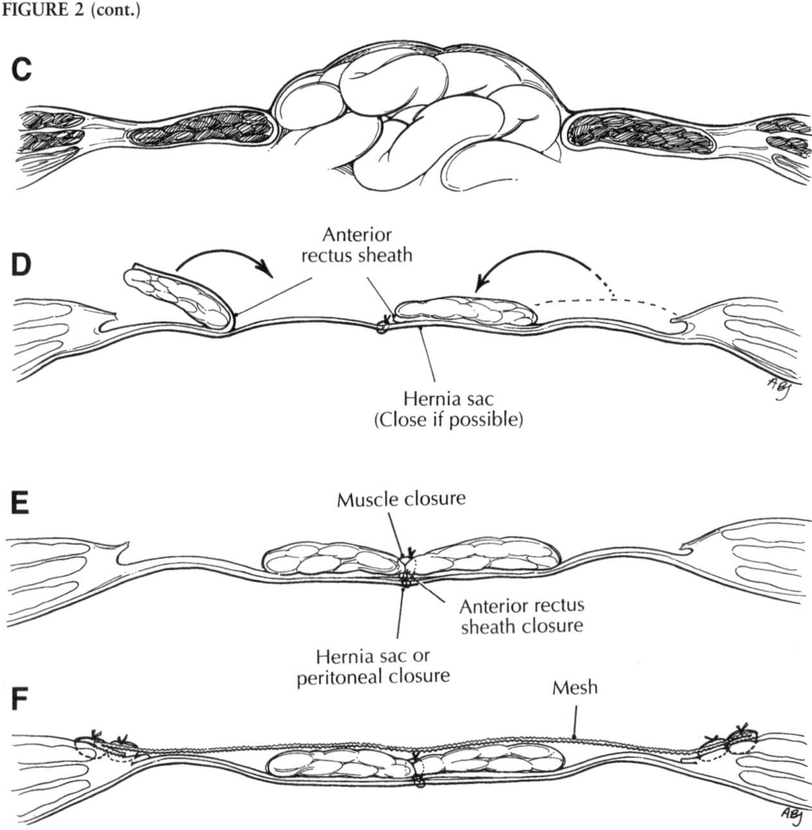

FIGURE 2.—A, a large midline abdominal hernia with fixed lateral retraction of the rectus muscles. **B,** rectus muscles with attached anterior rectus sheath create abdominal wall weakness when turned over below the arcuate line. **C,** rectus muscles are turned over with anterior rectus sheaths after reduction of the hernia. **D,** prolene (polypropylene) mesh is used to reinforce the repair. A double-row suture technique is done to fix the mesh to the external oblique aponeurosis. (Courtesy of DeFranzo AJ, Kingman GJ, Sterchi JM, et al: Rectus turnover flaps for the reconstruction of large midline abdominal wall defects. *Ann Plast Surg* 37:18–23, 1996.)

was attached from above the costal margin to the pubis and from the medial edge of the external oblique to the medial edge of the external oblique.

Methods.—Fifteen patients with large midline abdominal hernias underwent this procedure, with an average follow-up of 22 months. All hernias were repaired successfully. Seven patients had complications, including 4 with postoperative loss of the midline skin over the hernia sac. Two of these patients had only small areas of skin loss. The other 2 lost a large section of midline cover as a result of undermining of poor-quality midline skin, or attenuated scar tissue. Two patients had recurrent hernias necessitating redo surgery.

Conclusions.—Reconstruction of large midline abdominal hernias using a rectus abdominis turnover flap has been done. Although complications are common, overall morbidity is low and the patients' back and abdominal pain are much improved. Some ballooning of the abdominal wall occurs as a result of division of the segmental nerves.

▶ Plastic surgeons have become more interested in reconstruction of the anterior abdominal wall, probably because of experience with transverse rectus abdominis myocutaneous flap reconstruction of the breast and the resultant focus on the anatomy and pathology of the anterior abdominal wall defect created. As a result, their colleagues in general surgery have asked for plastic surgery involvement in more difficult anterior abdominal wall defects such as this series of cases.

Nevertheless, this reviewer has some substantial difficulties with the approach as described. First, by necessity, large amounts of skin are undermined to expose the lateral border of the rectus muscle, which is already displaced well laterally (at least greater than 15 cm in this series). The skin is thus devascularized because of the division of the blood supply perforating from the anterior rectus sheath. That problem, though, is a common denominator of many approaches to abdominal wall reconstruction. The other difficulty, perhaps considerably more problematic, is the denervation of the rectus muscles inherent in this technique. One has to assume that over a period of time, with a denervated anterior rectus and continuous intra-abdominal pressure, ballooning of the abdomen is an inevitable outcome.

Another approach to reconstruction of the anterior abdominal wall (alluded to by the authors) is the "components of separation."

E.A. Luce, M.D.

Grafting on Nude Mice of Living Skin Equivalents Produced Using Human Collagens

López Valle CA, Germain L, Rouabhia M, et al (Saint Sacrement Hosp, Quebec, Canada; Laval Univ, Sainte Foy, Quebec, Canada)

Transplantation 62:317–323, 1996 12–31

Background.—Although cultured epithelial autografts are available for permanent burn wound coverage, epithelial sheets lack some of the inherent qualities of dermis in vivo. Adding a dermal component would provide some of these properties, thus reducing delays in dermal organization, limiting scar tissue formation steps, and accelerating in situ skin regeneration. It may be possible to produce a clinically useful skin equivalent (SE) by isolating autologous living epidermal cells and dermal fibroblasts from a skin biopsy specimen, amplifying these cells, and seeding them in SE for growth in batches. The results of in vivo transplantation with an SE prepared with human and bovine collagen are reported.

Methods and Results.—Transplants were placed in athymic nude mice. Both human and bovine SE showed good adhesion onto the graft bed within the first week after transplantation. By 2 weeks, the graft "take" rate was 100%, with a well-organized stratum corneum that thickened progressively. The cuboidal morphology of basal cells was maintained in human SE grafts with and without additional dermal matrix components. Indirect immunofluorescence staining confirmed that the grafts were of human origin, and the 2 types of human SE grafts contained equal amounts of human type I collagen. Contraction over time was less with the human SE grafts than with the bovine SE grafts.

Conclusions.—Permanent transplantation of bioengineered SE may soon be an option for burn wound coverage. The experiments suggest that human epidermal cells seeded in SE undergo normal differentiation in situ and then retain their in vivo functional capacities after transplantation. Graft take and histologic evolution are better with anchored SE than with cultured epidermal sheets. A sequential approach to SE transplantation for use in patients with extensive burns is being investigated.

▶ This effort is a highly technical area of biological research, but the need for dermis with the use of large sheets of cultured epithelial keratinocytes (CEK) is now a widely accepted thesis, despite all the initial excitement for the use of CEK in large body burns. Clearly the problem is how to develop a viable dermis, although this experiment is steps away from that assumption. Certainly the results are promising, yet early. Besides...mice are not men.

E.A. Luce, M.D.

13 Vascular Surgery

Introduction

Published multicenter randomized trials have defined the role of the carotid endarterectomy in most patients with symptomatic carotid arterial disease. The one major exception is symptomatic patients with moderate carotid stenosis. Preliminary results from the European Carotid Surgery Trial (Abstract 13–1) suggest that carotid endarterectomy is of no value in such patients. However, differences in the method used to calculate the degree of internal carotid artery stenosis between the European Carotid Surgery Trial and the North American Symptomatic Carotid Endarterectomy Trial (NASCET) mean that this study only demonstrates carotid endarterectomy to be of no benefit for symptomatic stenoses or 50% smaller by NASCET criteria, which is not entirely unexpected. Assessment of the efficacy of carotid endarterectomy in symptomatic patients with carotid stenosis between 50% and 69% will probably await results from the NASCET study of such patients. Demonstration of the value of carotid endarterectomy in asymptomatic patients by the Asymptomatic Carotid Atherosclerosis Study has also raised the issue of screening patients for asymptomatic carotid stenosis. The incidence of significant asymptomatic carotid stenosis in the general population is too low to justify large-scale screening, but it is clear that the incidence of significant carotid artery disease in certain groups of patients, such as those with peripheral vascular disease (Abstract 13–2), may be high enough to justify such screening.

The most interesting and potentially controversial development in the treatment of patients with infrarenal abdominal aortic aneurysms has been endoluminal aneurysm repair using stent grafts. Although much excitement has accompanied publication of the preliminary results of the use of stent grafts to treat abdominal aortic aneurysms, much remains to be understood about the value of this approach. The study by White et al. (Abstract 13–5) questions whether this less invasive method of repairing abdominal aortic aneurysms will be associated with the presumed reduction in initial morbidity and mortality seen with standard surgical repair, at least when using currently available devices. Long-term problems with endoluminal aneurysm repair, including anastomotic leaks, which can lead to subsequent aneurysm rupture, also continue to be of concern, and the study by May et al. (Abstract 13–6) demonstrates that unless the aneurysm decreases in size after endoluminal repair, it is not isolated from the circulation, even if no leak at the graft fixation point is seen. Potentially more important, these authors also demonstrated that the neck of an aneurysm undergoing endoluminal repair continues to increase in size regardless of how the aneurysm itself reacts to endoluminal repair. Obviously, much remains to be learned about endoluminal aneurysm repair before this technique can be widely applied.

The role of endovascular techniques such as balloon angioplasty, arthrectomy, and thrombolysis in the treatment of peripheral arterial occlusive disease continues to evolve. Despite the widespread use of balloon angioplasty on infrainguinal arteries, the reported long-term success is limited at best (Abstract 13–10). Arthrectomy of infrainguinal arterial occlusive disease has also been associated with poor long-term results; however, the article by Porter et al. (Abstract 13–11) suggests that directional arthrectomy may have a role in the treatment of vein bypass graft stenosis. Finally, reanalysis of results from the study Surgery Versus Thrombolysis for Ischemia of the Lower Extremity (Abstracts 13–12 and 13–13), a prospective randomized comparison of catheter-directed thrombolysis and surgery, demonstrates that although catheter-directed thrombolysis may be of value in selected patients with acute infrainguinal arterial or bypass graft thrombosis, these benefits are achieved at the price of an increased risk of recurrent ischemia and/or subsequent amputation when compared with standard surgical therapy. Because of this, thrombolysis appears to be primarily useful in patients at high risk for surgical treatment and in those with few reconstructive alternatives. Therefore, arterial bypass remains the primary treatment in patients with infrainguinal arterial occlusive disease, but long-term bypass graft surveillance using duplex US is essential to achieve the best long-term patency for both vein grafts (Abstract 13–14) and potentially prosthetic grafts (Abstract 13–15).

The conventional wisdom is that deep venous thrombosis and valvular reflux and/or perforator incompetence in the deep veins of the lower extremity are the principal causes of acute and chronic venous disease. In contrast, the articles by Myers et al. (Abstract 13–19) and Chengelis et al. (Abstract 13–20) suggest that the superficial venous system may play a more important role in both acute and chronic venous disease than previously thought. Additionally, the recent introduction of low–molecular weight heparin has potentially simplified the treatment of acute deep venous thrombosis, and an analysis of published data by Siragusa et al. (Abstract 13–21) suggests that low–molecular weight heparin is more effective in preventing recurrent venous thrombosis, produces less bleeding, and potentially leads to decreased mortality when compared with standard, unfractionated heparin.

Finally, intraoperative heparinization during abdominal aortic aneurysm repair has now been shown to be of value by the prospective randomized trial of Thompson et al. (Abstract 13–22). Interestingly, the primary value of the use of heparin during aneurysm repair was not in decreasing the risk of distal thrombosis but rather decreasing the risk of perioperative myocardial infarction. Studies of catheter-directed thrombolysis in patients with acute lower extremity thrombosis and intraoperative thrombolysis during infrainguinal arterial reconstruction have reported similar results, which suggests that the observation that anticoagulation/thrombolysis may reduce the risk of myocardial infarction associated with the treatment of peripheral vascular disease may be real.

James M. Seeger, M.D.

Carotid Disease

Endarterectomy for Moderate Symptomatic Carotid Stenosis: Interim Results From the MRC European Carotid Surgery Trial

Slattery J, for the European Carotid Surgery Trialists' Collaborative Group (Western Gen Hosp, Edinburgh, Scotland)

Lancet 347:1591–1593, 1996 13–1

Introduction.—The desirability of performing a carotid endarterectomy depends on a balance between the benefit of avoiding an ipsilateral carotid territory stroke and the operative risk of immediate stroke or death. The appropriateness of treating patients with recent cerebrovascular events in the territory supplied by a moderately stenosed (30% to 69%) internal carotid artery was assessed.

Methods.—In a multicenter, randomized, controlled trial, 1,599 patients with moderate stenosis were treated in 97 hospitals in 15 countries. Sixty percent of patients were allocated to receive carotid endarterectomy, and 40% of patients were allocated to avoid the procedure.

Results.—Nine patients were dropped from the study because of the unavailability of follow-up data. In patients with 50% to 69% stenosis, an adverse effect of surgery on stroke-free survival was apparent at each time point between 0 and 2.3 years, whereas in patients with 30% to 49% stenosis, an adverse effect of surgery was apparent at each time point between 0 and 3.4 years. Beyond these time points, there were no between-group differences in stroke-free survival and no suggestion that the risk of disease recurrence was different between patients given surgery and those not operated upon.

Conclusion.—These findings demonstrate that carotid endarterectomy is not beneficial for most, and perhaps all, patients with moderate symptomatic carotid stenosis.

► This study of interim results from the European Carotid Surgery Trial found no benefit (and possible harm) from carotid endarterectomy in symptomatic patients with carotid stenosis of between 30% and 69%. However, the method used to calculate the degree of internal carotid artery stenosis in the European Carotid Surgery Trial is significantly different from that used in the North American Symptomatic Carotid Endarterectomy Trial (NASCET), so that symptomatic patients in this study who had no benefit from carotid endarterectomy had stenoses of 0% to 50% by NASCET criteria.

The revised conclusion—that symptomatic patients with stenoses under 50% will not benefit from carotid endarterectomy—is likely correct but remains to be confirmed. Assessment of the efficacy of carotid endarterectomy in symptomatic patients with carotid stenosis of between 50% and 69% (as measured by NASCET criteria) likely will await completion and publication of the NASCET study, which has just finished entering patients.

J.M. Seeger, M.D.

Carotid Artery Stenosis in Peripheral Vascular Disease

Alexandrova NA, Gibson WC, Norris JW, et al (Univ of Toronto)

J Vasc Surg 23:645–649, 1996 13–2

Introduction.—Peripheral vascular disease is associated with a high incidence of carotid atherosclerosis, and screening patients with such disease for carotid artery disease has been advocated to identify those at risk of stroke. The prevalence and severity of symptomatic and asymp-

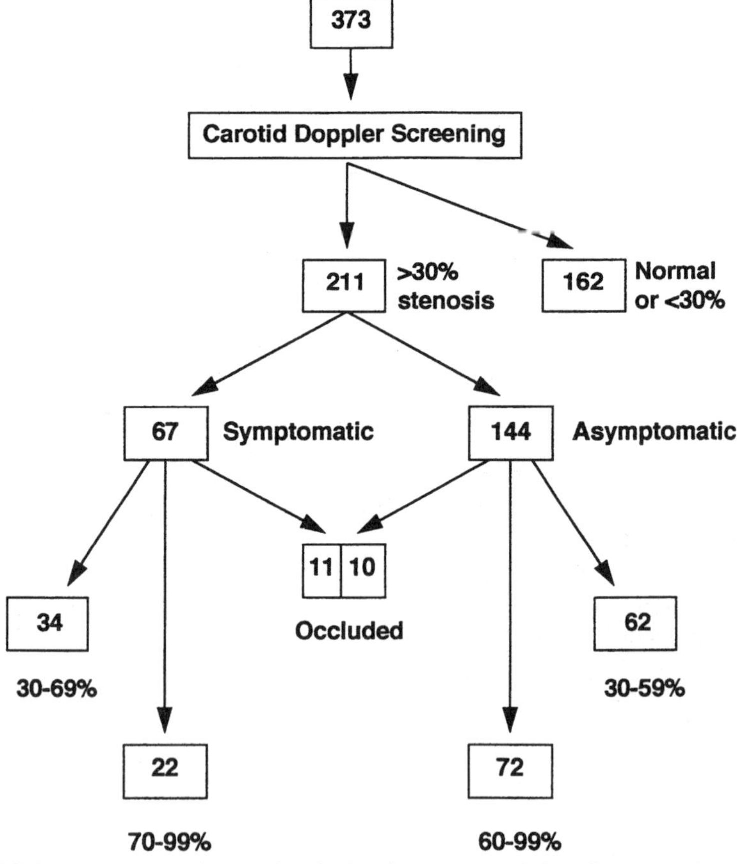

FIGURE 1.—Patient population and study algorithm. (Courtesy of Alexandrova NA, Gibson WC, Norris JW, et al: Carotid artery stenosis in peripheral vascular disease. *J Vasc Surg* 23:645–649, 1996.)

tomatic carotid artery disease was studied in patients with peripheral vascular disease so that operable carotid artery stenosis could be predicted.

Methods.—During 2 years, 372 consecutive patients with peripheral vascular disease, with a mean age of 70 ± 10 years, were studied. They were screened for the presence of carotid atherosclerosis with color-coded duplex ultrasonography. A vascular surgeon and radiologist graded the carotid artery stenosis. A questionnaire was used to record pre-existing risk factors including sex, age, diabetes mellitus, hypertension, history of smoking, coronary artery disease, and prior stroke/transient ischemic attacks.

Results.—In this group, 71% had a history of smoking, 47% had coronary artery disease, 43% had hypertension, and 21% had diabetes mellitus. Carotid artery duplex scanning detected 30% or greater carotid artery stenosis in 211 patients (57%). Symptoms of ischemic cerebral events were found in 67 patients (32%) of whom 22 had potentially operable carotid artery stenosis of 70% to 99% (Fig 1). Stenosis of 60% to 99% was found in 71 of 144 (49%) symptom-free patients. The strongest predictors of peripheral vascular disease and carotid artery disease were male sex and prior stroke/transient ischemic attack.

Conclusion.—The study found that 25% of the group with category I or greater peripheral vascular disease (22 with symptoms and 72 without symptoms) had sufficiently severe carotid disease to be potential surgical candidates.

► Now that the Asymptomatic Carotid Atherosclerosis Study has demonstrated benefit for carotid endarterectomy in patients with carotid stenoses of between 60% and 99%, the problem becomes how to identify such patients. Large-scale screening using carotid duplex ultrasound is far too costly and, thus, screening must be carefully directed toward high-risk populations. This paper shows that even mild peripheral vascular disease is a good marker for significant carotid artery disease, with 50% of the 144 asymptomatic patients in this study having carotid artery stenoses of 60% to 99%.

J.M. Seeger, M.D.

Management of Recurrent Carotid Stenosis: Should Asymptomatic Lesions Be Treated Surgically?

O'Donnell TF Jr, Rodriguez AA, Fortunato JE, et al (Tufts Univ, Boston; New England Med Ctr, Boston)

J Vasc Surg 24:207–212, 1996 13–3

Objective.—Recent trials have established the low morbidity and beneficial effect of carotid endarterectomy (CENDX). However, there is disagreement regarding performing the procedure on asymptomatic patients with hemodynamically significant recurrent carotid stenosis (RCS) which occurs after 2% to 5% of primary CENDX. A study was undertaken to investigate factors that may influence the decision to perform CENDX on asymptomatic patients with RCS and to contrast the results of primary and secondary CENDX with regard to morbidity and stroke prevention.

Methods.—Results of 48 operations performed on 44 patients for recurrent stenosis (RCS-OP group) were contrasted with results from a group of 35 patients (40 vessels) with RCS (greater than 50% stenosis on a subsequent duplex ultrasonogram) who did not undergo re-operation (RCS-NO-OP group). This latter group was derived from 348 patients who underwent 1,053 follow-up duplex ultrasonography studies. After primary CENDX, the results from each group were also compared with a meta-analysis of 6 previous key series.

Results.—No significant differences were seen in risk factors between the 2 groups except that the RCS-OP group had a significantly higher incidence of coronary artery disease (50% vs. 31%) and peripheral vascular disease (52% vs. 31%) than the RCS-NO-OP group. Twenty-seven percent of the repeat CENDX were done within 2 years of the primary CENDX, whereas 73% of the repeat CENDX were done after 2 years (similar to the meta-analysis). Repeat CENDX was done for symptomatic RCS in 56% of patients, with 39% of patients undergoing repeat CENDX within 2 years of being symptomatic, compared with 77% of those having repeat CENDX after 2 years. The operative-specific stroke and 30-day mortality rates were both 2.1% for the repeat CENDX. Seventy-five percent of the RCS-OP group had greater than 90% stenosis, whereas only 10% of the RCS-NO-OP group had greater than 80% stenosis. However, 1 of 21 vessels with 50% to 75% stenosis (4.7%) was associated with a transient ischemic attack (TIA), 3 of 9 vessels (33%) with 75% to 99% stenosis were associated with neurologic events (2 strokes and 1 TIA), and 6 of 10 occluded vessels (60%) were associated with neurologic events (3 strokes and 5 TIAs). Overall, 10 of 40 vessels progressed to sudden occlusion, 2 occlusions were associated with unheralded strokes, and 3 of 40 patients (7.5%) had unrelated strokes.

Conclusion.—Recurrent carotid stenosis of 75% or greater is associated with a surprisingly high incidence of neurologic events and unheralded strokes. Repeat CENDX may be indicated for these lesions as the stroke risk associated with the procedure is low.

▶ Repeat carotid endarterectomy can be done with only a slight increase in risk by those experienced in the procedure and should be done in patients with symptomatic RCS greater than 70% to 75%. This study also suggests repeat CENDX to be of benefit in patients with high grade (greater than 75%) *asymptomatic* stenoses, based on the finding of a high rate of progression of asymptomatic RCS to occlusion with a substantial associated stroke risk.

In contrast, previous studies (including 1 from the same institution) have suggested that the overall risk of stroke associated with asymptomatic RCS is so low that routine follow-up is not indicated. Obviously, the management of these recurrent lesions remains unclear, but repeat CENDX for high-grade asymptomatic RCS developing more than 2 years after the initial CENDX seems reasonable, as these lesions are usually atherosclerotic and likely have the same natural history as primary high-grade asymptomatic carotid lesions.

J.M. Seeger, M.D.

Long-term Prognosis and Effect of Endarterectomy in Patients With Symptomatic Severe Carotid Stenosis and Contralateral Carotid Stenosis or Occlusion: Results From NASCET

Gasecki AP, for the North American Symptomatic Carotid Endarterectomy Trial (NASCET) Group (Univ of Western Ontario, London, Canada)

J Neurosurg 83:778–782, 1995 13–4

Background.—Results from the North American Symptomatic Carotid Endarterectomy Trial clearly show that endarterectomy benefits patients having severe (70% or greater) carotid stenosis and either transient cerebral ischemia or a nondisabling stroke. The benefit appears to decline with the degree of carotid stenosis, however, as does the risk of stroke in patients receiving medical treatment. Possibly, the presence of disease in the contralateral carotid artery also modifies these effects.

Study Population.—The prognostic effects of contralateral carotid disease were examined in 659 patients with 70% to 99% stenosis of a carotid vessel and a recent ischemic event referable to this artery. The risk of ipsilateral stroke arising from the carotid artery associated with the index symptoms was compared in 559 patients with less than 70% stenosis of the contralateral carotid artery; 57 with 70% to 99% contralateral stenosis; and 42 patients in whom the contralateral carotid artery was occluded.

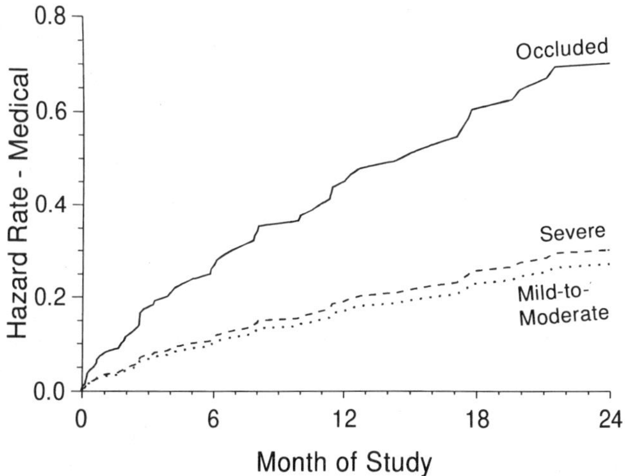

FIGURE 1.—Cumulative hazard curves show risk (hazard rate) of ipsilateral stroke for medically treated patients at 3 degrees of contralateral carotid artery disease. (Courtesy of Gasecki AP, for the North American Symptomatic Carotid Endarterectomy Trial [NASCET] Group. Long-term prognosis and effect of endarterectomy in patients with symptomatic severe carotid stenosis and contralateral carotid stenosis or occlusion: Results from NASCET. *J Neurosurg* 83:778–782, 1995.)

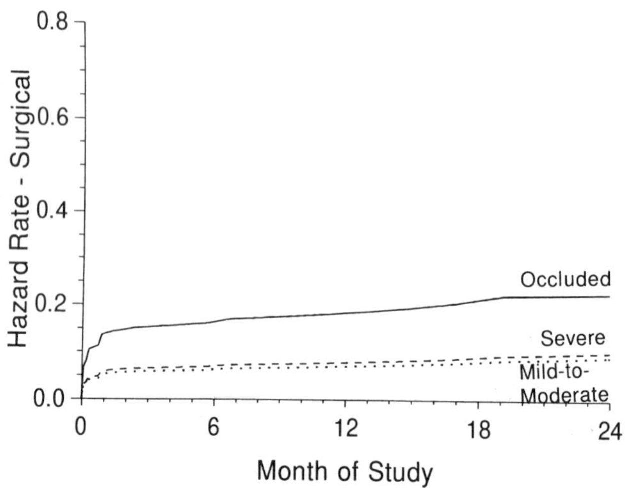

FIGURE 2.—Cumulative hazard curves show risk (hazard rate) of ipsilateral stroke for surgically treated patients at 3 degrees of contralateral carotid artery disease. (Courtesy of Gasecki AP, for the North American Symptomatic Carotid Endarterectomy Trial [NASCET] Group. Long-term prognosis and effect of endarterectomy in patients with symptomatic severe carotid stenosis and contralateral carotid stenosis or occlusion: Results from NASCET. *J Neurosurg* 83:778–782, 1995.)

Endarterectomy was done in 328 patients, whereas 331 were assigned to medical treatment. The average follow-up was 18 months.

Findings.—An occluded contralateral carotid artery significantly increased the risk of stroke associated with a severely stenosed index artery. The effect of an occluded contralateral carotid artery was much more evident for medically treated patients than for those undergoing endarterectomy (Figs 1 and 2). In addition, the risk of ipsilateral stroke during the first 30 days after endarterectomy was 14% if the contralateral carotid was occluded; 4% if it was severely stenosed but patent; and 5% if it was mildly to moderately narrowed. No strokes occurred in the region of the occluded contralateral vessel.

Conclusion.—Although an occluded contralateral carotid artery significantly increases the risk of stroke in patients with severe ipsilateral carotid stenosis, endarterectomy of the recently symptomatic vessel remains beneficial.

▶ Whether contralateral occlusion increases the risk of carotid endarterectomy remains controversial. This review of the North American Symptomatic Carotid Endarterectomy Trial data for patients with symptomatic stenosis of 70% to 99% suggests that it does increase the risk of perioperative stroke. However, despite this increased risk, the long-term benefit of carotid endarterectomy in this group of patients was evident, and the presence of a contralateral occlusion should not be used as a reason to withhold surgical treatment.

J.M. Seeger, M.D.

Aorto Iliac Disease

Historic Control Comparison of Outcome for Matched Groups of Patients Undergoing Endoluminal Versus Open Repair of Abdominal Aortic Aneurysms

White GH, May J, McGahan T, et al (Univ of Sydney, Australia)
J Vasc Surg 23:201–212, 1996 13–5

Introduction.—Transfemoral endoluminal graft repair of abdominal aortic aneurysms (AAA) appears to be a relatively safe management option for selected high-risk patients, but no studies have compared the morbidity and mortality of the open and endoluminal methods of AAA repair. Two matched groups of patients, each consisting of individuals who were fit and suitable to undergo either technique, were evaluated for outcome after open or endoluminal repair.

Patients and Methods.—The endoluminal repair group included 28 patients treated between May 1992 and November 1994. They were selected from a series of 62 consecutive patients; excluded were 28 at risk for open repair and 6 who failed endoluminal repair and were immediately converted to open operation. The open repair group (27 patients) was selected from a historical control cohort operated on between January 1991 and February 1992. Those in the open repair group underwent conventional AAA repair via midline transperitoneal approach (22 tube grafts and 5 bifurcated grafts). Twenty-two patients underwent a transfemoral approach for endoluminal repair (21 tube grafts and 2 bifurcated grafts), and 2 were treated with an iliac approach. The 2 groups were analyzed for length of operation, operative blood loss, type and size of the graft, duration of ICU admission, length of hospital stay, and complications.

Results.—Compared with open repair, endoluminal repair was associated with significantly less blood loss (873 vs. 1,422 mL) and shorter ICU stay (0.7 vs. 1.8 days). Local/vascular complications were more common in the endoluminal repair group (25% vs. 15%), but there were more remote/systemic complications in the open repair group (37% vs. 29%). Five patients who underwent endoluminal repair of AAA required early operative repair or late revision. When these failed procedures were included in the analysis, the incidence of local/vascular complications was significantly greater for endoluminal repair. Duration of operation and length of hospital stay were similar in the 2 groups.

Conclusion.—Patients with AAA who were medically suitable for either open or endoluminal repair did no worse when the endoluminal technique was used. However, this less invasive method yielded no advantages in terms of duration of operation, length of hospital stay, or perioperative morbidity and mortality. The benefits of endoluminal repair were decreased blood loss and shorter ICU stay.

▶ The presumed value of an endovascular, less invasive method to repair AAA has been a reduction in initial morbidity and mortality. This study questions whether that will be achieved, at least when currently available devices are used. Long-term problems with endoluminal aneurysm repair (such as anastomotic leaks, which can lead to subsequent aneurysm rupture) also continue to be reported. Clearly, endoluminal repair of AAA remains experimental and the place of this procedure in the management of patients with AAA is yet to be determined.

J.M. Seeger, M.D.

A Prospective Study of Anatomico-pathological Changes in Abdominal Aortic Aneurysms Following Endoluminal Repair: Is the Aneurysmal Process Reversed?

May J, White G, Yu W, et al (Univ of Sydney, Australia; Royal Prince Alfred Hosp, Australia)

Eur J Vasc Endovasc Surg 12:11–17, 1996 13–6

Background.—Endoluminal repair of abdominal aortic aneurysms (AAAs) is being increasingly performed. However, it is unknown whether an AAA will continue to grow around a graft placed transluminally and whether the natural progression of aneurysmal disease into the normal aortic wall proximal and distal to AAA will be arrested. Early anatomicopathologic changes in AAAs after endoluminal repair were analyzed prospectively to determine whether the natural history of continued AAA is reversed.

Methods.—Forty-seven patients undergoing AAA repair were divided into 2 groups based on the findings of serial contrast-enhanced CT. Thirty-nine patients (group 1) had a decrease and 8 (group 2) had an increase in the AAA maximum transverse diameter during follow-up.

Findings.—Contrast material leaks at the endoluminal graft attachment site were observed in 5 of group 2 patients and in none of group 1 patients. Additionally, in group 2 patients, change in the AAA maximum transverse diameter depended on whether the aneurysmal sac was isolated from the circulation. Regardless of this, the diameter of the proximal and distal necks increased in both groups, but the length of the necks did not shorten.

Conclusion.—During early follow-up after endoluminal repair, AAAs that decrease in diameter remain isolated from the general circulation. However, despite a decrease in the AAA diameter, the proximal and distal neck diameters increase but do not shorten.

▶ The critical question concerning endoluminal AAA repair is whether endoluminal grafting will exclude the AAA from the circulation and, thereby, prevent repair. This study, using serial CT scans, suggests that those aneurysms that decrease after endoluminal repair are isolated from the circulation, whereas those that increase are not, even if no leak at the graft fixation point is seen. What is potentially of more significance is that in this study, the neck of the repaired aneurysms continued to enlarge, regardless of how the aneurysms themselves changed size; this could lead to late leaks around the endoluminal graft. All of this means that endoluminal repair of AAAs using current devices is not as secure as surgical repair, and careful long-term observation will be necessary as aneurysm exclusion may not be permanent. Obviously, much remains to be learned about endoluminal aneurysm repair.

J.M. Seeger, M.D.

A Statewide, Population-based, Time-Series Analysis of the Outcome of Ruptured Abdominal Aortic Aneurysm

Rutledge R, Oller DW, Meyer AA, et al (Univ of North Carolina, Chapel Hill)
Ann Surg 223:492–505, 1996 13–7

Background.—The incidence of both abdominal aortic aneurysm (AAA) and ruptured AAA (RAAA) appears to be increasing with the aging population. The demographics and time course of RAAA and associations that might lead to a better or worse outcome were studied for a statewide population.

Methods.—Information was retrieved from 4 statewide medical data bases to determine the incidence; course; and associated patient, hospital, and physician characteristics for all patients admitted to any of North Carolina's 157 hospitals between 1988 and 1993 for AAA or RAAA. The effect on outcome of various independent variables was analyzed, with hospital survival serving as the dependent variable.

Results.—Of 14,138 admissions for AAA over the 6 years, 1,480 patients (10%) were found to have RAAA. Adjusted for population changes, the per capita rate of AAA rose 24.7% from 2.91 AAAs/10,000 population in 1988 to 3.63/10,000 population in 1993. The rate of RAAA increased over the same period from 0.31 RAAAs of 10,000 population in 1988 to 0.37 of 10,000 population in 1993. Overall, the mortality rate among hospitalized patients with RAAA was 54.9%, with most deaths occurring in the first 3 days. There was no significant improvement in the mortality rate over the 6 years. The death rate for the 307 women (20.7% of cases) was significantly higher (62.5%) than for men (52.9%). Survivors were significantly younger (mean, 69.2 years) than those who died (mean, 74.6 years). Shock, intestinal ischemia, and cardiac arrest were strongly associated with a poor outcome. Non–board-certified surgeons had a somewhat lower patient survival rate than those with board certification for RAAA. Physician experience with RAAA, but not experience with all AAAs, significantly affected patient survival. Surgery performed at smaller hospitals (< 100 beds) resulted in significantly greater mortality than at larger hospitals.

Conclusion.—Mortality in RAAA did not improve over 6 years, with women and older patients having the highest mortality rates. The experience of both physician and hospital affects the outcome.

Ruptured Abdominal Aortic Aneurysms: Who Should Be Offered Surgery?

Hardman DTA, Fisher CM, Patel MI, et al (Royal North Shore Hosp, St Leonards, Australia)

J Vasc Surg 23:123–129, 1996 13–8

Introduction.—Mortality remains high among patients who undergo surgery for ruptured abdominal aortic aneurysm (RAAA). (An increase in the elderly segment of the population and budgetary restraints on health care are factors that may influence the selection of patients for surgical intervention.) A retrospective study of patients with RAAA sought to identify admission characteristics predictive of surgical outcome.

Patients and Methods.—Between January 1985 and December 1993, 188 patients were admitted to a university teaching hospital with RAAA; 154 underwent surgery and had records available for review. Patients were prepared for operation as soon as RAAA was diagnosed. Surgery was not undertaken in cases of serious comorbidity, patient or guardian refusal, or when the attending surgeon judged the patient unsuitable. Mortality was defined as death, from any cause, within 30 days of operation or during the hospital stay.

Results.—Patients who did not undergo surgery had a mean age of 81.1 years, whereas those selected for surgery had a mean age of 71.4 years. Comorbidity was the most common reason for withholding surgical intervention. The hospital mortality rate was 39% for operated patients; 20 did not survive the operation and 34 died in-hospital. The median survival was 2 hours 10 minutes for 20 of the 21 patients who did not have surgical intervention. Preoperative variables that were significant independent risk factors for mortality were ECG ischemia, loss of consciousness after arrival, age > 76 years, creatinine level > 0.19 mmol/L, and hemoglobin < 9 g%. The likelihood of survival decreased as the number of risk factors in any individual patient increased (Table VI). No patient with all 5 risk

TABLE VI.—Mortality of Patients With Multivariate Model of 5 Equally Weighted Factors According to Number of Factors Present

No. of factors present	*No.*	*Deaths*	*Percent*
0	62	10	16%
1	52	19	37%
2	32	23	72%
3 or more	8	8	100%

Note: Missing data for individual patients given mean value for that variable.

(Courtesy of Hardman DTA, Fisher CM, Patel MI, et al: Ruptured abdominal aortic aneurysms: Who should be offered surgery? *J Vasc Surg* 23:123–129, 1996.)

factors survived. The subsequent mortality rate for survivors of surgery was particularly high among those in whom acute renal failure developed.

Conclusion.—The admission risk factors identified here may help to select patients with RAAA who are likely to benefit from surgery. Patients with none of the 5 significant risk factors had a mortality rate of 16%; a single risk factor more than doubled this rate to 37%. The rate of postoperative deaths, most of which are related to major organ failure, remains high.

▶ The mortality rate of RAAA remains high, and the cost associated with caring for patients with this problem is significant. As the incidence of RAAA is increasing, approaches such as regionalization of care of patients with RAAA and careful selection of patients with RAAA for treatment may soon be necessary. The first of these 2 studies (Abstract 13–7) shows survival after RAAA to be strongly influenced by the experience with the condition of the surgeon and hospital caring for the patient, whereas the second (Abstract 13–8) identifies clinical factors present before RAAA repair that may identify individual patients not likely to survive the disease.

J.M. Seeger, M.D.

Combined Aortic and Renal Artery Surgery: A Contemporary Experience

Benjamin ME, Hansen KJ, Craven TE, et al (Wake Forest Univ, Winston-Salem, NC)

Ann Surg 223:555–567, 1996 13–9

Background.—It is generally agreed that combined surgical treatment of aortic and renal artery disease should be performed in patients with symptomatic total aortic occlusion or a large aortic aneurysm in conjunction with renal artery stenosis or occlusion causing uncontrolled hypertension and azotemia. However, it is less clear whether simultaneous corrections should be undertaken in patients with either renal artery stenosis without functional significance or clinically silent aortoiliac disease. The risks and outcomes of combined aortic and renovascular procedures were compared with those associated with aortic or renal artery procedures alone.

Methods.—The records of 133 patients who underwent combined aortic and renovascular procedures, 182 patients who underwent isolated in situ renal artery repair, and 269 patients who underwent isolated aortic reconstruction were reviewed. The treatment groups were compared for perioperative and long-term survival, changes in hypertension status, and changes in renal function status. The significance of preoperative risk factors in predicting perioperative death was analyzed.

Results.—The perioperative mortality rate was 5.3% in the combined procedures group, 1.6% in the renal surgery group, and 0.7% in the aortic surgery group. No preoperative factors were found to have any significance in predicting perioperative death. There were no statistically significant differences in long-term survival among the 3 groups. Postoperatively, hypertension was cured or significantly reduced in 63% of the patients in the combined procedures group, which compared unfavorably with the 90% improvement rate in the renal surgery group. Renal function improved in 33% of the combined procedures group.

Conclusion.—Patients undergoing simultaneous aortic and renal artery reconstructions have a significantly higher risk of perioperative mortality than do patients undergoing aortic repair alone. These patients also have a lower rate of hypertension correction than do patients undergoing renal artery repair alone. Therefore, simultaneous aortic and renal artery repair should be reserved for patients with clinically significant disease.

▶ As the complexity of vascular reconstructive procedures increases, so does the risk of postoperative complications. In particular, combining aortic reconstruction with renal artery repair is associated with significantly increased morbidity and mortality, as shown here. This finding is similar to results of other recently reported studies (including a study of mortality after elective aortic reconstruction from our group). Thus, in these patients with extensive atherosclerosis, combined renal and aortic reconstruction should not be undertaken lightly and prophylactic repair of clinical "silent" renal artery disease during aortic procedures should probably be avoided.

J.M. Seeger, M.D.

Infrainguinal Occlusive Disease

Efficacy of Balloon Angioplasty of the Superficial Femoral Artery and Popliteal Artery in the Relief of Leg Ischemia

Stanley B, Teague B, Raptis S, et al (Univ of Adelaide, Australia)
J Vasc Surg 23:679–685, 1996 13–10

Background.—Because it is minimally invasive, percutaneous transluminal angioplasty (PTA) is often used to treat leg ischemia. However, its long-term efficacy has not been examined. The short- and long-term efficacy of PTA in treating severe ischemia or claudication caused by disease of the superficial femoral and popliteal arteries was studied.

Methods.—All patients undergoing PTA of the superficial femoral artery or popliteal artery during a 57-month period were re-evaluated for symptoms and signs of recurrent disease at 1, 3, and 6 months after the procedure and every 6 months thereafter. Duplex ultrasonography and arteriography were performed if indicated.

Results.—Patency, limb salvage, and patient survival were determined using life table analysis. One hundred seventy-six patients undergoing 200 angioplasties entered the study and were followed for a median of 25 months. Seventy-four percent of procedures were done for claudication relief and 26% for critical ischemia. Although 93% of procedures were technically successful, initially only 73% were clinically successful at 24 hours. Short occlusions and those with good distal runoff were significantly more likely to be associated with initial clinical successes. There were 51 complications (25%) in 45 procedures including 2 hemorrhages requiring surgical repair. Success rates were 69% at 1 month, 58% at 1 year, 46% at 2 years, and 26% at 5 years. Ten patients required amputation within 6 months after PTA and 1 at 63 months. Limb survival was 95% at 24 months, with significant predictors being good runoff and presentation with claudication instead of critical ischemia. Overall patient survival was 91% at 2 years, with those with claudication having significantly greater survival than those with severe ischemia.

Conclusion.—The use of PTA for claudication is not recommended, because the 2-year success rate is 49%, and the lesions most likely to remain patent are those that would be expected to do well with conservative management.

▶ This relatively large study with good long-term follow-up shows that balloon angioplasty of infrainguinal arteries is associated with only moderate long-term success. More importantly, *only* patients with short lesions and good runoff had patencies > 50% at 2 years. A recent study from another institution also found that the use of stents in infrainguinal arteries did not improve results in patients with longer lesions. Thus, endoluminal therapy of infrainguinal arterial disease is of only limited value at present.

J.M. Seeger, M.D.

Mid-term and Long-term Results With Directional Atherectomy of Vein Graft Stenoses

Porter DH, Rosen MP, Skillman JJ, et al (Beth Israel Hosp, Boston; Harvard Med School, Boston)

J Vasc Surg 23:554–567, 1996 13–11

Objective.—When stenoses develop in infrainguinal vein bypass grafts, they can be very difficult to treat by percutaneous transluminal angioplasty. These stenoses might respond better to directional atherectomy (DA) with potentially reduced restenosis rates and prolonged graft patency. An experience with DA for the treatment of stenoses in infrainguinal vein grafts was reported.

Methods.—The 6-year experience included 52 DA procedures performed in 42 patients. A total of 67 stenoses in 44 infrainguinal vein grafts were treated. The patients included 28 men and 14 women, mean age 72 years; the stenoses were asymptomatic in about half of patients, discovered only during routine follow-up. After DA, surveillance studies included ankle/brachial indexes, pulse volume recordings, and color-flow duplex ultrasonography. Eighteen patients had follow-up angiography; indications for angiography included recurrent symptoms, reduction in ankle/brachial index of greater than 0.15, a focal increase in peak systolic velocity, and incidental studies performed during evaluation of the opposite leg.

Results.—The initial technical success rate was 94%. Residual diameter stenosis of greater than 30% was left in 1 patient, and atherectomy could not be performed in another. The minor complication rate was 11% and the major complication rate 6%. The 3 major complications were 2 acute graft occlusions and 1 delayed pseudoaneurysm. None of the patients died within 30 days after surgery.

Eighty-two percent of grafts were patent and free of restenosis at a mean follow-up of 21 months. Eleven percent of grafts were patent but "failed" because of restenosis or pseudoaneurysm, and 5% were occluded. Seventy-five percent of extremities remained asymptomatic during follow-up. On life-table analysis of all 52 DA procedures, the cumulative primary atherectomy patency rate in the 44 grafts was 82% at 1 year, 78% at 2 years, and 78% at 3 years. For the 67 stenoses treated in the experience, cumulative patency rate was 86%, 83%, and 83%, respectively.

Conclusions.—Good results are achieved with DA for stenoses of infrainguinal vein grafts. Technical and clinical success rates are high, morbidity is acceptable, and patency rates are better than with percutaneous transluminal angioplasty. Additionally, the long-term patency rate of DA for vein graft stenoses appears comparable to that of surgical vein patch angioplasty.

▶ This study suggests that graft patency after treatment of a vein graft stenosis with DA is equivalent to patency after surgical repair of such lesions, and that DA should be used initially to treat such lesions because of lower costs. However, treated stenoses were short (<1 cm) and some were only 50%, which favorably influenced results. In addition, approximately one fourth of the patients in this study were lost to follow-up or died, which probably affected long-term patency rates. Thus, whether DA of vein graft stenoses will result in assisted graft patency equivalent to surgical repair remains to be determined. Furthermore, the argument for use of DA based on lower cost is likely no longer valid as surgical treatment of vein graft stenoses under local anesthesia, based on duplex ultrasound imaging alone, is more commonly done.

J.M. Seeger, M.D.

Results of a Prospective, Randomized Trial of Surgery Versus Thrombolysis for Occluded Lower Extremity Bypass Grafts

Comerota AJ, Weaver FA, Hosking JD, et al (Temple Univ, Philadelphia; Univ of Southern California, Los Angeles; Univ of North Carolina, Chapel Hill; et al)

Am J Surg 172:105–112, 1996 13–12

Background.—Leg bypass graft thrombosis usually requires surgical intervention. Some investigators have successfully restored graft patency using catheter-directed thrombolysis, but the value of thrombolysis in the management of bypass graft thrombosis remains unclear. Catheter-directed thrombolysis and surgical revascularization were compared in patients with leg bypass graft thrombosis in a prospective randomized study.

Methods.—After randomization, 124 patients (average age, 66.5 years) with ischemia as a result of thrombosed bypass grafts, were treated with intra-arterial catheter-directed thrombolysis using urokinase (250,000 U bolus followed by 4,000 U/min for 4 hours, then 2,000 U/min for as long as 36 hours, for 34 patients); recombinant plasminogen activator (rt-PA), 0.1 mg/kg/hr modified to 0.05 mg/kg/hr for as long as 12 hours (44 patients); or surgical revascularization (46 patients). Outcome was defined as failure to improve perfusion, repeat thrombosis, death, major amputation, or periprocedure or postoperative complications.

Results.—The average duration of graft occlusion was 34 days (14 days or less in 58 patients), and ischemia was limb threatening in 87 patients. In patients randomized to surgery, bypass grafts were replaced in 50% of patients, whereas 31% underwent thrombectomy and graft revision. In patients randomized to thrombolysis, catheter placement was successful in 61%, regardless of graft type; graft patency was restored in 84% of grafts in which catheter placement was successful; and the extent in the surgical procedure was reduced by 42%. Treatment with urokinase and rt-PA was equally successful. Overall, there was a better clinical outcome in the surgical group compared with the thrombolysis group. However, compared with surgery patients, patients receiving thrombolysis for ischemia present less than 14 days had a significantly lower amputation rate at 1 year, whereas those with ischemia for more than 14 days had a significantly higher rate of recurrent ischemia. Patients with occluded prosthetic grafts had more complications and a poorer outcome than those with occluded autogenous grafts, regardless of the type of treatment.

Conclusion.—Proper catheter positioning currently limits catheter-directed thrombolysis in the treatment of occluded bypass grafts. However, compared with patients treated surgically, patients with less than 14 days of ischemia and an occluded autogenous graft treated with thrombolysis have improved limb salvage.

Surgical Revascularization Versus Thrombolysis for Nonembolic Lower Extremity Native Artery Occlusions: Results of a Prospective Randomized Trial

Weaver FA, and the STILE Investigators (Univ of Southern California, Los Angeles)

J Vasc Surg 24:513–523, 1996 13–13

Background.—An initial report of the overall results of the STILE (Surgery Versus Thrombolysis for Ischemia of the Lower Extremity) trial for both lower extremity and graft occlusion was published in 1994. This report presents the final analysis of patients from that study who had native artery occlusion and were randomly assigned to either catheter-directed thrombolysis or surgical revascularization.

Methods.—In the subset of 237 patients reported here, 69 had iliac–common femoral artery (IF) occlusion and 168 had superficial femoral–popliteal artery (FP) occlusion; 150 were randomly assigned to thrombolysis and 87 to surgical revascularization. The optimal surgical procedure for each patient was determined before randomization. Of those receiving thrombolysis, 84 were randomly assigned to recombinant tissue plasminogen activator and 66 to urokinase. The primary study end point was the occurrence of at least 1 event of a composite clinical outcome (death, major amputation, ongoing or recurrent ischemia, major complications). Evaluations were performed at 30 days, 6 months, and 1 year.

Results.—The patients had a median age of 66 years; 68% were men. The median duration of ischemia was 59 days. Common risk factors for atherosclerotic occlusive disease were smoking history (79%), hypertension (57%), and diabetes mellitus (43%). At 30 days, a statistically significant increase was noted in ongoing or recurrent ischemia and composite clinical outcome for the thrombolytic group (both the IF and FP subgroups). No patient in the surgical revascularization group required amputation during follow-up, but 14 major amputations were performed in patients with FP occlusions who were treated with thrombolysis. One-year mortality rates were similar in the surgery and lysis groups. Among patients randomly assigned to lysis, this therapy allowed approximately 50% to have subsequent surgical procedures of lesser magnitude than the "best" surgical procedure as determined before randomization.

Discussion.—In these prospectively studied patients with lower extremity native artery occlusions, surgical revascularization was a more effective and durable treatment than thrombolysis, although lysis often allows a lesser surgical procedure to be performed. The long-term outcome after thrombolysis is also inferior to that of surgical revascularization. Factors associated with poor outcome after thrombolysis are FP occlusion, diabetes, and critical ischemia.

▶ The STILE study, a prospective randomized comparison of catheter-directed thrombolysis and surgery in patients with arterial or bypass graft occlusion, clearly demonstrated thrombolytic therapy to be inferior to surgical revascularization. However, an intent-to-treat analysis was used in the initial analysis of the data from the STILE study, which may have biased against thrombolytic therapy, because thrombolytic catheters could not be successfully placed in a significant number of patients randomly assigned to thrombolysis. These 2 subsequent analyses of the STILE data (Abstracts 13–12 and 13–13, separate studies for bypass graft occlusion and native arterial occlusion) include per protocol analysis, which includes only the patients who had a thrombolytic catheter successfully placed and longer follow-up. However, these studies do little to identify subgroups of patients with arterial or bypass graft occlusion who may benefit from thrombolytic therapy. From these 2 studies, it appears that patients with short durations of ischemia (less than 14 days), autogenous bypass graft occlusion, or iliofemoral native arterial occlusions may be those most likely to benefit from thrombolytic therapy. In addition, the magnitude of the planned surgical procedure and the mortality associated with treatment of a femoropopliteal occlusion may be reduced by thrombolysis. However, these benefits appear to be achieved at the price of an increased risk of recurrent ischemia and/or subsequent amputation compared with standard surgical therapy. Because of this, I think that thrombolysis is primarily useful in patients at high risk for surgical treatment and/or those with few reconstructive alternatives.

J.M. Seeger, M.D.

Ongoing Vascular Laboratory Surveillance Is Essential to Maximize Long-term in Situ Saphenous Vein Bypass Patency

Erickson CA, Towne JB, Seabrook GR, et al (Med College of Wisconsin, Milwaukee; Zablocki VA Med Ctr, Milwaukee, Wis)

J Vasc Surg 23:18–27, 1996 13–14

Introduction.—Up to one third of infrainguinal autogenous vein bypass grafts will require intervention during follow-up because of the development of lesions than can lead to graft failure. Some grafts, including those constructed with spliced vein segments and those injured and repaired during the initial procedure, may be at increased risk for subsequent problems. The records of a series of patients with autogenous vein grafts were reviewed to quantitate the length of time graft surveillance was required.

Methods.—From January 1981 to October 1994, 380 men and 119 women underwent 556 lower extremity autogenous vein bypasses at the study institution. The conduit used was in situ saphenous vein in 97% of cases; critical limb ischemia was the most common indication for grafting. A surveillance protocol for patient monitoring consisted of clinical evaluation and serial noninvasive hemodynamic testing. After initial postoperative studies, patients were evaluated every 3 months during the first 2 years and every 6 months therafter. Defined abnormal findings included the presence of postoperative arteriovenous fistulas, retained valves, structural abnormalities, and blood flow patterns that suggested 50% to 75% graft diameter reduction.

Results.—Cumulative patient survival was 91% after 1 year, 68% after 5 years, and 37% after 10 years. Serial hemodynamic data, available for analysis in 462 grafts, revealed 450 abnormalities in 236 grafts or limbs (51%). Most (65%) occurred within the first 2 years of follow-up, but 35% of abnormalities were detected after 2 years. In 50 of 169 grafts (30%) free of abnormalities at 24 months, at least 1 abnormality subsequently developed, and 11% of grafts free of abnormalities at 24 months went on to fail. The median interval from vascular surgery to detection of an abnormality varied with the location of the defect, with lesions occurring at a median of 6 months in the conduit, at a median of 8.5 months at the proximal anastomosis, and at a median of 7 months at the distal anastomosis. In addition, progression of inflow disease threatened the graft at a median of 15 months and outflow disease at a median of 29 months.

Conclusion.—The patency of infrainguinal autogenous vein bypass grafts is at risk even years after the initial procedure. Regular surveillance can identify lesions amenable to revision and ensure the best long-term outcome.

► The value of vein bypass graft surveillance using duplex scanning is clear. However, it is also expensive and the optimum frequency and duration of surveillance remain to be determined. This study shows that lesions that can threaten the patency of a bypass continue to develop years after bypass construction, suggesting that perpetual surveillance is necessary. Whether such a program will be cost effective remains to be determined, but repair of lesions before graft failure will likely be less expensive than repeat bypass procedures or amputations.

J.M. Seeger, M.D.

Duplex Ultrasonography to Diagnose Failing Arterial Prosthetic Grafts

Calligaro KD, Musser DJ, Chen AY, et al (Thomas Jefferson Med College, Philadelphia)

Surgery 120:455–459, 1996 13–15

Objective.—Duplex ultrasonography (DU) is a useful technique for diagnosing malfunctioning or failing autologous vein bypasses. The value of DU as a surveillance tool for prosthetic bypass grafts has not been established. The diagnostic value of DU compared with other noninvasive methods for diagnosing failing arterial prosthetic grafts was evaluated, and a cost-benefit analysis of the use of the noninvasive vascular laboratory for surveillance of such grafts was undertaken.

Methods.—Prospectively 59 patients (19 women), aged 51 to 91 years, with 85 prosthetic grafts were entered into a noninvasive vascular laboratory graft surveillance program. There were 35 femoropopliteal, 16 femorotibial, 15 iliofemoral, 13 axillofemoral, and 6 femorofemoral grafts, 75 of which were polytetrafluoroethylene and 10 of which were Dacron. Duplex ultrasonography and other noninvasive techniques were performed 1 week after surgery, at 3-month intervals for 1 year, and at 6-month intervals thereafter. Changes in symptoms or pulses, a decrease in ankle pulse of volume recordings > 50%, or a decrease in ankle/brachial index of > 0.15 were criteria for graft failure. Grafts that remained patent for 3 months and had < 50% stenosis were termed normal, and those that underwent thrombosis, required revision, or had > 50% stenosis were termed problem grafts. Patients were followed for 3 to 36 months.

Results.—Sensitivity for predicting problem grafts was significantly higher for DU (81%; 17 of 21) than for other methods (24%; 5 of 21). Specificity for normal grafts was similar for DU (93%; 54 of 58) and for other methods (94%; 60 of 64). The negative predictive values for the DU and non-DU methods were 93% (54 of 58) and 79% (60 of 76), and the positive predictive values were 63% (17 of 27) and 56% (5 of 9), respectively. The overall accuracies were 84% (71 of 85) and 77% (65 of 85) for DU and non-DU procedures, respectively. Thromboses developed in only 7% of grafts found to be normal by DU and in 21% of grafts found to be normal by other methods. Stenotic lesions that led to 21 graft failures were perianastomotic in 10 cases, in adjacent inflow or outflow arteries in 8, and within the graft in 3.

Conclusion.—Duplex ultrasonography is more accurate than non-DU techniques in predicting prosthetic graft failure and should be performed routinely for arterial prosthetic grafts survaillence.

▶ Routine surveillance using DU ultrasonography has been clearly shown to improve the patency of autologous vein bypass grafts, and this study suggests that similar improved results can be obtained when surveillance is done on prosthetic bypass grafts. We have also found that routine surveillance of prosthetic grafts detects lesions that threaten graft patency. However, in the study reported here, grafts were examined every 3 months to achieve this result, and a significant number of false positive studies occurred, prompting unnecessary arteriography. Thus, it is uncertain whether routine surveillance of prosthetic bypass grafts will prove to be cost-effective.

J.M. Seeger, M.D.

Results of a Policy With Arm Veins Used as the First Alternative to an Unavailable Ipsilateral Greater Saphenous Vein for Infrainguinal Bypass

Hölzenbein TJ, Pomposelli FB Jr, Miller A, et al (Harvard Med School, Boston)

J Vasc Surg 23:130–140, 1996 13–16

Objective.—The performance of an arm vein graft as the primary alternative to contralateral saphenous vein was assessed retrospectively in patients without a suitable ipsilateral saphenous vein.

Patients and Methods.—Patients were 143 men and 81 women with a mean age of 68.3 years; 82.6% had diabetes. Bypass grafts in this consecutive series were divided into 3 groups according to indication for operation. Eighty-five grafts were primary and involved patients whose first distal bypass procedure was performed on this extremity. There were 103 repeat grafts in patients who had failure of a previous graft on the same leg. The other 62 grafts were in patients who underwent revision of a previously placed distal arterial reconstructive operation on the ipsilateral leg. Vein configuration and orientation of the vein graft, quality of the vein as assessed by angioscopy, frequency and location of endoluminal disease, and subsequent surgical decisions were examined for impact on graft patency. Patients were followed for graft patency, limb salvage, and survival.

Results.—All but 2 procedures were performed for limb salvage. A total of 114 femorotibial-pedal, 62 jump or interposition, 41 femoropopliteal, and 33 popliteodistal grafts were constructed; 199 grafts were single vein and 51 were composite vein. The cephalic vein alone was the source in 50.4% of cases, the basilic vein alone in 14%, and both cephalic and basilic vein in 35.6%. Approximately half of the procedures required interventions guided by angioscopy to "upgrade" the graft. Early (≤30 days) patency, 94.5% overall, did not differ significantly among anatomic subgroups. At 1 year, cumulative primary patency was 70.6%, secondary patency was 76.9%, and limb salvage was 88.2%. Limb salvage at 3 years was 51.9% for primary grafts, 56.7% for revision grafts, and 42.4% for repeat grafts. In 22 of 97 (22.7%) procedures where the contralateral saphenous vein was available, it was used for contralateral limb revascularization during follow-up.

Conclusion.—Arm veins are easily accessible and can yield excellent patency rates in patients threatened with loss of the limb who lack an adequate ipsilateral saphenous vein. This allows the contralateral saphenous vein to be saved for subsequent contralateral revascularization which is commonly necessary at least in patients with diabetes mellitus.

▶ This article reports reasonable results with arm vein as conduit of choice for infrainguinal bypass when ipsilateral greater saphenous vein was absent. The results agree with several previous studies in which the long term patency of infrainguinal bypass with arm vein has been shown to be superior to the patency of prosthetic infrapopliteal bypass grafts, but inferior to the patency of greater saphenous vein infrainguinal bypass grafts. What is surprising is the justification of this approach based on a prediction that up to 60% of contralateral greater saphenous veins will subsequently be needed for reconstruction of that extremity. This contradicts previous reports, which found that the need for bypass in the opposite extremity was uncommon so that use of the contralateral saphenous did not compromise later limb salvage. However, this finding may be true in diabetics requiring infrainguinal bypass because of the relatively high incidence of subsequent contralateral ischemia in such patients.

J.M. Seeger, M.D.

Infrapopliteal Bypasses to Severely Calcified, Unclampable Outflow Arteries: Two-Year Results

Misare BD, Pomposelli FB Jr, Gibbons GW, et al (Harvard Med School, Boston)

J Vasc Surg 24:6–16, 1996 13–17

Objective.—Although calcification of distal outflow vessels can lead to poor results after distal infrapopliteal reconstruction, the prognostic value of such calcification on graft patency and limb salvage has not been thoroughly studied. Results of a retrospective study assessing the effects of

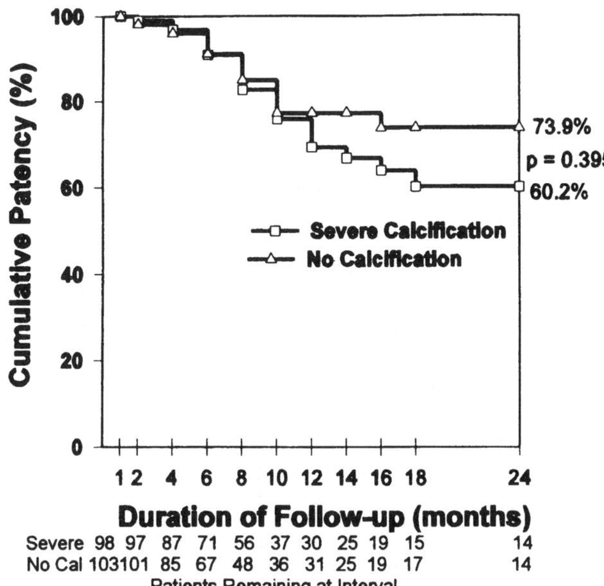

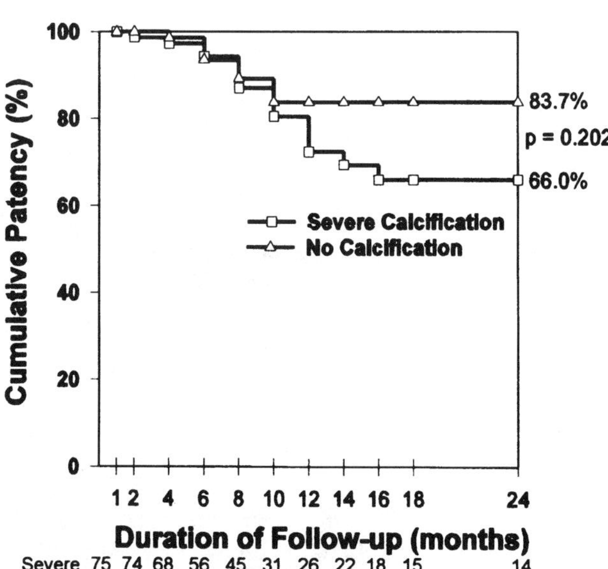

FIGURE 2.—Twenty-four-month primary graft patency rate for infrapopliteal bypasses by log-rank life-table analysis. **Top graph** summarizes data for all cases. **Bottom graph** includes data from bypasses performed as the primary procedure only. (Courtesy of Misare BD, Pomposelli FB Jr, Gibbons GW, et al: Infrapopliteal bypasses to severely calcified, unclampable outflow arteries: Two-year results. *J Vasc Surg* 24:6–16, 1996.)

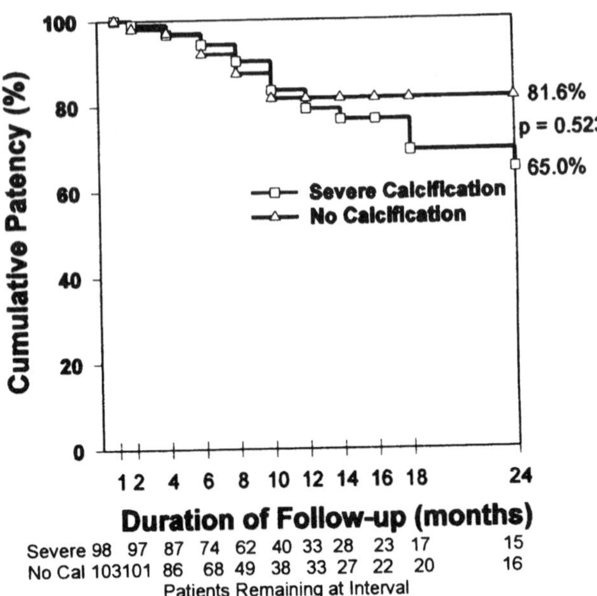

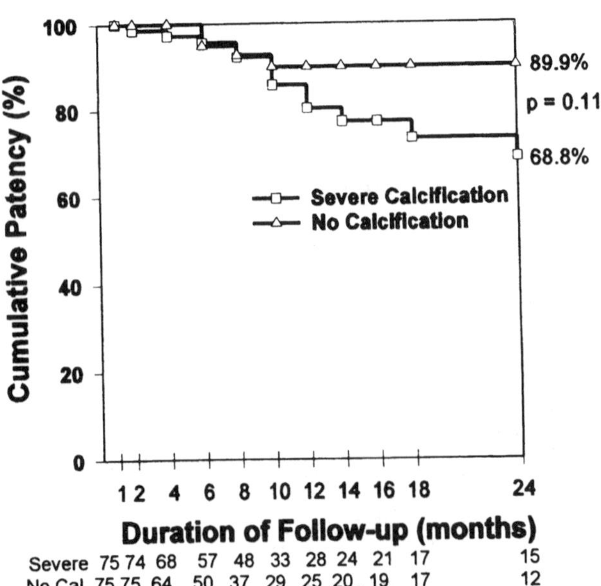

FIGURE 3.—Twenty-four-month secondary graft patency rate for infrapopliteal bypasses by log-rank life-table analysis. **Top graph** demonstrates patency rate for all cases. **Bottom graph** summarizes results, excluding secondary procedures. (Courtesy of Misare BD, Pomposelli FB Jr, Gibbons GW, et al: Infrapopliteal bypasses to severely calcified, unclampable outflow arteries: Two-year results. *J Vasc Surg* 24:6–16, 1996.)

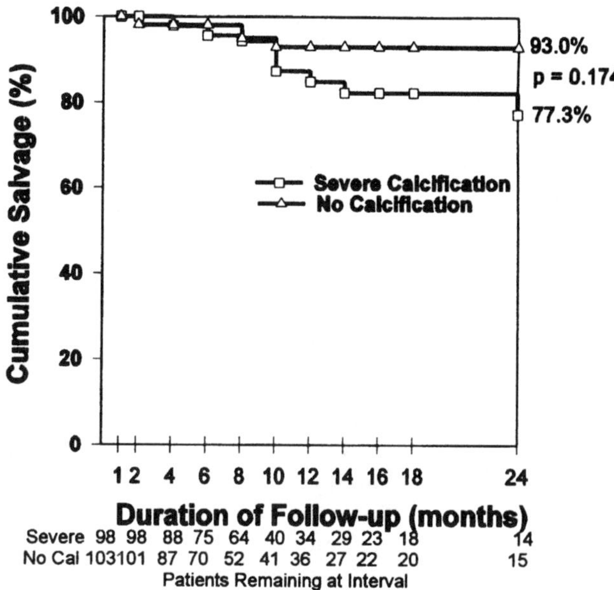

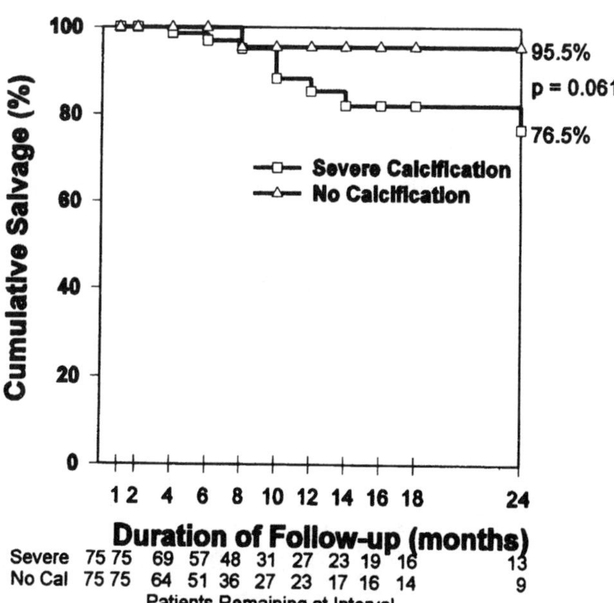

FIGURE 4.—Twenty-four-month foot salvage rates by log-rank life-table analysis. **Top graph** shows results for all cases included in the study. **Bottom graph** illustrates data for primary bypass procedures only. (Courtesy of Misare BD, Pomposelli FB Jr, Gibbons GW, et al: Infrapopliteal bypasses to severely calcified, unclampable outflow arteries: Two-year results. *J Vasc Surg* 24:6–16, 1996.)

circumferential crural and pedal arterial calcification on distal bypass graft patency and limb salvage rates were presented.

Methods.—A retrospective review was conducted of 93 patients (27 female) aged 29 to 90 years who underwent 101 infrapopliteal bypass operations to severely calcified and unclampable outflow arteries, and 99 patients (38 female) aged 37 to 91 years who underwent 105 similar bypass operations in which no calcification was present in the outflow arteries. The procedures were performed between 1990 and 1995 at 1 hospital. Patients with calcification were significantly more likely to have diabetes mellitus, renal failure, dependency on dialysis, and a transplanted kidney. In 90% of patients with calcification and 84% of patients without calcification, bypass surgery was performed for limb-threatening ischemia, nonhealing ulcers, or gangrene/cellulitis. Five surgeons performed all bypass operations in a similar manner. Patients with calcification were more likely to receive popliteal inflow grafts, whereas patients without calcification were more likely to receive femoral level inflow grafts. Autogenous veins were used in 90% of operations.

Results.—Patients were followed for an average of 12.7 months. The 30-day graft patency rates were similar for patients with and without calcification (99% vs. 98%). Primary patency rates at 24 months were similar for the 2 groups (Fig 2). Secondary patency rates were also similar between the 2 groups (Fig 3). For primary procedures, foot salvage rates tended to be higher in patients without calcification than in patients with calcification (Fig 4). The operative mortality rate at 30 days for both groups was 1%. The survival at 24 months was 84% in the group with calcification and 83% in the group without calcification.

Conclusion.—Severely calcified, unclampable outflow arteries can be used successfully as outflow sites for infrapopliteal bypass grafts with no increase in graft failure rate and only a slight decrease in long-term limb salvage.

▶ As this report shows, infrapopliteal arterial calcification alone does not preclude successful bypass, and severe calcification should not be an indication of an unreconstructable situation. Long-term limb salvage may be somewhat worse in patients with such arteries, but use of appropriate techniques will allow limb preservation in approximately 75% of patients for at least 2 years.

J.M. Seeger, M.D.

Prospective Comparison of Infrainguinal Bypass Grafting in Patients With and Without Antiphospholipid Antibodies

Lee RW, Taylor LM Jr, Landry GJ, et al (Oregon Health Sciences Univ, Portland)

J Vasc Surg 24:524–533, 1996 13–18

Introduction.—The association between autoantibodies to phospholipid (APLs) and leg arterial disease has been documented in numerous retrospective studies and case reports. In this prospective study, the results of infrainguinal revascularization in patients who were APL positive and patients who were APL negative were compared.

Methods.—From 1990 to 1994, all patients admitted to a vascular surgery service for elective leg revascularization procedures were evaluated for hypercoagulable states: anticardiolipin antibodies (ACLs), lupus anticoagulant (LA), protein C, protein S, and antithrombin III. Results of screening for hypercoagulable states were not known at the time of surgery and, thus, did not influence perioperative decisions. Patients were evaluated every 3 months for 1 year, then every 6 months for life. Data recorded included demographic information, medical history, primary patency, limb salvage, and survival.

Results.—Laboratory tests for the presence of a hypercoagulable state were obtained in 262 of 307 patients (85%); these 262 patients underwent 327 bypass procedures. Hypercoagulable states were identified in 84 patients (32%) (102 leg bypass procedures). Seventy of these patients had ACLs only, 11 had LA only, and 2 had both ACLs and LA. Patients who were APL-positive had postoperative warfarin therapy nearly twice as often as APL-negative patients, but the 2 groups were otherwise similar in demographics, patient characteristics, and operative factors. In the APL-positive group, rates for life-table 4-year primary patency, assisted primary patency, limb salvage, and survival rates were 43%, 72%, 79%, and 67%, retrospectively; in the APL-negative group, the corresponding values were 59%, 73%, 88%, and 66%. Only the difference in primary patency at 4 years was of borderline statistical significance. Within the APL-positive group, patients who received warfarin therapy had a lower 4-year primary patency rate (34%) than those who did not receive the therapy (52%).

Discussion.—Approximately one third of this group of patients scheduled for elective lower extremity bypass procedures were APL-positive, and most of the APLs identified were ACLs (87%). In contrast to findings of some previous studies, patients with APLs did not differ significantly from those without APLs in rates of graft primary patency, graft-assisted primary patency, limb salvage, or survival. Thus, APLs do not appear to be a contraindication to leg revascularization procedures.

▶ This study shows that patients with APLs can undergo infrainguinal bypass grafting with results that are similar to those of patients without this hypercoagulable state. However, from this study, it should not be concluded that hypercoagulable states such as APL do not affect bypass graft patency as there were many potentially confounding variables in this study, including unequal coumadin use in patients with APLs compared with controls as well as low bypass graft patency in controls. Regardless, as the authors appropriately state, the presence of APLs should not be regarded as a contraindication to indicated leg bypass procedures.

J.M. Seeger, M.D.

Venous Disease

Duplex Ultrasonography Scanning for Chronic Venous Disease: Patterns of Venous Reflux

Myers KA, Ziegenbein RW, Zeng GH, et al (Monash Univ, Melbourne, Australia)

J Vasc Surg 21:605–612, 1995 13–19

Background.—It is generally believed that lipodermatosclerosis and venous ulceration associated with chronic venous disease are caused by reduced valve function in the deep and perforating veins, leading to chronic congestion in the calf muscle venous plexuses. However, this belief has been challenged by recent findings suggesting that deep venous reflux is uncommon and that outward flow in perforators occurs commonly in healthy patients. Patterns of venous flow were studied by duplex ultrasonography in patients with both uncomplicated and complicated varicose veins.

Methods.—Duplex ultrasonography scanning was performed on 776 lower limbs with primary uncomplicated varicose veins, 70 limbs with lipodermatosclerosis, and 96 limbs with past venous ulceration. Venous flow was studied in the long and short saphenous veins; the common femoral, superficial femoral, and popliteal veins; the 3 sets of crural veins; and the medial calf perforators. Differences between the findings in the different patient groups were analyzed.

Results.—Deep venous obstruction was found in only 2 limbs, including 1 with lipodermatosclerosis and 1 with past venous ulceration. In patients with uncomplicated varicose veins, lipodermatosclerosis, or past ulceration, superficial venous reflux alone was seen in 55%, 39%, and 38%, respectively; deep venous reflux in 2%, 2%, and 8%, respectively; and combined superficial and deep reflux in 18%, 34%, and 48%, respectively. There was outward flow in the medial calf perforators in 57% of the limbs with uncomplicated varicose veins, 67% of the limbs with lipodermatosclerosis, and 66% of the limbs with past ulceration.

Conclusion.—Deep venous reflux caused by incompetent deep vein valves was rare in patients with and without complications of venous stasis disease, whereas outward flow through medial calf perforators was seen frequently in limbs without complications. These findings contradict the common belief that deep and perforator venous disease typically causes complications of venous disease and indicates the greater significance of superficial reflux.

▶ This study challenges the conventional wisdom that deep venous valvular reflux and perforator incompetence are the primary causes of complications of venous disease. If superficial venous reflux is a major contributor to the pathophysiology of lipodermatosclerosis and ulceration, as reported here, then procedures to interrupt this superficial reflux would be indicated, and the more complex procedures to repair deep venous reflux would be unnecessary.

J.M. Seeger, M.D.

Progression of Superficial Venous Thrombosis to Deep Vein Thrombosis

Chengelis DL, Bendick PJ, Glover JL, et al (William Beaumont Hosp, Royal Oak, Mich)

J Vasc Surg 24:745–749, 1996 13–20

Introduction.—Superficial venous thrombosis at the saphenofemoral junction is often treated with ligation to avoid the risk of progression to deep venous thrombosis (DVT) or embolization. However, little is known about the natural history of more distal superficial venous thrombosis without deep venous involvement. A group of patients with such findings were studied to determine the frequency of progression to DVT, including femoral popliteal involvement, and response to treatment.

Methods.—During a 4-year period, 263 patients referred to the vascular laboratory for lower extremity venous duplex examinations had superficial venous thrombosis without deep venous involvement. During initial and follow-up duplex scans, the femoropopliteal and deep calf veins were evaluated in their entirety. Follow-up studies, done at an average of 6.3 days, were compared with results of the initial examinations for evidence of disease progression into the deep veins.

Results.—Thirty patients (11%) had documented progression to deep venous involvement. Twenty-one patients (70%) had progression from the greater saphenous vein in the thigh to the common femoral vein. Eighteen of these extensions were nonocclusive, and 12 had a free-floating component. Three patients had extended above-knee saphenous vein thrombi into the femoral vein, 3 had extended below knee saphenous thrombi into the popliteal vein, and 3 had extended below-saphenous thrombi into the tibial perineal veins. Patients with progression to DVT had a mean age of 63 years; none had received anticoagulation therapy after the initial study. Risk factors included recent surgery in 7 cases, active malignancy in 9, lengthy immobilization in 2, and a history of superficial thrombophlebitis in 2. Common findings at physical examination were medial leg tenderness in 26 patients, a palpable cord in 20, erythematous streaking near the most proximal site of involvement in 15, and varicose veins in 11. The initial treatment was anticoagulation in 29 patients, 2 of whom subsequently underwent surgical ligation of the saphenofemoral junction. Nine of 10 patients observed for more than 1 month after DVT was diagnosed had some degree of resolution of the thrombus.

Discussion.—All but 3 of these 30 patients who progressed from untreated superficial venous thrombosis to DVT had progression into the femoropopliteal system, placing them at increased risk for significant pulmonary embolism. Anticoagulation and/or serial duplex evaluation should be used in cases of proximal saphenous vein thrombosis because of the risk of progression to DVT. When more distal superficial venous thrombosis is present, patients should be carefully followed clinically and examined with repeat duplex ultrasonography if symptoms worsen or progression occurs.

▶ This study is retrospective and uncontrolled so that all patients with lower extremity superficial venous thrombosis certainly did not undergo serial follow-up examinations. Thus, the true incidence of progression of superficial venous thrombosis to DVT cannot be determined. Regardless, this study shows that even distal superficial venous thrombosis should not be considered a benign condition, as it can progress to DVT. On the basis of this observation, it appears that, at a minimum, superficial venous thrombosis should be carefully followed with repeat venous duplex examinations. In addition, as suggested by the authors of this study, treatment with anticoagulation or saphenous ligation potentially should be considered for superficial venous thrombosis close to the saphenofemoral junction.

J.M. Seeger, M.D.

Low-Molecular-Weight Heparins and Unfractionated Heparin in the Treatment of Patients With Acute Venous Thromboembolism: Results of a Meta-Analysis

Siragusa S, Cosmi B, Piovella F, et al (IRCCS Policlinico S Matteo, Pavia, Italy; McMaster Univ, Hamilton, Ontario, Canada)

Am J Med 100:269–277, 1996 13–21

Background.—Use of low molecular weight heparins (LMWHs) has been shown to be at least as effective as unfractionated heparin (UFH) in treating venous thrombosis. In addition, their use does not require close monitoring. Estimates of the relative efficacy and safety of LMWH, compared to UFH, were developed by meta-analysis of published trials.

Methods.—A computerized search of MEDLINE and Excerpta Medica from 1980 to 1994 was conducted to identify studies of randomized treatment of documented venous thrombosis and/or pulmonary embolus with LMWH and UFH. Two investigators reviewed each identified study, using previously established criteria. Efficacy and safety of therapy were compared for days 1 to 15, a period reflecting immediate results of heparin therapy; days 16 to 90, a period of continued oral anticoagulant therapy; and overall (days 1 to 90).

Results.—Thirteen studies met criteria for inclusion. Studies reporting symptomatic recurrence of venous thrombosis showed a significant risk reduction of 68% for days 1 to 15 and of 50% overall (days 1 to 90), favoring LMWH. Low molecular weight heparin showed a significant advantage both in reducing thrombus size and in minimizing an increase in thrombus size. Furthermore, a significant reduction of risk for major bleeding (66%) was seen in favor of LMWH, and overall, LMWH was associated with significantly lower mortality (49% risk reduction) compared with UFH. For the subgroup of thrombosis patients with cancer, a significant decrease in mortality was seen with LMWH for the overall study period. Death caused by autopsy documented pulmonary emboli was equivalent for LMWH and UFH.

Conclusion.—Unmonitored LMWHs are at least as safe and effective as UFH for treating venous thromboembolism and are probably more effective and safer than UFH for the treatment of deep venous thrombosis.

▶ Multiple studies have shown LMWH to be equivalent to UFH in the management of venous thromboembolism. However, LMWH is considerably more expensive than UFH and, thus, must produce superior results to be cost-effective. This meta-analysis suggests that use of LMWH is actually more effective in preventing recurrent venous thromboembolism, produces less bleeding, and potentially leads to decreased mortality compared with UFH—at least in patients with cancer and acute deep venous thrombosis. Hopefully, large enough single studies will soon confirm or reject these conclusions based on pooled data and will also examine the cost-effectiveness of this new anticoagulant.

J.M. Seeger, M.D.

Miscellaneous

Intraoperative Heparinisation, Blood Loss and Myocardial Infarction During Aortic Aneurysm Surgery: A Joint Vascular Research Group Study

Thompson JF, Mullee MA, Bell PRF, et al (Royal Devon & Exeter Hosp, England)

Eur J Vasc Endovasc Surg 12:86–90, 1996 13–22

Background.—Patients who undergo vascular reconstructive surgery commonly receive intraoperative IV heparin to prevent thrombosis caused by stasis distal to blood vessel clamps. However, some surgeons avoid heparin for fear of increased bleeding, postoperative complications, and blood transfusions. Few data exist about the association between bleeding or thrombosis and intraoperative heparin. The effects of IV heparin on perioperative bleeding and thrombosis were studied in patients who underwent elective surgery for abdominal aortic aneurysm (AAA).

Methods.—The prospective, randomized trial included 284 patients who underwent primary surgery for elective repair of AAA. They were assigned to receive either IV heparin, 5,000 IU before aortic cross-clamping, or no heparin at all. The 2 groups were similar in age, sex, weight, aneurysm size, hemoglobin concentration, platelet count, and ankle/brachial indices.

Results.—There were no significant differences in blood loss or units of blood transfused. The incidence of distal thrombosis was also similar between groups. Surprisingly, there was a significant difference in the rate of fatal perioperative myocardial infraction (MI): 5.7% in the non-heparin group vs. 1.4% in the heparin group. The overall rate of MI, which included nonfatal MI, was 8.5% and 2.0%, respectively. Although the study was not designed to test this outcome, the 2 groups were believed to be comparable in their cardiac risk factors.

Conclusions.—Neither blood loss nor the need for blood transfusion is increased by IV heparin in patients who undergo AAA repair. Furthermore, heparin is not necessary to prevent distal thrombosis. However, if given before aortic cross-clamping, heparin does appear to reduce the incidence of perioperative MI, including fatal MI.

▶ The findings of this study that anticoagulation during AAA repair does not increase blood loss and that a decision not to use heparin does not increase the risk of distal thrombosis are not surprising. In contrast, the finding that heparinization may be protective against intraoperative MI is unexpected. A previous study of use of thrombolysis during peripheral arterial reconstruction also documented a decreased risk of perioperative MI, which suggests that this may be a real and important observation.

J.M. Seeger, M.D.

The Importance of Complete Follow-up for Results After Femoro-infrapopliteal Vascular Surgery

Jensen LP, Nielsen OM, Schroeder TV (Natl Univ, Rigshospitalet, Copenhagen)

Eur J Vasc Endovasc Surg 12:282–286, 1996 13–23

Background.—Vascular registries commonly used to determine bypass graft patency contain data on patients with variable length of follow-up. Because of this, analysis of registry data often uses life-table methods which assume that any withdrawn patients (shorter length of follow-up) have the same probability of events (such as graft failure) as patients with maximum follow-up. To examine the validity of this assumption in patients with peripheral vascular disease, graft patency rates calculated from registry data using life-table methods were compared with patency rates determined from complete follow-up of the same patients.

Methods.—Prospective data from 102 patients undergoing infrainguinal bypass between October 1990 and June 1992 were collected as part of a clinical trial of adjunctive medical treatment of femoral infrapopliteal bypass. All patients were examined at 3 and 12 months and follow-up was complete at 1 year. Graft patency, limb salvage, and patient survival determined from these data were then compared with similar results for the same patients calculated from registry data collected as part of a standard follow-up protocol at 6 weeks and 3, 6, 9, 12, 24, 36, 48, and 60 months.

Results.—The primary and secondary graft patency rates at 1 year were 68% and 90%, respectively, in the vascular registry and 52% and 63%, respectively, in the clinical trial. Similarly, limb survival and patient survival rates were 97% and 95% for the vascular registry data and 77% and 85% for data from the clinical trial study. These differences could be explained by the significant number of vascular registry patients (50) who did not complete follow-up and the fact that patients who did not complete follow-up were found to have a significant increase in amputation, graft thrombosis, and death.

Conclusion.—The life-table analysis assumption that patients who do not complete follow-up experience the same probabilities of events as patients who are observed for a long period of time is inaccurate. Because of this, the accuracy of life-table results is dependent on the completeness of follow-up, and life-table plots should be supplemented with information on the number of patients lost to follow-up.

▶ This interesting paper raises a very valid concern regarding the increasing use of the life-table method of analyzing follow-up data in the vascular surgical literature. The life-table method is based on the assumption that patients who do not complete follow-up will behave similarly to those who complete the follow-up period being studied. However, as is shown in this study, patients may have discontinued follow-up because of poor outcomes, and life-table analysis of registry data can make long-term results look better than actual results derived from complete follow-up. This means that life-table data must be carefully examined for completeness of follow-up and that, if follow-up is incomplete or information about follow-up is not available, conclusions drawn from such data must be taken with a grain of salt.

J.M. Seeger, M.D.

Role of Magnetic Resonance Imaging in the Diagnosis of Osteomyelitis in Diabetic Foot Infections

Croll SD, Nicholas GG, Osborne MA, et al (Lehigh Valley Hosp, Allentown, Pa)

J Vasc Surg 24:266–270, 1996 13–24

Introduction.—Precise diagnosis of osteomyelitis in diabetic foot infections could help prevent needless surgical exploration and guide appropriate treatment. Plain radiographs and nuclear scanning have traditionally been used to diagnose osteomyelitis. Magnetic resonance imaging has recently been used to successfully diagnose osteomyelitis in diabetic foot infections. The accuracy and cost of MRI in diagnosing osteomyelitis in diabetic patients' feet were evaluated and compared with traditional modalities.

TABLE 1.—Diagnostic Test Results for Osteomyelitis in 27 Patients

	n	*Sensitivity (%)*	*Specificity (%)*	*Accuracy (%)*	*Cost ($)*
MRI	27	89	100	95	785
Plain radiographs	27	22	94	70	76
Technetium bone scan	22	50	50	50	235
Indium leukocyte scan	19	33	69	58	1045

(Courtesy of Croll SD, Nicholas GG, Osborne MA, et al: Role of magnetic resonance imaging in the diagnosis of osteomyelitis in diabetic foot infections. *J Vasc Surg* 24:266–270, 1996.)

Methods.—Twenty-seven patients admitted with diabetic foot infections underwent history and physical examination, pertinent laboratory testing, MRI, and plain radiography. Technetium bone scans and indium scans were also performed in 22 and 19 patients, respectively. Patients were not included if they had obvious gangrene or fetid foot.

Results.—The diagnosis of osteomyelitis was confirmed or refuted by pathologic specimen, bone culture, or successful response to medical management in 18, 3, and 6 patients, respectively. Osteomyelitis was confirmed by pathologic specimen in 9 patients. For MRI, the diagnostic sensitivity, specificity, accuracy and cost were 88%, 100%, 95%, and $785, respectively. For plain radiographs, these numbers, were 22%, 94%, 70%, and $76, respectively. For technetium bone scans, they were 50%, 50%, 50%, and $235, respectively and for indium leukocyte scans, they were 33%, 69%, 58%, and $1,095, respectively (Table 1).

Conclusion.—Magnetic resonance imaging had significantly better diagnostic accuracy than plain radiographs. It was also less expensive than the frequently used indium scans. Magnetic resonance imaging is a sensitive and specific test for the diagnosis of osteomyelitis in patients with diabetic foot infections.

► The diagnosis of osteomyelitis in conjunction with diabetic foot infection remains difficult. This small study suggests that MRI may be valuable in patients with this problem as the accuracy of MRI is better than the accuracy of plain films, bone scans, and labeled white cell scans. However, MRI is expensive, so clinical judgment still must be used, and MRI likely will be most useful in determining which patients might benefit from long-term IV antibiotic therapy.

J.M. Seeger, M.D.

Long-term Outcome of Raynaud's Syndrome in a Prospectively Analyzed Patient Cohort

Landry GJ, Edwards JM, McLafferty RB, et al (Oregon Health Sciences Univ, Portland)

J Vasc Surg 23:76–86, 1996 13–25

Introduction.—Knowledge of the long-term clinical outcome in patients with Raynaud's syndrome (RS) is lacking in the medical literature. It would be helpful to be able to predict the clinical outcome of patients with RS so that monitoring of the disease process and patient education could be planned appropriately. One thousand thirty-nine patients with RS were monitored prospectively, including 118 (11.4%) who were followed for 10 years to determine prognostic variables present at the initial visit.

Methods.—When first seen, patients were assigned to 1 of 4 groups determined by vascular laboratory and serologic testing findings: vasospastic and serologically positive (spast, sero+), vasospastic and serologically negative (spast, sero−), obstructive and serologically positive (obst, sero+), and obstructive and serologically negative (obst, sero−).

Results.—Overall, 48.6% and 72.9% of patients, respectively, with spast, sero+ and obst, sero+ results had connective tissue disease (CTD) present at the initial visit. Progression to CTD in the remaining patients in these groups during follow-up occurred in 16.4% of patients with spast, sero+ results and 30.4% of patients with obst, sero+ results. Progression to CTD occurred in only 2% of patients in the spast, sero− group and 8.5% of patients in the obst, sero− group. Digital ulcers occurred in 15.5% of patients in the spast, sero+ group, 5.2% of patients in the spast, sero− group, and 55.6% of patients in the obst, sero+ group and 48.2% of patients in the obst, sero− group (Table 8). The respective rates of amputations for patients in each of these groups were 1.4%, 1.6%, 11.6%, and 19.0%.

Conclusion.—The long-term outcome of patients with RS can be predicted by initial serologic and vascular laboratory studies which divide patients into vasospastic and obstructive categories. In addition, the development of CTD can be strongly predicted in the presence of serologic

TABLE 8.—Presence of Digital Ulcerations

Initial classification	*All**	*> 10 yrs. follow-up†*
Spast, sero −	23/443 (5.2%)	2/32 (6.3%)
Spast, sero +	22/142 (15.5%)	5/18 (27.7%)
Obst, sero −	119/247 (48.2%)	15/28 (53.6%)
Obst, sero +	115/207 (55.6%)	21/40 (52.5%)

*$P < 0.001$ between all groups except C to D.
†$P < 0.001$ between A to C and A to D.
Abbreviations: Spast, sero −, vasospastic and serologically negative; *Spast, sero* +, vasospastic and serologically positive; *Obst, sero* −, obstructive and serologically negative; *Obst, sero* +, obstructive and serologically positive.
(Courtesy of Landry GJ, Edwards JM, McLafferty RB et al: Long-term outcome of Raynaud's syndrome in a prospectively analyzed patient cohort. *J Vasc Surg* 23:76–86, 1996.)

positivity. Digital ulcerations are more likely to occur in patients with obstructive RS, regardless of initial serology results, and 10% to 20% of patients with obstructive disease eventually needed amputation. In contrast, in patients initially seen with vasospastic RS, ulcerations and amputations were rare.

▶ The value of being able to predict long-term outcome in patients with RS using simple vascular laboratory evaluations and tests for CTD is obvious. Based on this excellent study, it is evident that patients with spastic disease do well and really do not need follow-up if their serology studies for CTD are initially negative, whereas ulcerations are likely to develop in those with digital arterial obstruction, particularly when CTD is present.

J.M. Seeger, M.D.

14 Noncardiac Thoracic Surgery

Introduction

A review of the general thoracic surgery literature in 1997 reflects several exciting new trends and developments in the field of general thoracic surgery. The practicing thoracic surgeon may have the opportunity to apply surgical therapy to one of the most common diseases in the United States. Specifically, emphysema, which afflicts more than 2 million Americans, may now fall into the category of diseases for which thoracic surgical therapy may be of benefit. Several reports in this year's review begin to provide further physiologic basis for the effectiveness of volume reduction surgery. The papers selected in this year's YEAR BOOK review may provide some new insight into the physiologic basis and ultimate application of this disease in a select group of patients with emphysema. Other literature involving advances in the staging of non–small-cell lung cancer are included. The continual progress in the field of video-assisted thoracic surgery (VATS) has also contributed articles to this year's YEAR BOOK. These studies continue to mature and the indications for VATS continue to evolve.

The role of age and gender in the treatment of patients with non–small-cell lung cancer is the subject of several articles in this year's YEAR BOOK. This is of great importance to the practicing thoracic surgeon inasmuch as more patients are seen later in life with this deadly disease. The rapid rise of lung cancer in women has also generated the need for specific reviews of the impact of gender on outcome of this disease.

Positron emission tomography (PET) holds great promise as a means of noninvasive staging of patients with pulmonary disease. Specifically, the role of PET scanning in patients with non–small-cell lung cancer is an area for the thoracic surgeon to watch. Earlier identification of malignancies with the use of PET scanning could dramatically alter the timing of surgical intervention. The articles abstracted in this year's YEAR BOOK regarding PET scanning will help introduce this new technology to the practicing thoracic surgeon. Although access to these scanners at the present time is quite restricted, evolution of this technology should be watched closely.

Lung cancer (including small cell) is the leading cause of cancer death. Non–small-cell lung cancer remains the leading cause of cancer-related death in both men and women in the United States. The use of adjuvant chemotherapy in this disease has not been supported by previous data. Combination therapies, including adjuvant chemotherapy and surgery, are included in this year's YEAR BOOK review.

Malignant pleural mesothelioma is becoming a significant source of mortality in the United States. The incidence of this disease continues to rise and has almost doubled in the last decade. Thus we have included in this year's YEAR BOOK a collection of abstracts that should enhance readers' understanding of appropriate diagnosis, staging, and various treatment options for one of the deadliest malignancies known.

The field of general thoracic surgery has come into its own as a surgical subspecialty. This author has enjoyed reviewing this year's literature, which has begun to reflect the energy of surgeons focused on the field of general thoracic surgery. The future of this endeavor appears bright as areas where thoracic surgical expertise can benefit patients continue to expand.

Lung Volume Reduction Surgery

Lessons From Lung Volume Reduction Surgery
Tonelli MR, Benditt JO, Albert RK (Univ of Washington, Seattle)
Chest 110:230–238, 1996 14–1

Background.—Despite the growing demand for evidence-based medicine, new treatments often are introduced and practiced before they have been studied thoroughly. An example is the recent introduction of lung volume reduction surgery (LVRS) for patients with emphysema. The use of this operation became widespread before appropriate scientific studies had been made of patient selection, outcome variables, risk-benefit ratios, or cost-effectiveness. Medicare stopped reimbursing for this procedure at the end of 1995. The situation with LVRS was discussed as an example of the problems encountered in evaluating innovative therapies.

Lung Volume Reduction Surgery.—Claims that LVRS "improves quality of life in emphysema patients" began to appear in 1994. Although the results were impressive, they were achieved in small groups of patients with short follow-up. Because of a billing technicality, third-party payers, including Medicare, covered the costs of the procedure at first. Patient demand grew, spurred by reports in the popular press, and hospitals began recruiting referral sources. At the end of 1995, Medicare announced that it would retroactively halt reimbursement for LVRS, and private payers are following suit. Patients protested, and lawsuits seem likely unless the Medicare decision is reversed.

Evaluation of Experimental Therapies.—The history of LVRS demonstrates the medical community's failure to evaluate new treatments adequately before their widespread utilization, in the absence of legal or reimbursement limitations. Practitioners must recognize new procedures as experimental, without being told so by the courts or by third-party payers. One test of a procedure's experimental nature is informed consent, which differs for experimental and standard treatments. If patients understand that there are few scientific data on the effects of LVRS and still agree to have the procedure—despite the inability to predict the results in probabilistic fashion—then they are granting consent for an experimental procedure. Comparison of the experience with LVRS with the scientific proof required for new drug therapies underscores the double standard for evaluating new surgical innovations. This double standard—which also applies to certain medical procedures, such as bone marrow transplantation for nonhematologic malignancies—is unjustifiable ethically or scientifically.

Discussion.—Even though LVRS seems likely to prove beneficial for many patients with emphysema, its widespread adoption before proper scientific evaluation raises concerns about current techniques of evaluating surgical and certain medical innovations. The way in which experimental therapies are introduced and disseminated should be changed, specifically, by creating oversight groups within the structure of existing medical organizations. If the objective of evidence-based medicine is to be fulfilled, all surgical and medical innovations must be evaluated thoroughly before they become the new standards of care.

▶ This editorial introduces the controversy regarding the way in which LVRS has been applied to patients with emphysema. It is precisely this controversy that led to the suspension of funding for this procedure by the Health Care Financing Administration and the development of the subsequent surgical trial.

D.J. Sugarbaker, M.D.

The Current Status of Lung Volume Reduction Operations for Emphysema

Naunheim KS, Ferguson MK (St Louis Univ, Mo; Univ of Chicago)
Ann Thorac Surg 62:601–612, 1996 14–2

Introduction.—Emphysema is a progressive, disabling disease that affects a large number of people and carries a high mortality (Fig 1). Conventional therapies have little effect on quality of life or survival. Recently, promising results have been reported with parenchymal resection, or lung volume reduction (LVR) surgery, for patients with emphysema. There is now a large body of data with which to evaluate the short-term results of these operations. The background, outcomes, and future of LVR surgery for emphysema were reviewed.

Techniques and Outcomes.—The idea behind LVR surgery is that reversing some of the pathophysiologic effects of emphysema can lead to improvements in symptoms and performance. The operation is regarded as best for patients with "pure" emphysema, not combined with other forms

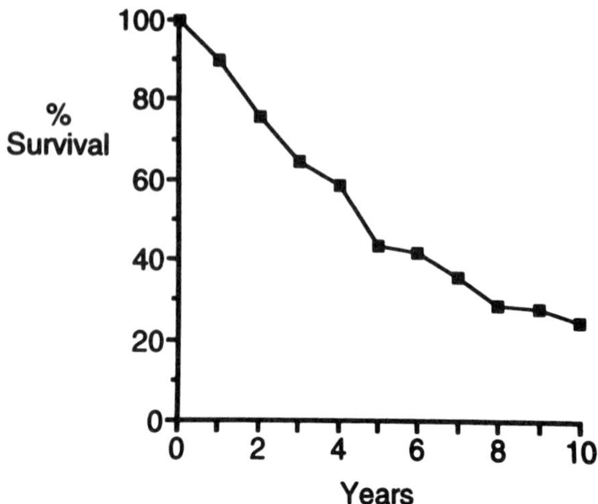

FIGURE 1.—Survival in patients with chronic obstructive pulmonary disease who have a forced expiratory volume in 1 second of less than 30% of predicted. (Courtesy of Naunheim KS, Ferguson MK: The current status of lung volume reduction operations for emphysema. *Ann Thorac Surg* 62:601–612, 1996. Reprinted with permission from the Society of Thoracic Surgeons.)

of chronic obstructive pulmonary disease. These patients usually have severe respiratory functional impairment, with desaturation during exercise and hypoxia at rest. Clinical and laboratory criteria for patient selection have been established; most patients referred for the procedure prove not to be appropriate candidates. Even after acceptance, many patients undergo preoperative pulmonary rehabilitation. The rationale for LVR is ablation or resection of the most diseased portions of the lungs. Patients with clear "target zones" on ventilation-perfusion scans (i.e., zones with markedly reduced perfusion limited to a single region in both lungs) are considered ideal for LVR. The rest of the lung also should have relatively good perfusion. The operation seeks to resect the "target zones" and thus reduce the amount of trapped gas. The mechanisms of improved respiratory function may involve elastic recoil, ventilation/perfusion mismatch, the respiratory musculature, and cardiovascular hemodynamics.

Several different techniques and approaches to LVR have emerged in the few years since its reintroduction. These include bilateral and unilateral procedures performed through various approaches, including sternotomy, thoracotomy, and thoracoscopy. Stapled excision of lung tissue is the favored method of parenchymal ablation; most practitioners have abandoned laser ablation. Although debate continues, simultaneous, bilateral LVR procedures may be the optimal approach. The use of a unilateral vs. bilateral procedure depends on the patient's individual situation.

Discussion.—Lung volume reduction surgery appears to provide significant short-term improvement in selected patients with emphysema. These benefits, including gains in spirometric indices and oxygen saturation, exceed those obtained with rehabilitation. The procedure must be carried out in an organized and systematic fashion, with the involvement of an experienced multidisciplinary team. Substantial resources must be committed, and the morbidity and mortality resulting from this aggressive approach must be borne in mind. More research is needed, particularly in the areas of patient selection, operative technique, and results.

► This article nicely summarizes the difficulties in assessing our progress in the area of LVR surgery. It is precisely the selection of patients, the selection of operative procedure, and the means of follow-up that have led to the controversies surrounding the introduction and efficacy of this procedure. We will learn a lot from the ongoing prospective trial. Operative mortality for this procedure ranges from 18% to 0%. The hospital lengths of stay also are significant, ranging from 11 to 17 days, indicating the effect this surgery will have on the consumption of health care resources in the United States.

D.J. Sugarbaker, M.D.

Economic Aspects of Lung Volume Reduction Surgery

Albert RK, Lewis S, Wood D, et al (Univ of Washington, Seattle)

Chest 110:1068–1071, 1996 14–3

Objective.—Emphysema has a serious effect on survival, exercise capacity, and quality of life for many people. Recent reports have suggested that lung volume reduction surgery (LVRS) can improve airflow limitation, gas exchange, exercise capacity, and quality of life for patients with emphysema. If the encouraging results are borne out, large numbers of patients will become candidates for LVRS. The costs and charges associated with LVRS at 1 hospital were analyzed.

Methods.—The study included 23 consecutive patients undergoing LVRS at an academic medical center during a 1-year period. The charges and costs associated with LVRS were analyzed, with the goal of identifying areas of potential savings.

Findings.—The patients spent a median of 8 days in the hospital; none died. Charges ranged from about $20,000 to $76,000, with a median of approximately $27,000. Seventy-three percent of charges were for medical center services and 27% for physician services. Of the medical center charges, 71% were for rooms and operating suite time. Seventy-seven percent of professional fees were charged by the surgeons and anesthesiologists. There was a direct correlation between total charges and length of stay. Median reimbursement for medical center services was approximately $22,000, a rate of 114%. For physician services, median reimbursement was $2,783, a rate of 34%. Overall, the median total reimbursement accounted for 94% of total charges. Compared to a median reimbursement-to-cost ratio of 1.05 for all medical services during the study year, the ratio for LVRS was 1.22.

Conclusions.—The substantial costs of LVRS must be weighed against the outcomes, including quality of life, patient function, and long-term survival. If just 10% of the 1.65 million Americans with emphysema are candidates for LVRS, the additional health care costs for this procedure will exceed $4.6 billion. Cost-benefit analyses of LVRS are needed.

▶ The economic impact of the evolution of this technique is nicely outlined by Dr. Albert and colleagues in this summary report. The cost of this procedure was significant, despite the fact that the length of stay and operative results reported by this group compare favorably to those of previous reports. Length of stay was the principal determinant of the economic effect of this procedure. The impact of LVRS also must be measured in terms of the patient's ability to return to work and the benefit to society of restoring a patient to a functional state. Long-term studies of these effects will need to be looked at in the context of the immediate medical and surgical therapy.

D.J. Sugarbaker, M.D.

Lung Volume Reduction Surgery: Case Selection, Operative Technique, and Clinical Results

Daniel TM, Chan BBK, Bhaskar V, et al (Univ of Virginia, Charlottesville)

Ann Surg 223:526–533, 1996 14–4

Purpose.—For patients with severe, disabling emphysema, lung volume reduction surgery (LVRS) may serve as a useful alternative or bridge to lung transplantation. The optimal techniques of this procedure have not been determined; questions also remain about the risks, benefits, and long-term results. The preoperative strategies and intraoperative techniques of LVRS that would lead to minimal morbidity and maximal physiologic improvement were determined.

Methods.—The study included 26 patients who underwent LVRS for disabling chronic obstructive pulmonary disease. The patients were 17 men and 9 women, with a mean age of 62 years. Patients who met selection criteria underwent a series of physiologic and anatomical studies. The effects of surgery on pulmonary function, quality of life, and oxygen requirements were analyzed.

Technique.—Thoracic epidural anesthesia is initiated, followed by inhalation anesthesia. The resection is performed through a median sternotomy with blunt dissection of the parietal pleura. The worst lung, identified on preoperative imaging studies, is resected first. The lung is deflated and adhesions are released carefully. Access to the posterior and basilar segments is aided by floating the partially inflated lower lobe with saline (Fig 1). Based on the preoperative single-photon emission scan, 20% to 30% of each lung is resected with a linear GIA stapler. The stapler is applied sequentially to provide a continuous line of excision. The pleural space is flooded with saline during lung inflation to check for leaks. Two chest tubes are placed in each pleural space and connected to

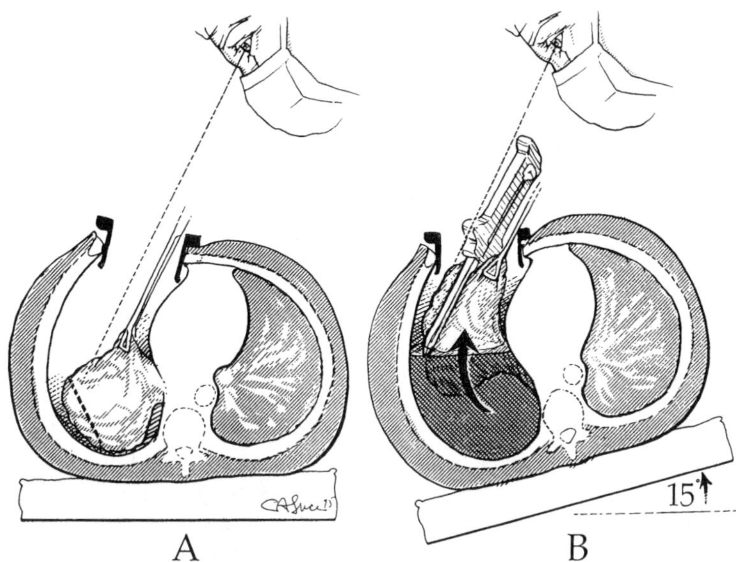

FIGURE 1.—A and B, intraoperative illustration of the saline float technique to facilitate exposure to the basilar segments of the lower lobe. (Courtesy of Daniel TM, Chan BBK, Bhaskar V, et al: Lung volume reduction surgery: Case selection, operative technique, and clinical results. *Ann Surg* 223:526-533, 1996.)

water seal or low suction. Extubation is performed immediately after the procedure.

Results.—The average length of hospital stay was 14 days. Seventeen patients underwent 3-month follow-up evaluations. The evaluations revealed a 49% rate of improvement in forced expiratory volume in 1 second and a 23% rate of improvement in forced vital capacity. More than 85% of patients who required supplemental oxygen before surgery no longer needed oxygen at all, or only with exercise. Seventy-nine percent of patients reported marked improvement in quality of life. There was 1 death, for a mortality rate of 3.8%. The rate of morbidity involving air leaks was 18%.

Conclusions.—In properly selected patients with end-stage emphysema, LVRS provides predictably good results. Both objective and subjective pulmonary function are improved, with low morbidity and mortality. Good results depend on careful patient selection, accurate preoperative localization of lung target areas, careful anesthetic and operative technique, and intensive postoperative care.

▶ This well-written article outlines very well the technique of volume reduction surgery by median sternotomy. The figure illustrated shows an interesting technique that can enhance a surgeon's ability to visualize basilar segments by floating the lung in a chest filled with saline. The study emphasizes the importance of preoperative pulmonary rehabilitation and a team approach to this procedure that includes the pulmonologist, anesthesiologist, and surgeon.

D.J. Sugarbaker, M.D.

Lung Volume Reduction in Patients With Severe Diffuse Emphysema: A Retrospective Study

Roué C, Mal H, Sleiman C, et al (Hôpital Beaujon, Clichy, France)

Chest 110:28–34, 1996 14–5

Introduction.—Next to pulmonary transplantation, resection of large bullae is usually considered the only type of effective surgery in patients with pulmonary emphysema. Most reports suggest that voluminous bullae occupy at least one third of the hemithorax before surgery is considered. Surgery can result in dramatic improvements in dyspnea and lung function that can last several years, even in the presence of advanced disease. There is a general belief that lung volume reduction is associated with poor results and high perioperative mortality and morbidity. Records of patients who underwent lung volume reduction from 1982 to 1992 for severe emphysema were examined. Of the more than 50 patients reviewed, all 13 patients with either no well-demarcated bullae or only small bullae (detected by CT scan and pulmonary angiography) were retrospectively studied.

Methods.—All 13 patients had severe diffuse emphysema with a dyspnea grade 4 or 5 and a mean forced expiratory volume in 1 second (FEV_1) of 18% of predicted. The partial pressure of carbon dioxide in arterial blood ($PaCO_2$) was greater than 42 mm Hg in 7 patients. Radiographic evaluation indicated either small bullae or, more frequently, areas of destroyed lung. Eleven and 2 patients underwent unilateral and bilateral procedures, respectively. Patients underwent a postoperative assessment at 6- to 12-month intervals that included dyspnea grading, FEV_1 measurement, and blood gas analysis.

Results.—Two patients died postoperatively at 30 and 48 months, respectively. Five patients were unavailable at follow-up, and the remaining patients were still alive. The mean hospital stay was 29 days. In the early postoperative period, 5 patients had an uneventful course, 6 had air leakage that persisted for more than 1 week, 1 patient had a pulmonary embolism that responded to anticoagulant therapy, 1 patient had a pleuropulmonary infection, and 1 patient had an ischemic stroke on postoperative day 1 from which he recovered slowly. He still had brachial and facial paralysis at follow-up. Postoperative follow-ups at 6, 12, 18, 24, and 36 months revealed symptomatic improvement in 92%, 85%, 54%, 31%, and 31% of patients, respectively, with FEV_1 increasing by at least 20% in 92%, 46%, 46%, 31%, and 24% of patients, respectively.

Conclusions.—Findings in this cohort of patients were contrary to general beliefs. These patients with diffuse emphysema benefited from resection of emphysematous lung, even in the absence of large bullae. Length of hospital stay was shorter in these patients, compared with patients who underwent lung volume reduction for large bullae. Many patients remained clinically improved 1 year after surgery. Emphysematous lung resection should be considered in patients with severe disease before considering lung transplantation.

► The authors have taken a very careful look at the way in which the palliative benefit of the surgical procedure is to be measured. Dyspnea is a clinical symptom. The therapeutic benefit of volume reduction surgery appears to focus around its palliative benefit for patients. At the present time there are no data to suggest that volume reduction surgery may enhance overall life expectancy. As noted by these authors, the durability of the palliative effect of volume reduction surgery may be in doubt. Specifically of note is that at 36 months, only 4 patients (or 31%) still had their dyspnea grade lower than before surgery, indicating that the palliative benefit for the majority of patients had disappeared. An objective benefit was present in only 3 patients at the 36-month interval. It is precisely this long-term effect that will need to be considered as we evaluate this procedure.

D.J. Sugarbaker, M.D.

Morbidity and Mortality After Thoracoscopic Pneumonoplasty

Fujita RA, Barnes GB (Chapman Med Ctr, Orange, Calif)

Ann Thorac Surg 62:251–257, 1996 14–6

Introduction.—Patients with bullous emphysema can be treated by video-assisted or open lung-reduction surgery. The surgical and anesthetic risk factors for these patients remain ill-defined. Risk factors for morbidity and mortality in patients undergoing thoracoscopic laser pneumonoplasty were analyzed.

Methods.—The experience included the first 339 cases of thoracoscopic laser pneumonoplasty performed at one institution. Twenty-two patients underwent bilateral lung-reduction surgery. Their mean age was 66.5 years, and all were American Society of Anesthesiologists physical status 3 or 4. The patients' mean forced expiratory volume in 1 second (FEV_1) was 750 mL, and their mean ratio of FEV_1 to forced vital capacity was 35%. Data on these patients were analyzed to identify risk factors associated with increased postoperative morbidity and mortality.

Findings.—The in-hospital mortality rate was 4.1% to 4.9% for men vs. 2.1% for women. There was a 0.9% incidence of myocardial infarction and a 3-month survival rate of 92.7%. About 3% of patients required tracheal intubation and re-institution of mechanical ventilation. Patient outcomes were no different for patients receiving inhalation anesthesia versus balanced anesthesia. Factors carrying an elevated risk of morbidity and mortality were advanced age, particularly over 75 years; male sex; and resting carbon dioxide retention, specifically an arterial carbon dioxide tension of greater than 55 mm Hg. Morbidity and mortality were increased at an FEV_1 of less than 700 mL in men and 500 mL in women. A maximum voluntary ventilation of less than 25% predicted and a residual volume/total lung capacity greater than 60% also were adverse risk factors.

Conclusions.—Age, sex, and lung function affect the risk of postoperative morbidity and mortality in patients undergoing thoracoscopic laser pneumonoplasty. Early extubation is an important objective.

▶ This report further highlights the controversy over the surgical technique that should be used to achieve volume reduction. The use of laser pneumonoplasty through the thoracoscope is outlined. The authors are anesthesiologists and, therefore, provide an alternative perspective in the evaluation of this procedure. The factors that led to increased mortality in this series were advanced age (greater than 65 years), sex (with men having a higher risk), and CO_2 retention in the resting state. An FEV_1 of less than 700 mL for men and 500 mL for women also was associated with increased mortality. This report is somewhat incomplete in that it does not contain any data regarding the therapeutic benefit of this approach. The reader must be mindful in evaluating this procedure that, without these data, it will be very difficult to establish the efficacy of this technique.

D.J. Sugarbaker, M.D.

Role of Lung Reduction in Lung Transplant Candidates With Pulmonary Emphysema

Zenati M, Keenan RJ, Sciurba FC, et al (Univ of Pittsburgh, Pa)

Ann Thorac Surg 62:994–999, 1996 14–7

Introduction.—For patients with end-stage pulmonary emphysema who are candidates for lung transplantation (LTx), waiting time can average up to 2 years. The mortality rate during this time is 15%. Lung reduction surgery can provide significant improvement in pulmonary mechanics and function in patients with coronary obstructive pulmonary disease. Lung reduction surgery was evaluated as a means of decreasing mortality during the waiting period for LTx, or as a possible alternative to LTx.

Methods.—Ninety-five patients were evaluated by an LTx program over a 1½-year period. All had severe impairment in quality of life and disabling dyspnea. After evaluation, 45 patients were considered eligible for both LTx and lung reduction surgery. Thirty-five of these patients underwent lung reduction; most had unilateral thoracoscopic lung reduction with a stapler, laser, or both. The lung reduction procedure sought to reduce lung volume by 25%. The patients were 21 men and 14 women, with a mean age of 58 years. Follow-up was at least 3 months in 30 patients.

Results.—The patients' mean forced expiratory volume in 1 second (FEV_1) improved from 0.64 to 0.97 L. Significant improvement also was observed in forced vital capacity, from 2.12 to 2.76 L; residual volume,

5.62 to 4.26 L; maximum voluntary ventilation, 28.1 to 38.5 L/min; 6-minute walking distance, 904 to 1,012 ft; Borg dyspnea index, 3.7 to 2.4; and arterial carbon dioxide tension, 44.9 to 41.6 mm Hg. The improvement was sufficient to remove 20 patients (group A) from the LTx waiting list. Compared to the 10 patients who remained on the waiting list (group B), the group A patients had a greater percent increase in FEV_1, 70% vs. 27%. The group A patients also had a significantly greater increase in forced vital capacity, 41% vs. 18%, and a greater decrease in residual volume, 26% vs. 1.5%. Seven of the group B patients went on to LTx. Eighty-six percent of these patients had hypercarbia before lung reduction surgery, compared with 40% of group A patients. All 7 patients were alive after LTx, with a mean FEV_1 of 53% and a forced vital capacity of 64% predicted.

Conclusions.—For properly selected patients with end-stage emphysema who are awaiting LTx, lung reduction is a safe and effective surgical procedure. It may serve as a bridge or an alternative to transplantation. The best surgical choice can be selected on the basis of an extensive emphysema workup. Hypercarbia may be a risk factor for relatively poor results. The long-term results of lung reduction in this patient population remain to be determined.

▶ This excellent report illustrates one of the potentially valuable applications of lung volume reduction surgery (LVRS). Emphysema has become one of the principal indications for LTx. Lung volume reduction surgery, as illustrated in this report, may provide an alternative therapy for a significant percentage of patients referred for LTx. In addition, in some patients, it may provide enough palliative and physiologic improvement to allow them to sustain the long wait required for this donor-limited procedure. It is precisely in this subgroup of patients that LVRS may find its earliest routine application.

D.J. Sugarbaker, M.D.

Unilateral Volume Reduction After Single-lung Transplantation for Emphysema

Kroshus TJ, Bolman RM III, Kshettry VR (Univ of Minnesota, Minneapolis)

Ann Thorac Surg 62:363–368, 1996 14–8

Background.—End-stage emphysema can be treated successfully by single-lung transplantation. However, the native lung may become hyperinflated, causing mediastinal shifting with compression and impaired ventilation of the transplanted lung. Lung volume reduction surgery (pneumonectomy) has been proposed as an alternative to lung transplantation. Unilateral volume reduction surgery of the native lung was described in 3 single-lung transplant recipients with hyperinflation of the native lung.

Patients.—Sixty-six patients underwent single-lung transplantation for emphysema over a 6-year period. In 3 of these patients, the native lung hyperexpanded, causing mediastinal shifting and compression of the transplanted lung. This complication developed from 12 to 42 months after transplantation. Each patient underwent unilateral volume reduction through a median sternotomy incision. Multiple wedge resections were performed with bovine pericardium-reinforced staplers, for an overall resection of 25% to 30% of lung volume.

Results.—There were no complications of lung-reducing surgery. The chest radiographic findings improved in all patients, with return of the mediastinum to the midline and resolution of native lung herniation. Dyspnea was relieved. Exercise tolerance improved in 2 patients, and the third was able to be taken off mechanical ventilation. Pulmonary function studies showed improvement in the 1 patient in whom they were performed.

Conclusions.—Unilateral volume reduction surgery can be performed successfully in single-lung transplant recipients with symptomatic hyperinflation of the native lung. This operation may be done from months to years after lung transplantation. It provides both objective and subjective improvement, with gains in respiratory mechanics.

▶ The use of a single-lung transplant to treat a patient with end-stage emphysema has presented significant problems for the lung transplant surgeon. The mismatch in lung compliance between the native, emphysematous, overly compliant lung and the newly transplanted, normal lung may lead to significant hyperinflation of the native lung and physiologic impairment of the newly transplanted lung. Lung volume reduction surgery (LVRS) would appear to have an immediate application in this subgroup of patients. Although it reduces the native lung, mediastinal shifts occur that restore normal physiologic functioning of the newly transplanted lung. It is the technique of LVRS that will be most important. Minimizing trauma and subsequent air leaks will be the key to keeping operative mortality and morbidity low in this group of patients. The timing of LVRS in this subgroup of patients also will need to be considered. The case could be made for volume reduction before transplantation, although this may limit the possibility of using either lung in this donor-limited procedure. More likely, either simultaneous or subsequent volume reduction will be the appropriate sequence for this procedure.

D.J. Sugarbaker, M.D.

Combined Operations for Lung Volume Reduction Surgery and Lung Cancer

McKenna RJ Jr, Fischel RJ, Brenner M, et al (Hosp of the Good Samaritan, Los Angeles; Lakewood Regional Med Ctr, Calif; Beckman Laser Inst, Los Angeles; et al)

Chest 110:885–888, 1996 14–9

Introduction.—Lung cancer in a patient with poor pulmonary function poses difficult problems. The pulmonary problems may preclude an attempt at surgical cure; even if radiation therapy can be done, the results are poor. Some patients undergoing evaluation for lung volume reduction surgery (LVRS) will have both lung cancer and emphysema. In this situation, LVRS may permit resection of lung cancer in a patient who otherwise would be inoperable. An experience with combined LVRS and lung cancer surgery was described, including an evaluation of the incidence of benign and malignant lung masses in candidates for LVRS.

Patients.—Three hundred twenty-five patients with emphysema underwent LVRS over a 1½-year period. Fifty-one of these patients (16%) had lung masses resected. Forty-two patients (13%) had benign lung masses, mainly calcified nodules and granulomas. Eleven had clinical stage I non–small-cell lung cancer. Three of these patients were referred specifically for combined LVRS and lung cancer surgery. The other cancers were detected during the workup for LVRS or on pathologic examination. Thus, 2% of patients undergoing LVRS had previously undiagnosed lung cancer.

Outcomes.—The patients undergoing cancer resection were 8 men and 3 women, with an average age of 69 years. All cancers were clinical stage I and 10 were pathologic stage I. The cancer operation consisted of lymph node dissection with wedge resection in 8 patients and lobectomy in 3. None of the patients died or experienced a major complication, although 45% had prolonged air leakage. The patients stayed in the hospital an average of 9 days. Their mean forced expiratory volume in 1 second improved from 22% of predicted before surgery to 49% of predicted after surgery. In 5 patients, the cancer was in the target area for LVRS; these patients all had major improvement in pulmonary function after surgery.

Conclusions.—The availability of LVRS permits surgical treatment of patients whose poor pulmonary function otherwise would have made their lung cancer inoperable. Chest CT scans of patients being evaluated for LVRS should be examined carefully for unsuspected lung cancer.

► The use of LVRS in patients with a solitary lung mass and emphysema is the subject of this interesting report. The thoracic surgeon needs to become more mindful of the potential benefits of LVRS in patients referred on the basis of other lung pathology. Conversely, patients evaluated for LVRS will have a significant incidence of malignant tumors found in the lung at the time of evaluation. The 16% overall incidence of lung masses in this group is of interest. In this group, 11 of the 51 lesions proved to be malignant. Although the authors state that lobectomy was performed when possible in this series, our experience has been that most of these patients require a parenchyma-sparing procedure. The evaluation of patients with severe end-stage emphysema for both lung transplantation and LVRS has caused many pulmonologists and surgeons to re-think the limitations imposed by the patients' severely limited respiratory reserve on the ability to perform a successful resection. It seems clear that this subgroup of patients undergoing evaluation for LVRS because of their severe pulmonary dysfunction will provide the greatest challenge for surgical oncologists to successfully resect potentially curable cancers in this high-risk population.

D.J. Sugarbaker, M.D.

Effect of Surgical Lung Volume Reduction on Respiratory Muscle Function in Pulmonary Emphysema

Teschler H, Stamatis G, El-Raouf Farhat E-R, et al (Ruhrlandklinik, Essen, Germany)

Eur Respir J 9:1779–1784, 1996 14–10

Objective.—Severe pulmonary emphysema causes harmful abnormalities of ventilatory mechanics, including increased airway resistance, diaphragmatic inefficiency, and dynamic hyperinflation. Lung volume reduction surgery (LVRS) is increasingly recognized as beneficial for selected patients with severe emphysema. By reducing lung volume, LVRS may improve the performance of the respiratory muscles and reduce dyspnea. Various indicators of respiratory muscle strength and respiratory drive were measured to investigate the hypothesis that LVRS has beneficial effects on the respiratory pump.

Methods.—The study included 17 patients, mean age 53 years, who had severe emphysema with dyspnea on minimal exertion. The patients performed a battery of tests before and 1 month after LVRS. In addition to pulmonary function tests, the patients underwent measurement of maximal inspiratory mouth pressure (MIP), sniff nasal inspiratory pressure (SNIP), sniff transdiaphragmatic pressure (P_{di}), and inspiratory mouth occlusion pressure ($P_{0.1}$).

Results.—After LVRS, mean forced expiratory volume in 1 second increased significantly, from 0.82 to 1.12 L. Residual volume decreased from 337% to 250% of predicted, functional residual capacity from 210% to 159% of predicted, and total lung capacity from 138% to 110% of predicted. All measures of respiratory muscle strength increased: on average, MIP increased by 52%, SNIP by 66%, and P_{di} by 28%. As a measure of respiratory drive, $P_{0.1}$ decreased by 24% on average. None of these measurements was significantly correlated with the results of pulmonary function tests, 6-minute walk distance, or dyspnea score.

Conclusions.—Part of the clinical improvement seen after LVRS for severe emphysema is related to an increase in the force-generating capacity of the inspiratory muscles. At the same time, there is a parallel decrease in the central respiratory drive, probably related to a reduction in the work of breathing. Improved pulmonary function as a result of increased elastic recoil is not the only factor involved in the clinical success of LVRS.

► The long-term clinical value of LVRS will depend on the establishment of a sound physiologic basis for the symptomatic improvement reported by patients and surgeons. This very interesting and well-performed study begins to lay a foundation for the concept that LVRS improves muscle function and reduces central respiratory drive in patients with severe pulmonary emphysema. We should be cautioned, however, to continue to rely on the clinical and symptomatic outcomes in tandem with the physiologic improvement that appears to result from LVRS. It is clear that our understanding of pulmonary function will be significantly enhanced by the rigorous physiologic investigations that need to surround patients undergoing LVRS.

D.J. Sugarbaker, M.D.

Bilateral Volume Reduction Surgery for Diffuse Pulmonary Emphysema by Video-assisted Thoracoscopy

Bingisser R, Zollinger A, Hauser M, et al (Univ Hosp of Zurich, Switzerland)

J Thorac Cardiovasc Surg 112:875–882, 1996 14–11

Purpose.—There is renewed interest in bilateral lung volume reduction surgery for patients with severe pulmonary emphysema. This procedure can be performed through a median sternotomy. Good results have been achieved with video-assisted thoracoscopy (VAT) for various types of lung surgery. The surgical technique, results, and complications of lung volume reduction performed by VAT were reported.

Methods.—The prospective study included 20 patients with diffuse pulmonary emphysema. There were 15 men and 5 women, with a mean age of 64 years. All had substantial impairment of daily activity because of severe airflow obstruction and hyperinflation. All patients underwent bilateral lung volume reduction surgery using VAT. Twenty to thirty percent of lung volume was resected using endoscopic staplers and, in the latter part of the experience, a 45-mm thoracoscopic linear cutter. The patients were assessed thoroughly before and 3 months after surgery by pulmonary function studies, dyspnea assessment, and exercise performance.

Results.—There were no perioperative deaths. The median length of hospitalization was 15 days. Perioperative and postoperative recovery was uneventful in 12 of 20 patients; 6 patients had bacterial pneumonia and 2 had pneumothorax. Seven patients required more than 7 days of chest tube drainage. Forced expiratory volume in 1 second (FEV_1) improved from 0.80 before surgery to 1.09 3 months after surgery, while residual volume decreased from 5.8 to 4.4L. The improvement in FEV_1 was apparent even before the patients left the hospital. Twelve-minute walking distance increased from a median of 495 to 688 min, while mean maximal oxygen consumption improved from 10 to 13 mL/kg/min. The mean Medical Research Council dyspnea score decreased from 3.4 to 1.8. The improvement in shortness of breath was moderately correlated with surgically induced alterations in lung mechanics.

Conclusions.—Bilateral lung volume reduction surgery using VAT produced good resutls. The VAT technique provided good access to all parts of the lungs, allowing precise dissection of adhesions that can be difficult to reach through sternotomy. It also permitted wedge resection without overmanipulation of the lungs. The thoracoscopic approach also may permit earlier functional recovery than with sternotomy.

▶ Patients with severe emphysema would appear to be the ideal group to benefit from the reduced operative trauma afforded by a thoracoscopic approach. The controversy continues, however, as to whether a median sternotomy or a unilateral or staged thoracoscopic procedure represents the best operative approach to the chest. Median sternotomy allows surgeons to palpate both lungs and to perform a speedy and well-controlled volume reduction procedure. Limitations in visibility do occur, particularly in the apices and posterior paravertebral areas of the lung. The left lower lobe is especially difficult to visualize in selected patients. The thoracoscopic approach allows excellent visualization of the posterior lung fields and may prove to be the superior technique in the final analysis.

The appropriate sequence of thoracoscopic surgery has yet to be established. Initial reports of unilateral and then bilateral procedures have contributed to an ongoing debate. Data that may help in the resolution of this question have come from some long-term reports that show a decrease in the palliative benefit over time. Therefore, it may be that if significant palliative benefit and physiologic improvement can be achieved with unilateral volume reduction, the second-stage procedure could be performed at the time when the palliative benefit is beginning to decline. Thus, patients could have longer total palliation by undergoing the staged thoracoscopic approach. The data to firmly establish these conclusions are currently lacking.

D.J. Sugarbaker, M.D.

Lung Volume Reduction Surgery in Ventilator-dependent COPD Patients

Criner GJ, O'Brien G, Furukawa S, et al (Temple Univ, Philadelphia)
Chest 110:877–884, 1996 14–12

Introduction.—Reports conflict regarding appropriate candidates for lung volume reduction surgery. Patients with ventilator-dependent chronic obstructive pulmonary disease (COPD) have an exceptionally poor prognosis and severe limitations on quality of life. The outcomes of 3 patients with ventilator-dependent COPD who underwent lung volume reduction surgery in an attempt to improve their respiratory and functional status were reported.

Methods.—All 3 patients had severe COPD and respiratory failure requiring 11 to 16 weeks of ventilator support, despite high-dose bronchodilatory therapy. All 3 patients were unable to be weaned from mechanical ventilation. Spirometry, arterial blood gas analysis, and bedside measurements of maximum inspiratory pressure (MIP) and ventilation were compared before and after lung volume reduction surgery.

Results.—The patients ranged in age from 53 to 60. Compared to presurgical values, the patients had substantial increases (nearly doubled lung volumes) in spirometric values at 3 to 5 months after surgery. Before surgery, all patients had mild hypoxemia and moderate to severe hypercapnia. At 3 to 5 months after surgery, all patients showed stability or moderate improvement in oxygenation and moderate decreases in hypercapnia. The MIP was greater after surgery in all patients, compared to preoperative measurements. Minute ventilation was higher after surgery, compared to preoperative values, because of increased tidal volume. The respiratory rate changed from rapid, shallow breathing before surgery to slower, deeper breathing after surgery. Two patients experienced persistent air leaks for 2 weeks or more. One patient had a tension pneumothorax and the other had a persistent, but asymptomatic, left apical pneumothorax. All patients were ventilator independent at 10 to 21 days after surgery and were discharged home. At prolonged follow-up, all patients had continued significant improvements in gas exchange and functional status. All patients were living independently and 1 returned to work.

Conclusions.—Select patients with ventilator-dependent COPD can benefit from lung volume reduction surgery, as evidenced by improved gas exchange, spirometry, and respiratory function. Longer follow-up is needed to determine whether these physiologic improvements can be sustained.

► For many patients with end-stage emphysema, ventilator dependency becomes an unavoidable consequence of their progressive disease. Ventilator-dependent patients with emphysema present one of the most frustrating and recalcitrant clinical scenarios for the surgeons, pulmonologists, and internists who care for them. The potential value of lung volume reduction surgery (LVRS) in improving respiratory function to the degree that patients could be weaned from the ventilator could represent an important application of this developing technique. This particular application remains unproven, despite the experience with 3 patients outlined in this report. Nevertheless, it does point up the potential impact that LVRS could have on a variety of critical pulmonary situations.

D.J. Sugarbaker, M.D.

► In summary, lung volume reduction surgery remains an unproven but intriguing approach to the treatment of end-stage emphysema. As summarized in these reports, the clinical experience with this technique varies greatly. The operative mortality, postoperative morbidity, and cost of the widespread use of this treatment strategy for patients with end-stage emphysema supports careful evaluation of this procedure. Surgeons have an exciting opportunity to again contribute to the advances in operative technique that will be required to lower perioperative morbidity and mortality and bring the procedure into the mainstream of treatment for these patients.

D.J. Sugarbaker, M.D.

Advances in Staging of Non–Small-Cell Lung Cancer

Detection of Disseminated Lung Cancer Cells in Lymph Nodes: Impact on Staging and Prognosis

Passlick B, Izbicki JR, Kubuschok B, et al (Central Hosp Gauting, Germamy; Ludwig-Maximilians Universität, Munich)

Ann Thorac Surg 61:177–183, 1996 14–13

Purpose.—Early tumor cell dissemination probably plays a major role in the high incidence of tumor recurrence in patients with apparently resectable non–small-cell lung cancer (NSCLC). A newly developed immunohistochemical assay can detect individual disseminated NSCLC cells in the lymph nodes. Patients with operable NSCLC who were tumor free by conventional histopathologic studies were studied to determine the frequency and prognostic significance of disseminated cancer cells in the lymph nodes.

Methods.—One hundred twenty-five patients treated by lobectomy or pneumonectomy with systematic mediastinal lympadenectomy for NSCLC were studied. Resected tumor specimens and 565 lymph nodes were studied by the new immunohistochemical assay, which used the monoclonal antibody Ber-Ep4. The frequency of nodal tumor cell dissemination was assessed, along with the prognostic significance of this finding.

Results.—Twenty-two percent of patients and 6% of lymph nodes were found to have Ber-Ep4–positive cells. Of the 27 patients with a positive immunohistochemical finding, 24 were upstaged as a result. Sixteen percent of patients who had been staged as pN0 had tumor cells detected by the immunohistochemical assay. Disease-free survival was reduced in patients with minimal tumor cell dissemination to lymph nodes.

Conclusions.—The immunohistochemical assay used in this study can identify many NSCLC patients with regional lymphatic tumor cell dissemination at the time of surgery. Many of these cancers may not be curable by surgery alone, so the immunohistochemical results could be helpful in risk stratification and selection of patients for adjuvant therapy. For example, epithelial-specific antibodies could be a useful approach in this group of patients.

▶ The disappointing survival in patients with stage I and stage II NSCLC is caused by the relatively high rate of distant failure. This report from Munich illustrates beautifully the role of immunohistochemistry in the detection of disseminated disease not apparent through conventional histologic staging procedures. Correlation of Ber-Ep4 markers with the presence of metastatic disease causes a significant number of these patients to be upstaged.

Current therapy in carcinoma of the breast and in colon cancer relies on adjuvant chemotherapy to improve survival of patients with metastatic disease detected at the time of surgery. Regardless of the malignancy that has been studied, response rates to chemotherapy escalate as tumor bulk or stage is reduced at the time of treatment. That is, patients with stage I disease are more likely to respond to chemotherapy than are patients with stage IV disease. The identification of patients with metastatic disease on the basis of micrometastatic immunohistochemical methods allows the use of conventional chemotherapeutic agents in this early-stage disease, with improved survival.

D.J. Sugarbaker, M.D.

Blood Vessel and Lymphatic Vessel Invasion in Resected Nonsmall Cell Lung Carcinoma: Correlation With TNM Stage and Disease Free and Overall Survival

Bréchot J-M, Chevret S, Charpentier M-C, et al (Hôtel-Dieu, Paris; Hôpital Saint-Louis, Paris; Hôpital Antoine Béclère, Clamart, France)

Cancer 78:2111–2118, 1996 14–14

Introduction.—Blood vessel invasion (BVI) and lymphatic vessel invasion (LVI) have been associated with poor outcome in several types of cancer. The prognostic value of BVI and LVI in non–small-cell lung carcinoma (NSCLC) was evaluated at a median of 69 months in 96 patients with resected stage I to IV disease.

Methods.—All patients underwent pulmonary resection and lymph node dissection. No patients received chemotherapy or radiation therapy before surgery. The histologic tumor types were 45 squamous cell carcinomas, 40 adenocarcinomas, 7 large-cell carcinomas, and 4 carcinomas of other histologic types. Hematoxylin and eosin stains were used to identify BVI and LVI in surgical specimens.

Results.—Blood vessel invasion was identified in 50 patients (52%) and LVI was observed in 57 patients (59%). Twenty patients had both venous and arterial invasion, 26 patients had only venous invasion, and 4 patients had only arterial invasion. Fifty patients with BVI had concomitant LVI. There was a correlation between the prevalence of BVI and TNM stage and lymph node involvement; 47% of 58 N0 tumors showed LVI, compared with 81% of N2 tumors. Both venous and lymphatic tumor emboli were observed in all 3 patients with metastases at diagnosis. The estimated overall 3- and 5-year survival rates were 52% and 43%, respectively. The disease-free interval was correlated with the pathologic TNM (pTNM) stage, T and N classification, and LVI. Survival was significantly influenced by pTNM stage, T and N factors, and LVI in univariate analysis. In multivariate analysis, pTNM and LVI were predictors for poor disease-free and overall survival. Compared to patients without LVI, patients with lymphatic tumor emboli had a relative risk of death of 3.2. The presence of BVI was not associated with poor survival; arterial invasion had a relative risk of 1.2 and venous invasion showed a stronger trend toward an association with poor outcome.

Conclusions.—The prevalence of BVI and LVI was prominent in patients with NSCLC, particularly those with advanced pTNM stages. Lymphatic vessel invasion, but not BVI, was predictive of poor outcome in terms of disease-free and overall survival.

▶ The use of conventional hematoxylin and eosin staining to further predict this group of patients at high risk for subsequent recurrence in stage I lung cancer is the basis of this report. The correlation of BVI and LVI as observed on hematoxylin and eosin stains with subsequent TNM stage and disease-free and overall survival was evaluated in this cohort of patients with resectable NSCLC of various stages. Of interest is the fact that BVI was not correlated with survival but LVI was. This probably was due to the fact that patients in more advanced disease stages were examined in this study. To accurately assess the importance of BVI, one probably would need to look principally at patients with stage I disease. This most likely is due to the fact that BVI and LVI are the 2 principal mechanisms of tumor spread. One might expect that LVI would be more common in patients with more advanced disease, and this would simply amplify the current staging system, which is driven principally by node status.

D.J. Sugarbaker, M.D.

Angiogenesis and Molecular Biologic Substaging in Patients With Stage I Non–Small-cell Lung Cancer

Harpole DH Jr, Richards WG, Herndon JE II, et al (Harvard Med School, Boston)

Ann Thorac Surg 61:1470–1476, 1996 14–15

Introduction.—Non–small-cell lung cancer (NSCLC) is the most common cause of cancer mortality in both men and women. The cancer recurrence rate of pathologic stage I disease has been reported at 25% to 50%. Survival might be affected by adjuvant therapy if the subset of patients with stage I disease who were likely to have recurrence and die of NSCLC could be identified. Recent advances in molecular biology may help identify markers of metastatic propensity. The value of angiogenesis was evaluated to determine whether a molecular biological substaging system could be predictive of survival in patients with NSCLC.

Methods.—Archived paraffin-embedded blocks of tumor and normal lung were reviewed in 275 consecutive patients with stage I NSCLC. Two paraffin blocks of resected lung tissue for each patient underwent immunohistochemical analyses. Angiogenesis was measured with factor viii immunostaining of microvessels and was recorded as the number of microvessels per 10 200× microscopic fields. These measurements were

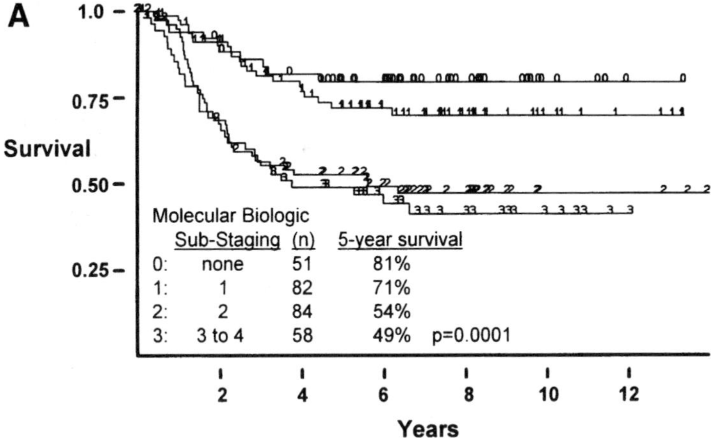

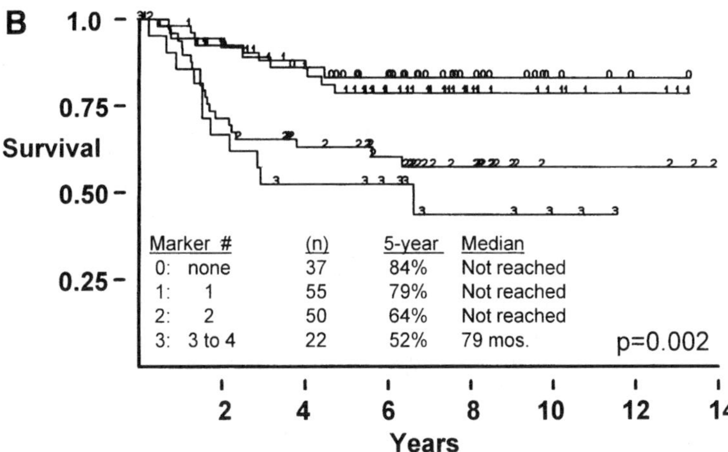

FIGURE 4.—Molecular biological substaging for pathologic stage I disease is demonstrated for the expression of 4 molecular tumor markers: hottest area angiogenesis greater than 4, proliferation marker KI-67 greater than 7%, expression of proto-oncogene *erb*B-2, and expression of tumor suppressor gene p53. **A**, each patient (n = 275) was ranked from 0 to 4 by the number of markers expressed, and a significant decrement in survival was observed for an increasing number of markers. Numbers denote censored observations at last follow-up. **B**, this curve demonstrates a similar survival analysis for the 164 patients with T1 lesions (3 cm or less in diameter). (Courtesy of Harpole DH Jr, Richards WG, Herndon JE II, et al: Angiogenesis and molecular biologic substaging in patients with stage I non–small cell lung cancer. *Ann Thor Surg* 61:1470–1476, 1996. Reprinted with permission from the Society of Thoracic Surgeons.)

taken at the center, the periphery, and the 200× microscopic field, with the highest microvessel number considered to be the "hottest" area.

Results.—Angiogenesis data gathered at the central area of the tumor were inconsistent because of prominent necrosis, so these measurements were excluded from further analyses. The microvessel numbers recorded at both the periphery and the hottest area were well correlated. Decreased survival was associated with increasing angiogenesis scores at the peripheral and hottest areas. In multivariate survival analysis comparing angiogenesis, proto-oncogene *erb*B-2, tumor suppressor gene p53, and the proliferation marker KI-67, angiogenesis was the most significant prognostic factor in stage I NSCLC. Molecular biological substaging for pathologic stage I used 4 molecular tumor markers: hottest area angiogenesis greater than 4, proliferation marker KI-67 greater than 7%, expression of proto-oncogene *erb*B-2, and expression of tumor suppressor gene p53. With each patient ranked from 0 to 4 according to the number of markers expressed, a significant decrease in survival was observed for an increasing number of markers expressed (Fig 4).

Conclusions.—The measurement of tissue molecular markers more directly evaluates the aggressiveness of an NSCLC tumor, compared to traditional histopathologic examinations. The biological markers used in this molecular biological substaging system were independent of routine histopathologic factors and revealed an additive adverse effect on survival with the expression of several biological markers.

▶ This article lays the groundwork for a molecular staging system in NSCLC. As discussed previously, the identification of patients after surgical resection who are at highest risk for both distant and local recurrence would allow the routine use of conventional chemotherapeutic agents in the adjuvant setting. This group has systematically applied molecular substaging to a group of carefully observed patients with resected stage I disease. Four molecular substages predicted survival ranging from 84%, with a median survival not reached but a substage where 3 to 4 markers were present and only a 79-month median survival and a 52% 5-year survival were recorded. This analysis needs to be duplicated in large, multi-institutional trials so that molecular substaging in NSCLC can be used productively in the design of clinical trials that would assess the efficacy of conventional chemotherapeutic agents in this deadly disease.

D.J. Sugarbaker, M.D.

Progress in Video-Assisted Thoracic Surgery

Complications of Video-assisted Thoracic Surgery: A Five-year Experience

Jancovici R, Lang-Lazdunski L, Pons F, et al (Hôpital du Val de Grace, Paris; Hôpital Purpan, Toulouse, France; Hôpital Avicenne, Bobigny, France)
Ann Thorac Surg 61:533–537, 1996 14–16

Introduction.—The advent of video-assisted thoracic surgery (VATS) and endoscopic equipment allows the performance of standard thoracic surgical procedures by a less invasive approach. These procedures are being performed with increased frequency, and sometimes without data demonstrating their benefits. Because of this trend, a 5-year experience at 4 separate institutions with more than 900 VATS procedures was investigated to determine high-risk procedures, inappropriate indications for VATS intervention, and patients at high risk for the procedure.

Methods.—Data were collected at the time of hospital discharge on 937 patients undergoing a thoracoscopic or VATS procedure regarding demographics, indications for and type of procedure, type of anesthesia, type of analgesia, and perioperative or postoperative complications. Video-assisted lobectomy was performed in 4.4% of patients and several different VATS procedures were performed in 95.6% of patients. Five patients (0.5%) died in the postoperative period. Of these, 4 patients had undergone surgery for malignant pleural effusion and died within the first postoperative month. The overall incidence of postoperative complications was 10.9% in 35 patients (3.7%). The most common complications were prolonged air leak (6.7%) and pleural effusion (0.7%). Other complications included infectious, neurologic, neoplastic, trocar-related, or port-related complications; chylothorax; and postoperative deep-vein thrombosis. A total of 116 procedures (12.4%) were converted to thoracotomies. A thoracotomy was the decision of choice in 20 patients for economic reasons or because of equipment failure.

Conclusions.—The incidence of complications associated with VATS procedures was acceptable. With the exception of prolonged air leak, the incidence of complications for VATS did not differ significantly from that for analogous open procedures. Only qualified thoracic surgeons should perform VATS procedures because of the ever-present possibility of dramatic life-threatening perioperative complications that could require emergency conversion to thoracotomy.

Complications of Thoracoscopy

Krasna MJ, Deshmukh S, McLaughlin JS (Univ of Maryland, Baltimore)

Ann Thorac Surg 61:1066–1069, 1996 14–17

Objective.—The safety and efficacy of thoracoscopy have not been studied thoroughly. The incidence of postoperative complications and the ability of preoperative imaging to predict intraoperative complications associated with thoracoscopy were assessed in a retrospective study.

Methods.—Between July 1990 and March 1995, 348 thoracoscopic procedures were performed in 321 patients for solitary pulmonary nodules (n=121); pulmonary infiltrates (n=25); lung cancer staging (n=16); esophageal cancer staging (n=49); pleural diseases (n=57); emphysema, bullae, and blebs (n=41); biopsy of mediastinal masses and nodes (n=13); sympathectomy and splanchinectomy (n=7); and other indications (n=19). Preoperative complications and morbidity and mortality were recorded within 30 days of the procedures or during the same hospitalizations.

Results.—Conversion to open thoracotomy was necessary in 27 patients, and postoperative complications occurred in 14 patients. There were no deaths from the procedure. Twelve patients required further resection after a diagnosis of lung cancer; 6 were converted to open thoracotomy because of adhesions, 2 because the lesion could not be found, 3 because the lesion was too large to remove through the thoracoscopy port, and 2 because of inadequate 1-lung ventilation; and 1 patient required exploratory surgery for bleeding and 1 for a missing needle from a preoperative needle biopsy. Ten patients experienced early postoperative complications, including excessive drainage (n=2); prolonged air leaks (n=3); emphysema (n=2); recurrent pneumothorax (n=1); pulmonary edema (n=1); and pneumonia (n=1). Late postoperative complications included tumor recurrence (n=2); malignant pleural effusion (n=1); and large parenchymal recurrence (n=1). Computed tomography failed to detect adhesions in 33% of patients.

Conclusion.—Thoracoscopy has a low incidence of perioperative and postoperative complications and is a safe alternative for certain thoracic surgery indications.

▶ The technique of video-assisted thoracic surgery and thoracoscopy continues to be applied to more patients with reduced operative morbidity and mortality. It always should be considered in the context of potential conversion to open thoracotomy. Abstract 14–17 suggests that with this integrated approach to patients, a large number of procedures can be performed with acceptable operative morbidity and mortality. Specifically, the conversion rate of 12.4% in the first study (Abstract 14–16) is in line with our own experience. This report emphasizes that patients should have the possibility of thoracotomy explained carefully to them as part of the consent procedure for thoracoscopy or video-assisted resection.

D.J. Sugarbaker, M.D.

Resection of Pulmonary Nodules Using Video-assisted Thoracic Surgery

Bernard A, and the Thorax Group (Hôpital du Bocage, Dijon, France)
Ann Thorac Surg 61:202–205, 1996 14–18

Objective.—Peripheral nodules located within 3 cm of visceral pleura are difficult to diagnose using bronchoscopy or transthoracic needle aspiration biopsy. Thoracotomy is associated with significant morbidity. Video-assisted thoracic surgery has been used for the resection of pulmonary nodules, but competency among thoracic surgeons has not been assessed. Failures, accidents, and complications using this technique and its success in the diagnosis and treatment of peripheral nodules were evaluated.

Methods.—A voluntary registry was sent to 29 French surgeons. The 20 centers that responded provided data on 388 patients (113 women), aged 17 to 85. Nodules were located by CT-guided methylene blue injection in 59 patients and by the hook wire technique in 17 patients.

Results.—Methylene blue localization failed in 8 patients (13%) and the hook wire technique failed in 8 (47%). Conversion to thoracotomy was required in 67 patients (17%), because of bleeding or air leak (n=4); inability to localize the nodule (n=29); carcinoma (n=30); dense pleural adhesions (n=2); lack of pulmonary exclusion (n=1); and poor tolerance of pulmonary exclusion (n=1). The conversion rate for teams with 30 patients or more (8.5%) was significantly lower than for teams with 10 patients or less (28%), 11 to 20 patients (22%), and 21 to 30 patients (39%). Wedge resection was performed in 300 patients and lobectomy in 21. There were no perioperative deaths. Two patients died postoperatively. The complication rate was 8% and included air leak (n=11), pneumonia (n=12), lack of pulmonary re-expansion (n=2), and hemothorax (n=2). The average chest tube placement lasted 3.3 days. The average hospitalization was 6 days. Video-assisted thoracic surgery was performed diagnostically in 226 patients and therapeutically in 162.

Conclusions.—Video-assisted thoracic surgery is a safe technique with a low incidence of perioperative complications. The individual complication rate is dependent on the competency of the surgeon. The primary reason for conversion to thoracotomy is failure to localize the nodule.

▶ The clinical management of solitary pulmonary nodules appears to be an area in transition. Previous approaches to solitary pulmonary nodules have included operative resection, but based on a large number of patients followed up in many centers, clinical follow-up with continued radiographic imaging has been the preferred approach. This approach has the potential problem of patients being lost to clinical follow-up, with rapid disease progression in the interim. It also is plagued by the continuous need for expensive imaging studies, which may be required at regular intervals. In addition, the psychological difficulties that many patients experience with the continued uncertainty regarding diagnosis can make this approach less preferable. Improvements in operative techniques and instrumentation and the growing experience of surgeons with thoracoscopic surgery have reduced significantly the operating time and hospital stays of patients undergoing diagnostic resection of solitary pulmonary nodules. This report demonstrates the utility of such an approach. The low complication rate and short hospital stay for all patients support the continued evaluation of this new approach to the management of solitary pulmonary nodules, particularly for patients in a high-risk clinical setting.

D.J. Sugarbaker, M.D.

Role of Video-assisted Thoracic Surgery in the Treatment of Pulmonary Metastases: Results of a Prospective Trial

McCormack PM, Bains MS, Begg CB, et al (Mem Sloan-Kettering Cancer Ctr, New York)

Ann Thorac Surg 62:213–217, 1996 14–19

Objective.—There is controversy regarding whether video-assisted thoracic surgery (VATS) can identify all metastatic tumors in the lung. In 1 study, the missed lesion rate was 28%. The accuracy of CT scanning and VATS compared to open thoracotomy in patients with 2 or fewer presumed pulmonary metastases was examined prospectively.

Methods.—Computed tomographic scans were performed in 50 patients with suspected pulmonary metastases 3 weeks or less before resection. Scans were reviewed and nodules were graded on a 5-point scale, with 0 = normal, 1 = probably normal, 2 = indeterminate, 3 = probably abnormal, and 4 = abnormal. Resected nodules underwent pathologic examination.

Results.—Computed tomography located 1 lesion in each of 14 patients and 2 lesions in each of 4. Thoracoscopy located all nodules in 15 patients, no nodules in 2 patients, and 1 of 2 nodules in 1 patient. The missing lesions, subsequently found at thoracotomy, were not detected by VATS because of deep locations or adhesions. Thoracotomy detected no new lesions in 4 patients, additional benign lesions in 4, and additional malignancies in 10. An additional lesion was detected by VATS in 1 patient. In 14 patients with solitary lesions detected by CT, 7 had 14 additional malignant lesions found at thoracotomy. Five patients had 5 additional benign lesions discovered at thoracotomy. The results of CT and VATS were the same in 8 patients. Thoracoscopy missed 2 malignant lesions in 2 patients that subsequently were located by thoracotomy. In the other 2 patients with 2 malignancies, both were removed by VATS, but additional malignancies were identified at thoracotomy. Seven of 12 CT scans were overread (n=3) or underread (n=4).

Conclusions.—Neither CT nor VATS detects all pulmonary metastases. Video-assisted thoracic surgery is useful only for diagnostic purposes in these patients. Thoracotomy and manual palpation are superior for the detection of pulmonary metastases.

▶ Thoracoscopy has met with certain obstacles in its application to a variety of thoracic surgical procedures. Inability of the surgeon to palpate lung tissue by the thoracoscopic approach led these authors to perform an excellent study of the efficacy of thoracoscopy in the treatment of metastatic disease. Based on the principle that complete resection has been shown in previous studies to be an indicator of long-term survival, the need for surgeons to remove all palpable tumor appears to present a major obstacle to the use of thoracoscopy in resecting metastatic lesions in the lung.

The use of helical CT scanners in a growing number of institutions may help to render the results of this trial invalid. It is principally the discrepancy between the surgeon's palpating hand and the preoperative CT evaluation that is the underlying basis for the recommendation of the authors to disregard thoracoscopic surgery in the treatment of metastatic disease. Helical CT scans were used in only 2 patients in the current study.

In addition, the lack of a recommendation to perform a median sternotomy in all cases in which ipsilateral metastatic lesions are documented would seem to contrast with the authors' stated recommendation that a thoracotomy be performed in all patients to enable careful palpation of the ipsilateral lung. This is because the mechanism for metastases to the lungs is, of course, hematogenous dissemination. Therefore, once one has determined that there are 1 or more metastatic lesions in the lung, it would appear that the recommendation that both lungs be palpated would be a logical extension from the principles outlined in this article.

Further, because complete resectability in previous studies could be achieved only in patients with a resectable number of lesions, the conclusion that complete resectability in cases where there were 2 or 3 lesions is as important as in cases where there were 50 lesions may be flawed. That is to say, if one chooses to believe that the inability to resect all tumor leads completely leads to the patient's ultimate demise, one is characterizing the situation in which there is an overwhelming amount of tumor in the lung. It may not be appropriate to extend that logic to a situation where there is a limited amount of disease in the lung. Indeed, a prospective trial with survival as the end point would need to be performed between median sternotomy and ipsilateral thoracoscopies to answer the question as to whether the morbidity of thoracotomy or sternotomy is justified by the end result of survival.

D.J. Sugarbaker, M.D.

Thoracoscopic Surgery for Lung Cancer Using the Two Small Skin Incisional Method: Two Windows Method

Iwasaki M, Nishiumi N, Maitani F, et al (Tokai Univ, Bohseidai, Isehara Kanagawa, Japan)

J Cardiovasc Surg 37:79–81, 1996 14–20

Objective.—Thoracoscopic surgery performed using the 2-window approach is comparable to conventional thoracotomy for lung cancer, including mediastinal lymph node dissection. The results of pulmonary lobectomy and mediastinal lymph node dissection in patients with stage I lung cancer were evaluated.

Methods.—Thoracoscopy was performed in 25 patients (10 women), aged 42 to 72, using a 3-cm posterior incision and a 2-cm lateral incision made in the 4th intercostal space, centering on the inferior angle of the scapula. The close site was used for direct vision and the far site was used for the scope.

Results.—The average operative times for lymph node dissection and pulmonary lobectomy were 70 minutes and 65 minutes, respectively. The average number of nodes dissected was 32. Average blood loss was 82.6 mL. The duration of hospitalization ranged from 5 to 17 days. Most patients did not require analgesics 6 days after surgery.

Conclusions.—The 2-incision method leaves minimal scarring and impairment of respiratory muscle function and permits the best 3-dimensional visual field and most accurate lymph node dissection. This method is as good or better than the standard thoracotomy technique for stage I lung cancer.

▶ The authors present an interesting technique of thoracoscopic resection. The continued drive to reduce operative morbidity and decrease the number of incisions is illustrated by the technique used. The authors are to be congratulated for their technical expertise in performing mediastinal lymph node dissection and pulmonary lobectomy through the described incision. This article is included simply to illustrate the continued pressure to reduce further operative morbidity and mortality without compromising the oncologic principles regarding the resection of intrathoracic malignancies.

D.J. Sugarbaker, M.D.

Age and Gender Considerations in the Surgical Treatment of Lung Cancer

Video-assisted Thoracic Surgery in the Elderly: A Review of 307 Cases

Jaklitsch MT, DeCamp MM Jr, Liptay MJ, et al (Brigham and Women's Hosp, Boston; Dana Farber Cancer Inst, Boston; Univ of Minnesota, Minneapolis)

Chest 110:751–758, 1996 14–21

Objective.—Because of the increasing number of thoracic procedures performed in elderly patients, age-related morbidity and mortality are important considerations. Thoracoscopic surgery is associated with fewer operative risks than open thoracotomy. The clinical benefits of video-assisted thoracic surgery were evaluated prospectively in elderly patients.

Methods.—Data on death, morbidity, conversion to open procedures, and duration of hospital stay were collected for 307 procedures performed on 296 patients. Patients were followed up at 1 and 6 weeks after surgery. Patients who underwent parenchymal resections for malignant disease were followed up every 4 months for 3 years. Groups were compared using Fisher's Exact Test.

Results.—There were 188 operations for lung disease, 88 for pleural disease, 27 for mediastinal disease, and 14 for pericardial windows. Mean forced expiratory volume in 1 second tended to decrease with age. There were 109 procedures performed on patients aged 65 to 69, 110 on patients aged 70 to 74, 55 on patients aged 75 to 79, and 33 on patients aged 80 to 90. Hospitalization averaged 4 days for the groups aged 65 to 79 and 5 days for the group aged 80 to 90. Rates of mortality, morbidity, and conversion to thoracotomy were low (Table 2).

Conclusions.—The results of video-assisted thoracic surgery were superior to those of open thoracotomy, with a low 30-day mortality rate and a low morbidity rate that was not related to age. The duration of hospitalization also was reduced.

TABLE 2.—Mortality, Conversion, and Morbidity as Functions of Age

	Age, yr				
	65–69	70–74	75–79	80–90	Totals
No. of procedures	109	110	55	33	307
Death (% group)	0	3 (3)	0	0	3 (<1)
Conversion (% group)	1 (1)	2 (2)	0	1 (3)	4 (1)
Procedures associated with morbidity (% group)	15 (14)	19 (17)	7 (13)	4 (12)	45 (15)
Procedures with major morbid events (%)	4 (4)	13 (12)	4 (7)	1 (3)	22 (7)
No. of events					
Prolonged air leak	1	7	2	0	10
Respiratory failure/pneumonia	1	2	2	1	6
Reoperation for bleeding	1	1	0	0	2
Other	1	4	0	0	5
Procedures with minor morbid events (%)	13 (12)	8 (7)	3 (5)	3 (9)	27 (9)
No. of events					
Dysrhythmia					
Supraventricular	6	5	1	1	13
Ventricular	2	1	0	0	3
Confusion	3	2	2	1	8
Other	5	1	0	1	7

(Courtesy of Jaklitsch MT, DeCamp MM Jr, Liptay MJ, et al: Video-assisted thoracic surgery in the elderly: A review of 307 cases. *Chest* 110:751–758, 1996).

Surgical Treatment of Non–Small-cell Lung Cancer in Patients Older Than Seventy Years

Harvey JC, Erdman C, Pisch J, et al (Beth Israel Med Ctr, New York)
J Surg Oncol 60:247–249, 1995 14–22

Introduction.—About one third of all cancer deaths in men are from lung cancer. Preventive measures, such as discouraging smoking, using early detection methods, and extending treatments, would help improve cancer statistics. Increased mortality has been associated with the surgical treatment of non–small-cell lung cancer, particularly with the use of pneumonectomy. The surgical management of elderly patients with non–small-cell lung cancer over a 9-year period was described.

Methods.—Eighty-one patients were included in the study. All the patients had complete medical histories and physical examinations, blood counts, and blood chemistries performed. For patients with reversible airways disease, bronchodilators were prescribed. Except for 1 thoracoscopic wedge resection, operations were performed through posterolateral thoracotomies. Procedures included brachytherapy only, wedge or segmental resection, lobectomy, lobectomy with adjacent segmental or wedge resection, lobectomy with brachytherapy, lobectomy with chest wall resection, and pneumonectomy.

Results.—There was an overall surgical mortality rate of 4.9%, with 3 of the 4 deaths occurring among patients aged 80 or older. The operative mortality rate of those younger than 70 was 1.6%. Myocardial infarction, stroke, and pulmonary embolus were the causes of perioperative mortality. There were 5-year survival rates of 42% overall, 65% for stage I, and 24%

TABLE 2.—Survival Table for Patients With Lung Cancer Who Are Older Than 70

Study group	Year	No. of patients	Operative mortality (%)	5-Year survival (%)
Harviel et al. [4]	1978	32	18.2	NA
Breyer et al. [5]*	1981	213	3	27
Ginsberg et al. [6]*	1983	58	14	30
Deneffe et al. [7]	1988	71	11.2	NA
Ishida et al. [8]	1990	185	3	48
Thomas et al. [10]	1993	47	12.8	29.8
Harvey et al. [present study]	1995	81	4.9	42

*Includes patients with disease other than primary non–small-cell lung cancer.
(Courtesy of Harvey JC, Erdman C, Pisch J, et al: Surgical treatment of non–small-cell lung cancer in patients older than seventy years. *J Surg Oncol* 60:247–249, copyright 1995. Reprinted by permission of Wiley-Liss, Inc., a subsidiary of John Wiley & Sons, Inc.)

for stages II to IIIB. Patients with brachytherapy as part of their treatment had a 5-year survival rate of 14% compared with patients who had resection alone, in whom the 5-year survival rate was 46%.

Conclusions.—Among the elderly, mortality rates for pulmonary resection have been reported as greater than 10% (Table 2). Selected patients between the ages of 70 and 80 can have surgical treatment with results that are similar to those expected among younger patients. The risks of surgical treatment increase at age 80, and heparin prophylaxis is important in this age group. Alternative therapies for patients in this age group who cannot tolerate lobectomy or pneumonectomy also result in a better 5-year survival rate.

▶ The population of the United States is aging. Life expectancies are increasing at a slow but consistent rate. The widespread practice of cigarette smoking by individuals who are currently in their 70s and 80s has caused an increasing number of surgeons to face the decision regarding operative therapy in patients of advanced age. These 2 reports (Abstracts 14–21 and 14–22) suggest that patients of advanced age, including those older than 80, can have successful therapy, and that age alone should not be used as a contraindication to surgery. However, age is a consistent predictor of increased perioperative mortality, particularly when conventional surgery is used, as it was in the report by Harvey and colleagues. Patients older than 80 had a mortality rate of 17.6%, which approaches a rate that may dishearten a surgeon from proceeding in this subgroup of patients. The mortality rate for patients older than 70 has been substantial in previous reports. Five-year survival rates appear to justify an aggressive approach in this subgroup of patients.

The use of video-assisted thoracic surgery in this select subgroup of patients would appear to be an appropriate approach. Reduced operative morbidity and mortality in this group, which is at high risk, may be afforded by a more aggressive thoracoscopic and video-assisted approach. The surgeon is reminded never to compromise oncologic principles of resection unless they are justified by a substantial reduction in operative risk. The continued advance of video-assisted and thoracoscopic techniques would appear to have a significant potential for improving the outcome of elderly patients undergoing operative therapy.

D.J. Sugarbaker, M.D.

Influence of Age on the Treatment of Limited-stage Small-cell Lung Cancer

Siu LL, Shepherd FA, Murray N, et al (Toronto Hosp; British Columbia Cancer Agency, Vancouver; Princess Margaret Hosp, Toronto; et al)

J Clin Oncol 14:821–828, 1996 14–23

Introduction.—For both sexes in North America, the leading cause of cancer mortality is lung carcinoma. In the geriatric population, few studies have been conducted to examine systemic antineoplastic treatment, particularly because many of the elderly are excluded from the studies for a variety of reasons, such as a decline in organ function, decreased bone marrow tolerance to myelosuppressive agents, and diminished overall life expectancy. Twenty percent of all cases of bronchogenic carcinoma are accounted for by small-cell lung cancer. The prognostic importance of age on response rate and survival was evaluated in patients with limited-stage small-cell lung cancer, and the effect of age on chemotherapy dose delivery and toxicity was determined.

Methods.—There were 608 patients with small-cell lung cancer who had limited disease, who all received the same chemotherapy, and who were part of this retrospective analysis from randomized trials conducted by the National Cancer Institute of Canada. The chemotherapy was administered in a delayed alternating or immediate fashion, and included etoposide plus cisplatin, vincristine, cyclophosphamide, and doxorubicin. Cranial and thoracic irradiation also was administered.

Results.—In baseline characteristics, there were no differences among the 520 patients younger than 70 and the 88 patients who were 70 or older, including performance status, serum lactate dehydrogenase level, and treatment protocol. Response rates were comparable between the 2 groups, being 78% in the younger group and 82% in the older group. The 5-year survival rates were similar, with 8% alive in the older group and 11% alive in the younger group. When analyzed as a continuous variable in a univariate model, age was a significant predictor of overall survival; however, in the multivariate regression analysis, it was no longer an independent prognostic factor. Patients in the older group received lower total doses of each drug, primarily as a result of dose omissions, than patients in the younger group. The frequency of dose delays between the 2 groups was similar, and there were no significant differences in the incidence of hematologic or most nonhematologic toxicities.

Conclusions.—In limited-stage small-cell lung cancer, age is not a significant adverse prognostic variable. In older patients, moderately aggressive chemotherapy can be delivered safely, but it may be modestly attenuated through dose reduction or omission.

▶ Small-cell lung cancer carries a uniformly poor prognosis. This interesting study, however, documents well that age should not be an independent factor in determining the extent of therapy. Age was not a significant adverse prognostic variable in patients with limited small-cell lung cancer. Comparable 5-year survival rates were achieved, supporting the concept of aggressive treatment based on performance study and independent of age.

D.J. Sugarbaker, M.D.

Differences in Lung Cancer Risk Between Men and Women: Examination of the Evidence

Zang EA, Wynder EL (American Health Found, New York)

J Natl Cancer Inst 88:183–192, 1996 14–24

Introduction.—The principal cause of lung cancer is cigarette smoking. There has been a 500% increase in lung cancer among women since 1950, and the disease has surpassed even breast cancer as the leading cause of cancer deaths among women since 1987. Within the next 3 decades, lung cancer rates among women are expected to surpass those among men because of the slower decline in smoking prevalence among women. Women also may be more susceptible to tobacco carcinogens than men. An in depth evaluation of the differences in lung cancer risk between men and women was conducted.

Methods.—Data from 1,108 male and 781 female smokers with lung cancer of small-cell/oat cell, large-cell, squamous/epidermoid, and adenocarcinoma types were compared with data from 1,122 male and 948 female control subjects with diseases unrelated to smoking (Table 2). Unconditional multiple logistic regression analyses were used to estimate odds ratios and 2-sided tests were used to determine statistical significance. Increasing levels of exposure to cigarette smoke were used to estimate the odds ratios for major histologic types.

Results.—Men were more likely to have been smokers than women, as there were more never-smoking women (8.3% aged 55 or older) than men (2.9% aged 55 or older), particularly those with the squamous/epidermoid type of cancer. Women started smoking later, reported inhaling less deeply, and smoked fewer cigarettes than men. Dose-response odds ratios over cumulative exposure to cigarette smoking were 1.2- to 1.7-fold higher in women than in men for major histologic types (Fig 1). In small-cell/oat cell carcinomas and adenocarcinomas, these differences were more pronounced than in squamous/epidermoid carcinomas. The odds ratios were not altered by adjustments for height, weight, or body mass index.

Conclusions.—Women have consistently higher odds ratios for major lung cancer types than men at every level of exposure to cigarette smoking. Differences in baseline exposure, body size, or smoking history did not

TABLE 2.—Characteristics of the Study Population

Characteristic	Males				Females			
	Squamous/ epidermoid carcinoma (n = 397), %	Adenocarcinoma (n = 418), %	Small-cell/ oat cell carcinoma (n = 182), %	Controls (n = 1122), %	Squamous/ epidermoid carcinoma (n = 165), %	Adenocarcinoma (n = 384), %	Small-cell/ oat cell carcinoma (n = 142), %	Controls (n = 948), %
Age, y								
<45	6.6	14.1	5.5	10.6	6.7	10.2	7.7	10.0
45–54	22.2	24.6	22.0	18.5	27.3	26.8	21.1	21.4
55–64	40.3	38.0	47.8	39.0	29.7	32.8	45.8	35.9
≥65	31.0	23.2	24.7	31.8	36.4	30.2	25.4	32.7
Marital status								
Single	7.8	8.6	6.6	8.0	9.1	5.5	4.9	8.0
Married	74.8	79.0	73.1	81.0	53.3	63.5	62.7	61.0
Separated/divorced	9.8	8.6	14.3	6.8	9.7	10.7	11.3	9.5
Widowed	7.6	3.8	6.0	4.2	27.9	20.3	21.1	21.5
Education, y								
<12	34.3	25.7	33.5	21.0	18.8	18.5	30.3	19.5
12	28.8	25.5	36.3	27.1	46.7	47.4	38.7	41.8
13–16	25.5	34.1	27.5	32.0	28.5	28.1	28.2	29.2
>16	11.4	14.7	2.7	19.9	6.1	6.0	2.8	9.6
Occupation								
Professional	27.0	36.1	22.5	40.1	17.0	13.3	14.1	21.6
Skilled	44.8	43.5	47.3	41.9	47.9	43.8	42.3	40.8
Unskilled	28.2	20.3	30.2	18.0	9.1	13.5	22.5	12.9
Housewife	—	—	—	—	26.1	29.4	21.1	24.7

(Courtesy of Zang EA, Wynder EL: Differences in lung cancer risk between men and women: Examination of the evidence. *J Natl Cancer Inst* 88:183–192, 1996.)

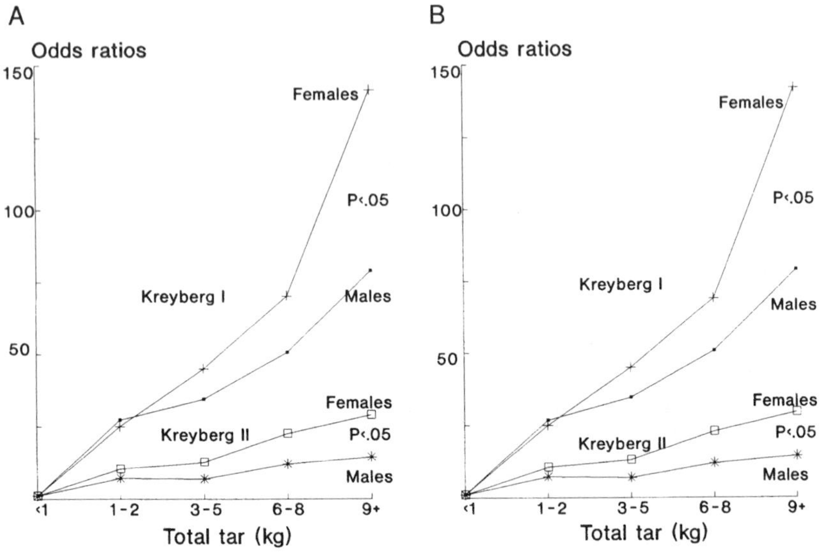

FIGURE 1.—Sex-specific odds ratios for Kreyberg I–type (690 male and 397 female case subjects) versus Kreyberg II–type (435 male and 414 female case subjects) lung cancer, adjusted for age only (**A**) or adjusted for age plus prediagnostic body weight (**B**). *P* values are based on overall gender differences in odds ratios. (Courtesy of Zang EA, Wynder EL: Differences in lung cancer risk between men and women: Examination of the evidence. *J Natl Cancer Inst* 88:183–192, 1996.)

explain the gender differences; however, women may be more susceptible to tobacco carcinogens than men. This may be explained by variations in physiologic mechanisms, such as detoxification of lung carcinogens and metabolic activation.

▶ Lung cancer continues to escalate as the primary cancer killer in women. Multiple studies have suggested that the cancer risk from smoking is greater in women than in men. This study beautifully demonstrated that, at all levels of tobacco smoke exposure, women have a higher incidence of squamous and epidermoid carcinoma than men. The same is true for the development of adenocarcinoma. Women demonstrated a higher risk for the development of adenocarcinoma at each level of smoke exposure. The authors carefully discuss whether the observed difference in susceptibility to the effects of tobacco carcinogens by women could result from external factors. They conclude that it does not result from differences in occupational exposure or smoking behavior and is not related to body size or lung size. They propose that a more plausible explanation would be variations in physiologic mechanisms, such as a difference in metabolic activation or lung detoxification of carcinogens. The continued high smoking prevalence and growing incidence of lung cancer among women, coupled now with this observation of an increased susceptibility to carcinogens, should be cause for significant discussion of a national public health policy regarding smoking.

D.J. Sugarbaker, M.D.

New Advances in Staging Therapy for Chest Malignancies

INTRODUCTION

Positron emission tomography (PET) has taken radiographic imaging one step beyond conventional anatomical characterization of intrathoracic structures. By detecting the increased rates of glucose metabolism in tumor cells and measuring uptake of the positron-emitting glucose analogue 2-^{18}F-fluoro-2-deoxy-D-glucose, protection of tumor cells is now combined with imaging. This dramatic breakthrough for radiographic imaging may hold promise for significant improvement in our understanding of the clinical stage of patients with non–small-cell lung cancer for definitive diagnosis and therapy.

David J. Sugarbaker, M.D.

Thoracic Nodal Staging With PET Imaging With ^{18}FDG in Patients With Bronchogenic Carcinoma

Patz EF Jr, Lowe VJ, Goodman PC, et al (Duke Univ, Durham, NC)
Chest 108:1617–1621, 1995 14–25

Background.—Computed tomography is only 60% sensitive in detecting nodal metastases of bronchogenic carcinoma, and it is not very specific. In addition, CT does not reliably predict the histologic type of cancer. Positron emission tomography (PET) using 18-fluoro-2-deoxyglucose (^{18}FDG) provides both anatomical and physiologic information.

Patients.—Positron emission tomography was performed in 42 adults with newly diagnosed bronchogenic carcinoma before planned sampling of the thoracic nodes. Adenocarcinomas were most prevalent. A total of 62 node stations, 40 in the hilar/lobar region and 22 in mediastinal sites, were sampled. Thoracic CT scanning also was performed in 14 cases with IV contrast enhancement.

Findings.—Imaging with PET was 83% sensitive and 82% specific in detecting thoracic node metastases. The respective percentages for CT were 43% and 85%. Positron emission tomography imaging accurately predicted the presence or absence of metastases in 75% of hilar/lobar node stations (Fig 1). There were 7 false positive node stations, 3 of which were normal on CT scanning. None of the 3 false negative stations were positive on CT. There was only 1 false negative PET study of the mediastinal nodes. In contrast, CT was only 58% sensitive in detecting mediastinal metastases.

Conclusions.—A normal ^{18}FDG-PET study nearly eliminates the need to sample the mediastinal nodes preoperatively. An abnormal study result probably represents spread of bronchogenic cancer to the mediastinum.

▶ This interesting study suggests that PET scanning may develop as an important method for staging the mediastinum in patients with non–small-cell lung cancer. Mediastinoscopy has been the "gold standard" for determining whether mediastinal lymph node involvement has occurred. Tradi-

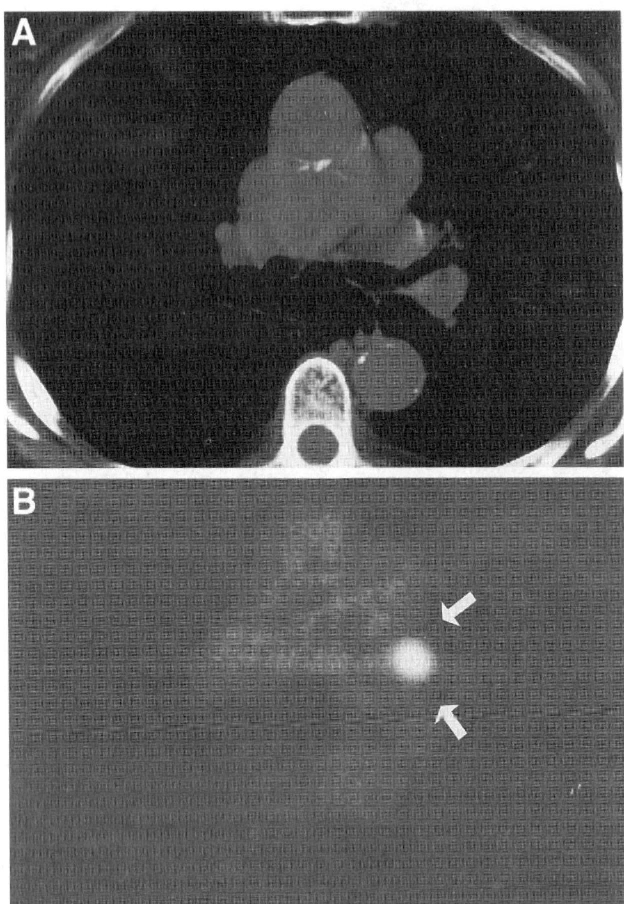

FIGURE 1.—Woman aged 72 years with a 1.6-cm left upper lobe nodule. Surgery demonstrated stage II (T1N1) adenocarcinoma. **Top,** CT at the level of the left hilum is normal. **Bottom,** axial positron emission tomography with 18-fluoro-2-deoxyglucose (^{18}FDG-PET) image at the same level demonstrates a focal area of increased uptake in the left hilum (*arrow*). At surgery there was metastatic adenocarcinoma in a hilar lymph node. (Courtesy of Patz EF Jr, Lowe VJ, Goodman PC, et al: Thoracic nodal staging with PET imaging with ^{18}FDG in patients with bronchogenic carcinoma. *Chest* 108:1617–1621, 1995.)

tionally, this was done to determine whether patients were to be offered operative therapy. However, with the advent of induction chemotherapy and 2 prospective randomized trials showing its positive impact on long-term survival, the detection of metastatic disease in mediastinal lymph nodes becomes more crucial if these patients are to be offered these therapeutic strategies. Use of PET scanning may allow detection of mediastinal nodes for a larger number of patients, particularly if mediastinoscopy is not available. We will watch with great interest as Dr. Patz and his colleagues further develop the applications and establish the sensitivity and specificity of this technology. As noted in Figure 1 for lobar/hilar or mediastinal node stations,

PET scanning improved the sensitivity and specificity over that obtained with conventional CT scans.

D.J. Sugarbaker, M.D.

Mediastinal Lymph Node Staging of Non–Small-cell Lung Cancer: A Prospective Comparison of Computed Tomography and Positron Emission Tomography

Scott WJ, Gobar LS, Terry JD, et al (Creighton Univ, Omaha, Neb; Omaha Veterans Affairs Med Ctr, Neb)

J Thorac Cardiovasc Surg 111:642–648, 1996 14–26

Introduction.—CT is commonly used for the preoperative assessment of the mediastinum in patients with non–small-cell lung cancer. However, the specificity and sensitivity of CT for detecting mediastinal lymph node metastases is low. By measuring the uptake of a positron-emitting glucose analogue, fluoro-2-deoxy-D-glucose, positron emission tomography detects increased rates of glucose metabolism, which are characteristic of malignant cells. The ability of positron emission tomography to detect lymph node metastases in patients with non–small-cell lung cancer was examined, and was compared to that of CT.

Methods.—A total of 27 patients underwent CT, positron emission tomography, and surgical staging. They had a total of 75 lymph node stations, or 2.8 per person. Separate radiologists who were blinded to surgical staging results read the CT and positron emission tomographic scans. Lymph nodes were considered positive by CT if they were larger than 1 cm in short-axis diameter. Lymph nodes were considered positive by positron emission tomography if they were greater than 4.2, as the standardized uptake values were recorded from areas that corresponded to those from which biopsy specimens were taken.

Results.—In 3 patients, the mediastinum was incorrectly staged as positive for metastases by CT, and in 3 patients, it was incorrectly staged as negative for metastases. Computed tomography resulted in a sensitivity of 67% and a specificity of 83%. In all 27 patients, the mediastinum was correctly staged by positron emission tomography. Computed tomography resulted in 4 false-positive and 4 false-negative findings, when analyzed by individual node station. One node station was mislabeled as positive with positron emission tomography. Computed tomography had a sensitivity of 60%, a specificity of 93%, and a positive predictive value of 60% for individual node stations. Positron emission tomography had a sensitivity of 100%, a specificity of 98%, and a positive predictive value of 91% for individual node stations.

Conclusions.—Positron emission tomography combined with CT is more accurate than CT alone in detecting mediastinal lymph node metastases from non–small-cell lung cancer. Further research will help determine the most appropriate use of positron emission tomography technology in the treatment of patients with malignant disease of the thorax.

▶ This report provides further data to suggest that positron emission tomography (PET) is substantially better than conventional CT of the chest. Integration of tumor biology into tumor imaging as is done by the PET scanner provides the explanation for this substantial improvement in imaging capabilities.

D.J. Sugarbaker, M.D.

Staging Non–Small-cell Lung Cancer by Whole-body Positron Emission Tomographic Imaging

Valk PE, Pounds TR, Hopkins DM, et al (Northern California PET Imaging Ctr, Sacramento; Radiological Associates of Sacramento, Calif)

Ann Thorac Surg 60:1573–1582, 1995 14–27

Background.—An accurate, noninvasive method for staging non–small-cell lung cancer (NSCLC) is needed so that the morbidity and cost of surgical staging can be avoided. The role of regional and whole-body positron emission tomography (PET) imaging in this setting was studied prospectively.

Methods.—Ninety-nine patients were studied. In 76 patients, mediastinal PET and CT findings were compared with the results of surgical staging. Findings of possible distant metastasis on PET and CT were checked against biopsy results and findings on clinical and imaging follow-up.

Findings.—The sensitivity of PET for the diagnosis of N2 disease was 83%, with a specificity of 94%. For CT, these values were 63% and 73%, respectively. Previously unsuspected distant metastasis were identified by PET in 11% of the patients. There were no false positive findings. In 19% of the patients, normal PET findings were obtained at distant sites of CT abnormality. In 14 of these patients, clinical and imaging follow-up showed no evidence of metastasis. One PET result was falsely negative.

Conclusions.—In the diagnosis of mediastinal and distant metastasis, PET was more accurate than CT. The number of thoracotomies done for nonresectable disease may be reduced by the detection of unsuspected metastatic disease by PET.

▶ This is the third study (Abstracts 14–25 to 14–27) to document the superiority of PET scanning over CT of the chest. The application of PET scanning in this study was for whole-body imaging. The use of PET scanning for the detection of distant metastatic disease may further enhance our ability to accurately stage patients before therapy. These 3 papers represent a spectrum of the application of PET technology and have provided data for its approved diagnostic accuracy over conventional CT scanning. Unfortunately, this technology remains largely inaccessible to the majority of practicing physicians and surgeons.

D.J. Sugarbaker, M.D.

Adjuvant Chemotherapy After Complete Resection in Non–Small-cell Lung Cancer

Wada H, and the West Japan Study Group for Lung Cancer Surgery (Kyoto Univ, Japan)

J Clin Oncol 14:1048–1054, 1996 14–28

Introduction.—For patients with stage I non–small-cell lung cancer, even when complete resection is possible, the 5-year survival rate is only 50% to 60%. Therefore, postoperative adjuvant therapy should be viewed as a means of prolonging survival. Because multidrug chemotherapy is the treatment of choice in these cases, the efficacy of concomitant administration of uracil (UFT) with cisplatin (CDDP) and vindesine (VDS) vs. single therapy was evaluated prospectively in a randomized, nonblind study of 5-year survival. The efficacy of UFT therapy for non–small-cell lung cancer was also examined.

Methods.—From 37 Japanese institutions, 323 patients aged 15–75 years with stage I to III primary non–small-cell lung cancer were studied. The CVU (multidrug) group (n = 115) received CDDP, 50 mg/m^2 body surface, and VDS, 2–3 mg/kg 1–3 weeks after surgery, and VDS, 2–3 mg/kg twice at 1- to 2-week intervals, followed 2 weeks later by oral administration of UFT, 400 mg/day for 1 year. The UFT group (n = 108) received 400 mg/day for 1 year beginning 1–3 weeks after surgery. The control group (n = 100) received surgical treatment only. Five-year survival rates were compared.

Results.—There were 109 CVU patients, 103 UFT patients, and 98 control patients available for evaluation at 5 years. Five-year survival rates were higher in the CVU (60.6%) and UFT (64.1%) groups than in the control (49.0%) group, and significantly higher in the UFT group than in the control group (Fig 2). Multivariate analysis showed that older age was significantly associated with a poorer prognosis and postoperative adjuvant chemotherapy significantly associated with an improved prognosis in the CVU and UFT groups. The incidence of hematologic adverse events was significantly lower in the UFT group (11.7%) than in the CVU group (29.4%); the UFT group also had lower incidences of fatigue, nausea/vomiting, and anorexia. Recurrence rates were 38.6% in the CVU group, 39.9% in the UFT group, and 42.9% in the control group. Deaths from primary lung cancer were 31.2% in the CVU group, 28.2% in the UFT group, and 38.8% in the control group. Deaths from nonrecurrent second primary carcinomas were 2.8%, 1.9%, and 5.1%, respectively.

Conclusions.—Postoperative adjuvant therapy with CVU and UFT significantly increased the survival of patients with non–small-cell lung can-

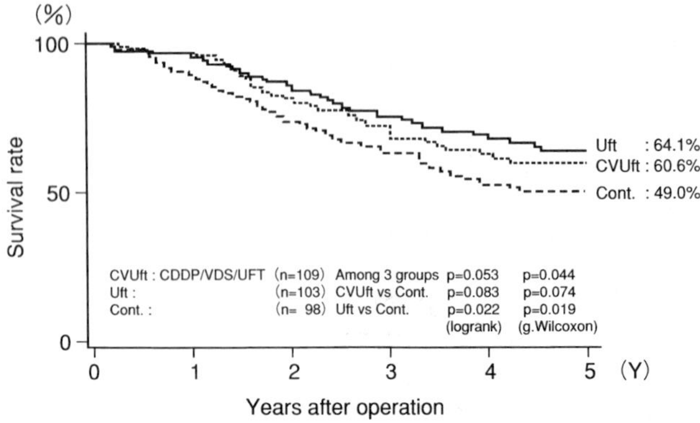

FIGURE 2.—Survival curves for all patients. *Abbreviations: Uft,* uracil; *CVUft,* multidrug; *Cont,* control. (Courtesy of Wada H, and the West Japan Study Group for Lung Cancer Surgery: Adjuvant chemotherapy after complete resection in non–small-cell lung cancer. *J Clin Oncol* 14:1048–1054, 1996.)

cer. Low-dose oral UFT was at least as effective as the more conventional type of adjuvant chemotherapy.

▶ As shown in Figure 2, this trial demonstrated a statistically significant improvement in survival for patients undergoing adjuvant chemotherapy compared with the control group. The importance of this study is that it is the first to suggest a survival advantage for patients receiving adjuvant chemotherapy. The survival advantage of 10% to 15% is relatively small. This may be because a large number of patients treated were in advanced stage II or III disease. Indeed, a small cohort of treated patients had stage IIIB disease. As previously mentioned, the observation that patients with lower tumor bulk or earlier stage will respond to chemotherapy at higher fractions may account for the relatively poor effect on survival noted in this trial.

D.J. Sugarbaker, M.D.

Chest Wall Invasive Non–Small-cell Lung Cancer: Patterns of Failure and Implications for a Revised Staging System

Harpole DH Jr, Healey EA, DeCamp MM Jr, et al (Brigham and Women's Hosp, Boston; Harvard Med School, Boston)

Ann Surg Oncol 3:261–269, 1996 14–29

Introduction.—Less than 5% of patients with non–small-cell lung cancer have chest wall invasion. However, as the incidence of non–small-cell lung cancer increases, more patients with chest wall invasion will be seen. The mainstay of therapy for superior sulcus tumors has been operative resection after preoperative radiation therapy. Resection followed by radiation therapy for positive margins or positive lymph nodes has been used for chest wall invasion outside the superior sulcus. Chest wall invasion has been classified as a subset of stage IIIA by the new international staging

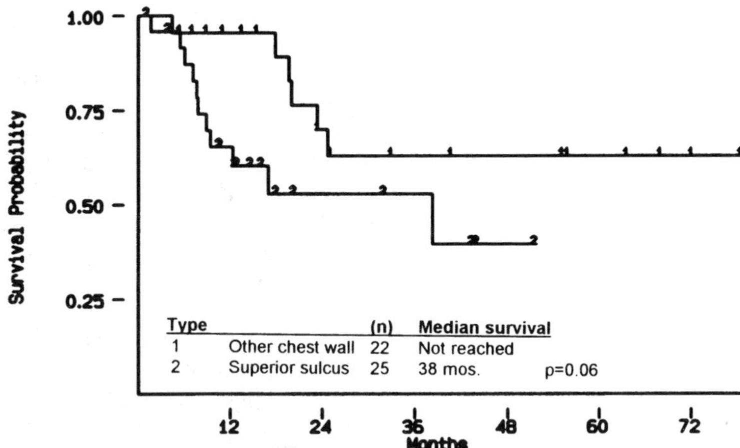

FIGURE 2.—Overall survival by resection type is demonstrated. Notice that the superior sulcus tumors relapse sooner. Tic markers (numbers on the curve) indicate censored data points. (Courtesy of Harpole DH Jr, Healey EA, DeCamp MM Jr, et al: Chest wall invasive non–small-cell lung cancer: Patterns of failure and implications for a revised staging system. *Ann Surg Oncol* 3:261–269, 1996.)

system. There has been evidence to indicate that patients with T3N0 cancers have an improved outcome compared to patients with IIIA disease and positive N2 lymph nodes. Patients with documented chest wall–invasive non–small-cell lung cancer were evaluated prospectively to determine whether there is a difference in outcome between those with superior sulcus tumors and those with chest wall invasion outside the superior sulcus.

Methods.—In 47 patients with non–small-cell lung cancer, pre-resectional stagings were made by bone scan, head and chest/abdominal CT, and mediastinoscopy. The patients had histologically proven chest wall–invasive non–small-cell lung cancer, 25 with superior sulcus tumors and 22 with chest wall invasion outside the superior sulcus. Clinical data included smoking history, serum laboratory test results, and initial physical examination. Neoadjuvant therapy was prescribed for all patients with superior sulcus tumors. Resection alone was given to those with chest wall invasion outside the superior sulcus. Three of these patients also had platinum-based chemotherapy and radiation therapy before their operations.

Results.—An operative complication occurred in 17 patients (36%) and their median length of stay increased from 7 to 12 days; however, there were no perioperative deaths. For 44 of 47 patients (94%), a complete pathologic resection was achieved. There was a median survival time of 38 months, with a 2-year survival rate of 62% and a 5-year survival rate of 50%. For superior sulcus tumors, the median length of survival was 36 months, and for other chest wall tumors, the median length of survival was more than 60 months (Fig 2). Poor performance status, positive margins, and positive lymph nodes were the significant univariate predictors of decreased overall and cancer-free survival. In 22 of 47 patients (46%), recurrence was observed at a median of 8 months.

Conclusions.—Even after neoadjuvant therapy, the operative risk for chest wall–invasive non–small-cell lung cancer was acceptable. However, despite the use of more neoadjuvant therapy, there was the suggestion that patients with superior sulcus tumors may have recurrence sooner, and more intensive systemic therapy is worth investigating. A reappraisal of the international staging system is warranted with the survival of this subset (T3N0) of patients with stage IIIA disease when compared with the survival of patients with positive N2 lymph nodes.

▶ The current staging system for non–small-cell lung cancer includes stages I to IV. Stage IIIA has been the focus of considerable interest as innovative induction therapeutic strategies have been developed. Evaluation of the effects of therapy in stage IIIA disease is somewhat confounded by the subdivision of IIIA, which includes T3N0 tumors and tumors with N2 mediastinal node involvement. As seen in this series, patients with T3N0 stage IIIA lung cancer fare significantly better with surgical resection than do patients with IIIA disease on the basis of N2 mediastinal adenopathy, for whom survival rates are diminished. This finding is consistent with numerous previous reports. Downstaging patients with T3N0 disease to a stage IIB category may be justified on the basis of overall survival in this subgroup. More accurate staging based on prognosis inevitably will lead to improved survival as therapeutic strategies are targeted more specifically to biologic subtypes of tumor.

D.J. Sugarbaker, M.D.

Successful Treatment of Solitary Extracranial Metastases From Non–Small-cell Lung Cancer

Luketich JD, Martini N, Ginsberg RJ, et al (Mem Sloan-Kettering Cancer Ctr, New York)

Ann Thorac Surg 60:1609–1611, 1995 14–30

Background.—Patients with recurrent tumor after resection of non–small-cell lung carcinoma usually have poor outcomes. Such recurrences are treated with either systemic agents or palliative irradiation. Long-term survival after resection of isolated brain metastases from non–small-cell lung carcinoma has recently been reported, but resection of other metastatic sites has not been investigated.

Methods.—Fourteen patients with solitary extracranial metastases treated aggressively after curative surgery for non–small-cell lung carcinoma were reviewed. Five patients had squamous carcinoma; 8, adenocarcinoma; and 1, large-cell carcinoma. Initially, disease stage was I in 3 patients, II in 5, and IIIa in 6. Metastases occurred in the extrathoracic lymph nodes in 6 patients, skeletal muscle in 4, bone in 3, and small bowel in 1.

Findings.—The median disease-free period before metastases was 19.5 months. Twelve patients had complete resection of metastatic sites. The remaining 2 patients underwent curative irradiation alone, which produced complete responses in both. The overall actuarial survival rate was 86% at 10 years. Eleven patients are currently alive and well 17 months to 13 years after treatment of metastases. One patient is alive with recurrent disease. Another patient died of recurrent widespread metastases, and 2 died of unrelated causes.

Conclusions.—Long-term survival can be achieved with treatment of isolated metastases from non–small-cell lung carcinoma to various sites. However, appropriate patient selection is critical.

▶ This study represents a retrospective review of patients treated for extrathoracic, extracranial metastases. The long-term survival rate noted in this group of 86% should be considered in the context of a retrospective review of highly selected patients. There appears to be no solid evidence for the surgical resection of extracranial, extrathoracic metastases in non–small-cell lung cancer. The resection of isolated cranial metastases remains the only established indication for resection of M1 disease in non–small-cell lung cancer.

D.J. Sugarbaker, M.D.

Predictors of Survival in Malignant Tumors of the Sternum

Martini N, Huvos AG, Burt ME, et al (Mem Sloan-Kettering Cancer Ctr, New York; Cornell Univ, New York)

J Thorac Cardiovasc Surg 111:96–106, 1996 14–31

Background.—Primary malignant tumors of the sternum are uncommon. One type is solid tumors, which include primary bony or cartilaginous tumors and soft-tissue sarcomas. The other type is small-cell tumors, including Ewing's sarcomas, plasmacytomas, and lymphomas, which are usually systemic but may initially appear as a localized sternal mass. The outcomes with these tumors were reviewed and predictors of survival were identified.

Methods and Findings.—Fifty-four patients with primary malignant tumors of the sternum were treated between 1930 and 1994. Fifty initially had a mass. Half also had pain in the sternal region. Two patients were initially asymptomatic. The 39 solid tumors included 26 chondrosarcomas, 10 osteosarcomas, 1 fibrosarcoma, 1 angiosarcoma, and 1 malignant fibrous histiocytoma. Twenty-five of these were low grade and 14, high grade. The 15 small-cell tumors included 8 plasmacytomas, 6 malignant lymphomas, and 1 Ewing's sarcoma. Thirty-seven patients underwent partial or subtotal sternectomy, and 3, total sternectomy. Ten of the remaining 14 patients had external radiation, or chemotherapy without surgery, or both; 3 had local excision; and 1, no treatment. Some form of skeletal reconstruction of the chest wall defect was present in all but 1 patient treated by wide resection. Seventy-eight percent of the patients underwent Marlex mesh repair. In 25 of these 31 patients, this was combined with methyl methacrylate. Skin edges were closed per primum in 32 patients. Eight needed muscle, omentum, or skin flaps. The 5-year survival rate in patients undergoing chondrosarcoma resection was 80%. Those with osteosarcomas had a 5-year survival rate of 14%. Resection was curative in 64% of the patients with low-grade sarcomas but in only 7% of those with high-grade sarcomas. Resection and radiation were beneficial for local control in patients with small-cell tumors. All failures in this group resulted from distant metastases.

Conclusions.—Primary sarcomas of the sternum are potentially curable by wide surgical excision. The surgical complication rates are low when rigid prostheses are used to repair skeletal defects. Overall survival after complete surgical resection is associated with the histologic type and grade of the tumor.

▶ This large series of resected sternal tumors provides the basis for the surgical approach to the majority of these neoplasms. The authors emphasize that CT scanning is an important component in the workup, as is the MRI. The high distant failure rate suggests that the use of routine bone scanning and distant metastatic disease surveys are also warranted. The majority of these tumors, as is recommended, should be reconstructed with Marlex mesh and methyl methacrylate to provide an adequate reconstruction.

D.J. Sugarbaker, M.D.

Surgical Treatment of Lung Metastases: The European Organization for Research and Treatment of Cancer—Soft Tissue and Bone Sarcoma Group Study of 255 Patients

van Geel AN, Pastorino U, Jauch KW, et al (Daniel den Hoed Cancer Ctr, Rotterdam, The Netherlands; Instituto Nazionale por lo studio e la cura dei tumori, Milano, Italia; Ludwig-Maximilian Universität München, Grosshadern, Germany; et al)

Cancer 77:675–682, 1996 14–32

Background.—Although surgical treatment of pulmonary metastases from soft-tissue sarcomas has been reported to prolong survival, the prognostic factors that predict a favorable outcome are still unclear. Significant prognostic factors were analyzed in a multicenter trial.

Methods.—Two hundred fifty-five patients undergoing complete resection of lung metastases from soft-tissue sarcomas were studied retrospectively. Patients with chondrosarcoma and small round-cell sarcomas such as Ewing sarcoma were excluded.

Findings.—Survival rates after metastasectomy were 54% and 38% at 3 and 5 years, respectively. The corresponding disease-free rates were 42% and 35%, respectively. Disease-free intervals of 2.5 years or more occurred when a resection had microscopically free margins, patients were younger than 40 years, and tumors were grade I or II. These prognostic variables were found to independently affect overall survival in a multivariate Cox regression model.

Conclusions.—When preoperative assessment indicates that complete clearance of metastases is possible, surgical excision of lung metastases from soft-tissue sarcomas should be considered the first-line treatment. Additional research is needed before chemotherapy can be recommended as additional treatment.

► Aggressive surgical management of metastatic soft-tissue sarcomas to the lung is supported in this prospective study. Of interest is that the disease-free interval, whether a radical resection was performed, and age were the significant prognostic variables for this subgroup of patients.

D.J. Sugarbaker, M.D.

Mesothelioma Update

Malignant Mesothelioma: Immunohistochemistry and DNA Ploidy Analysis as Methods to Differentiate Mesothelioma From Benign Reactive Mesothelial Cell Proliferation and Adenocarcinoma in Pleural and Peritoneal Effusions

Friedman MT, Gentile P, Tarectecan A, et al (Albert Einstein College, New Hyde Park, NY)

Arch Pathol Lab Med 120:959–966, 1996 14–33

Introduction.—It is difficult to diagnose malignant mesothelioma, an aggressive neoplasm of adults, because its clinical and histopathologic features overlap extensively with those of metastatic adenocarcinoma to the pleura and peritoneum. Good markers have been found for carcinomas, lymphomas, and melanomas, but one remains to be found for tumors of mesothelial origin. Immunohistochemical analysis with DNA ploidy analysis was used to determine whether malignant mesotheliomas could be differentiated from adenocarcinomas and benign reactive mesothelial cells in pleural and peritoneal fluids.

Methods.—Sixteen patients with malignant mesotheliomas, ranging in age from 10 to 85 years, were studied. Their tumors were of the epithelial, sarcomatous, and biphasic types. There also were 7 patients with adenocarcinomas and 7 with benign reactive mesothelial cells. DNA analysis using flow cytometry or image analysis was performed on the mesothelioma group. Cytospin cell preparations were performed on the adenocarcinoma and reactive mesothelial cell groups. Immunohistochemical studies also were conducted.

Results.—All the malignant mesotheliomas tested stained positive for prekeratin. However, stains for carcinoembryonic antigen, B72.3, Leu-M1, and Ber-EP4 were negative. In 75% of the patients tested for vimentin and epithelial membrane antigen, stains were positive. In 25% of the patients tested for CA125, stains were positive. Stains for patients with benign reactive mesothelial cell tumors were similar. Patients with adenocarcinomas were more likely to test negative with vimentin, and positive with B72.3, Ber-EP4, and carcinoembryonic antigen. All patients with benign tumors were diploids, according to DNA analysis, whereas all those with adenocarcinomas were nondiploid. Fifty-three percent of malignant mesotheliomas were nondiploid. Image analysis had greater sensitivity in detecting nondiploidy than did flow cytometry (100% versus 75%).

Conclusions.—To differentiate malignant mesotheliomas from adenocarcinomas, B72.3, Ber-EP4, carcinoembryonic antigen, and vimentin were useful. However, immunohistochemistry did not reliably distinguish benign from malignant hyperplastic mesothelial cells; the addition of DNA ploidy studies was useful for that purpose. For the diagnosis of malignant mesothelioma, no single test or marker alone is entirely adequate. A combination of studies must be relied on.

► The increasing incidence of malignant mesothelioma in the United States has caused a larger number of surgeons to face the diagnostic challenge of this disease. Benign disorders such as fibrothorax and post-empyema fibrosis with mesothelial proliferation often can confound the diagnosis of mesothelioma. Other malignant tumors, particularly metastatic adenocarcinoma, frequently are confused with malignant pleural mesothelioma. The principles of open biopsy with incisions placed in the line of subsequent thoracotomy should be followed to make the diagnosis effectively and accurately. The principal contribution of this study is to reaffirm that the presence of carcinoembryonic antigen in adenocarcinomas and its absence in mesotheliomas can help confirm the diagnosis. This disease presents another instance in which close collaboration and cooperation in communication between the surgeon and the pathologist is mandatory if the patient is to benefit.

D.J. Sugarbaker, M.D.

Mineral Fiber Content of Lungs in Patients With Mesothelioma Seeking Compensation in Québec

Dufresne A, Bégin R, Churg A, et al (McGill Univ, Montréal; CHU Sherbrooke, Québec; Univ of British Columbia, Vancouver, Canada)

Am J Respir Crit Care Med 153:711–718, 1996 14–34

Introduction.—Determination of past occupational exposure to airborne contaminants, such as dust particles, is sometimes difficult. For asbestos, interlaboratory variations in the analysis and reporting of lung fiber concentrations are significant problems, making interpretation of results difficult. Additionally, without a reference population, true elevations of fiber concentrations in individuals with work-related conditions, such as mesothelioma, cannot be determined. The mineral fiber content of lung specimens from workers with occupation-related mesothelioma was determined and compared with that of a reference population.

Methods.—Lung tissue specimens from 50 workers who sought compensation for work-related mesothelioma were obtained. Forty-one lung specimens were obtained at autopsy and the remainder from lung resections. Twenty-three of the 50 workers had been exposed to asbestos through mining or milling activities. Workers were from 2 different mining regions; 11 from the chrysotile mining region of Thetford Mines and 12 from Asbestos Township. The remainder had exposure from other nonmining industries (such as asbestos factories or shipyards). Lung tissue specimens were also obtained at autopsy from 49 men from a local population who had no occupational exposure to asbestos (the reference group). Lung specimens from both groups were analyzed for the presence of ferruginous bodies, mineral fibers, fiber type, and fiber length and diameter.

Results.—Tremolite, chrysotile, crocidolite, and amosite fibers were found in the lung specimens of workers with mesothelioma from Asbestos Township. Only tremolite and chrysotile asbestos fibers were found in the lung specimens of workers from Thetford Mines. Primarily amosite and crocidolite fibers were found in the lung specimens of workers exposed through other industries. Lung specimens from the reference group contained very few amosite and crocidolite fibers. Lung specimens from individuals who worked as miners or millers had higher concentrations of short and long chrysotile and tremolite fibers compared with lung specimens from individuals who worked in other industries. The concentrations of ferruginous bodies were not significantly different between the workers but were significantly higher than the concentrations found in the reference group. Overall, the mean concentrations of all asbestos fibers were higher in the lung specimens from workers with mesothelioma as compared with the reference group. For the reference group, 507 fibers per milligram of dry lung were found, compared with 2,497 fibers per milligram for workers from other industries, 27,342 fibers per milligram for those from Asbestos Township, and 89,680 fibers per milligram for those from Thetford Mines. The corresponding concentrations of ferruginous bodies were 83 per milligram dry lung, 3,925 per milligram, 11,226 per milligram, and 2,697 per milligram, respectively.

Conclusions.—The occupational exposure of the workers who sought compensation for work-related mesothelioma was confirmed. Workers with mesothelioma had significantly higher concentrations of asbestos fibers and ferruginous bodies in lung specimens than did specimens from an unexposed reference population. Different fiber types were also found in the 3 different groups of workers.

▶ The rise in the incidence of mesothelioma in the United States is undoubtedly caused by the prevalent use of asbestos as an insulator in industry and construction. Although cases were previously clustered in areas of occupational exposure primarily in shipyards, an expanding number of patients do not have a known history of asbestos exposure. This most likely results from the exposure that one gets during daily living in a society where this material was used in building construction and insulation. This study is interesting in that it further confirms that occupational exposure of asbestos can be traced based on the exact fiber type. It is possible to trace specific fiber types to specific locations and therefore document exposure.

D.J. Sugarbaker, M.D.

Mesothelioma, Asbestos, and Reported History of Cancer in First-degree Relatives

Heineman EF, Bernstein L, Stark AD, et al (Natl Cancer Inst, Bethesda, Md; Univ of Southern California, Los Angeles; New York State Dept of Health, Albany)

Cancer 77:549–554, 1996 14–35

Introduction.—Asbestos exposure is the major risk factor for mesothelioma, a rare cancer of the lining of the pleural and peritoneal cavities. With familial or genetic factors, little is known about the role of mesothelioma, and it has been difficult to rule out carry-home exposure to asbestos. Data from one of the largest case-control studies of mesothelioma were analyzed to determine whether mesothelioma risk was increased among individuals with a family history of cancer and whether the association of mesothelioma with asbestos exposure varied according to the absence or presence of a family history of cancer.

Methods.—Reported history of cancer in first-degree relatives was compared. The histories were obtained from telephone interviews with the next-of-kin of 196 patients who had a pathologic diagnosis of mesothelioma. These were compared to 511 deceased control subjects.

Results.—There was a statistically significant 2-fold increase in the risk of mesothelioma for patients reporting cancer in 2 or more first-degree relatives among the men exposed to asbestos. Among the women or among the the men without asbestos exposure, there was no significant increased risk. A possible mesothelioma in a first-degree relative was reported by the next-of-kin of 3 patients, and asbestos exposure could not be ruled out in those relatives. Among the men with a reported family history of cancer, the association of asbestos with pleural mesothelioma was stronger than among the men without a family history of cancer. No statistical evidence of an interaction was found.

Conclusion.—A family history of cancer may be a risk factor for mesothelioma. For most patients with mesothelioma, asbestos is a major risk factor, particularly among men, in whom the attributable risk ranges from 45% to 75% for occupational exposure.

► Studies in lung cancer have suggested that a genetic or inherited susceptibility to non–small-cell lung cancer may put certain smokers at high risk for the development of this disease. This study is interesting in that it suggests, for the first time, a potential link between the development of malignant pleural mesothelioma and a reported cancer history in first-degree relatives. This epidemiologic factor may be important in explaining the increasing incidence of this disease in the United States.

D.J. Sugarbaker, M.D.

Post-irradiation Malignant Mesothelioma

Cavazza A, Travis LB, Travis WD, et al (Mayo Clinic, Scottsdale, Ariz; NIH, Bethesda, Md; Armed Forces Inst of Pathology, Washington, DC; et al)

Cancer 77:1379–1385, 1996 14–36

Introduction.—Although the relation between malignant mesothelioma and asbestos exposure is well known, it is not known why all patients with malignant mesothelioma do not have a history of asbestos exposure. Other causes may be non-asbestos mineral fibers, radiation, viruses, organic chemicals, and chronic inflammation. Patients in whom malignant mesothelioma developed after radiation therapy were described.

Methods.—Files of patients with malignant mesothelioma of the pleura were examined, and all had had a previous cancer and had undergone radiation therapy in the region where the malignant mesothelioma developed. Data from the National Cancer Institute's Surveillance, Epidemiology and End Results Program and from the Connecticut Tumor Register for patients with a previous cancer in whom a malignant mesothelioma of the pleura developed were reviewed. The literature on post-irradiation malignant mesotheliomas also was reviewed.

Results.—Four men and 4 women with malignant mesothelioma who had undergone radiation therapy for a prior tumor were identified (Table 1). The average interval between the radiation therapy and the development of the mesothelioma was 21 years (range 11 to 29 years) and the mean age at diagnosis of the mesothelioma was 45 years (range 22 to 78 years). Three patients also had received chemotherapy. The mesotheliomas were epithelial in 5 patients, sarcomatous in 1 patient, and biphasic in 1 patient. The epidemiologic survey identified 142 patients, with a median latency between the first cancer and the mesothelioma of 4.3 years (range 2 months to 29.9 years).

Conclusions.—In about 20% of occurrences in men and most occurrences in women, there has been no history of asbestos exposure, and radiation therapy appears to induce a small, but significant, number of second malignancies in organs more remote from the target area and in heavily irradiated tissues. The relation of second malignancies should be clarified by additional studies.

► Previous radiation has been identified as an alternate cause of malignant mesothelioma. Previous therapy for Hodgkin's disease is the most common prior malignancy leading to the subsequent development of pleural mesothelioma.

D.J. Sugarbaker, M.D.

TABLE 1.—Post-irradiation Mesotheliomas: Clinicopathologic Findings

		First cancer	Treatment		Malignant mesothelioma of pleura (second cancer)			
Case no.	Age*/Sex (Yrs).	Diagnosis	Radiotherapy (year)	Chemotherapy	Interval between 1st cancer and mesothelioma (yrs)	Chest X-ray/ CT findings	Asbestos exposure	Outcome after diagnosis
1	28/M	Hodgkin's disease	Mantle (1973, details na)	None	21	Pleural thickening and effusion	None	DOD†
2	21/M	Hodgkin's disease	Supraclavicular (1968) (Left: 40 Gy, Right: 32 Gy); Mediastinal (22 Gy)	None	22	Pleural thickening and effusion	None	DOD
3	20/M	Hodgkin's disease (nodular sclerosis)	Mantle (1976) (42 Gy)	COPP for first relapse 3 yrs. after diagnosis. CCNU, bleomycin, Velban, adriamycin for second relapse 8 yrs. after diagnosis.	11	Pleural thickening and effusion	None	DOD, 4 mos.
4	7/M	Hodgkin's disease (mixed cellularity)	Mantle (1969) (35 Gy)	Chlorambucil and MOPP for histologically confirmed relapse 22 years after initial therapy, with CR.	24	Pleural thickening and effusion	Unk.	Extrapleural pneumonectomy followed by RT (20 Gy). Patient alive 9 mos. after surgery. No active tumor.

5	55/F	Left breast carcinoma (mastectomy)	Left chest (1959; details n/a)	None	21	Pleural effusion; opacified left hemithorax with mediastinal shift	Unk.	n/a
6	5/M	Mediastinal Hodgkin's disease	Mediastinum (1968; details n/a)	None	17	Intrathoracic mass with pleural studding	Unk.	DOD (3 yrs.)
7	1/F	Cervical/ supraclavicular Hodgkin's disease-1962 (initially had only surgery)	Mantle RT (18 Gy) for recurrent Hodgkin's disease (1965)	None	24	Pleural effusion	Unk.	DOD (4 yrs).
8	49/F	Right breast carcinoma (mastectomy)	Right chest wall and supraclavicular region (1966; details n/a)	None	29	Pleural effusion	None	Alive with disease 1 week after diagnosis

*Age at diagnosis of first cancer.
†Autopsy diagnosis.
Abbreviations: *COPP,* cyclophosphamide, vincristine, procarbazine, and prednisone; *CR,* complete remission; *DOD,* dead of disease; *F,* female; *Gy,* Gray; *M,* male; *MOPP,* mechlorethamine, vincristine, procarbazine, and prednisone; *n/a,* not available; *RT,* radiation therapy; *Unk,* unknown.
(Courtesy of Cavazza A, Travis LB, Travis WD, et al: Post-irradiation malignant mesothelioma. *Cancer* 77:1379–1385, copyright © 1996, American Cancer Society. Reprinted by permission of Wiley-Liss, Inc., a subsidiary of John Wiley & Sons, Inc.)

Calcification as a Sign of Sarcomatous Degeneration of Malignant Pleural Mesotheliomas: A New CT Finding

Raizon A, Schwartz A, Hix W, et al (George Washington Univ, Washington, DC)

J Comput Assist Tomogr 20:42–44, 1996 14–37

Introduction.—The development of the serous membrane tumor, malignant pleural mesothelioma, is associated with exposure to asbestos. In such lesions, osteosarcomatous degeneration also may occur, usually in the form of focal areas within the primary malignancy. Two patients with histories of occupational asbestos exposure who had densely calcified pleural masses that developed in association with diffuse pleural mesothelioma were described.

Case 1.—Man, 69, worked in a U.S Navy shipyard and was exposed to asbestos dust, and had a 4-week history of shortness of breath. His chest radiograph showed a large right pleural effusion. A CT scan showed calcified masses adjacent to the pleura in the right upper hemithorax (Fig 1). On the right, there was evidence of pleural nodularity and visceral pleural thickening adjacent to the right hemidiaphragm. The tumor was biphasic, diffuse malignant mesothelioma with a tubular papillary pattern and a sarcomatous component with malignant spindle cells.

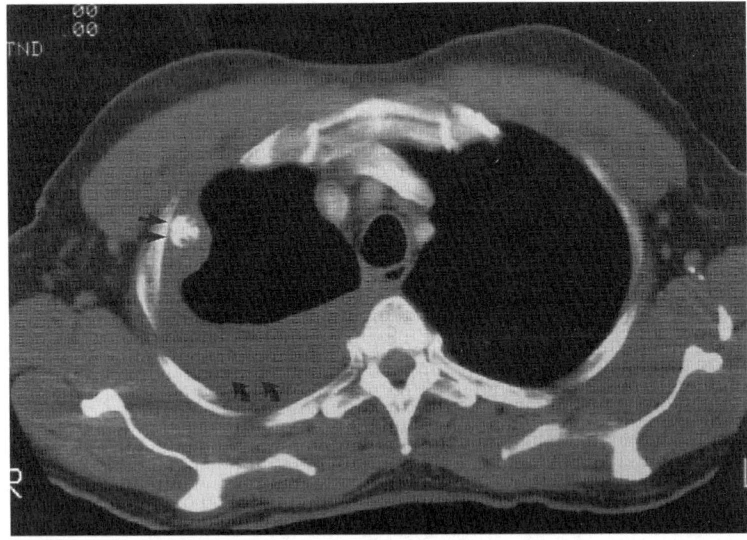

FIGURE 1.—Computed tomograph showing a calcified pleura-based mass (*straight arrows*) and right pleural effusion (*curved arrows*). (Courtesy of Raizon A, Schwartz A, Hix W, et al: Calcification as a sign of sarcomatous degeneration of malignant pleural mesotheliomas: A new CT finding. *J Comput Assist Tomogr* 20:42–44, 1996.)

Case 2.—Man, 68, worked in a shipyard for 9 months and was exposed to asbestos. The patient complained of "fullness" in his chest and a radiograph revealed a large pleura-based mass and large pleural effusion. His CT scan showed a calcified mass contiguous with the left posterior pleura. A thoracotomy revealed an ossified mass arising from the posterior parietal pleura with several very firm satellite nodules and several more nodular masses. The malignant tumor invaded the underlying lung.

Conclusions.—Both these patients had diffuse malignant mesothelioma and areas of dense collagenous pleural plaques, which were typical of asbestos exposure. They also had areas of tumor-associated chondro-osseous differentiation. The clinical history of asbestos exposure, the typical radiographic encasing pleural tumor, the features of biphasic and monophasic patterns of malignant mesothelioma with malignant chondro-osseous differentiation, and the absence of any chondrosarcoma or osteogenic sarcoma anywhere else led to the diagnosis of diffuse malignant mesothelioma with osteocartilaginous differentiation.

▶ This report documents the diagnosis of osteogenic sarcomatous degeneration within pre-existing mesotheliomas. This is displayed on the CT scan by the identification of a calcified pleura-based mass, along with the fusion characteristic of malignant pleural mesothelioma. Malignant pleural mesothelioma is made up of 3 principal histologic subtypes: epithelial tumors, mixed tumors, and pure sarcomatous lesions. These tumors characteristically are variegated, with combinations of tumor subtypes within the same specimen. Thus, an osteogenic sarcomatous degeneration is identified at the extreme of the continuum of pathology in these tumors.

D.J. Sugarbaker, M.D.

Prospective Study of Combination Chemotherapy With Cyclophosphamide, Doxorubicin, and Cisplatin for Unresectable or Metastatic Malignant Pleural Mesothelioma

Shin DM, Fossella FV, Umsawasdi T, et al (Univ of Texas, Houston)

Cancer 76:2230–2236, 1995 14–38

Introduction.—The incidence of malignant mesothelioma is rising because of a long latency interval from the time of initial asbestos exposure to the onset of disease 20 to 40 years later. The inception of preventive measures in industry has decreased new exposure, but there is a large population of workers whose exposure preceded preventive measures. Surgery and radiation have had limited roles in the treatment of unresectable or metastatic malignant pleural mesothelioma. Response rates have been improved with systemic chemotherapy. The efficacy of a chemotherapy combination of cyclophosphamide (C), doxorubicin (D), and cisplatin (P) in patients with inoperable, unresectable, or metastatic malignant pleural mesothelioma was evaluated, and the quantitative and qualitative toxic effects of this regimen were analyzed.

Methods.—The histologic tumor types of 23 patients with unresectable or metastatic malignant pleural mesothelioma were 14 epithelial, 4 sarcomatoid, 4 unclassified, and 1 mixed type. Twenty patients had known asbestos exposure and 3 had no known asbestos exposure. Patients were treated with a starting chemotherapy dose of C, 500 mg/m^2 IV on day 1; D, 50 mg/m^2 IV on day 1; and P, 80 mg/m^2 IV on day 1. This regimen was repeated every 3 weeks for 3 courses, then the P dose was decreased to 50 mg/m^2 as a fixed dose for remaining courses. The doses of C and D were modified in response to the nadir granulocyte and platelet counts. Patients underwent CT scans of the chest after every 3 cycles of chemotherapy and chest radiographs and physical examinations after each course of therapy.

Results.—Seven, 3, and 14 patients, respectively, had partial responses, mild responses, and stable or progressive disease. Three patients with partial responses and minimal to moderate amounts of pleural effusion had a significant reduction in fluid during treatment. One patient with a partial response underwent surgical resection and no viable tumor cells were detected in the pathologic specimen. The overall duration of median survival was 60 weeks and 8 patients were still alive. Responses ranged from 25 to more than 258 weeks (median 45 weeks). Chemotherapy doses were increased in 3 patients and decreased in 14 patients. The most frequent hematologic toxic effects were neutropenia, mild thrombocytopenia, and anemia. Grade 4 and grade 3 granulocytopenia were observed in 59% and 17% of patients, respectively. Anemia and thrombocytopenia were mild for all cycles in 8% and 3% of patients, respectively. The most common non-hematologic side effects were nausea and vomiting. Other side effects included neutropenic fever (3 patients), peripheral neuropathy (1 patient), and congestive heart failure (1 patient).

Conclusion.—The CDP chemotherapy combination was generally well tolerated and resulted in significant antitumor activity. The overall and median survival rates were as good as or better than those associated with other reported multimodality approaches. The median duration of response of 60 weeks is still far from satisfactory. There remains a need for new strategies for combating this disease, greater understanding of the tumorigenesis of these tumors, and testing of new agents for patients with unresectable or metastatic malignant pleural mesothelioma.

▶ Intravenous chemotherapy in combination has been used in previous studies of malignant pleural mesothelioma. This study using CDP demonstrates that combination chemotherapy can be delivered with acceptable toxicity in this group of patients. Its role as an adjuvant to surgery has not been established. The data presented here may form the basis for the application of this combination chemotherapy into a more aggressive regimen, which would include surgical resection. However, the overall long-term outlook for these patients is still measured in weeks.

D.J. Sugarbaker, M.D.

Intrapleural Chemotherapy for Patients With Incompletely Resected Malignant Mesothelioma: The UCLA Experience

Lee JD, Perez S, Wang H-J, et al (Univ of California, Los Angeles)

J Surg Oncol 60:262–267, 1995 14–39

Introduction.—Most therapies for malignant pleural mesothelioma, including surgery, systemic chemotherapy, and radiation therapy, have largely been shown to be ineffective. Intrapleural administration of chemotherapy would provide higher local concentrations at the tumor site, with potentially less systemic toxicity. The outcomes of patients with intrathoracic malignant pleural mesothelioma treated with intrapleural chemotherapy after surgery were studied.

Methods.—Patients with malignant pleural mesothelioma with no extrathoracic disease who were previously untreated were included in the study. After surgical resection of gross disease, 250 mL of normal saline containing cisplatin, 100 mg/m^2, and cytosine arabinoside, 1,200 mg, was instilled into the hemithorax. The chemotherapeutic agents remained in the pleural cavity for 4 hours, after which dependent drainage and −20 cm H_2O suction was used to drain the cavity. Hydration and diuresis were used to maintain a urine output of greater than 100 mL/hr for 12 hours after surgery and greater than 50 mL/hr for the subsequent 12 hours. Additional systemic chemotherapy or radiation was administered at the individual physician's discretion. Chest roentgenograms, CT, or both were used to assess the efficacy of treatment.

Results.—Seventeen patients underwent intrapleural chemotherapy; 2 patients were found to have metastatic pleural adenocarcinoma and were not evaluated. Eighty percent of the remaining patients had a history of asbestos exposure, and 64% had a history of smoking. Thirteen percent of patients (2 of 15) experienced grade 3 or 4 hemorrhage, infection, or cardiopulmonary or renal toxicity. There was no treatment-related mortality. Of the 15 patients, 7 received adjuvant systemic chemotherapy and 11 received radiation therapy. Disease recurred in all patients; 14 patients have died since the procedure, with a median survival of 11.5 months. Survival varied with the histologic subtype of the malignancy (Fig 2). For patients with the epithelial subtype, the median survival was 12 months; for the mixed-biphasic type, 10.5 months; and for the sarcomatoid type, 5.9 months. Univariate analysis found the histologic subtype to be a significant predictor of survival. The survival of patients with the epithelial subtype was significantly longer than that of patients with a sarcomatoid malignancy.

Conclusions.—The use of intrapleural chemotherapy after pleurectomy and decortication for the treatment of malignant pleural mesothelioma was associated with low morbidity and no mortality. However, disease progression was observed in all patients, and adjuvant chemotherapy and radiation had no effect on survival.

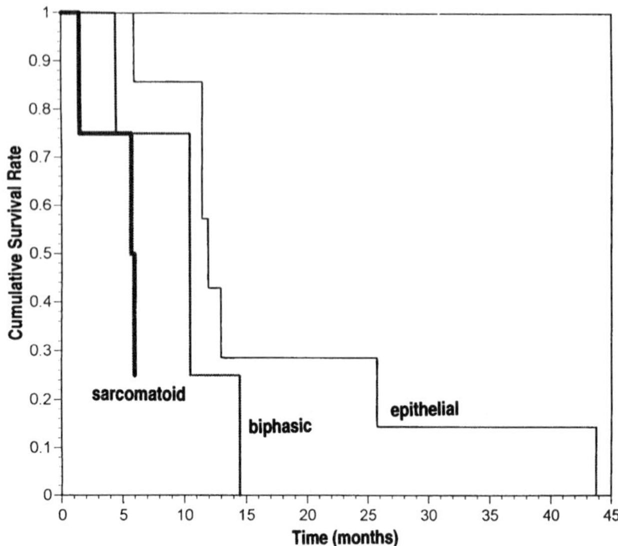

FIGURE 2.—Survival curves of the patients with different histologic subtypes of malignant pleural mesothelioma treated by pleurectomy and decortication and intrapleural cisplatin (100 mg/m^2) and cytosine arabinoside (1,200 mg). Median survival: epithelial (n = 7), 12 months; biphasic (n = 4), 10.5 months; sarcomatoid (n = 4), 5.9 months. (Courtesy of Lee JD, Perez S, Wang H-J, et al: Intrapleural chemotherapy for patients with incompletely resected malignant mesothelioma: The UCLA experience. *J Surg Oncol* 60:262–267, copyright 1995. Reprinted by permission of Wiley-Liss, Inc., a subsidiary of John Wiley & Sons, Inc.)

▶ The use of regional chemotherapy has been investigated in several malignant tumors. Its application to malignant pleural mesothelioma has been described in previous reports. This retrospective review of 15 patients with malignant pleural mesothelioma does not show a significant long-term survival in this group. In our experience, the difficulty of performing pleurectomy in most patients has relegated it to a purely palliative procedure in which significant cytoreduction is not the goal. Pleurectomy can be used in some patients with malignant pleural mesothelioma as an excellent way of causing pleural synthesis and preventing recurrence of the symptomatic pleural effusion. Extrapleural pneumonectomy in selected patients will yield a significantly better cytoreduction, which may affect long-term survival. As noted in Figure 2, the epithelial subgroup fared better than either the biphasic or pure sarcomatoid groups, which is consistent with previous reports.

D.J. Sugarbaker, M.D.

Extrapleural Pneumonectomy in the Multimodality Therapy of Malignant Pleural Mesothelioma: Results in 120 Consecutive Patients

Sugarbaker DJ, Garcia JP, Richards WG, et al (Dana-Farber Cancer Inst, Boston; Brigham and Women's Hosp, Boston)

Ann Surg 224:288–296, 1996 14–40

Introduction.—Malignant pleural mesothelioma is a fatal disease, with a median survival time of 4 to 12 months if untreated. However, single modality therapy, using either surgery, chemotherapy, or radiation, has not been shown to increase the survival of patients with this malignancy. A less aggressive surgical approach has been tried in combination with chemotherapy and radiation to reduce treatment mortality and morbidity and improve survival. The outcomes of patients with malignant pleural mesothelioma who were classified using a previously published revised staging system and treated with a trimodal approach were assessed.

Methods.—One hundred twenty patients with malignant pleural mesothelioma underwent extrapleural pneumonectomy followed by chemotherapy and radiation. Four to 6 weeks after surgery, patients received chemotherapy with doxorubicin 50 to 60 mg/m^2 and cyclophosphamide 600 mg/m^2 for 4 to 6 cycles. Cisplatin 70 mg/m^2 was added to the regimen after 1985. Chemotherapy was followed by external-beam radiation therapy. Patient survival and factors associated with survival were assessed.

Results.—A history of asbestos exposure was present in 78% of patients, and 77% had a history of smoking. Major complications of treatment occurred in 15 patients and included intrathoracic hemorrhage, respiratory failure, pneumonia, disrupted diaphragmatic patch, perforated duodenal ulcer, empyema, upper gastrointestinal bleeding, and deep-vein thrombosis. Overall, the morbidity rate associated with the treatment was 22%. The survival rate was 45% at 2 years and 22% at 5 years. The range of survival in months was 1 to 96, with a median overall survival of 21 months. Prolonged survival was significantly associated with epithelial cell type, as was lack of involvement of hilar, mediastinal, or pulmonary nodes. Survival rates were higher in 59 patients with epithelial cell–type tumors, with 2- and 5-year rates of 65% and 27%, respectively. Patients who had both epithelial cell–type tumors and no nodal involvement had 74% 2-year and 39% 5-year survival rates, as compared with rates of 52% and 10%, respectively, for patients with nodal involvement. Patients with mixed or sarcomatous cell–type tumors had 2- and 5-year survival rates of 20% and 0%, respectively. Significant differences in survival also were found when patients were stratified by stage of disease. Patients with stage I disease had a median survival time of 22 months, whereas patients with stage II and III disease had median survival times of 17 and 11 months, respectively.

Conclusions.—Extrapulmonary pneumonectomy followed by chemotherapy and radiation treatment improved survival in some patients with malignant pleural mesothelioma. Both tumor cell type and node involvement were found to be predictive factors in determining survival. Survival was highest in patients with epithelial cell–type tumors and no nodal involvement.

▶ Malignant pleural mesothelioma has a unique tumor biologic behavior. Local recurrence is the principal cause of death for most patients with this disease. This study demonstrates that extrapleural pneumonectomy can be performed with acceptable morbidity and mortality, and may be the preferred surgical debulking procedure for carefully selected patients with this disease. Specifically, the use of MRI of the chest to determine transdiaphragmatic or transmediastinal involvement of tumor and the use of preoperative echocardiography to assess pericardial invasion and myocardial function, along with standard pulmonary function testing, are guidelines for patient selection. Prognostic factors included node status and cell type. Of note is the fact that patients with epithelial tumors and node-negative status had a 41-month median survival time. The use of adjuvant chemotherapy after maximal cytoreduction in combination with well-tolerated whole ipsilateral chest radiation therapy may be responsible for this enhanced survival. When applied to this group of 120 consecutive patients, the previously published staging system stratified patients by stage with statistical significance. Establishing the efficacy of this approach as the primary therapy for patients with resectable disease still awaits prospective, multi-institutional trials.

D.J. Sugarbaker, M.D.

Subject Index*

A

* *All entries refer to the year and page number(s) for data appearing in this and the previous edition of the* YEAR BOOK.

C

D

E

F

G

H

I

N

O

P

Q

R

S

T

W

Z

Author Index

A

B

C

D

E

F

G

H

I

J

K

L

M

N

O

P

Q

R

S

T